Decision Making in Anesthesiology

An Algorithmic Approach

4th Edition

Lois L. Bready, MD
Associate Dean for Graduate Medical Education
Professor and Vice Chair
Department of Anesthesiology
University of Texas Health Sciences Center in San Antonio
San Antonio, Texas

Dawn Dillman, MD
Department of Anesthesiology and Perioperative Medicine
Oregon Health Sciences University
Portland, Oregon

Susan H. Noorily, MD
Clinical Professor
Department of Anesthesiology
University of Texas Health Sciences Center in San Antonio
San Antonio, Texas

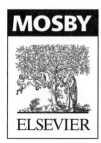

MOSBY

ELSEVIER

MOSBY
ELSEVIER

1600 John F. Kennedy Blvd.
Ste 1800
Philadelphia, PA 19103-2899

DECISION MAKING IN ANESTHESIOLOGY:
AN ALGORITHMIC APPROACH, FOURTH EDITION   ISBN: 978-0-323-03938-3

Previous editions copyrighted 1987, 1992, 2007

Library of Congress Cataloging-in-Publication Data

Decision making in anesthesiology : an algorithmic approach / [edited by] Lois L. Bready, Susan H. Noorily, Dawn Dillman. — 4th ed.
    p. ; cm

  Includes bibliographical references and index.
  ISBN 978-0-323-03938-3

  1. Anesthesia—Decision making. 2. Algorithms. I. Bready, Lois L. II. Noorily, Susan H. (Susan Helene) III. Dillman, Dawn.
  [DNLM: 1. Anesthesia—methods. 2. Decision Trees. 3. Perioperative Case—methods.
  WO 200 D294 2007]

RD82.D43 2007
617.9'6–dc22

                                                2007018660

Acquisitions Editor: Natasha Andjelkovic
Editorial Assistant: Isabel Trudeau
Project Manager: David Salzberg
Design Direction: Ellen Zanolle

Printed in the United States of America

9 8 7 6 5 4 3 2 1

CONTRIBUTORS

Stacey Allen, MD
Department of Anesthesiology
University of Texas Health Sciences Center
  in San Antonio,
San Antonio, Texas

D.M. Anderson, MD
Department of Anesthesiology
University of Texas Health Sciences Center
  in San Antonio
San Antonio, Texas

Franklin L. Anderson, MD
Department of Anesthesiology
University of Texas Health Sciences Center
  in San Antonio
San Antonio, Texas

J. Jeff Andrews, MD
Department of Anesthesiology
University of Texas Health Sciences Center
  in San Antonio
San Antonio, Texas

William P. Arnold III, MD
Department of Anesthesia
University of Virginia
Charlottesville, Virginia

Patrick Bakke, MD
Department of Anesthesiology and Perioperative Medicine
Oregon Health Sciences University
Portland, Oregon

Joanne Baust, MD
Department of Anesthesiology
University of Texas Health Sciences Center
  in San Antonio
San Antonio, Texas

Jonathan L. Benumof, MD
Department of Anesthesia
University of California at San Diego
San Diego, California

Lauren Berkow, MD
Department of Anesthesiology and Critical Care
  Medicine
The Johns Hopkins Medical Institutions
Baltimore, Maryland

Arnold J. Berry, MD, MPH
Department of Anesthesiology
Emory University School of Medicine
Atlanta, Georgia

Daniel Martin Bitner, MD, MS
Department of Anesthesiology
University of Texas Health Sciences Center
  in San Antonio
San Antonio, Texas

Mary Blanchette, MD
Department of Anesthesiology and Perioperative
  Medicine
Oregon Health Sciences University
Portland, Oregon

Erik A. Boatman, MD
San Antonio Uniformed Services Health Education
  Consortium
San Antonio, Texas

Gwendolyn L. Boyd, MD
Department of Anesthesiology
University of Alabama at Birmingham School
  of Medicine
Birmingham, Alabama

Christopher A. Bracken, MD, PhD
Department of Anesthesiology
University of Texas Health Sciences Center
  in San Antonio
San Antonio, Texas

Carol R. Bradford, MD
Department of Otolaryngology
University of Michigan Medical Center
Ann Arbor, Michigan

Kevin M. Brady, MD
Department of Anesthesiology and Critical Care
  Medicine
The Johns Hopkins Medical Institutions
Baltimore, Maryland

Ansgar M. Brambrink, MD, PhD
Department of Anesthesiology and Perioperative
  Medicine
Oregon Health Sciences University
Portland, Oregon

Darin Brandt, DO
Department of Anesthesiology and Perioperative Medicine
Oregon Health Sciences University
Portland, Oregon

Lois L. Bready, MD
Department of Anesthesiology
University of Texas Health Sciences Center
  in San Antonio
San Antonio, Texas

Russell C. Brockwell, MD
Department of Anesthesiology
University of Alabama at Birmingham
Birmingham, Alabama

David M. Broussard, MD
Department of Anesthesiology
Ochsner Clinical Foundation
New Orleans, Louisiana

Allan C.D. Brown, MD
Department of Anesthesiology
University of Michigan Medical Center
Ann Arbor, Michigan

Carol E. Campbell, MD
Department of Anesthesiology
University of Texas Health Sciences Center
   in San Antonio
San Antonio, Texas

A. Sue Carlisle, MD, PhD
Department of Anesthesia and Perioperative Care
University of California San Francisco and San Francisco
   General Hospital
San Francisco, California

Bonny Carter, MD
Department of Anesthesiology
University of Texas Health Sciences Center
   in San Antonio
San Antonio, Texas

Lydia Cassorla, MD, MBA
Department of Anesthesia and Perioperative Care
University of California San Francisco
San Francisco, California

Harold D. Cline, MD
Department of Anesthesiology
University of Maryland Medical Center
Baltimore, Maryland

Corey Collins, DO
Medford, Massachusetts

Sally Combest, MD
Department of Anesthesiology
University of Texas Health Sciences Center
   in San Antonio
San Antonio, Texas

Saundra E. Curry, MD
Department of Anesthesiology
Columbia University College of Physicians and
   Surgeons
New York, New York

Myrdalis Diaz-Ramirez, MD
Department of Anesthesiology and Perioperative Care
Oregon Health Sciences University
Portland, Oregon

John A. Dilger, MD
Department of Anesthesiology
Mayo Clinic
Rochester, Maryland

Dawn Dillman, MD
Department of Anesthesiology and Perioperative Medicine
Oregon Health Sciences University
Portland, Oregon

Stephen Donahue, MD
Anesthesiologists for Children
Dallas, Texas

Nivine H. Doran, MD
Department of Anesthesiology and Critical Care
   Medicine
University of New Mexico
Albuquerque, New Mexico

M. Joanne Douglas, MD
Department of Anesthesia
University of British Columbia
Vancouver, British Columbia, Canada

George A. Dumitrascu, MD
Ottawa, Ontario, Canada

Lynn A. Fenton, MD
Department of Anesthesiology and Perioperative Medicine
Oregon Health Sciences University
Portland, Oregon

Juergen Fleisch, MD
Department of Anesthesiology and Perioperative Medicine
Oregon Health Sciences University
Portland, Oregon

Judith A. Freeman, MD, CHB
Department of Anesthesiology and Perioperative Medicine
Oregon Health Sciences University
Portland, Oregon

Thomas Frietsch, MD
Department of Anesthesiology and Perioperative Medicine
Oregon Health Sciences University
Portland, Oregon

William R. Furman, MD
Department of Anesthesiology
University of North Carolina
Chapel Hill, North Carolina

Susan Garwood, MD, ChB, BSc, FRCA
Department of Anesthesiology
Yale School of Medicine
Yale-New Haven Hospital
New Haven, Connecticut

Ethan Gaumond, MD
Department of Anesthesiology and Perioperative Medicine
Oregon Health Sciences University
Portland, Oregon

Kevin B. Gerold, DO, JD
Department of Anesthesiology and Critical Care
    Medicine
The Johns Hopkins Medical Institutions
Johns Hopkins Bayview Medical Center
Baltimore, Maryland

James D. Griffin, MD
Department of Anesthesiology and Pain Management
University of Texas Southwestern Medical Center at
    Dallas
Dallas, Texas

Mary Ann Gurkowski, MD
Department of Anesthesiology
University of Texas Health Sciences Center
    in San Antonio
San Antonio, Texas

Charles B. Hantler, MD
Department of Anesthesiology
Washington University
St. Louis, Missouri

Jinny Kim Hartman, MD
Department of Anesthesiology
Dartmouth-Hitchcock Medical Center
Lebanon, New Hampshire

Joy L. Hawkins, MD
Department of Anesthesia
University of Colorado Health Sciences Center
Denver, Colorado

Eugenie Heitmiller, MD
Department of Anesthesiology and Critical Care
    Medicine
The Johns Hopkins Medical Institutions
Baltimore, Maryland

Antonio Hernandez, MD
Department of Anesthesiology
University of Texas Health Sciences Center
    in San Antonio
San Antonio, Texas

Rosemary Hickey, MD
Department of Anesthesiology
University of Texas Health Sciences Center
    in San Antonio
San Antonio, Texas

Joseph R. Holahan, MD
South Texas Oncology and Hematology PA
San Antonio, Texas

W. Corbett Holmgreen, MD, DDS
Department of Anesthesiology
University of Texas Health Sciences Center
    in San Antonio
San Antonio, Texas

Vivian Hou, MD
Department of Anesthesiology and Perioperative Medicine
Oregon Health Sciences University
Portland, Oregon

Michael P. Hutchens, MD, MA
Department of Anesthesiology and Perioperative Medicine
Oregon Health Sciences University
Portland, Oregon

Per-Olof Jarnberg, MD, PhD
Department of Anesthesiology and Perioperative Medicine
Oregon Health Sciences University
Portland, Oregon

Wendy B. Kang, MD, JD
Department of Anesthesiology
University of Texas Health Sciences Center in San Antonio
San Antonio, Texas

Suzanne B. Karan, MD
Department of Anesthesiology
University of Rochester School of Medicine
    and Dentistry
Rochester, New York

Celia I. Kaye, MD, PhD
Department of Pediatrics
University of Colorado Health Sciences Center
Denver, Colorado

Angela Kendrick, MD
Department of Anesthesiology and Perioperative Medicine
Oregon Health Sciences University
Portland, Oregon

Jeffrey R. Kirsch, MD
Department of Anesthesiology and Perioperative Medicine
Oregon Health Sciences University
Portland, Oregon

Kevin K. Klein, MD
Department of Anesthesiology and Pain Management
University of Texas Southwestern Medical Center at
    Dallas
Dallas, Texas

Ines P. Koerner, MD
Department of Anesthesiology and Perioperative
    Medicine
Oregon Health Sciences University
Portland, Oregon

Hector LaCassie, MD
Department of Anesthesiology
Duke University Health System
Durham, North Carolina

Kirk Lalwani, MD
Department of Anesthesiology and Perioperative Medicine
Oregon Health Sciences University
Portland, Oregon

Marilyn Green Larach, MD, FAAP
Owing Mills, Maryland

Catherine K. Lineberger, MD
Department of Anesthesiology
Duke University Health System
Durham, North Carolina

John J. Liszka-Hackzell, MD, PhD
Department of Anesthesiology
University of Arizona College of Medicine
Tucson, Arizona

Robert Loeb, MD
Department of Anesthesiology
University of Arizona College of Medicine
Tucson, Arizona

Gaelan B. Luhn, MD
Department of Anesthesiology
University of Texas Health Sciences Center
   in San Antonio
San Antonio, Texas

Colin F. Mackenzie, MD, ChB, FCCM
Department of Anesthesiology
University of Maryland Medical Center
Baltimore, Maryland

T. Philip Malan, Jr., MD, PhD
Department of Anesthesiology
University of Arizona College of Medicine
Tucson, Arizona

Vinod Malhotra, MD
Department of Anesthesiology
Weill Medical College of Cornell University
New York, New York

David C. Mayer, MD
Department of Anesthesiology
University of North Carolina
Chapel Hill, North Carolina

Kathryn E. McGoldrick, MD
Department of Anesthesiology
New York Medical College
Valhalla, New York

Katherine R. McGuire, MD
Department of Anesthesiology
University of Texas Health Sciences Center in San Antonio
San Antonio, Texas

William T. Merritt, MD, MBA
Department of Anesthesiology and Critical Care Medicine
The Johns Hopkins Medical Institutions
Baltimore, Maryland

Sara M. Metcalf, MD
Department of Anesthesiology and Perioperative Medicine
Oregon Health Sciences University
Portland, Oregon

Kimberly D. Milhoan, MD
Department of Anesthesiology
University of Texas Health Sciences Center in San Antonio
San Antonio, Texas

Tobias Moeller-Bertram, MD
Department of Anesthesiology
University of California at San Diego
San Diego, California

Joseph J. Naples, MD
Department of Anesthesiology
The Methodist Hospital
Houston, Texas

David V. Nelson, PhD
Department of Psychology and Philosophy
Sam Houston State University
Huntsville, Texas

Christopher D. Newell, MD
Department of Anesthesiology and Perioperative Medicine
Oregon Health Sciences University
Portland, Oregon

Victor Ng, MD
Department of Anesthesia and Perioperative Care
University of California San Francisco
San Francisco, California

Dolores B. Njoku, MD
Department of Anesthesiology and Critical Care Medicine
The Johns Hopkins Medical Institutions
Baltimore, Maryland

Susan H. Noorily, MD
Department of Anesthesiology
University of Texas Health Sciences Center
   in San Antonio
San Antonio, Texas

J. Russell Norton, MD
Department of Anesthesiology
University of Rochester School of Medicine and
   Dentistry
Rochester, New York

Steven C. Onstad
Department of Anesthesiology and Perioperative Medicine
Oregon Health Sciences University
Portland, Oregon

James C. Opton, MD
Department of Anesthesiology and Perioperative Medicine
Oregon Health Sciences University
Portland, Oregon

Malcolm D. Orr, MD, PhD
Department of Anesthesiology
University of Texas Health Sciences Center in San Antonio
San Antonio, Texas

Robert H. Overbaugh, MD
Department of Anesthesiology
Penn State Milton S. Hershey Medical Center
Hershey, Pennsylvania

Fred G. Panico, MD
Seaford, Delaware

Cathleen L. Peterson-Layne, MD, PhD
Department of Anesthesiology
Duke University Health System
Durham, North Carolina

Michael G. Phillips, BHS, PA-C
University of Alabama at Birmingham
    School of Medicine
Birmingham, Alabama

Jorge Pineda, MD
Department of Anesthesiology and Perioperative
    Medicine
Oregon Health Sciences University
Portland, Oregon

Anthony S. Poon, MD, DDS, PhD
Department of Oral and Maxillofacial Surgery
University of Texas Health Sciences Center
    in San Antonio
San Antonio, Texas

Marcelo Quezado, MD
Department of Anesthesiology and Critical Care
    Medicine
The Johns Hopkins Medical Institutions
Baltimore, Maryland

Rajam S. Ramamurthy, MD
Department of Anesthesiology
University of Texas Health Sciences Center
    in San Antonio
San Antonio, Texas

Somayaji Ramamurthy, MD
Department of Anesthesiology
University of Texas Health Sciences Center
    in San Antonio
San Antonio, Texas

Deborah K. Rasch, MD
Department of Anesthesiology
University of Texas Health Sciences Center
    in San Antonio
San Antonio, Texas

Jeffrey M. Richman, MD
Department of Anesthesiology and Critical Care Medicine
The Johns Hopkins Medical Institutions
Baltimore, Maryland

Kerri M. Robertson, MD
Department of Anesthesiology
Duke University Health System
Durham, North Carolina

Marco S. Robin, DO
Department of Anesthesiology and Perioperative Medicine
Oregon Health Sciences University
Portland, Oregon

Stephen T. Robinson, MD
Department of Anesthesiology and Perioperative Medicine
Oregon Health Sciences University
Portland, Oregon

James N. Rogers, MD
Department of Anesthesiology
University of Texas Health Sciences Center
    in San Antonio
San Antonio, Texas

Mark A. Rosen, MD
Department of Anesthesia and Perioperative Care
University of California San Francisco
San Francisco, California

Renata Rusa, MD
Department of Anesthesiology and Perioperative Medicine
Oregon Health Sciences University
Portland, Oregon

Andrew S. Rushton, MD
Department of Anesthesiology and Perioperative
    Medicine
Oregon Health Sciences University
Portland, Oregon

Susan M. Ryan, MD
Department of Anesthesia and Perioperative Care
University of California San Francisco
San Francisco, California

Lauren L. Salgado, MD
Department of Anesthesiology
University of Texas Health Sciences Center in San Antonio
San Antonio, Texas

Jamie McElrath Schwartz, MD
Department of Anesthesiology and Critical Care Medicine
The Johns Hopkins Medical Institutions
Baltimore, Maryland

Jaydeep S. Shah, MD
Department of Anesthesiology
University of Texas Health Sciences Center
    in San Antonio
San Antonio, Texas

David I. Shapiro, MD
Department of Anesthesiology
Erie County Medical Center
Buffalo, New York

Aarti Sharma, MD
Department of Anesthesiology
Weill Medical College of Cornell University
New York, New York

Nicholas R. Simmons, MD
Department of Anesthesiology
Washington University
St. Louis, Missouri

Gary D. Skrivanek, MD
Department of Anesthesiology and Pain Management
University of Texas Southwestern Medical Center at
    Dallas
Dallas, Texas

Tod B. Sloan, MD, PhD
Department of Anesthesiology
University of Colorado Health Sciences Center
Denver, Colorado

Fred J. Spielman, MD
Department of Anesthesiology
University of North Carolina
Chapel Hill, North Carolina

Louis A. Stool, MD
Department of Anesthesiology and Pain Management
University of Texas Southwestern Medical Center at
    Dallas
Dallas, Texas

Vijayendra Sudheendra, MD
Department of Surgery
Brown University
Providence, Rhode Island

Melba W.G. Swafford, MD
Department of Anesthesiology
Baylor College of Medicine
Houston, Texas

Veronica C. Swanson, MD
Department of Anesthesiology and Perioperative Medicine
Oregon Health Sciences University
Portland, Oregon

Jeffrey E. Terrell, MD
Department of Anesthesiology
University of Michigan Medical Center
Ann Arbor, Michigan

John E. Tetzlaff, MD
Division of Anesthesiology
Cleveland Clinic
Cleveland, Ohio

Mohamed Tiouririne, MD
Department of Anesthesiology
University of Virginia Health System
Charlottesville, Virginia

Irena Vaitkeviciute, MD
Department of Anesthesiology
Yale University School of Medicine
New Haven, Connecticut

Michael Verber, MD
Department of Anesthesiology
University of Texas Health Sciences Center
    in San Antonio
San Antonio, Texas

Jennifer F. Vookles, MD
Department of Anesthesiology and Perioperative
    Medicine
Oregon Health Sciences University
Portland, Oregon

David B. Waisel, MD
Department of Anesthesiology
Boston Children's Hospital
Boston, Massachusetts

Tessa L. Walters, MD
Burlingame, California

Denham S. Ward, MD, PhD
Department of Anesthesiology
University of Rochester School of Medicine and
    Dentistry
Rochester, New York

Leila G. Welborn, MD
Department of Anesthesiology
Children's National Medical Center
Washington, DC

Gary Welch, MD
Mico, Texas

Lynda T. Wells, MD
Department of Anesthesiology
University of Virginia Health System
Charlottesville, Virginia

James R. Zaidan, MD, MBA
Department of Anesthesiology
Emory University School of Medicine
Atlanta, Georgia

Angela Zimmerman, MD
Department of Anesthesiology and Perioperative
    Medicine
Oregon Health Sciences University
Portland, Oregon

Marcos A. Zuazu, MD
Department of Anesthesiology
University of Texas Health Sciences Center
    in San Antonio
San Antonio, Texas

PREFACE

The purpose of *Decision Making in Anesthesiology* is to present the process of anesthetic management during the perioperative period in a decision-tree format. Thus, this work is not intended to replace major anesthesia textbooks but rather to illustrate how to employ the information they contain. This format encourages the reader to think systematically and to follow a logical sequence through preoperative evaluation and preparation, intraoperative management, and postoperative considerations. Our goal was to construct decision trees that were easy to follow, demonstrated decision points clearly, and were simple but not simplistic. The comments are keyed to designated decision points for further information, supported by references. It has been most interesting to reformulate and reorganize our knowledge and clinical experiences in order to construct these algorithms.

Although we would like to suppose that our practices are evidence-based, many decisions in the "real world" are influenced by patient preferences, availability of equipment or supplies, and medicolegal considerations, as well as the current limitations of the science of anesthesia. Despite these constraints, we all strive daily for precision in our decision making and for optimal outcomes in our patient care. We have attempted to ensure that the algorithms are accurate and realistic. In controversial areas, they may reflect the preferences and thinking of the individual contributors. In some cases there may be valid alternative techniques that are not described.

As educators involved in university training programs, we have consciously targeted the work for **anesthesiology residents.** In learning the practice of anesthesiology or reviewing an unfamiliar procedure, it is very helpful to have immediate access to an experienced consultant who can suggest a reasonable approach and review special surgical requirements (and potential pitfalls). That is what is proposed in our book—to suggest reasonable anesthetic management schemes and to serve as a clinical reference. Just as advice rendered by the experienced consultant must be individualized for the patient in question, so must our suggestions be considered in light of special patient needs. We hope that anesthesia providers and others involved in the perioperative care of surgical patients may also find this a refreshing method of review. Feedback from those who have used the book has been very helpful, and we encourage you to communicate your concerns to us.

Many thanks to our authors, who shared their clinical expertise generously and enthusiastically tackled this rather unusual format. Thanks to Natasha Andjelkovic for her help and support, without which this book would have been impossible. Special thanks to Katharine Holahan, editorial assistant extraordinaire, who coordinated the editorial processes for the manuscript and kept everything organized. And as always, our profound gratitude to the many anesthesiology residents with whom we have worked and learned over the years—you make us proud.

Lois L. Bready, MD
Dawn Dillman, MD
Susan H. Noorily, MD

CONTENTS

PRINCIPLES OF ANESTHESIA

GENERAL ANESTHESIA

REGIONAL ANESTHESIA (RA)

PREMEDICATION OF ADULTS

PREMEDICATION OF CHILDREN

ANESTHESIA BREATHING SYSTEMS

TRACHEAL INTUBATION (TI)

DIFFICULT AIRWAY: RECOGNIZED

DIFFICULT AIRWAY: UNRECOGNIZED,
CAN VENTILATE

DIFFICULT AIRWAY: UNRECOGNIZED, CANNOT
VENTILATE, CANNOT INTUBATE

MONITORING IN ANESTHESIA

CAPNOGRAPHY

PULSE OXIMETRY

OXYGENATION

INTRAOPERATIVE HYPOXEMIA

DECREASED INSPIRED OXYGEN
CONCENTRATION

INCREASED PEAK AIRWAY PRESSURE

RESPONSE TO LOW-PRESSURE ALARM

NEUROMUSCULAR BLOCKING AGENTS

THE FULL STOMACH PATIENT

ELDERLY PATIENT

INFORMED CONSENT FOR THE
ANESTHESIOLOGIST

ADVANCE DIRECTIVES (AD)

DO NOT RESUSCITATE ORDERS IN THE OR

General Anesthesia

DAWN DILLMAN, M.D.

General anesthesia is defined by the American Society of Anesthesiologists (ASA):

General anesthesia is a drug-induced loss of consciousness during which patients are not able to be aroused, even by painful stimulation. The patient's ability to independently maintain ventilatory function is often impaired. Patients often require assistance in maintaining a patent airway, and positive pressure ventilation may be required because of depressed spontaneous ventilation or drug-induced depression of neuromuscular function. Cardiovascular function may be impaired.[1]

Drugs are administered to produce a patient who is unconscious to the point of being nonresponsive to painful stimulus. Amnesia is expected. Unfortunately, the drugs used to induce and maintain general anesthesia almost always cause profound physiological effects on the body, including cardiovascular, respiratory, and by definition, neurological depression. For this reason, many investigators have hypothesized that regional anesthesia should be associated with less serious morbidity and mortality, although there has been little evidence to support that claim across broad populations.

A. Because of the physiological changes anticipated with general anesthesia, any patient for whom deep sedation or general anesthesia is planned should have a preoperative evaluation, including a review of his or her medical record, medical history including previous anesthetic exposures, last oral intake, physical examination (with emphasis on the airway, the cardiopulmonary system, and neurological status), and appropriate laboratory tests and studies. It is also essential that informed consent is obtained and that documentation of this process occurs.[2]

B. Preparation and monitoring should be consistent with the amount of information required to ensure cardiovascular and respiratory stability during the surgery. The standards of the ASA for basic monitoring include cardiovascular function by continuous ECG monitoring; arterial pressure and pulse monitoring; level of oxygenation and ventilation via pulse oximetry; capnometry or capnography; and for general anesthetics utilizing an anesthesia machine, an oxygen analyzer and disconnect sensor.[3]

C. The type of induction of anesthesia will be influenced by the age and physical status of the patient, the NPO status of the patient, the general anesthetic agent(s) to be used, and whether intubation of the trachea is required. Although IV and mask inductions are most common, anesthesia may also be induced via IM injection for an uncooperative patient. Unique aspects of each agent should be considered to avoid deleterious

responses and potential morbidity (e.g., the use of barbiturates in the patient with acute intermittent porphyria and propofol in the patient with egg allergy).

D. The necessity for tracheal intubation should be assessed. If intubation is not required, a facemask or extraglottic device, such as a laryngeal mask airway, may be used. However, the adequacy of ventilation must constantly be assessed. If problems arise (airway obstruction, hypoventilation, or aspiration), tracheal intubation should be performed.

E. Maintenance of a stable course of anesthesia with minimal alteration in physiological status requires constant assessment of the adequacy of anesthesia for the level of consciousness, muscle relaxation, and hemodynamic stability. Adjustment of the anesthetic dose (inhalational or intravenously) and the addition of an analgesic agent (inhalational or intravenously) or a neuromuscular blocking agent (depolarizing or nondepolarizing) ensure this stable course. If additional amnestic agents are required, benzodiazepines or scopolamine can be added.

F. The postoperative course after the use of general anesthesia is related to the operative procedure and the technique and agents used to manage the associated anesthesia. After any general anesthetic, the patient will be transported to either a PACU or its equivalent by a member of the anesthesia team, who will report to the accepting care team. Monitoring of cardiovascular status and respiration is essential, especially in patients who were given muscle relaxants or narcotics during the surgery.[4]

REFERENCES

1. American Society of Anesthesiologists: *Continuum of depth of sedation: definition of general anesthesia and levels of sedation/analgesia,* available at: http://www.asahq.org/publications andservices/standards/20.pdf, 2004.
2. American Society of Anesthesiologist Task Force on Preanesthesia Evaluation: Practice advisory for preanesthesia evaluation: a report by the American Society of Anesthesiologists Task Force on Preanesthesia Evaluation, *Anesthesiology* 96 (2):485-496, 2002.
3. American Society of Anesthesiologists: *Standards for basic anesthetic monitoring,* available at: http://www.asahq.org/publicationsand services/standards/02.pdf, 2005.
4. American Society of Anesthesiologist Task Force on Postanesthetic Care: Practice guidelines for postanesthetic care: a report by the American Society of Anesthesiologists Task Force on Postanesthetic Care, *Anesthesiology* 96 (3):742–752, 2002.

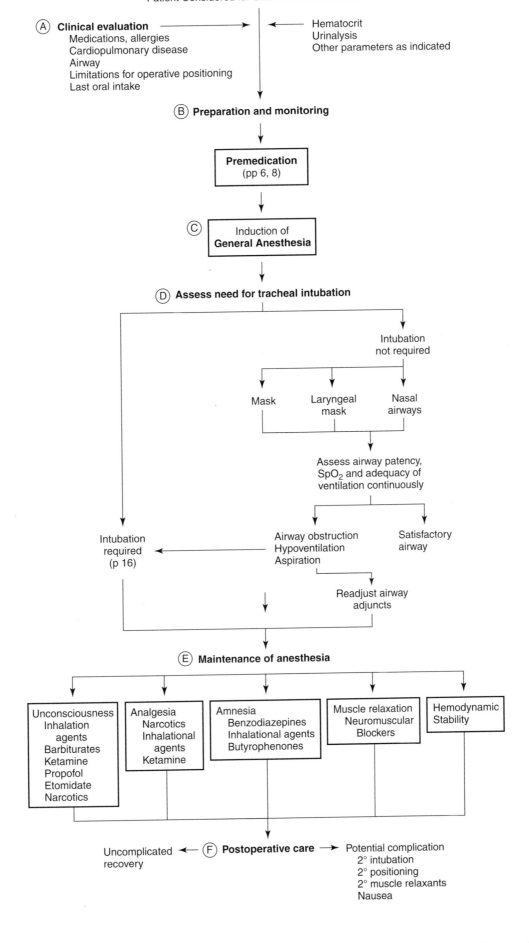

Patient Considered for GENERAL ANESTHESIA

Ⓐ **Clinical evaluation**
    Medications, allergies
    Cardiopulmonary disease
    Airway
    Limitations for operative positioning
    Last oral intake

Hematocrit
Urinalysis
Other parameters as indicated

Ⓑ **Preparation and monitoring**

Premedication
(pp 6, 8)

Ⓒ Induction of
General Anesthesia

Ⓓ **Assess need for tracheal intubation**

Intubation
not required

Mask   Laryngeal   Nasal
            mask   airways

Assess airway patency,
SpO_2 and adequacy of
ventilation continuously

Airway obstruction   Satisfactory
Hypoventilation   airway
Aspiration

Intubation
required
(p 16)

Readjust airway
adjuncts

Ⓔ **Maintenance of anesthesia**

Unconsciousness
Inhalation
    agents
Barbiturates
Ketamine
Propofol
Etomidate
Narcotics

Analgesia
Narcotics
Inhalational
    agents
Ketamine

Amnesia
Benzodiazepines
Inhalational agents
Butyrophenones

Muscle relaxation
Neuromuscular
Blockers

Hemodynamic
Stability

Uncomplicated   ◄—   Ⓕ **Postoperative care**   —►   Potential complication
recovery   2° intubation
                                                         2° positioning
                                                         2° muscle relaxants
                                                         Nausea

Regional Anesthesia (RA)

ROSEMARY HICKEY, M.D.

JAMES N. ROGERS, M.D.

Regional anesthesia (RA) using local anesthetic (LA) prevents nociceptive impulses from reaching the central nervous system. Efferent signals to blood vessels, muscle, and viscera are thus blocked, protecting against reflex responses to operative pain and the phenomenon of "wind-up." Advantages of RA include reduced physiological derangement with surgery, less risk of pulmonary aspiration (airway reflexes are not obtunded), and the provision of postoperative analgesia. In addition, RA reduces the incidence of deep vein thrombosis (DVT) and blood loss after orthopedic surgery.[1]

A. Contraindications to RA include active infection or tumor at the site of needle insertion, untreated sepsis, anticoagulation, and lack of patient cooperation or consent. Preexisting neurological deficit, although not an absolute contraindication, dissuades some anesthetists from the use of RA because of medicolegal considerations. Carefully document any neurological deficits prior to performance of the block.

B. Use of aspirin, nonsteroidal antiinflammatory drugs (NSAIDs), and subcutaneous heparin do not appear to represent significant risks for neuraxial block if conventional guidelines are followed.[2] The safety of newer, more potent antiplatelet drugs (ticlopidine and clopidogrel) in the presence of neuraxial blockade has not been established and various time delays have been recommended (14 days ticlopidine and 7 days clopidogrel.)[2] Use of low molecular weight heparin (LMWH) prophylaxis is associated with a significant risk of epidural hematoma, particularly with concomitant use of other anticoagulants.[2] LMWH does not alter the partial thromboplastin time (PTT). If neuraxial anesthesia is employed, use a single injection spinal anesthetic > 10 to 12 hours after the last LMWH dose.[3] If an epidural catheter must be removed in a patient in who LMWH has been initiated, wait > 10 to 12 hours after the last dose of LMWH (single daily dosing regimen) and 2 hours before a subsequent dose.[3]

C. Premedicate the patient to alleviate anxiety and reduce pain of block placement (particularly if paresthesias will be sought). Benzodiazepines raise the seizure threshold. Do not sedate the patient so heavily that cooperation is lost.

D. Use axillary block (AB) or Bier block (BB) for surgery on the distal forearm, hand, and wrist. Subclavian perivascular block (SCPB), supraclavicular block (SCB), and infraclavicular block are most suitable for the mid portion of the upper extremity. Interscalene block (ISB) is best for the proximal upper extremity and shoulder. ISB may not block the C8, T1 distribution (ulnar, medial brachial, cutaneous). If prolonged analgesia is desired, continuous catheters can be inserted and connected to an infusion pump that is programmed to deliver a constant infusion plus incremental supplemental boluses. The infraclavicular technique is well suited to a catheter (ease of fixation to the skin and lower likelihood of dislodgement postoperatively).

E. In spinal anesthesia, motor block level is usually two dermatomal segments below the sensory level, and sympathetic block is two above. Knowledge of the baricity of the LA solution compared to CSF allows control of spinal level. Hyperbaric solutions are prepared by adding glucose and allowing it to settle to the most dependent aspect of the subarachnoid space. Hypobaric solutions are prepared by adding sterile water, and allowing the solution to rise to nondependent areas in the subarachnoid space. Isobaric solutions are prepared by diluting local anesthetic with CSF and do not produce as high a block level as hyperbaric solutions.

F. In epidural anesthesia, motor block may be about six dermatomal segments below the sensory level, with sympathetic block the same as sensory. Catheter techniques allow repeated bolus injections, continuous infusion, and patient-controlled analgesia. Recovery from spinal and epidural anesthesia regresses from the highest dermatome in a caudad direction.

G. Addition of epinephrine to LA produces more profound anesthesia, shortens the time of onset, prolongs duration (most marked in shorter acting agents), and serves as a marker of IV injection. It reduces peak blood levels and toxicity. Systemic absorption occurs; therefore, consider avoiding the use of epinephrine in patients who are sensitive to it (i.e., hypertensive, hyperthyroid, beta-blocked, or prone to arrhythmias). It should not be used for blocks of the finger, toe, or penis.

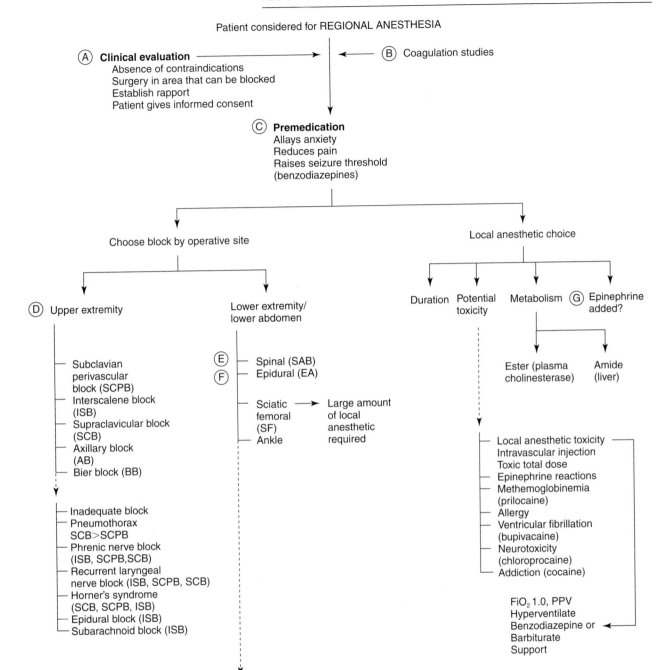

Patient considered for REGIONAL ANESTHESIA

Ⓐ **Clinical evaluation** ⟶ ⟵ Ⓑ Coagulation studies
    Absence of contraindications
    Surgery in area that can be blocked
    Establish rapport
    Patient gives informed consent

Ⓒ **Premedication**
    Allays anxiety
    Reduces pain
    Raises seizure threshold
    (benzodiazepines)

Choose block by operative site   Local anesthetic choice

Ⓓ Upper extremity   Lower extremity/   Duration Potential   Metabolism Ⓖ Epinephrine
                               lower abdomen   toxicity   added?

                        Ⓔ ⟶ Spinal (SAB)
                        Ⓕ ⟶ Epidural (EA)   Ester (plasma   Amide
    Subclavian   cholinesterase)   (liver)
    perivascular
    block (SCPB)   Sciatic ⟶ Large amount
    Interscalene block   femoral   of local
    (ISB)   (SF)   anesthetic
    Supraclavicular block Ankle   required
    (SCB)
    Axillary block   Local anesthetic toxicity
    (AB)   Intravascular injection
    Bier block (BB)   Toxic total dose
                                                                Epinephrine reactions
                                                                Methemoglobinemia
    Inadequate block   (prilocaine)
    Pneumothorax   Allergy
    SCB>SCPB   Ventricular fibrillation
    Phrenic nerve block   (bupivacaine)
    (ISB, SCPB,SCB)   Neurotoxicity
    Recurrent laryngeal   (chloroprocaine)
    nerve block (ISB, SCPB, SCB)   Addiction (cocaine)
    Horner's syndrome
    (SCB, SCPB, ISB) FiO_2 1.0, PPV
    Epidural block (ISB)   Hyperventilate
    Subarachnoid block (ISB)   Benzodiazepine or ⟵
                                                                Barbiturate
                                                                Support

(Cont'd on p 7)

TABLE 1
Maximal Safe Doses of Local Anesthetics

Local anesthetic	Duration (mins)	Total doses (mg/70 kg)	With epinephrine 1:200,000
Procaine	60–90	500	600 mg
Chloroprocaine	30–60	600	650 mg
Mepivacaine	120–240	300	500 mg
Prilocaine	120–240	400	600 mg
Lidocaine	90–200	300	500 mg
Tetracaine	180–600	100	—
Bupivacaine	180–600	175	250 mg
Ropivacaine	180–600	175	250 mg
Etidocaine	180–600	300	400 mg

H. Systemic effects of toxic blood levels of LAs may cause dizziness, metallic taste, tinnitus, nystagmus, facial twitching, seizures of the CNS, respiratory depression, and cardiovascular collapse. If toxic levels are rapidly reached (as in IV injection), CNS, respiratory, and cardiovascular depression may occur immediately without premonitory symptoms. IV injection may be avoided by using proper technique, aspiration in all quadrants, and test doses. True allergic reactions to LAs are rare and are far more common with esters than with amides. Some reactions may be caused by the use of methylparaben and could be avoided with preservative-free preparations.

Bupivacaine binds to the myocardium, thereby causing ventricular fibrillation; cardiac resuscitation is difficult and prolonged. The newer LAs, ropivacaine and levobupivacaine, contain only the S-isomer rather than the more cardiotoxic R-isomer. Standard bupivacaine is a mixture of both the R- and S- isomers. The neurotoxicity of intrathecal chloroprocaine appears to result from a combination of the antioxidant (sodium bisulfite) and the low pH of the solution. Potential complications of the block relate to the site of placement. Neuraxial blocks result in hypotension, headache, and backache. Transient neurologic symptoms (TNS), in which pain develops in the lower extremities after an initial full recovery, is more common with lidocaine than bupivacaine or procaine.[4]

REFERENCES

1. Breen P, Park KW: General anesthesia versus regional anesthesia, *Int Anesthiol Clin* 40 (1):61, 2002.
2. Mulroy M: Indications for and contraindications to regional anesthesia, *American Society of Anesthesiologists Annual Meeting Refresher Course Lectures* 135:1–5, 2003.
3. Horlocker TT, Wedel DJ, Benzon H, et al.: Regional anesthesia in the anticoagulated patient: defining the risks, *Reg Anesth Pain Med* 29 (2 Suppl):1, 2004.
4. Zaric D, Christiansen C, Pace NL, et al.: Transient neurologic symptoms (TNS) following spinal anaesthesia with lidocaine versus other local anaesthetics, *Cochrane Database Syst Rev* 2:CD003006, 2003.

Patient considered for REGIONAL ANESTHESIA
(Cont'd from p 5)

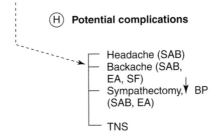

Ⓗ **Potential complications**

— Headache (SAB)
— Backache (SAB,
EA, SF)
— Sympathectomy,↓ BP
(SAB, EA)

— TNS

Premedication of Adults

KATHERINE R. McGUIRE, M.D.

The most common goals of premedication are anxiolysis, sedation, amnesia, analgesia, prophylaxis against aspiration pneumonitis, postoperative nausea and vomiting (PONV), drying of airway secretions, and maintenance of hemodynamic stability. Other indications include the need for corticosteroid supplementation, bronchodilator therapy, and prophylaxis against surgical wound infection, endocarditis, and allergic reactions.

A. Perform a thorough preoperative evaluation. Choose appropriate premedication, individualizing choices to each patient's particular needs and remembering that not all patients require premedication. In fact, an informative and reassuring preoperative visit by the anesthesiologist can effectively calm fear and anxiety.[1] The anesthetic plan, surgical procedure and its urgency, and inpatient status versus ambulatory status of the patient influence premedication choices, as do the pharmacokinetics and pharmacodynamics of the drugs themselves.

B. Consider the need for sedatives, narcotics, PONV prophylaxis, or antibiotic prophylaxis in most patients undergoing anesthesia. Obtain informed consent prior to administering sedating drugs. Benzodiazepines (midazolam, diazepam, and lorazepam) produce anxiolysis, sedation, and anterograde amnesia and are among the most commonly used premedicants. Although relatively free of side effects, they can cause respiratory and CNS depression, especially if combined with other sedatives. Diazepam and lorazepam can cause prolonged sedation. Opiates (morphine, meperidine, and fentanyl) provide preoperative analgesia and sedation. Use caution when administering these drugs to patients with renal failure. Side effects include respiratory depression, orthostatic hypotension, nausea and vomiting, delayed gastric emptying, choledochoduodenal sphincter spasm, and pruritus. Administer sedating drugs with caution to the elderly, and to patients with intracranial pathology, altered mental status, limited cardiac or pulmonary reserve, impending airway obstruction, hemodynamic instability, and full-stomach status.[2] Nonsteroidal anti-inflammatory drugs (NSAIDs) or cyclooxygenase-2 (COX-2) inhibitors given preemptively will decrease supplemental analgesic consumption in the perioperative period.[3] However, use of NSAIDS carries the risk of platelet dysfunction. Prophylaxis against PONV often includes a combination of selective 5-HT$_3$ receptor antagonists (ondansetron and dolasetron), metoclopramide, dexamethasone, promethazine, or scopolamine patch. Droperidol use has declined since the Food and Drug Administration (FDA) issued its black box warning in 2001.[4] Anticholinergic use is not recommended for aspiration prophylaxis. Glycopyrrolate is given primarily for its antisialagogue effect; it is particularly useful in airway surgery or planned fiberoptic intubation. Many patients will be scheduled to receive antibiotics for surgical site infection prophylaxis; administer these within 1 hour of incision for maximal antibiotic levels and activity.

C. Premedication may be appropriate for specific comorbid conditions including gastroesophageal reflux, coronary artery disease, congenital/structural heart disease, reactive airway disease, and latex allergy. Consider prophylaxis against aspiration pneumonitis in at-risk patients.[5] Proton pump inhibitors (omeprazole and lansoprazole) and histamine-2 (H$_2$) receptor antagonists (ranitidine and famotidine) take 30 minutes to have full effect. Oral nonparticulate antacids (sodium citrate) increase gastric pH immediately. Metoclopramide speeds gastric emptying. Consider perioperative beta-blockade in patients at risk for myocardial ischemia; perioperative beta-blockade decreases cardiovascular morbidity and mortality.[6] Clonidine and dexmedetomidine are alpha-2-adrenergic agonists that provide sedation and anxiolysis as well as hemodynamic stability via reduced central sympathetic outflow. Consider bacterial endocarditis prophylaxis in patients with structural heart defects, valve replacements, or pacemakers who are scheduled to undergo certain surgical procedures.[7] Consider preoperative nebulized albuterol and/or ipratropium in patients with reactive airway disease. Administer antihistamines and corticosteroids to patients with a history of life-threatening allergic reaction to latex. Avoid use of latex products when caring for these patients.

D. Administer most premedication via oral or IV routes. IM injection may be painful and transmucosal absorption unpredictable. Nebulized drugs act within minutes. Appropriate timing of administration ensures maximum benefit. In general, give PO drugs 60 to 90 minutes, IM drugs 30 to 60 minutes, and IV drugs 1 to 5 minutes preoperatively.

REFERENCES

1. Morgan GE, Mikhail MS, Murray MJ: Nonvolatile anesthetic agents. In *Clinical anesthesiology*, ed 4, New York, 2006, McGraw-Hill.
2. Kumar S: Preoperative medication. In Duke J, editor: *Anesthesia secrets*, ed 3, Philadelphia, 2006, Elsevier.
3. Ong CK, Lirk P, Seymour RA, et al.: The efficacy of preemptive analgesia for acute postoperative pain management: a meta-analysis, *Anesth Analg*, 100 (3):757-773, 2005.
4. Schell RM, Bowe EA: Anesthetics and anesthetic adjuvants. In Cole DJ, Schlunt M, editors: *Adult perioperative anesthesia*, Philadelphia, 2004, Elsevier.

PREMEDICATION OF ADULTS

(A) Preoperative evaluation
  • History and physical exam
  • Reassurance of patient

(B) General premedication concerns → (C) Patient specific concerns

Ensure valid surgical consent before administering sedatives

— PONV prophylaxis – single agent or multi-modal

— Surgical site prophylaxis – as indicated by surgery and allergy

— Pain – opiates, NSAIDs/COX2 inhibitors

— Anxiety – benzodiazepines

Aspiration risk – PPI/H2 blocker, metoclopramide, Na citrate

Reactive airway – albuterol +/− ipratroprium MDI/nebulizer

Coronary disease – beta blocker or clonidine

Structural heart disease – endocarditis prophylaxis

Life-threatening allergy – H1 and H2 blocker, corticosteroid

(D) Consider route of administration and drug effect times when planning

5. American Society of Anesthesiologists Task Force on Preoperative Fasting: Practice guidelines for preoperative fasting and the use of pharmacologic agents to reduce the risk of pulmonary aspiration: application to healthy patients undergoing elective procedures: a report by the American Society of Anesthesiologists Task Force on Preoperative Fasting, *Anesthesiology* 90:896-905, 1990.

6. Stier GR: Preoperative evaluation and testing. In Cole DJ, Schlunt M, editors: *Adult perioperative anesthesia*, Philadelphia, 2004, Elsevier.

7. Dajani AS, Taubert KA, Wilson W, et al.: Prevention of bacterial endocarditis. Recommendations by the American Heart Association, *JAMA* 277 (22):1794–1801, 1997.

Premedication of Children

JOANNE BAUST, M.D.

Goals for premedication include anxiolysis, amnesia, analgesia, nausea and aspiration prophylaxis, reduction of airway secretions, perioperative stress reduction, and blocking of autonomic reflexes. Consider the patient's age, weight, drug history, allergies, medical history, level of anxiety of the patient and parents, and maturity. Most children present without an IV line; most premedications are given by alternative routes. Oral medications are generally well tolerated, but many institutions routinely use the rectal route. Nasal medications are less well tolerated. IM injections are painful, but may be useful in the uncooperative patient.[1–5]

A. Children between the ages of 6 months and 6 years may have anxiety regarding separation from parents or fears related to their surgery (e.g., pain). Children over 6 years old are concerned with mutilation and are afraid of being "put to sleep" like a pet. Adolescents are concerned with their physical appearance and fear lack of control. Psychological preparation (preoperative visit to the hospital or induction of anesthesia with parental presence) may enable avoidance of an anxiolytic. Children who have had anesthesia before and remember the experience can be particularly difficult to manage and may require more intensive sedation. Patients with significant cardiopulmonary disorders may not be candidates for sedation.

B. Midazolam usually produces a calm child who separates easily from parents within 10 to 15 minutes. Sedative effects are short-lived, although midazolam may be partially responsible for the emergence delirium seen with sevoflurane. Diazepam has a much longer duration. Barbiturates cause hyperalgesia and may intensify preoperative pain. Thiopental and methohexital are short acting but may not be appropriate for day surgery. Ketamine provides sedation and analgesia but may cause dysphoria and excess salivation. Given orally, it is useful in the child who is resistant to midazolam alone; given intramuscularly, it is excellent in the uncooperative patient. It is usually given in combination with midazolam and atropine. Clonidine, an alpha-2 agonist, has anxiolytic and sedative properties. A fall in perioperative BP, HR, hr, anesthetic requirements, postoperative pain, and nausea and vomiting are seen, but they may cause prolonged sedation and delayed emergence.[6] Antihistamines, such as hydroxyzine, diphenhydramine, and chlorpheniramine, can be used for sedation in hyperactive children.

C. Fentanyl, morphine, meperidine, and sufentanil are narcotics that have been used for sedation and analgesia, but their use is limited by side effects. The oral transmucosal fentanyl lozenge may cause pruritus, nausea and vomiting, and respiratory depression. Oral nonopioid analgesics (acetaminophen, ibuprofen, ketorolac, and dextromethorphan) given preoperatively can reduce postoperative pain.

D. Children with a history of reflux or a full stomach may require aspiration prophylaxis. Nonparticulate antacid (sodium citrate) raises gastric pH. Histamine-2 (H_2) receptor antagonists (cimetidine and ranitidine) also increase gastric pH. Metoclopramide speeds gastric emptying, increases lower esophageal sphincter tone (may be blocked by atropine), relaxes the pyloric sphincter, and possesses antiemetic properties.

E. Anticholinergics (glycopyrrolate, atropine, and scopolamine) are administered to prevent bradycardia (due to laryngoscopy and intubation, surgical manipulation, or succinylcholine) or to reduce airway secretions. All can cause tachycardia, dry mouth, and hyperthermia.

PREMEDICATION FOR CHILDREN

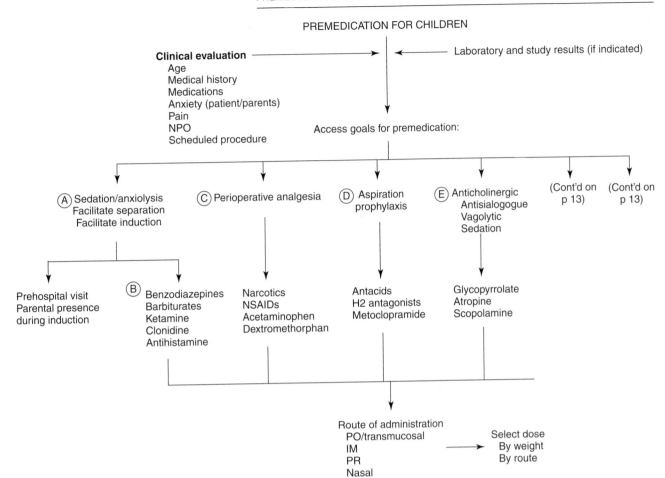

F. Antiemetics target postoperative nausea and vomiting (PONV). The 5-HT antagonists, metoclopramide and dexamethasone, are more effective when used in combinations than when used alone.

G. Children with cardiopulmonary disorders may require SBE prophylaxis per American Heart Association guidelines. Consider perioperative steroids for patients who have received steroids for >7 days in the past 6 months. Asthmatic children may benefit from preanesthetic albuterol nebulizer treatments.

REFERENCES

1. Cote CJ, Todres ID, Ryan JF, et al.: *A practice of anesthesia for infants and children*, ed 3, Philadelphia, 2001, W.B. Saunders.
2. Binstock W, Rubin R, Bachman C, et al.: The effect of premedication with OTFC, with or without ondansetron, on postoperative agitation, and nausea and vomiting in pediatric ambulatory patients, *Pediatr Anesth* 14:759–767, 2004.
3. Kain ZN, Caldwell-Andrews AA, Krivutza DM, et al.: Trends in the practice of parental presence during induction of anesthesia and the use of preoperative sedative premedication in the United States, 1995-2002: results of a follow-up national survey, *Anesth Analg* 98 (5):1252–1259, 2004.
4. Shende D, Bharti N, Kathirvel S, et al.: Combination of droperidol and ondansetron reduces PONV after pediatric strabismus surgery more than single drug therapy, *Acta Anaesthesiol Scand* 45: 756–760, 2001.
5. Weber F, Wulf H, el Saeidi G: Premedication with nasal s-ketamine and midazolam provides good conditions for induction of anesthesia in preschool children, *Can J Anaesth* 50 (5):470–475, 2003.
6. Yaguchi Y, Inomata S, Kihara S, et al.: The reduction in minimum alveolar concentration for tracheal extubation after clonidine premedication in children, *Anesth Analg* 94 (4):863–866, 2002.

TABLE 1
Pediatric Premedication

	Drug	Route of administration	Time of onset (mins)	Dose (mg/kg) (Usual dose)
Sedatives/Hypnotics	Midazolam	PO	15	0.25–0.75 (0.5)
		Nasal	5–10	max 20
		PR	45	0.2–0.3 (0.2)
		IM		0.3–1 (0.5) max 20
	Diazepam	PO	60–120	0.1–0.5 (0.2)
		PR		1
	Lorazepam	PO	—	0.05–0.1 max 4
		PR		0.1–0.2 (0.1)
	Ketamine	PO	—	3–10 (6)
		Nasal		3
		PR		6–10 (6)
		IM		2–10 (7)
	Pentobarbital	PO/PR	60–120	3–5 (3) max 200
		IM	30	2–5 (2) max 150
	Methohexital 10%	PR	10–15	20–35 (25)
		IM		5–10 (10)
	Thiopental	PR	10–15	20–40 (30)
	Secobarbital	PO/IM	60–120	3–5
	Chloral hydrate	PO/PR	90–120	15–100 (50) max 1 g
	Clonidine	PO	45–120	2–4 µg/kg
	Hydroxyzine	PO/IM		0.5–1 max 50 mg
	Diphenhydramine	PO/IM		0.5–1 max 50 mg
	Chlorpheniramine	PO		0.5
Narcotics	Morphine	IM	60	0.1–0.3 (0.1)
	Sufentanil	Nasal	5–10	0.0015–0.004
	Fentanyl	PO, transmucosal	—	0.005–0.015, max 0.015
	Meperidine	IM	30–60	1–2 (2)
Non-narcotic Analgesics	Tylenol	PO	15	30–40
		PR	40	10–15
	Ibuprofen	PO	—	10–15
	Ketorolac	IM/IV	—	1
	Dextromethorphan	PO	—	1
H2 Blockers	Cimetidine	PO/IM	60	5–10 (10)
		PR		30
	Ranitidine	PO	60	1–2.5 (2)
		IM		1–2 (1)
	Famotidine	PO	—	0.3–1
Antacid	Sodium Citrate	PO		0.4 ml/kg
Gastric stimulant	Metoclopramide	PO/IM	30	0.05–0.15 (0.1)
Anticholinergics	Atropine	PO/PR/IM	30–60	0.01–0.06 (0.02) min 0.1 mg, max 0.6 mg
	Scopolamine	PO/PR/IM	—	0.005–0.02 (0.01)
	Glycopyrrolate	PO/PR/IM	—	0.01
Beta-2 agonists	Albuterol	Nebulized	—	0.1–0.15
Antiemetics	Ondansetron	PO	—	0.15 max 4
	Droperidol	PO	—	0.3
	Promethazine	PO/IM/PR	30–60	0.25–1
	Dexamethasone	PO/IM	60	0.05–0.15

PREMEDICATION FOR CHILDREN

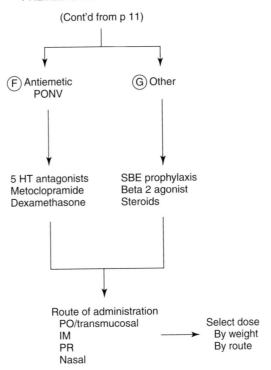

(Cont'd from p 11)

(F) Antiemetic
    PONV

(G) Other

5 HT antagonists
Metoclopramide
Dexamethasone

SBE prophylaxis
Beta 2 agonist
Steroids

Route of administration
   PO/transmucosal
   IM
   PR
   Nasal

Select dose
  By weight
  By route

Anesthesia Breathing Systems

RUSSELL C. BROCKWELL, M.D.

J. JEFF ANDREWS, M.D.

The anesthesia breathing circuit is the portion of the anesthesia workstation that delivers oxygen (O_2) and inspired gases to the patient while removing carbon dioxide (CO_2), minimizing waste of costly anesthetic agents, preserving patient airway heat and moisture, and preventing accumulation of undesirable or toxic by-products. The most widely used breathing system in the United States remains the *circle system* (Figure 1). Because of improvements in the circle system's reliability and design, Mapleson type breathing circuits have been less popular but continue to be sporadically used (Figure 2). The relative

efficiency of different Mapleson systems, with respect to prevention of rebreathing during *spontaneous ventilation*, can be summarized as: A > DFE > CB and during *controlled ventilation*, DFE > BC > A.[1,2] The Mapleson A, B, C systems are rarely used today, but the D, E, F systems are still employed. In the United States, the most popular representative from the D, E, F group is the Bain Circuit (modified Mapleson D).[1,2] There are no strict guidelines dictating the best breathing circuit for a given patient. For most contemporary anesthesia workstations, the anesthesia care provider should select the breathing

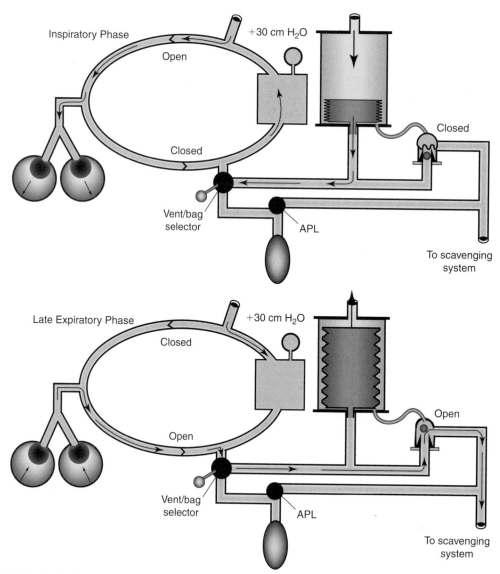

FIGURE 1 **A,** Inspiratory and **B,** expiratory phase gas flows of a generic ascending bellows pneumatic ventilator.

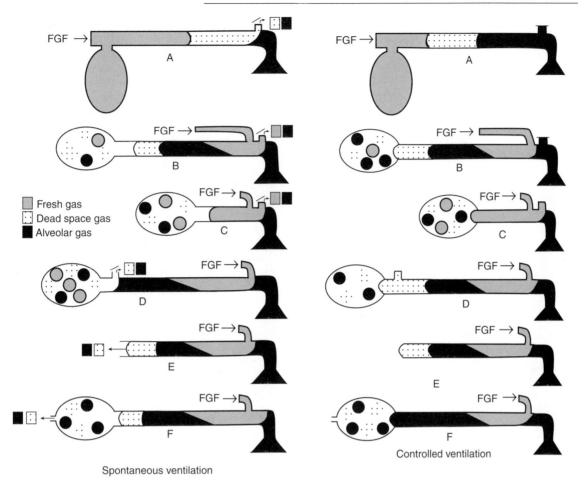

Fresh gas

Dead space gas

Alveolar gas

Spontaneous ventilation

Controlled ventilation

FIGURE 2 Mapleson-type breathing circuits.

system that he or she is most familiar with—in most cases this will be the circle system. In pediatric patients weighing less than 25 to 30 kg, either a neonatal or pediatric circle system or a Bain circuit is generally recommended. Consistently utilize the 1993 Food and Drug Administration (FDA) checklist; although there are some newer machines that incorporate integrated self-test systems, which make all or parts of the checklist unnecessary. The anesthesia machine manufacturer's preuse recommendations should be followed closely by all anesthesia care providers. If automated machine preuse checks are employed, it is incumbent on anesthesia care providers to understand what exactly is being checked and to know the limitations of these automated tests.

A. *Breathing circuit disconnection*, complete or partial (leaks), is a leading cause of critical incidents in anesthesia.[3,4] Preexisting undetected leaks can be present in compressed, corrugated, or disposable anesthetic circuits. Therefore, fully expand the circuit preoperatively to check for leaks. Breathing circuit disconnections and leaks manifest more readily with the ascending bellows type ventilator, because the bellows will not refill when volume is lost through the leak. CO_2 monitors, pneumatic and electronic pressure monitors, and respiratory volume monitors are helpful in diagnosing disconnections.

B. *Occlusion (obstruction) of the breathing circuit* produces increased peak inspiratory pressures or total failure of ventilation and may occur in the tracheal tube, elbow connector, "y"-piece, unidirectional valves (completely or partially stuck shut), hoses (external compression), or bacterial filter in the expiratory limb (associated with development of bilateral tension pneumothorax[5]). Incorrect insertion of components that are sensitive to flow direction (some PEEP valves and cascade humidifiers) can result in a no-flow state. Depending on the location of the occlusion relative to the pressure sensor, a high-pressure alarm may or may not alert the anesthesiologist to the source of the problem.

C. *Excess inflow to the breathing circuit* from the anesthesia machine during the inspiratory phase can cause barotrauma. The best example of this phenomenon is oxygen flushing. Excess volume cannot be vented from the system during the inspiratory phase, because the ventilator relief valve is closed and the APL valve is either out-of-circuit or closed. A high-pressure alarm, if present, may be activated when the pressure becomes excessive. With Dräger systems, both audible and visual alarms are actuated when the high-pressure threshold is exceeded.[6–15] In the Modulus II Plus System with the Datex-Ohmeda 7810 and later Datex-Ohmeda workstations, the ventilator either automatically switches from the inspiratory to the expiratory phase or a pressure release valve is opened when the adjustable peak pressure threshold is exceeded. This minimizes the possibility of barotrauma if the peak pressure threshold is set appropriately by the anesthesiologist.

D. *Malfunctioning valves* can cause serious problems and can even result in the death of a patient. Rebreathing can occur if the valves stick in the open position; total occlusion of the circuit can occur if they are stuck closed. If the expiratory valve is stuck shut, breath stacking and tension pneumothorax can occur. Be sure to perform a functional assessment of the unidirectional valves during any preuse machine check. The flow test (described in step 12 of the 1993 FDA Anesthesia Apparatus Pre-use Checklist), which is performed in addition to the static leak testing, is necessary to evaluate the functional integrity of these valves.

E. *Scavenging systems* probably represent the most neglected portion of the circle system. Scavenging systems are designed to minimize operating room pollution, yet they add complexity to the anesthesia system. A scavenging system functionally extends the anesthesia circuit all the way from the anesthesia machine to the ultimate disposal site. This extension increases the potential for problems. Obstruction of scavenging pathways can cause excessive positive pressure in the breathing circuit, resulting in barotrauma. Excessive vacuum applied to a scavenging system can cause negative pressures in the breathing system.

REFERENCES

1. Andrews JJ: Inhaled anesthetic delivery systems. In Miller RD, editor: *Anesthesia*, ed 5, Philadelphia, 2000, Churchill Livingstone.
2. Andrews JJ, Brockwell RC: Delivery systems for inhaled anesthetics. In Barash PG, Stoelting RK, editors: *Clinical anesthesia*, ed 4, Philadelphia, 2000, Lippincott.
3. Caplan RA, Vistica MF, Posner KL, et al.: Adverse anesthetic outcomes arising from gas delivery equipment: a closed claims analysis, *Anesthesiology* 87:741–748, 1997.
4. Cooper JB, Newbower RS, Kitz RJ: An analysis of major errors and equipment failures in anesthesia management: considerations for prevention and detection, *Anesthesiology* 60:34–42, 1984.
5. McEwan AI, Dowell L, Karis JH: Bilateral tension pneumothorax caused by a blocked bacterial filter in an anesthesia breathing circuit, *Anesth Analg* 76:440–442, 1993.
6. Dräger Medical, Inc.: *Narkomed 2A anesthesia system: technical service manual*, ed 6, Telford, PA, 1985, North American Dräger.
7. Fabius GS: *Anesthesia workstation: operator's instruction manual*, Telford, Pa, 2002, Dräger Medical, Inc.
8. Dräger Medical Inc.: *Narkomed GS anesthesia workstation: setup and installation manual*, Telford, PA, 2002, Dräger Medical, Inc.
9. Dräger Medical Inc.: *Narkomed 6000 anesthesia workstation: service manual*, Rev. H, Telford, PA, 2000, Dräger Medical, Inc.
10. Dräger Medical Inc.: *Narkomed 6000 anesthesia workstation: setup and installation manual*, Rev. F, Telford, PA, 2000, Dräger Medical, Inc.
11. Dräger Medical Inc.: *Narkomed 2A anesthesia system: instruction manual*, ed 7, Telford, PA, 1985, North American Dräger.
12. Dräger Medical Inc.: *Narkomed 2B anesthesia system: operator's manual*, Telford, PA, 1988, North American Dräger.
13. Dräger Medical Inc.: *Narkomed 3 anesthesia system: operator's instruction manual*, Telford, PA, 1986, North American Dräger.
14. Dräger Medical Inc.: *Narkomed 4 anesthesia system: operations instruction manual*, Telford, PA, 1990, North American Dräger.
15. The BOC Group: *Modulus II plus anesthesia system: operation and maintenance manual*, Madison, Ohmeda, 1988, The BOC Group, Inc.

BREATHING SYSTEM PROBLEM

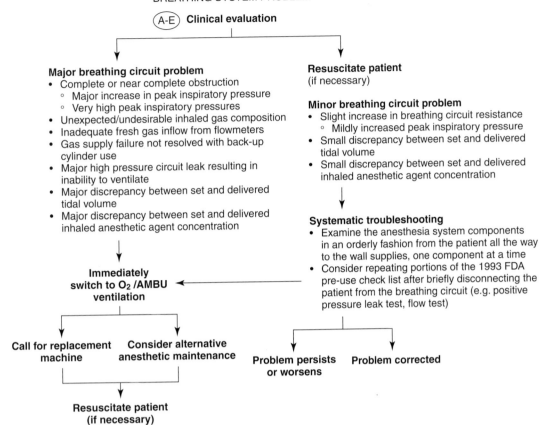

(A-E) **Clinical evaluation**

Major breathing circuit problem
- Complete or near complete obstruction
  - Major increase in peak inspiratory pressure
  - Very high peak inspiratory pressures
- Unexpected/undesirable inhaled gas composition
- Inadequate fresh gas inflow from flowmeters
- Gas supply failure not resolved with back-up cylinder use
- Major high pressure circuit leak resulting in inability to ventilate
- Major discrepancy between set and delivered tidal volume
- Major discrepancy between set and delivered inhaled anesthetic agent concentration

Immediately switch to O$_2$/AMBU ventilation

Call for replacement machine   **Consider alternative anesthetic maintenance**

Resuscitate patient (if necessary)

Resuscitate patient (if necessary)

Minor breathing circuit problem
- Slight increase in breathing circuit resistance
  - Mildly increased peak inspiratory pressure
- Small discrepancy between set and delivered tidal volume
- Small discrepancy between set and delivered inhaled anesthetic agent concentration

Systematic troubleshooting
- Examine the anesthesia system components in an orderly fashion from the patient all the way to the wall supplies, one component at a time
- Consider repeating portions of the 1993 FDA pre-use check list after briefly disconnecting the patient from the breathing circuit (e.g. positive pressure leak test, flow test)

Problem persists or worsens   **Problem corrected**

Tracheal Intubation (TI)

DAWN DILLMAN, M.D.

Many options are available for airway management, ranging from noninvasive (e.g., face mask) to surgically invasive (e.g., tracheostomy). Definitive airway management implies provision of an airway that will allow positive pressure ventilation and protect the airway from aspiration. This is most commonly accomplished by tracheal intubation (TI).

A. There are multiple indications for TI. In an emergency setting they include respiratory failure secondary to hypoventilation or hypoxemia, decreased mental status or inability to protect the airway from aspiration or bleeding, and predicted airway compromise. TI is also absolutely indicated for airway maintenance in patients who are at risk for aspiration when undergoing general anesthesia, including but not limited to patients with full stomachs or known delayed gastric emptying, including autonomic neuropathy, obstruction, and hiatal hernia. Relative indications for TI include general anesthetics in which patients may be positioned such that the anesthesiologist does not have access to the airway, prolonged procedures, patients predicted to require postoperative ventilation, or patients who have fixed reductions in lung compliance who may need high peak inspiratory pressures to maintain ventilation. If general anesthesia is required, but TI is not necessary, consideration should be given to either mask ventilation or alternate supraglottic airway device. Laryngeal mask airways (LMA) now enjoy widespread use and may be used with positive pressure ventilation up to 20 cm H_2O when well seated, and the Proseal LMA may be used at pressures up to 40 cm H_2O.[1] Use of the LMA may reduce complications, such as hoarseness and sore throat, compared to TI.[2,3] Although there are reports of patients who have had an LMA left in situ for up to 8 hours without sequelae, they are not currently appropriate for prolonged use.[4]

B. Planning for TI should include whether the surgical procedure will require an approach via the nasal or oral route. Also requirements for specific types of endotracheal tubes for a given procedure should be considered. For example, intrathoracic procedures may require double-lumen endobronchial tubes, or surgery involving laser use in the airway may require a laser-resistant tube.

C. Prior to any airway management, perform an airway examination to predict whether difficulty may be expected.[5] See the Chapters 7, 8, and 9 on difficult airway management.

D. Prior to TI, perform either induction of general anesthesia or topicalization of the airway to prevent gagging, potential aspiration, and the hemodynamic stimulation associated with intubation. Better quality of intubation conditions may correlate with reduced frequency of complications of intubation.[6]

E. After TI has been performed, it is essential to confirm placement of the endotracheal tube using clinical signs, such as breath sounds, and capnometry whenever possible. Esophageal intubation and endobronchial intubation are usually not life-threatening unless unrecognized.[5]

REFERENCES

1. Brain AI, Verghese C, Strube PJ: The LMA "ProSeal"—a laryngeal mask with an oesophageal vent, *Br J Anaesth* 84:650–654, 2000.
2. Tanaka A, et al.: Laryngeal resistance before and after minor surgery: endotracheal tube versus laryngeal mask airway, *Anesthesiology* 99:252–258, 2003.
3. Higgins PP, Chung F, Mezei G: Postoperative sore throat after ambulatory surgery, *Br J Anaesth* 88 (4):582–584, 2002.
4. Ferson D, Brimacombe JR, Brain AI: The intubating laryngeal mask airway, *Int Anesthesiol Clin* 36:183–209, 1998.
5. American Society of Anesthesiologists Task Force on Management of Difficult Airway: Practice guidelines for management of the difficult airway: an updated report by the American Society of Anesthesiologists Task Force on Management of the Difficult Airway, *Anesthesiology* 98:1269–1277, 2003.
6. Mencke T, Echternach M, Kleinschmidt S, et al.: Laryngeal morbidity and quality of tracheal intubation: a randomized controlled trial, *Anesthesiology* 98:1049–1056, 2003.

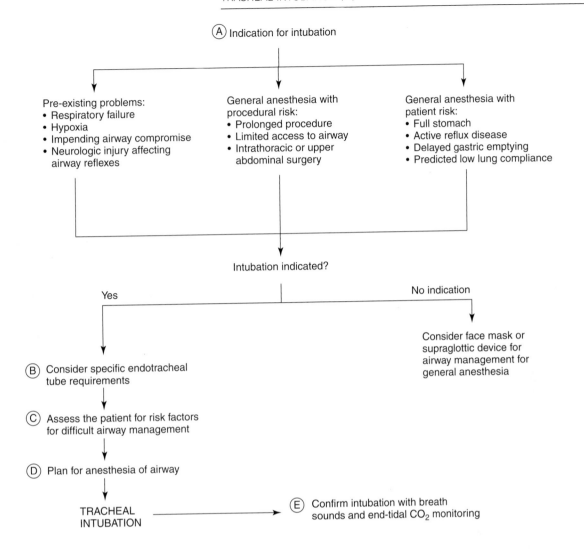

(A) Indication for intubation

Pre-existing problems:
• Respiratory failure
• Hypoxia
• Impending airway compromise
• Neurologic injury affecting
  airway reflexes

General anesthesia with
procedural risk:
• Prolonged procedure
• Limited access to airway
• Intrathoracic or upper
  abdominal surgery

General anesthesia with
patient risk:
• Full stomach
• Active reflux disease
• Delayed gastric emptying
• Predicted low lung compliance

Intubation indicated?

Yes

No indication

Consider face mask or
supraglottic device for
airway management for
general anesthesia

(B) Consider specific endotracheal
    tube requirements

(C) Assess the patient for risk factors
    for difficult airway management

(D) Plan for anesthesia of airway

TRACHEAL
INTUBATION ⟶ (E) Confirm intubation with breath
                   sounds and end-tidal CO_2 monitoring

Difficult Airway: Recognized

TOBIAS MOELLER-BERTRAM, M.D.

JONATHAN L. BENUMOF, M.D.

An algorithm for the management of the patient with a difficult airway was first created by the American Society of Anesthesiologists (ASA) in 1993 and then updated in 2003.[1] The updated algorithm is used as the basis for this chapter and the following two. The shaded portion of the decision tree represents the material presented in this chapter.

A. Perform a comprehensive airway examination on all patients undergoing an anesthesia. The ASA difficult airway algorithm[1] recommends an 11-step preoperative airway evaluation. Focus first on the teeth (steps 1–4), then the oropharynx (steps 5 and 6), the mandibular space (steps 7 and 8), and the neck (steps 9–11). (See Table 1, Figure 1.) In addition, note the presence of a beard, large breasts, and various pathological states (e.g., cancer, abscess, hemorrhage, or tracheal disruption). If the airway is recognized to be difficult, strongly consider safely securing the airway while the patient is awake using a tracheal intubation.

B. Prepare the patient for a tracheal intubation while he or she is awake by providing psychological support and administering necessary medications, such as an antisialagogue, a sedative, a mucosal vasoconstrictor, and, most importantly, local anesthetic, both topically and via nerve blocks. Deliver supplemental oxygen throughout the process.

C. Techniques for intubation while the patient is awake include fiberoptic bronchoscopy; direct laryngoscopy; blind orotracheal or nasotracheal intubation; retrograde intubation; or the use of an illuminated stylet, a rigid bronchoscope, or a percutaneous dilating tracheal entry device.

D. If tracheal intubation while the patient is awake fails, consider repreparation for intubation while the patient is awake using a new technique, employing regional anesthesia, creating a surgical airway, inducing general anesthesia, or rescheduling the surgical procedure for a different day.

E. Performing regional anesthesia in a patient with a difficult airway does not solve the airway problem. Consider regional anesthesia only if the operation is conducive to this technique and may be easily terminated if necessary. The airway must be easily accessible during the procedure.

TABLE 1
Eleven-Step Airway Evaluation, Adopted from the Practice Guidelines for Management of the Difficult Airway*

Airway examination component	Nonreassuring findings
1. Length of upper incisors	Relatively long
2. Relation of maxillary and mandibular incisors during normal jaw closure	Prominent overbite (maxillary incisors anterior to mandibular incisors)
3. Relation of maxillary and mandibular incisors during voluntary protrusion	Patient cannot bring mandibular incisors anterior to maxillary incisors
4. Interincisor distance	Less than 3 cm
5. Visibility of uvula	Not visible when tongue is protruded with patient in sitting position
6. Shape of palate	Highly arched or very narrow
7. Compliance of mandibular space	Stiff, indurated, occupied by mass, or nonresilient
8. Thyromental distance	Less than 5 cm
9. Length of neck	Short
10. Thickness of neck	Thick
11. Range of motion of head and neck	Patient cannot touch tip of chin to chest or cannot extend neck

*American Society of Anesthesiologists Task Force on Management of the Difficult Airway: Practice guidelines for management of the difficult airway: an updated report by the American Society of Anesthesiologists Task Force on Management of the Difficult Airway, *Anesthesiology* 98: 1269–1277, 2003.

DIFFICULT AIRWAY

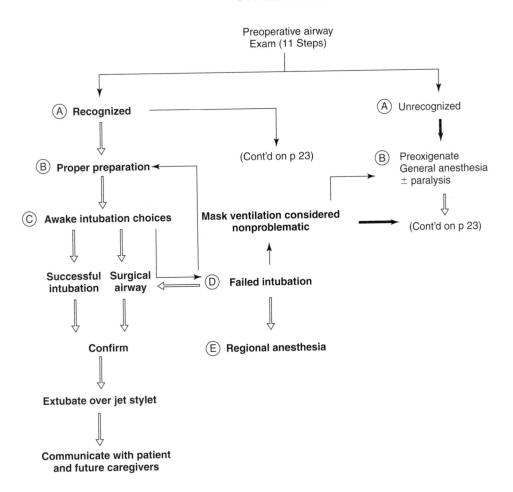

Preoperative airway
Exam (11 Steps)

(A) **Recognized**

(A) Unrecognized

(B) **Proper preparation**

(Cont'd on p 23)

(B) Preoxigenate
General anesthesia
± paralysis

(C) **Awake intubation choices**

**Mask ventilation considered
nonproblematic**

(Cont'd on p 23)

**Successful
intubation**   **Surgical
airway**

(D) **Failed intubation**

Confirm

(E) **Regional anesthesia**

Extubate over jet stylet

**Communicate with patient
and future caregivers**

F. Induce general anesthesia if ventilation via mask is considered unproblematic and if the patient is uncooperative (i.e., the reason for failure of intubation while the patient is awake). Fully preoxygenate prior to induction of general anesthesia.[2] Consider maintaining spontaneous ventilation during and after the induction of general anesthesia. The management of the patient from this point on essentially becomes the same as the management of the unrecognized difficult airway; see Chapters 8 and 9 involving the unrecognized difficult airway.

REFERENCES

1. American Society of Anesthesiologists Task Force on Management of the Difficult Airway. Practice guidelines for management of the difficult airway: an updated report by the American Society of Anesthesiologists Task Force on Management of the Difficult Airway, *Anesthesiology* 98:1269–1277, 2003.
2. Benumof JL: Preoxygenation. Best method for both efficacy and efficiency, *Anesthesiology* 91:603–605, 1999.

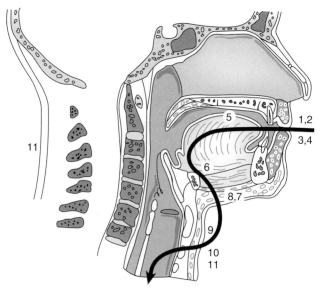

FIGURE 1 Eleven-step preoperative airway evaluation along the line of sight. **1–4:** focus eyes on teeth, **5–6:** focus eyes inside the mouth on the pharynx, **7–8:** complete a mandibular space examination, and **9–11:** complete a neck examination.

DIFFICULT AIRWAY

(Cont'd from p 21)

(F) **Uncooperative patient** ⟹ (B) Preoxigenate
General anesthesia
± paralysis

⟱

Mask ventilation

(C) Possible
(nonemergency path)

(A) Not possible
(emergency path)

(D) Optimal/best intubation attempt

(B) Consider/attempt LMA

(E) Other intubation choices ⟸ Success   Failure

(F) FAILED INTUBATION ⟹

(D) Awaken (C) Combitube
TTJV
rigid bronch

(E) Surgical airway ⟸ Success   Failure

(Cont'd from p 21)

Confirm ⟵

⟱

Extubate over jet stylet

⟱

**Communicate with patient
and future caregivers**

Difficult Airway: Unrecognized, Can Ventilate

TOBIAS MOELLER-BERTRAM, M.D.

JONATHAN L. BENUMOF, M.D.

The shaded portion of the decision tree represents the material presented in this chapter.

A. Analyses of the American Society of Anesthesiologists (ASA) Closed Claims database in 1990 revealed that as many as "30% of deaths totally attributable to anesthesia" were a result of the "inability to successfully manage very difficult airways."[1] A more recent closed claims analysis suggests that development of management strategies as presented in ASA practice guidelines may improve patient safety.[2] In the event of an unrecognized difficult airway (i.e., difficulty with mask ventilation or tracheal intubation), always consider calling for medical, surgical, and technical help, returning to spontaneous ventilation, or waking the patient.

B. Always preoxygenate the patient before the induction of general anesthesia, if possible. In the setting of this chapter, the patient is usually paralyzed. See C in Chapter 9 for discussion of recovery from neuromuscular blockade.

C. The ability to ventilate with a mask puts one on the nonemergency pathway of the ASA difficult airway algorithm. A two-person effort achieves better mask seal, jaw thrust, and tidal volume than a one-person effort.[3] Have a helper trained in managing airways perform bilateral jaw thrust and mask seal with both hands while the primary person does both these maneuvers unilaterally with the left hand and squeezes the bag with the right hand. Have an untrained helper squeeze the bag while the primary person uses both hands to achieve optimal jaw thrust and mask seal. Use oral or nasal airways to increase airway patency.

D. The optimal attempt at laryngoscopy is one performed by a reasonably experienced (2 years minimum) laryngoscopist in the absence of significant resistive muscle tone using an optimal sniff position.[4] The sniff position (slight flexion of the neck on the chest and extension of the head on the neck at the atlantooccipital joint) aligns the oral, pharyngeal, and laryngeal axes. In obese patients, obtaining optimal sniff position may require elevating the scapulae, shoulders, nape of the neck, and head before the induction of anesthesia. Optimal external laryngeal manipulation (OELM) can improve the laryngoscopic view by a full grade. To perform OELM, exert posterior and cephalad pressure on the thyroid cartilage with the free (right) hand. The length and type of blade may be changed once. The risk of airway trauma, edema, bleeding, and secretions increases with each attempt, and subsequent mask ventilation and fiberoptic bronchoscopy may become difficult or impossible.

E. Other choices for intubating the trachea include, but are not limited to, fiberoptic bronchoscopy; laryngeal mask airway (LMA) as an intubating conduit; blind orotracheal or nasotracheal intubation; retrograde technique; and use of the illuminating stylet, the rigid bronchoscope, or percutaneous dilational tracheal entry. Ventilate via mask between attempts at intubation (see bold arrow in Figure 8-1), and as outlined in Chapter 7 (B), "one should actively pursue opportunities to deliver supplemental oxygen throughout the process of difficult airway management."[5] Inability to ventilate via mask at any time puts one in the "cannot ventilate cannot intubate" (CVCI) emergency portion of the ASA difficult airway algorithm (see Chapter 9).

F. When repeated attempts at endotracheal intubation (as described in D and E) fail but ventilation via mask is still possible, cease intubation attempts and proceed with (1) waking the patient and, at a later date, using the recognized difficult airway algorithm; (2) providing anesthesia with ventilation via mask; or (3) establishing a surgical airway (i.e., cricothyrotomy or tracheotomy).

G. Surgery may proceed with anesthesia and ventilation via mask in the patient who is not at risk for aspiration. The surgery must be appropriate for ventilation via mask.

H. If one of the intubation choices results in the insertion of an endotracheal tube, confirm tracheal placement.[5] Traditional fail-safe signs of tracheal intubation are directly visualizing the endotracheal tube (ETT) to pass between the vocal cords (sometimes possible) and fiberoptic visualization of tracheal cartilagenous rings via the ETT (sometimes possible). The new ASA practice guidelines for management of the difficult airway also state "capnography or end-tidal carbon dioxide detection verifies tracheal intubation and leads to fewer adverse outcomes."[5] (always possible to use with a portable capnometer) and that other confirmatory tests, i.e., "esophageal detectors or self-inflating bulbs verify tracheal intubation and lead to fewer adverse outcomes."[5] (always possible to use with a portable esophageal detector device). Also helpful is observing for clinical signs of inhalation and exhalation (watching the chest rise and fall, observing fogging in the tube, auscultating bilateral breath sounds) and palpating the cuff of the endotracheal tube in the suprasternal notch.

DIFFICULT AIRWAY

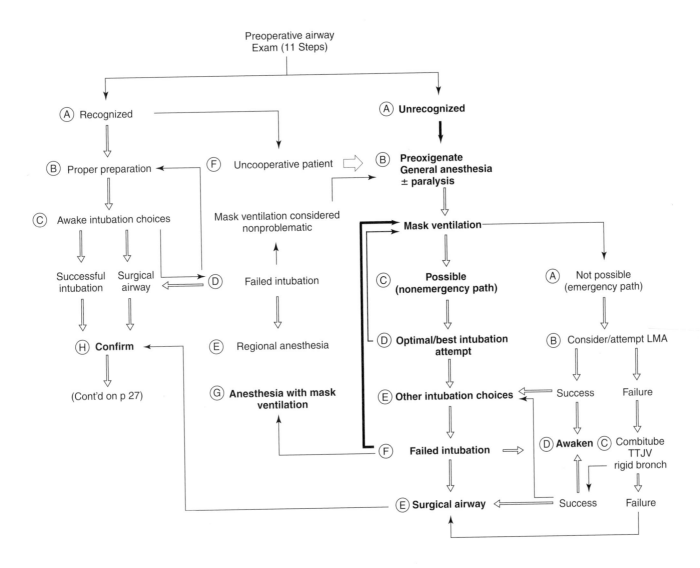

(Cont'd on p 27)

I. Extubate only when the patient is completely awake, spontaneously breathing, has airway reflexes, and has completely recovered from neuromuscular blockade. Consider giving IV steroids to decrease airway edema and an inhaled beta$_2$-agonist to decrease bronchospasm. Consider extubating over a jet ventilating stylet passed through the endotracheal tube or over a bronchoscope.[6]

J. See Chapter 9.

REFERENCES

1. Caplan RA, Posner KL, Ward RJ, et al.: Adverse respiratory events in anesthesia: a closed claims analysis, *Anesthesiology* 72:828–833, 1990.
2. Peterson GN, Domino KB, Caplan RA, et al.: Management of the difficult airway: a closed claims analysis, *Anesthesiology* 103:33–39, 2005.
3. Benumof JL: Management of the difficult airway. With special emphasis on awake tracheal intubation, *Anesthesiology* 75:1087–1110, 1991.
4. Benumof JL: The ASA management of the difficult airway algorithm, *ASA Refresher Course Lecture Manual* 25:241, 1997.
5. American Society of Anesthesiologists Task Force on Management of the Difficult Airway: Practice guidelines for management of the difficult airway: an updated report by the American Society of Anesthesiologists Task Force on Management of the Difficult Airway, *Anesthesiology* 98: 1269–1277, 2003.
6. American Society of Anesthesiologists Task Force on Management of the Difficult Airway: Practice guidelines for management of the difficult airway. A report by the American Society of Anesthesiologists Task Force on Management of the Difficult Airway, *Anesthesiology* 78:597–602, 1983.

DIFFICULT AIRWAY
(Cont'd from p 25)

(I) Extubate over jet stylet

(J) Communicate with patient
and future caregivers

Difficult Airway: Unrecognized, Cannot Ventilate, Cannot Intubate

TOBIAS MOELLER-BERTRAM, M.D.

JONATHAN L. BENUMOF, M.D.

The shaded portion of the decision tree represents the material presented in this chapter.

A. The combination of "cannot ventilate (by mask) cannot intubate" (CVCI) in a patient with apnea is imminently life-threatening and rare; the incidence has been estimated at 0.01 to 2.0 of 10,000 patients.[1] It is imperative that the anesthesiologist have a well-thought-out plan (the American Society of Anesthesiologists (ASA) difficult airway algorithm) and available equipment to deal with this circumstance.

B. The laryngeal mask airway (LMA) has become familiar to anesthesiologists in recent years and is an excellent CVCI option.[2] The LMA can be inserted quickly, blindly, and with a relatively low level of skill. The LMA serves as an excellent conduit to the larynx for a fiberscope. It is associated with few complications. *In fact, the updated version of the ASA practice guidelines for the management of the difficult airway[3] now suggests that the practitioner should consider attempting the insertion of an LMA as the first rescue option for CVCI.* Successful placement of the LMA leads one back to the nonemergency pathway (see Chapter 8, E) or allows awakening (see D).

C. Another good CVCI option is placement of the Combitube.[4] The Combitube can also be inserted quickly, blindly, and with a relatively low level of skill. It will enter the esophagus 99% of the time. In this position the inflated esophageal balloon protects against air insufflation of the stomach and isolates the esophagus from the trachea. Inflation of the large oropharyngeal balloon allows positive pressure ventilation through the pharyngeal holes into the lungs. Auscultation over the stomach and lungs and end-tidal carbon dioxide (CO_2) monitoring confirm proper placement. Transtracheal jet ventilation (TTJV) is instituted by inserting a 14- or 16-gauge IV catheter through the cricothyroid membrane in the caudad direction.[5] Correct placement is confirmed by aspiration of free air through the needle and catheter; the latter remains in the trachea. To minimize the risk of barotrauma, (1) reconfirm tracheal catheter position by reaspiration of air just before TTJV, (2) continuously hold the catheter at the skin line, (3) use an additional inline regulator to decrease the 50-psi wall pressure to 30 psi, (4) use a 0.5-second inspiratory time, and (5) have a second person ensure maximal upper airway patency (exhalation is through the natural airway) by maintaining bilateral jaw thrust and placing oropharyngeal or nasopharyngeal airways (see C of Chapter 8). Both the LMA and the Combitube are supraglottic ventilatory mechanisms and cannot solve a glottic (spasm, edema, tumor, abscess, or hematoma) or subglottic problem. A ventilatory mechanism below the lesion (e.g., TTJV, endotracheal tube [ETT], or surgical airway) will solve a glottic or subglottic problem.

D. Consider waking the patient. In the setting of this chapter, the patient is normally paralyzed. The mean time to recovery of 50% of control twitch height after 1 mg/kg of succinylcholine is 8.6 minutes. After 8.6 minutes of apnea, the SpO_2 of a fully preoxygenated, normal, 70-kg adult will be 75% (the SpO_2 of a moderately ill 70-kg adult will be below 50% in 8.6 minutes, the SpO_2 of an obese 127-kg adult will be below 50% in 4 minutes).[6] Therefore, waking the patient can be pursued as an option only if the patient can be ventilated (see B and C) or after small doses of succinylcholine.

E. If other CVCI options are unsuccessful, obtain an emergency surgical airway (cricothyroidotomy or tracheotomy). To perform a scalpel cricothyrotomy, widely spread the tissues with a clamp and insert a cuffed breathing tube into the trachea. When the alternative is death, the risk of cricothyrotomy is preferable. Try to oxygenate or ventilate while surgical access to the airway is being obtained.

F. See Chapter 8.

G. See Chapter 8.

H. After a difficult airway experience, write a detailed note in the patient's chart, give a note to the patient, and discuss the situation so that the gravity of the problem is understood. The best way to transmit the information that a patient has a difficult airway to future caregivers is to dispense a medical alert bracelet. Call to enter the patient in the Medic-Alert system (800-344-3226).

I. See Chapter 8.

J. See Chapter 8.

DIFFICULT AIRWAY

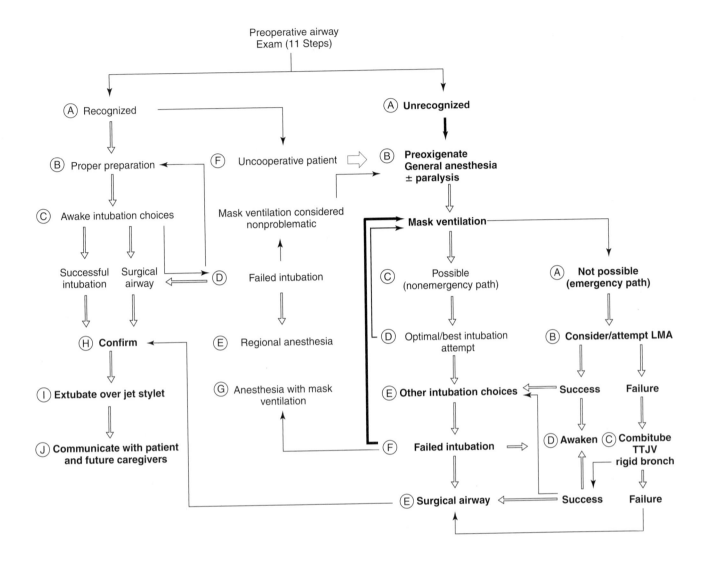

REFERENCES

1. Benumof JL, Scheller MS: The importance of transtracheal jet ventilation in the management of the difficult airway, *Anesthesiology* 71:769–778, 1989.
2. Brain AI: The laryngeal mask: a new concept in airway management, *Br J Anaesth* 55:801–805 1983.
3. American Society of Anesthesiologists Task Force on Management of the Difficult Airway: Practice guidelines for management of the difficult airway: an updated report by the American Society of Anesthesiologists Task Force on Management of the Difficult Airway, *Anesthesiology* 98: 1269–1277, 2003.
4. Frass M, Frenzer R, Ilias W, et al.: The esophageal tracheal Combitube (ETC): animal experiment results with a new emergency tube, *Anasth Intensivther Notfallmed* 22:142–144, 1987.
5. Benumof JL: Transtracheal jet ventilation via a percutaneous catheter and high-pressure source. In: Benumof JL, editor: *Airway management: principles and practice*, St. Louis, 1996, Mosby.
6. Benumof JL, Dagg R, Benumof R: Critical hemoglobin desaturation will occur before return to an unparalyzed state following 1 mg/kg intravenous succinylcholine, *Anesthesiology* 87:979–982, 1987.

Monitoring in Anesthesia

D.M. ANDERSON, M.D.

Monitoring refers to the acquisition of information and can be performed directly using the senses and indirectly using an increasingly complex array of instruments. In either case, the productive use of this information relies on proper interpretation. Once interpreted, the information becomes the basis for taking action.

A. The "standard" American Society of Anesthesiologists (ASA) monitors have proven to be useful for routine care of anesthetized patients (see Table 1).[1] There is a good deal of information that can be obtained from these monitors in addition to the data they were designed to provide. For example, the pulse oximeter is valuable for trending a patient's arterial oxygen saturation and detecting hypoxemia during surgery, but it also is useful for detecting hypovolemia. A substantial decrease in pulse ox waveform size and area under the curve during the inspiratory portion of a mechanical breath reliably suggests that the patient would respond to IV fluid with a significant increase in cardiac output.[2] Similarly, end-tidal carbon dioxide (CO_2) monitoring provides information about the cardiac output. If a patient's minute ventilation remains the same, over a short period of time, an increase of cardiac output will be reflected in an increase in end-tidal CO_2.[3] Change in pulse pressure noted during routine blood pressure measurement indicates a corresponding change in stroke volume as a result of fluid administration or intravascular volume loss. ECG and ST segment analysis appears to be among the best indicators of myocardial ischemia.

B. Some monitors, such as the pulmonary artery (PA) catheter, have evoked controversy.[4,5] This controversy includes debate over when, if ever, it should be used and whether or not its use actually increases patient morbidity and mortality. Keep in mind that saying a patient *needs* a PA catheter really implies that the *health care provider* believes that a PA catheter would be helpful in guiding patient therapy. There is little risk from inserting the PA catheter and allowing it to remain in place for a few days. Although most health care providers can be taught to safely insert a PA catheter with little morbidity, few health care providers know how to correctly interpret and use the data from PA catheters to make decisions about patient care. The risk of PA catheters primarily comes from misinterpretation of hemodynamic data and incorrect therapy based on that misinterpretation. Today many devices are available that serve as alternatives to the PA catheter. For example, the transthoracic electrical impedance instruments provide continuous cardiac output, cardiac contractility, and SVR data. Routine intravascular catheters have been adapted to new uses. Sophisticated computer algorithms enable radial arterial lines to yield information about stroke volume and cardiac output in a beat-to-beat fashion. Older tools, such as the CVP catheter, have gained new respect.[6] New CVP catheters provide continuous digital central venous oxygen saturation data analogous to mixed venous oxygen saturation data, measuring the adequacy of oxygen delivery to the tissues.

C. Although there is an extraordinary array of technology available for patient monitoring, human cognition remains the most important factor. It is essential for health care providers to acquaint themselves with the proper use and correct interpretation of all data acquired from monitors.

TABLE 1
ASA Standards for Basic Monitoring

1. Qualified anesthesia personnel present in the OR at all times.
2. Continuous evaluation of oxygenation, ventilation, circulation, and temperature.
   a. Oxygenation
      i. Inspired gas oxygen (O_2) analyzer, low O_2 alarm
      ii. Pulse oximetry
   b. Ventilation
      i. Observation
      ii. End-tidal carbon dioxide (CO_2) analysis
      iii. Disconnect alarm
   c. Circulation
      i. Continuous ECG
      ii. BP and HR every 5 minutes
      iii. Monitoring by at least one of the following: palpation, auscultation, arterial waveform, ultrasound, plethysmography, or oximetry
   d. Body temperature

REFERENCES

1. American Society of Anesthesiologists: *Guidelines for office-based anesthesia,* available at: http://www.asahq.org/publicationsandservices/standards/12.pdf, 2004.
2. Murray WB, Foster PA: The peripheral pulse wave: information overlooked, *J Clin Monit* 12 (5): 365–377, 1996.
3. Dubin A, Murias G, Estenssoro E, et al.: End-tidal CO2 pressure determinants during hemorrhagic shock, *Intensive Care Med* 26 (11):1619–1623, 2000.
4. Sandham JD, Hull RD, Brant RF, et al.: Canadian Critical Care Clinical Trials Group. A randomized, controlled trial of the use of pulmonary-artery catheters in high-risk surgical patients, *N Engl J Med* 348 (1):5–14, 2003.
5. Rhodes A, Cusack RJ, Newman PJ, et al.: A randomised, controlled trial of the pulmonary artery catheter in critically ill patients, *Intensive Care Med* 28 (3):256–264, 2002.
6. Magder S: More respect for the CVP, *Intensive Care Med* 24 (7):651–653, 1998.

MONITORING IN ANESTHESIA

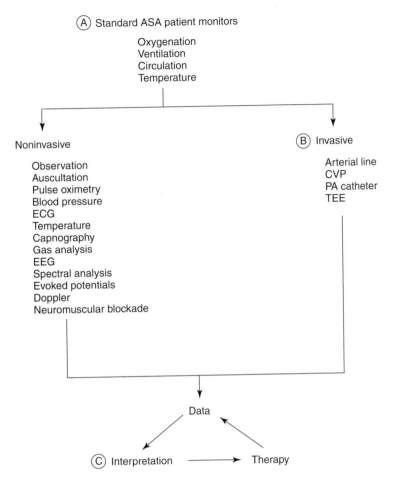

Capnography

D.M. ANDERSON, M.D.

Capnography, the visual display of exhaled carbon dioxide (CO_2) versus time, has several important uses in the OR, ICU, and emergency room. It yields valuable information beyond the end-tidal PCO_2 ($ETCO_2$). The shape of the capnogram gives information about the integrity of the breathing system and the physiology of the patient.

The terminology for capnography has been standardized.[1] The inspiratory portion of the respiratory cycle is called *phase 0*. The expiratory portion consists of three phases (see Figure 1): (1) *phase I*—the portion representing gas contained in the anatomical dead space with little CO_2; (2) *phase II*—the portion representing a mixture of anatomical and alveolar dead space; and (3) *phase III*—the portion representing exhaled alveolar gas. The angle between phases II and III, referred to as the α *angle*, increases with an increase in the slope of phase III. The α angle is an indirect indication of V/Q status.[1] The angle between phase III and the descending limb is referred to as the β *angle* and can be used to assess the extent of rebreathing.[2]

The $ETCO_2$ concentration is the peak exhaled CO_2 concentration. The normal gradient between the $PaCO_2$ and $ETCO_2$ is 5 mm Hg, because the $ETCO_2$ measures CO_2 from both well perfused and poorly perfused alveoli.

Physiological dead space can be estimated by comparing the $ETCO_2$ to the arterial PCO_2.

$$Vd/Vt = (PaCO_2 - ETCO_2)/PaCO_2$$

Several studies have evaluated the use of $ETCO_2$ for assessment of respiratory depression during conscious sedation or for postoperative respiratory monitoring. A modified or specially designed, commercially available nasal cannula can accurately monitor $ETCO_2$.[3,4]

Patients ventilated via laryngeal mask airway but not a face mask can be accurately monitored using exhaled CO_2.[5,6]

Certain factors have been noted in pediatric patients to interfere with the correlation between $ETCO_2$ and $PaCO_2$. These include mouth breathing, airway obstruction, delivery of oxygen via the ipsilateral nasal cannula, and congenital heart disease.

A. Each portion of the capnogram can become abnormal. For example, the $ETCO_2$ can increase, decrease, and be too high or too low. The $ETCO_2$ baseline, normally zero, can increase. The α and β angles can change. Use a systematic approach to determine the cause of the abnormality.[2]

B. Check for the CO_2 waveform. Diagnose esophageal intubation after the sixth breath.[2] Exhaled CO_2 is produced during an esophageal intubation when room air is forced into the stomach or if the patient recently had a carbonated drink. In this case, the $ETCO_2$ is usually less than 10 and decreases with each breath.

C. Problems with the breathing circuit, such as exhausted CO_2 absorbent and incompetent valves, are apparent on the capnogram. Check the baseline. An elevation indicates equipment problems. Check CO_2 absorber, gas flow, and valves. An incompetent inspiratory valve causes exhaled gas containing CO_2 to enter the inspiratory limb of the breathing circuit during expiration; the capnogram will have an increased β angle, prolonged phase III, and gradually rising baseline (see Figure 2).[2]

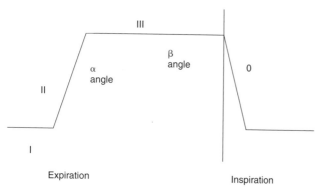

FIGURE 1 The normal capnogram.

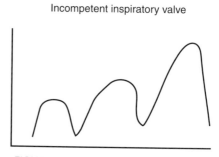

Incompetent inspiratory valve

FIGURE 2 Incompetent inspiratory valve.

CAPNOGRAPHY

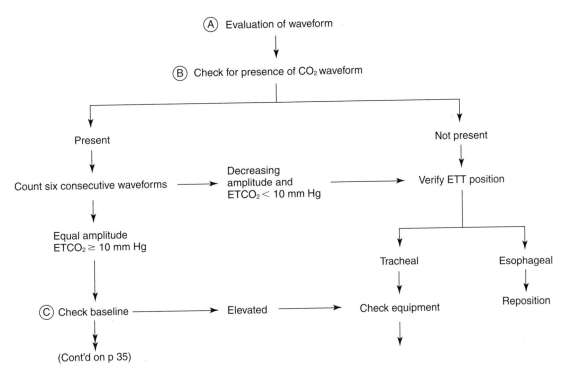

Ⓐ Evaluation of waveform

Ⓑ Check for presence of CO₂ waveform

Present

Not present

Count six consecutive waveforms → Decreasing amplitude and ETCO₂ < 10 mm Hg → Verify ETT position

Equal amplitude ETCO₂ ≥ 10 mm Hg

Tracheal   Esophageal

Ⓒ Check baseline → Elevated → Check equipment   Reposition

(Cont'd on p 35)

Bronchospasm

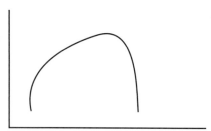

FIGURE 3 Bronchospasm.

D. Several pulmonary abnormalities can be diagnosed by capnography. Check the plateau (phase III), upstroke (phase II), and angles. Hypoventilation results in an elevated $ETCO_2$ with the baseline remaining at zero. To distinguish hypoventilation from increased CO_2 production, correlate the $PaCO_2$ with the minute ventilation. If the minute ventilation seems appropriate and the $PaCO_2$ is high, consider the presence of a hypermetabolic state. Uneven V/Q relationships appear as a gradually rising phase III instead of the normal flat plateau. This usually reflects bronchospasm (see Figure 3).

E. Reduced cardiac output is often overlooked as a cause for low $ETCO_2$. When all other factors (e.g., minute ventilation and alveolar dead space) remain constant, the $ETCO_2$ varies in direct proportion to the cardiac output. Therefore, a reduction in cardiac output and pulmonary blood flow results in a decreased $ETCO_2$ and an increased (α-ET) PCO_2. Cardiac arrest produces a sudden absence of $ETCO_2$. The probability of return of spontaneous circulation and the adequacy of CPR can be assessed with $ETCO_2$.[7,8]

The prognosis of critically ill patients can be predicted by monitoring $ETCO_2$. In one study, a persistent $ETCO_2$ of 28 mm Hg or less was associated with a mortality rate of 55%, compared to patients with a higher $ETCO_2$ who had a mortality of only 17%.[9] The mortality rate was also increased in patients with a persistent $PaCO_2$–$ETCO_2$ difference of 8 mm Hg or more.

REFERENCES

1. Bhavani-Shankar K, Kumar AY, Moseley HS, et al.: Terminology and the current limitations of time capnography: A brief review, *J Clin Monit* 11 (3):175–182, 1995.
2. Kumar AY, Bhavani-Shankar K, Moseley HS, et al.: Inspiratory valve malfunction in a circle system: pitfalls in capnography, *Can J Anaesth* 39 (9):997–999, 1992.
3. Bowe EA, Boysen PG, Broome JA, et al.: Accurate determination of end-tidal carbon dioxide during administration of oxygen by nasal cannulae, *J Clin Monit* 5 (2):105–110, 1989.
4. Roth JV, Barth LJ, Womack LH, et al.: Evaluation of two commercially available carbon dioxide sampling nasal cannulae, *J Clin Monit* 10 (4):237–243, 1994.
5. Chhibber AK, Kolano JW, Roberts WA: Relationship between end-tidal and arterial carbon dioxide with laryngeal mask airways and endotracheal tubes in children, *Anesth Analg* 82 (2):247–250, 1996.
6. Loughnan TE, Monagle J, Copland JM, et al.: A comparison of carbon dioxide monitoring and oxygenation between facemask and divided nasal cannula, *Anaesth Intensive Care*, 28 (2):151–154, 2000.
7. Garnett AR, Ornato JP, Gonzalez ER, et al.: End-tidal carbon dioxide monitoring during cardiopulmonary resuscitation, *JAMA* 257 (4):512–515, 1987.
8. White RD, Asplin BR: Out-of-hospital quantitative monitoring of end-tidal carbon dioxide pressure during CPR, *Ann Emerg Med* 23 (1):25–30, 1994.
9. Domsky M, Wilson RF, Heins J: Intraoperative end-tidal carbon dioxide values and derived calculations correlated with outcome: prognosis and capnography, *Crit Care Med* 23 (9):1497–1503, 1995.

CAPNOGRAPHY
(Cont'd from p 33)

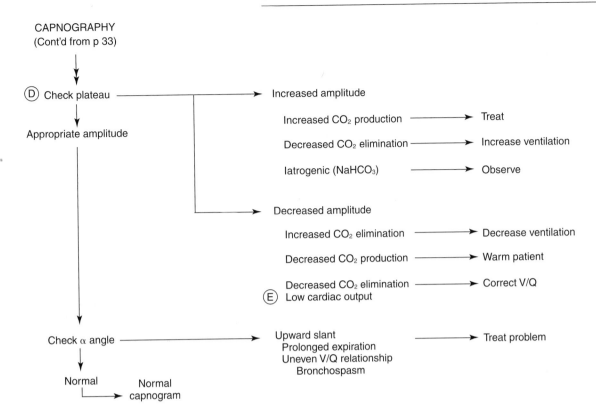

Pulse Oximetry

GEORGE A. DUMITRASCU, M.D.

Monitors are not capable of replacing a vigilant health care provider. As devices become more sophisticated, the potential for artifact and misinterpretation increases. It is important to understand how different monitors work before attempting to memorize protocols designed to address changes in various measured parameters.

Pulse oximetry relies on detecting the difference in absorption of particular wavelengths of light by oxygenated and reduced hemoglobin. A pair of high-intensity light-emitting diodes (LEDs) emits narrow wavelength bands of light; the chosen wavelengths are usually 660 and 940 nm, because reduced hemoglobin absorbs more at 660 nm and oxygenated hemoglobin absorbs more at 940 nm. The light is transmitted through well-perfused tissue and detected with a silicon photo diode. Saturation is measured as the percentage of oxygenated hemoglobin divided by the sum of oxygenated plus reduced hemoglobin. Early in the 1970s, Aoyagi had the seminal idea to use the pulsatility of the arterial system to discriminate between arterial blood saturation and background noise. The oximeter may thus give unreliable information if it is not sensing a pulse waveform or if it senses a rhythmical artifact.

The operating principle behind pulse oximetry can be found in the Lambert-Beer law of absorption. In vivo, light scattering by different tissues causes a deviation from theory; to compensate for this effect, empiric calibration from healthy volunteer studies is employed. Because these studies provided the majority of data within the 70% to 100% SpO_2 range, the accuracy of most devices is greater (within 5% of in vitro oximetry) in the aforementioned range.

Computers within the oximeters average calculations over several seconds' worth of measurements; there may be a time lag before changes in desaturation are displayed.

The accuracy of pulse oximeters has been investigated numerous times and various interferences have been reported. Intravascular dyes, ambient light, electromagnetic radiation, motion artifacts, and fingernail polish may underestimate SpO_2, while skin pigmentation, carboxyhemoglobin, and methemoglobin may cause falsely reassuring readings.

Desaturation is an early indicator of problems in patients breathing air but a late indicator in patients breathing higher concentrations of oxygen (i.e., a patient on 60% FiO_2 with severely impaired respiratory function may have a low PaO_2, yet SpO_2 will still read 100%).

Recent developments include the introduction into clinical practice of reflectance pulse oximeters. They reportedly have the advantage of faster response times and immunity to the effects of vasoconstriction; in addition, by placing the probe close to the central compartment (for example in the esophagus) one can potentially avoid the deleterious effects of low cardiac output on measurements.

REFERENCES

1. Eichhorn JH: Pulse oximetry as a standard of practice in anesthesia, *Anesthesiology* 78:423–426, 1993.
2. Longnecker DE, Tinker JH, Morgan GE, editors: *Principles and practice of anesthesiology*, ed 2, St. Louis, 1998, Mosby-Year Book.
3. Bickler PE, Feiner JR, Severinghaus JW: Effects of skin pigmentation on pulse oximeter accuracy at low saturation, *Anesthesiology* 102:715–719, 2005.
4. Hinkelbein J, Genzwuerker HV, Fiedler F: Detection of a systolic pressure threshold for reliable readings in pulse oximetry, *Resuscitation* 64:315–319, 2005.
5. Shelley KH, Tamai D, Jablonka D, et al. The effect of venous pulsation on the forehead pulse oximeter wave form as a possible source of error in SpO_2 calculation, *Anesth Analg* 100:743–747, 2005.

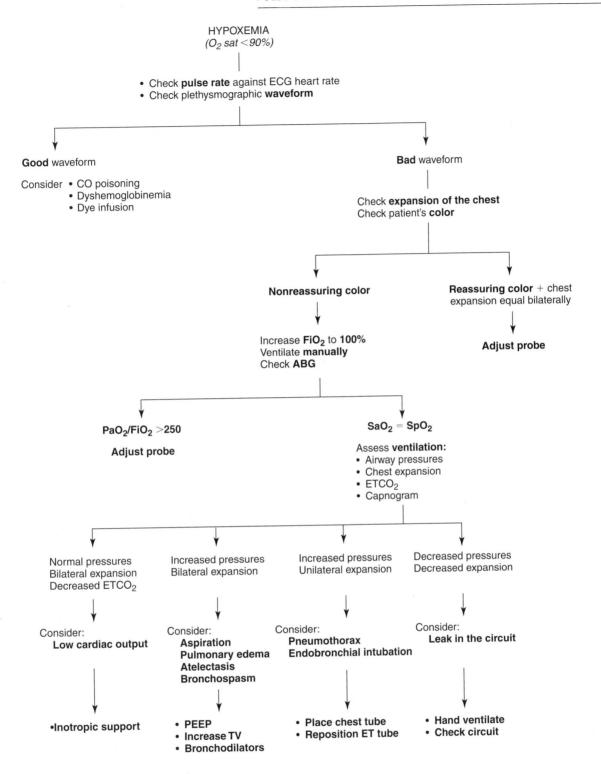

HYPOXEMIA
(O₂ sat <90%)

- Check **pulse rate** against ECG heart rate
- Check plethysmographic **waveform**

Good waveform

Consider • CO poisoning
        • Dyshemoglobinemia
        • Dye infusion

Bad waveform

Check **expansion of the chest**
Check patient's **color**

Nonreassuring color

Reassuring color + chest
expansion equal bilaterally

Increase **FiO₂** to **100%**
Ventilate **manually**
Check **ABG**

Adjust probe

PaO₂/FiO₂ >250

Adjust probe

SaO₂ = **SpO₂**

Assess **ventilation**:
- Airway pressures
- Chest expansion
- ETCO₂
- Capnogram

Normal pressures
Bilateral expansion
Decreased ETCO₂

Increased pressures
Bilateral expansion

Increased pressures
Unilateral expansion

Decreased pressures
Decreased expansion

Consider:
Low cardiac output

Consider:
**Aspiration
Pulmonary edema
Atelectasis
Bronchospasm**

Consider:
**Pneumothorax
Endobronchial intubation**

Consider:
Leak in the circuit

•Inotropic support

- **PEEP**
- **Increase TV**
- **Bronchodilators**

- **Place chest tube**
- **Reposition ET tube**

- **Hand ventilate**
- **Check circuit**

Oxygenation

DAVID M. BROUSSARD, M.D.

The oxygen delivery system must provide oxygen (O_2) at a rate adequate to support the O_2 consumption and survival of body tissues.[1–3] Essential features of O_2 delivery include (1) pulmonary function (adequate O_2 must be presented to hemoglobin [Hb]), (2) Hb function and concentration (sufficient to carry O_2), and (3) cardiac function (for delivery of oxyhemoglobin to tissues). The route taken by O_2, which is delivered to body tissues, can be divided into the following stages:

A. Mass transport of gases to the lungs. With a tidal volume of 450 ml and a dead space of 150 ml, alveolar ventilation is 300 ml/breath. Assuming a respiratory rate of 16 breaths per minute, alveolar ventilation would be 4800 ml/min. In the healthy patient, room air supplies an excess of oxygen to meet a resting O_2 consumption of 250 ml/min.

B. Alveolar capillary diffusion. Alveolar to capillary oxygen diffusion takes only 0.25 second for 90% equilibration across the membrane. Pulmonary capillary transit time (0.75 second) is longer than the time needed for oxygen diffusion to occur. A result of the relatively long pulmonary capillary transit time is that oxygen uptake is normally limited by pulmonary blood flow and the binding of oxygen to Hb not by O_2 diffusion across the alveolar capillary membrane. In fact, diffusion defects as a cause of arterial hypoxemia are rare and only occur with extensive destruction of the alveolar-capillary membrane. The most common cause of arterial hypoxemia is intrapulmonary shunt (lung that is perfused but poorly ventilated).

C. Oxygen transport in the blood. The majority of the oxygen that is transported in blood to body tissues is Hb-bound. One gram of fully saturated Hb will bind with 1.34 ml of O_2. In a healthy patient breathing room air with an arterial oxygen saturation of 98% (PaO_2 of 100), 15 g of Hb in 100 ml of arterial blood will carry approximately 20 ml of O_2. The Hb in returning venous blood is normally 75% saturated (PvO_2 of 40) and contains 15 ml of O_2 per 100 ml of blood. With a cardiac output of 5000 ml/min and an a-v O_2 content difference of approximately 5 ml of O_2 per 100 ml of blood, 250 ml of oxygen per minute is delivered to body tissues ($VO_2 = CO \times [CaO_2 - CvO_2]$). A number of important factors can affect O_2 binding to Hb. Conditions facilitating binding include alkalosis, hypocapnia (Bohr effect), hypothermia, low 2,3 diphosphoglycerate (2,3 DPG [ACD bank blood]), fetal Hb, and carboxyhemoglobin. Conditions facilitating O_2 unloading include acidosis, hypercapnia, hyperthermia, and high 2,3 DPG (hypoxia, anemia, and thyrotoxicosis[2]).

Only a small fraction of the total oxygen content of blood is physically dissolved. In solution, blood carries 0.003 ml of O_2 in each 100 ml for every 1 mm Hg of O_2 (0.3 ml O_2/100 ml blood at a PaO_2 of 100 mm Hg). With an arteriovenous PO_2 difference of 60 mm Hg (100 to 40 mm Hg), only 0.18 ml of O_2 is delivered to tissues from solution by each 100 ml of blood compared to about 5 ml from Hb. With hyperbaric oxygen therapy, O_2 is administered at three atmospheres resulting in a PaO_2 of 2025 mm Hg. Dissolved O_2 in blood is significantly increased from 0.3 ml (at a PaO_2 of 100 mm Hg) to 6.075 ml/100ml of blood (see Figure 13-1).

D. Capillary to cell diffusion. Mean systemic capillary PO_2 is approximately 50 mm Hg. Diffusion from capillaries to tissues can be calculated using the O_2 diffusion coefficient, capillary PO_2, capillary radius, and capillary domain size.

REFERENCES

1. Nunn JF: *Applied respiratory physiology*, ed 5, Woburn, 2000, Butterworth-Heinemann.
2. Levitzky MG: *Pulmonary physiology*, ed 6, Crawfordsville, 2002, McGraw-Hill.
3. Azami T, Preiss D, Somogyi R, et al.: Calculation of O2 consumption during low-flow anesthesia from tidal gas concentrations, flowmeter, and minute ventilation, *J Clin Monit Comput* 18:325, 2004.

Pathway of Oxygen Transport   **Clinical Variables**

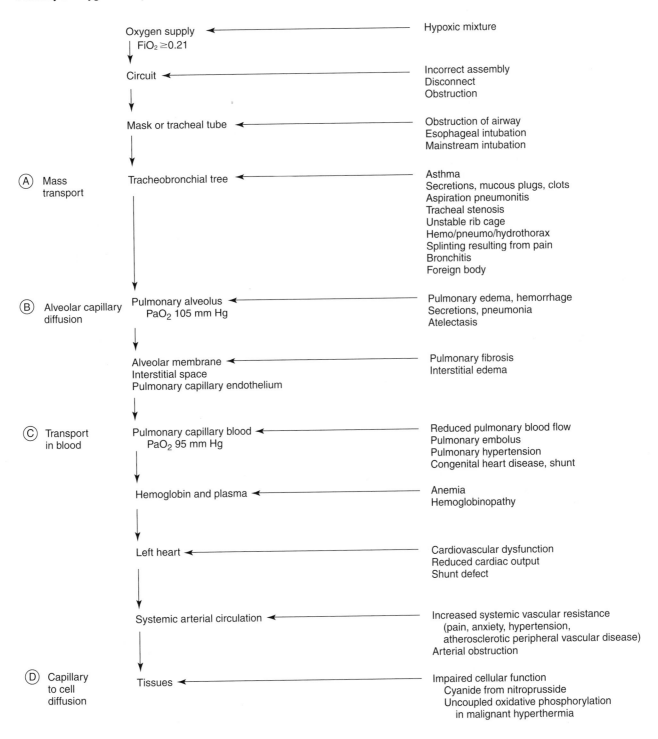

Oxygen supply ◀──────────────────────── Hypoxic mixture
│ FiO$_2$ ≥0.21

Circuit ◀──────────────────────── Incorrect assembly
Disconnect
Obstruction

Mask or tracheal tube ◀──────────────────────── Obstruction of airway
Esophageal intubation
Mainstream intubation

(A) Mass   Tracheobronchial tree ◀──────────────── Asthma
transport   Secretions, mucous plugs, clots
Aspiration pneumonitis
Tracheal stenosis
Unstable rib cage
Hemo/pneumo/hydrothorax
Splinting resulting from pain
Bronchitis
Foreign body

(B) Alveolar capillary   Pulmonary alveolus ◀──────────── Pulmonary edema, hemorrhage
diffusion   PaO$_2$ 105 mm Hg   Secretions, pneumonia
Atelectasis

Alveolar membrane ◀──────────────── Pulmonary fibrosis
Interstitial space   Interstitial edema
Pulmonary capillary endothelium

(C) Transport   Pulmonary capillary blood ◀────────── Reduced pulmonary blood flow
in blood   PaO$_2$ 95 mm Hg   Pulmonary embolus
Pulmonary hypertension
Congenital heart disease, shunt

Hemoglobin and plasma ◀──────────────── Anemia
Hemoglobinopathy

Left heart ◀──────────────────────── Cardiovascular dysfunction
Reduced cardiac output
Shunt defect

Systemic arterial circulation ◀──────────── Increased systemic vascular resistance
(pain, anxiety, hypertension,
atherosclerotic peripheral vascular disease)
Arterial obstruction

(D) Capillary   Tissues ◀──────────────────────── Impaired cellular function
to cell   Cyanide from nitroprusside
diffusion   Uncoupled oxidative phosphorylation
in malignant hyperthermia

Intraoperative Hypoxemia

D.M. ANDERSON, M.D.

Intraoperative abnormalities of pulmonary physiology leading to arterial hypoxemia are common. The ratio of alveolar V/Q is the ultimate determinant of alveolar gas exchange.[1] The major factors affecting alveolar PO_2 are the FiO_2, alveolar ventilation, and the rate of oxygen uptake.

A. Search for the cause of hypoxemia. It is useful to classify the causes of intraoperative hypoxemia according to when they occur during the anesthesia process.[2]

B. If hypoxemia occurs during induction, verify adequate oxygen delivery and ventilation. Check the FiO_2. Listen to breath sounds. Confirm that the chest rises during manual bag ventilation. Verify patency of the endotracheal tube (ETT) and circuit. Study the capnograph. Make adjustments if the patient is hypoventilating. Determine the SpO_2 trend. Feel for a pulse.

C. During anesthetic maintenance, determine the A-a gradient. If it is abnormally wide, than a V/Q mismatch or shunt is occurring. If the SpO_2 rises with an increase in FiO_2, then the problem is V/Q mismatch. Correct simple mechanical problems, such as ETT malposition.

D. Shunt is a common intraoperative problem and is usually the result of atelectasis, the most common cause of hypoxemia. Atelectasis occurs in 90% of patients under general anesthesia regardless of the type of anesthetic (e.g., IV or inhalational), technique of airway management (i.e., intubated or not), or type of ventilation (i.e., controlled or spontaneous).[3] Several factors contribute to loss of lung volume, including compression of dependent lung regions, absorption of gas in poorly ventilated or occluded alveoli, and abnormalities of surfactant. High FiO_2 promotes rapid absorption of gas in poorly ventilated lung regions. Surfactant abnormalities are postulated to contribute to atelectasis because when a patient develops atelectasis, it rapidly reoccurs if preventive measures are not taken.

E. Treat atelectasis by employing a recruitment maneuver. Apply pressure to the ETT, usually 40 cm H_2O for 7 to 8 seconds. Repeat the maneuver after a few minutes. Although PEEP will partially reopen collapsed alveoli, blood is diverted from normal lung to residual collapsed lung, and the shunt and hypoxemia will not improve. To prevention recurrent atelectasis, administer the lowest FiO_2 possible (preferably <40%) or add 10 cm H_2O of PEEP.

F. Rarely, patients develop intermittent shunt across a patent foramen ovale, leading to severe, refractory hypoxemia.[4] This occurs even when chronic pulmonary hypertension is not present. These patients are also at risk for paradoxical emboli and stroke.

REFERENCES

1. Calzia E, Radermacher P: Alveolar ventilation and pulmonary blood flow: the V(A)/Q concept, *Intensive Care Med* 29:1229–1232, 2003.
2. Bamber J: Airway crises, *Curr Anaesth Crit Care* 14 (1):2–8, 2003.
3. Hedenstierna G, Rothen HU: Atelectasis formation during anesthesia: causes and measures to prevent it, *J Clin Monit* 16:329–335, 2000.
4. Godart G, Rey C, Prat A, et al.: Atrial right-to-left shunting causing severe hypoxaemia despite normal right-sided pressures. Report of 11 consecutive cases corrected by percutaneous closure, *Eur Heart J* 21 (6):483–489, 2000.

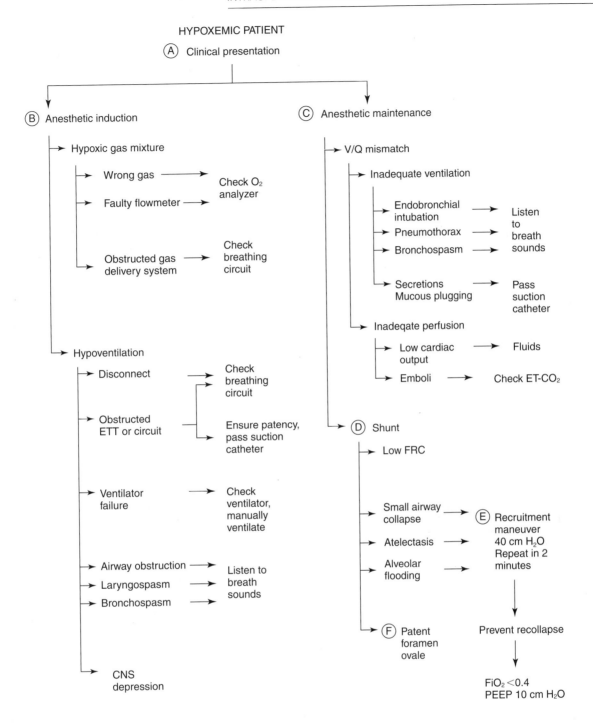

Decreased Inspired Oxygen Concentration

ROBERT LOEB, M.D.

Hypoxemia due to inhalation of hypoxic gases has historically been a significant cause of preventable death or morbidity during anesthesia. An oxygen analyzer with a low-oxygen-concentration limit alarm is required during all general anesthesia.[1] The oxygen analyzer must be calibrated before use. It may be calibrated to 21% with room air or to 100% with oxygen from an anesthesia machine. Calibration against room air is preferable to guard against hypoxia, because the analyzer is most accurate near the calibration value. Also room air is a more reliable calibration gas, because the oxygen from the anesthesia machine may be contaminated. The low-oxygen-concentration limit alarm has a threshold that can be set by the user. The alarm is most sensitive if it is set slightly below the calculated oxygen concentration being delivered from the anesthesia machine. Many health care providers leave the setting at its lowest value or at the lowest oxygen concentration that is safe for the patient. However at such low settings early problems, such as partial contamination of the oxygen supply,[2] will not be detected. Also, the available time for response to a rapidly falling oxygen concentration will be decreased. When the oxygen concentration is significantly less than expected on the basis of the anesthesia machine flow settings, the cause must be determined.

A. The initial response to a low oxygen concentration is to increase the oxygen flow rate. If the oxygen concentration increases to the expected value, there was either an incorrect oxygen flow setting or entrainment of room air into the circuit. Incorrect low flow settings can be classified as "low relative to other gas flows" and "low relative to the patient's oxygen consumption." The former is extremely unlikely, because modern anesthesia machines have oxygen-ratio protection devices that prevent the user from setting an oxygen flow that is too low relative to the flow of nitrous oxide. An oxygen flow that is less than the patient's oxygen consumption will cause a decline in the circuit oxygen concentration even though the fresh gas is not hypoxic.[3] Entrainment of room air into the breathing circuit is especially likely with the piston drive ventilators found on some newer anesthesia machines.[4] If the oxygen concentration increases when the oxygen flow is turned up but is still lower than expected, one of the flowmeters may be miscalibrated. This may occur during machine maintenance if the wrong float is inserted into the flow tube.

B. If the oxygen concentration does not increase with a higher oxygen flow rate, engage the oxygen flush. The oxygen flush is a separate system within the anesthesia machine that bypasses most of the internal tubing, flowmeters, and vaporizers (Figure 1). Even if there is an obstruction or disconnection within the anesthesia machine, the oxygen flush should operate properly. If the reservoir bag fills and the oxygen concentration increases, the problem is a disconnection or obstruction within the anesthesia machine.[5] If the reservoir bag does not fill, either the oxygen supply is depleted or the anesthesia machine is disconnected from the breathing circuit at the fresh gas hose. If the reservoir bag fills but the oxygen concentration remains low, the oxygen supply is contaminated.

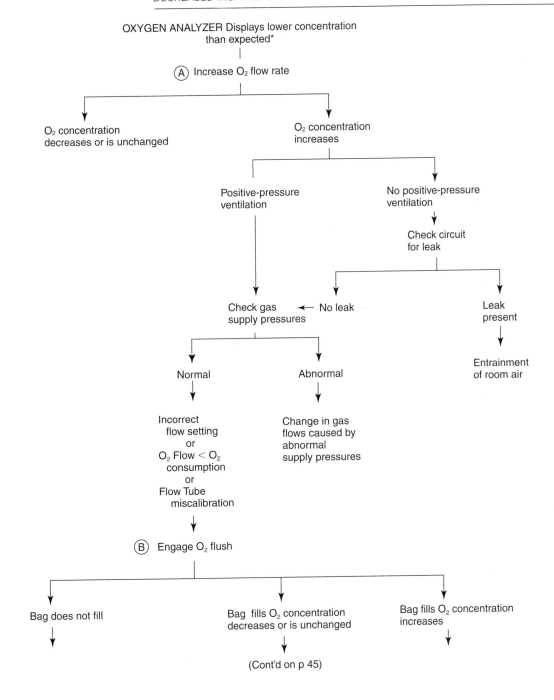

OXYGEN ANALYZER Displays lower concentration
than expected*

(A) Increase O₂ flow rate

O₂ concentration
decreases or is unchanged

O₂ concentration
increases

Positive-pressure
ventilation

No positive-pressure
ventilation

Check circuit
for leak

Check gas   ← No leak
supply pressures

Leak
present

Normal   Abnormal   Entrainment
of room air

Incorrect
flow setting
or
O₂ Flow < O₂
consumption
or
Flow Tube
miscalibration

Change in gas
flows caused by
abnormal
supply pressures

(B) Engage O₂ flush

Bag does not fill

Bag fills O₂ concentration
decreases or is unchanged

Bag fills O₂ concentration
increases

(Cont'd on p 45)

C. When it appears that the oxygen is contaminated, select a new source of oxygen by opening the reserve oxygen cylinder and disconnecting the hose to the oxygen pipeline. The hospital central supply may be contaminated by a central tank that has been filled with the wrong gas,[6] by a cross-connection in the central piping system, or by a cross-connection within a piece of equipment attached to the central piping system.[2] If the low oxygen condition persists, despite switching to the reserve cylinder, a cross-connection exists within the anesthesia machine or the oxygen analyzer is miscalibrated. In that event, ventilate the patient with another system (i.e., bag-valve circuit and a fresh oxygen cylinder).

REFERENCES

1. American Society of Anesthesiologists: *Guidelines for office-based anesthesia*, available at: http://www.asahq.org/publicationsand services/standards/12.pdf, 2004.
2. Thorp JM, Railton R: Hypoxia due to air in the oxygen pipeline: a case for oxygen monitoring in theatre, *Anaesthesia* 37:683, 1982.
3. Schreiber P: *Safety guidelines for anesthesia system.* Telford, PA, 1985, North American Drager.
4. Olympio MA: Modern anesthesia machines offer new safety features, *APSF Newsletter* 18:24, 2003.
5. Nuttall GA, Baker RD: Internal common gas line disconnect, *Anesthesiology* 79:605, 1993.
6. Sprague DH, Archer GW: Intraoperative hypoxia from an erroneously filled liquid oxygen reservoir, *Anesthesiology* 42:360, 1975.

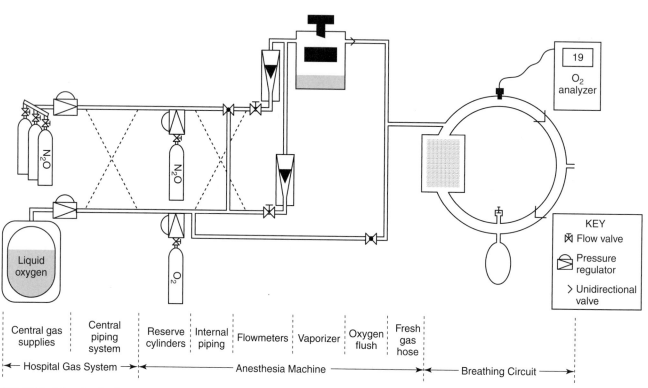

FIGURE 1 A low inspired oxygen concentration can result from problems anywhere along the path from the central gas supplies to the breathing circuit. The central or reserve oxygen supplies may be contaminated. Cross-connections (dashed *X's*) can occur within the hospital's central piping or the anesthesia machine internal piping. Oxygen flow may be disrupted owing to leaks, obstructions, or regular failures. Air may be entrained into the breathing circuit. Note that the oxygen flush system bypasses the anesthesia machine's internal piping, flowmeters, and vaporizers.

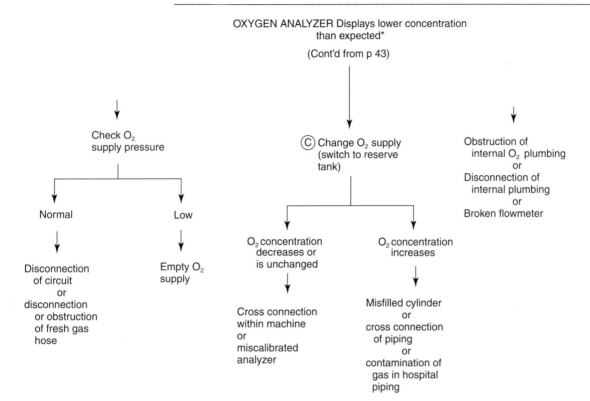

OXYGEN ANALYZER Displays lower concentration than expected*

(Cont'd from p 43)

Check O_2 supply pressure

Normal

Low

Disconnection of circuit or disconnection or obstruction of fresh gas hose

Empty O_2 supply

(C) Change O_2 supply (switch to reserve tank)

O_2 concentration decreases or is unchanged

O_2 concentration increases

Cross connection within machine or miscalibrated analyzer

Misfilled cylinder or cross connection of piping or contamination of gas in hospital piping

Obstruction of internal O_2 plumbing or Disconnection of internal plumbing or Broken flowmeter

Increased Peak Airway Pressure

ROBERT LOEB, M.D.

Airway pressure (AP) is a sensitive monitor during mechanical ventilation. AP may be sensed within the ventilator, within the CO_2 absorber canister, or at the y-piece, on the patient side of the inspiratory valve (best). At the latter site, abnormally high, low, or continuing pressures will be detected that might be missed at the other two locations. At the y-piece, an obstruction in the inspiratory limb of the circle system decreases the peak AP, and an obstruction in the expiratory limb increases the nadir and peak APs. For convenience, AP is often measured at the carbon dioxide (CO_2) absorber canister in a circle system. At this location, obstruction in the inspiratory or expiratory limb causes an increase in the peak AP without affecting the measured nadir pressure.

A. Peak AP is increased by coughing, circuit obstruction (usually at the endotracheal tube [ETT]), and increased tidal volume. On many older anesthesia machines, increasing the anesthesia machine fresh gas flow (FGF) causes a larger tidal volume to be delivered,[1] especially when the dialed tidal volume is small (e.g., in pediatric patients).

B. Obstruction of the inspiratory tubing may occur (e.g., due to improperly placed humidifiers or other equipment with unidirectional flow). Inspiratory tubing obstructions increase peak AP when measured proximal to the obstruction (e.g., CO_2 absorber canister) and decrease AP when measured distal to the obstruction (e.g., at the y-piece).

C. The inspiratory pause pressure (static AP during an inspiratory volume hold) helps to differentiate between increased airway resistance and decreased thoracic compliance (Figure 1, upper tracings). Decreased thoracic compliance elevates the pause pressure, whereas increased airway resistance lowers or does not change the pause pressure. The difference between the pause pressure and the peak airway pressure, normally 4 to 8 cm H_2O, is higher with increased airway resistance, because the peak pressure increases without concomitant increase in the pause pressure. An inspiratory pause can be delivered by some anesthesia ventilators or can be delivered manually by occluding the expiratory tubing briefly at the beginning of exhalation. This manual method can only be used if the AP is measured at the y-piece. The expiratory flow rate (EFR) can also help to differentiate resistance from compliance problems. EFR can be qualitatively assessed by observing the ventilator bellows' rate of rise or by auscultating the duration of expiratory flow. Better, it can be measured with a spirometer located at the airway or on the expiratory limb of the breathing circuit (Figure 1, lower tracings).

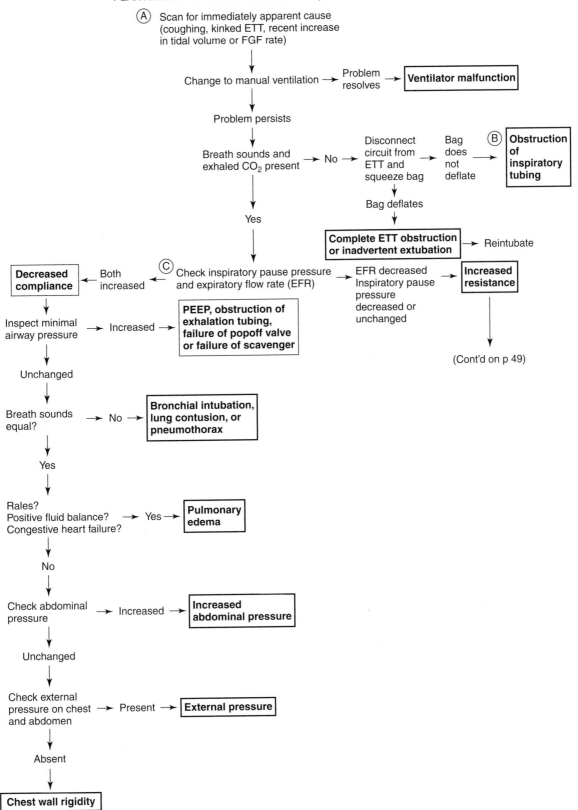

PEAK AIRWAY PRESSURE Increased from previous value*

(A) Scan for immediately apparent cause
(coughing, kinked ETT, recent increase
in tidal volume or FGF rate)

Change to manual ventilation → Problem resolves → **Ventilator malfunction**

Problem persists

Breath sounds and exhaled CO_2 present → No → Disconnect circuit from ETT and squeeze bag → Bag does not deflate → (B) **Obstruction of inspiratory tubing**

Bag deflates

Complete ETT obstruction or inadvertent extubation → Reintubate

Yes

Decreased compliance ← Both increased ← (C) Check inspiratory pause pressure and expiratory flow rate (EFR) → EFR decreased Inspiratory pause pressure decreased or unchanged → **Increased resistance**

Inspect minimal airway pressure → Increased → **PEEP, obstruction of exhalation tubing, failure of popoff valve or failure of scavenger**

(Cont'd on p 49)

Unchanged

Breath sounds equal? → No → **Bronchial intubation, lung contusion, or pneumothorax**

Yes

Rales?
Positive fluid balance?
Congestive heart failure? → Yes → **Pulmonary edema**

No

Check abdominal pressure → Increased → **Increased abdominal pressure**

Unchanged

Check external pressure on chest and abdomen → Present → **External pressure**

Absent

Chest wall rigidity

*Boxed information represents diagnoses, not recommended actions.

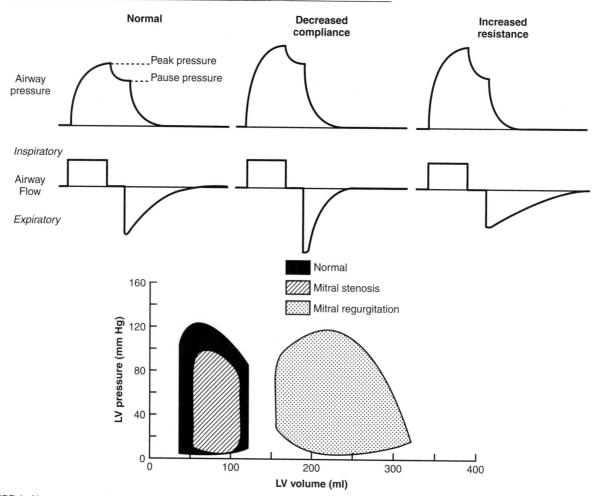

FIGURE 1 Airway pressure (upper tracings) and flow (lower tracings) can help to differentiate high resistance problems from low compliance problems. There is normally a 4- to 8-cm H_2O difference between the airway peak pressure and the pause pressure. A decrease in compliance causes a proportional increase in both pressures, while an increase in resistance only increases the peak airway pressure.[3] A decrease in thoracic compliance results in higher peak expiratory flows and shorter expiratory flow duration. Conversely, an increase in airway resistance decreases peak expiratory flow and increases exhalation duration.

D. Decreased cross-sectional area of small or large airways, or of the ETT, increases resistance to flow. Listen for expiratory wheezes and observe the shape of the capnogram to determine the location of the obstruction. Small airway obstruction (bronchospasm or chronic obstructive pulmonary disease [COPD]) is associated with expiratory wheezes and a sloping alveolar plateau of the capnogram,[4] which is due to maldistribution of alveolar ventilation.[5] Large airway obstruction (foreign body in the bronchus) or ETT obstruction (kinking of the ETT) is not associated with expiratory wheezing or maldistribution of alveolar ventilation. Mucus or blood in the airway may cause audible rhonchi but will not cause a sloping alveolar plateau on the capnogram.

REFERENCES

1. Gravenstein N, Banner MJ, McLaughlin G: Tidal volume changes due to the interaction of anesthesia machine and anesthesia ventilator, *J Clin Monit* 3:187, 1987.
2. Schreiber P: *Safety guidelines for anesthesia systems,* Telford, PA, 1985, North American Drager.
3. Bone RC: Monitoring respiratory and hemodynamic function of the patient with respiratory failure. In: Kirby RR, Smith RA, Desautels DA, editors: *Mechanical ventilation,* New York, 1985, Churchill Livingstone.
4. Paulus DA: Capnography, *Int Anesthesiol Clin* 27:167, 1989.
5. Nunn JF: *Applied respiratory physiology,* ed 5, Woburn, 2000, Butterworth-Heinemann.

PEAK AIRWAY PRESSURE Increased from previous value*
(Cont'd from p 47)

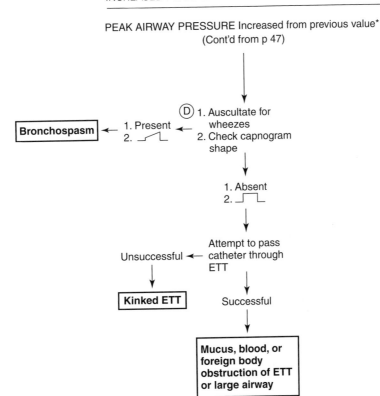

Response to Low-Pressure Alarm

J. RUSSELL NORTON, M.D.

DENHAM S. WARD, M.D., PH.D.

Problems with gas delivery to anesthetized patients continue to cause morbidity and mortality. Equipment misuse is three times more frequent than equipment failure.[1] Use of alarms to alert practitioners of potential or real problems is commonplace in anesthesia practice. Using them effectively is not.[2,3] Combining these human elements with the ever-increasing complexity of modern anesthesia machines makes it imperative for health care providers to learn how to use their equipment properly to protect patients from injury.

In understanding and using any alarm, health care providers must know exactly to which measurement the alarm is responding and what the variety of conditions are that can cause the alarm to operate. The low-pressure alarm connects to the breathing circuit (e.g., the circle system) and signals if a preset pressure is not exceeded for a certain period of time. Because flow resistance determines the pressure measured, a low-pressure alarm responds to decreases in either resistance or flow. Although frequently called and thought of as a disconnect alarm, the low-pressure alarm will not necessarily detect a disconnection and will respond to other conditions such as low pressure, sustained pressure, excessive pressure, subambient pressure, and PEEP. It can also detect the respiratory rate.[1] This information is primarily useful in the manually or mechanically ventilated patient. In the spontaneously breathing patient, a low-pressure alarm is not useful, but it may still be important to monitor some of the other airway pressure conditions (e.g., excessive pressure from a closed pressure release valve).

The low-pressure alarm is ideally positioned at the y-connection of the endotracheal tube. However, the connection tubing is inconvenient, and the moisture condensation may make the alarm less reliable. A more common point of connection is on the machine side of the exhalation valve, although the patient side of the valve may be theoretically better. Some alarms are internal to the ventilator, but this is not as acceptable as a direct connection to the breathing circuit. Common problems contribute to airway pressure monitoring alarm malfunction: failing to turn on the alarm; inappropriate threshold settings (either too low or use of PEEP causing a value above the alarm threshold); any partial or complete obstruction of a breathing system connection (e.g., by a pillow or heat exchanger) when it is disconnected from a patient; entrance of air into the system (e.g., partial extubation or a leak in the flow sensor tubing); moisture build up in the flow sensor tubing; and interference from bright and infrared light sources.[4–6]

The response algorithm must systematically isolate which of the three main elements of the system (fresh gas flow; gas conducting system; and pressure generator) is at fault.[7]

A. For the alarm to be useful, turn it on and check its operation. Many low-pressure alarms automatically turn on when the anesthesia ventilator is started. However, during manual ventilation, a low-pressure alarm can also be useful in reminding the operator to apply positive pressure ventilation.

B. Many alarms allow the activation threshold to be set. Set the threshold to the highest pressure that does not exceed the observed peak airway pressure. This will permit the greatest sensitivity to detect a low-pressure condition.

C. On detection of an alarm condition, have a systematic plan to detect and correct the cause of the alarm.[7] First switch to manual ventilation and attempt to ventilate the patient with the breathing circuit bag. If the bag is empty, check the fresh gas flow meters visually. Use the oxygen flush valve to refill the bag. If the bag cannot be refilled with the oxygen flush, check the connections from the machine to the circuit. During manual compression of the bag, auscultate for breath sounds and observe the patient's chest movement and airway pressure. Confirm the presence of airway carbon dioxide (CO_2) on exhalation. If appropriate manual ventilation can be accomplished, check the connections from the ventilator to the circuit. Ensure correct ventilator settings and operation.

D. If manual ventilation cannot be delivered, check for obvious sources of a leak, such as hose disconnects and full or partial extubation.

E. If no obvious leak sources are apparent, obtain a means of ensuring adequate ventilation while further investigations are carried out. Always have an appropriately sized resuscitation bag immediately available to provide positive pressure ventilation independent of the anesthesia machine. Figure 17-1 shows some common sites for disconnections to occur, but there are many possible sites for leaks (e.g., poorly sealed CO_2 absorption canister or malfunction of the scavenging system). Only a systematic checking of all hoses and connections will solve the problem.[4–8]

REFERENCES

1. Caplan RA, Vistica MF, Posner KL, et al.: Adverse anesthetic outcomes arising from gas delivery equipment: a closed claims analysis, *Anesthesiology* 87:741–748, 1997.
2. Cohen A, Roberts DJ, McInode A: An audit of the use of alarms in anesthetic monitoring, *Br J Anaesth* 83:525, 1999.
3. Morris RW, Montano SR: Response times to visual and auditory alarms during anaesthesia, *Anaesth Intensive Care* 24:682–684, 1996.
4. Dorsch JA, SE Dorsch: *Understanding anesthesia equipment*, ed 4, Baltimore, 1999, Williams & Wilkins.
5. Dhar P, George I, Mankad A, et al.: Flow transducer gas leak detected after induction, *Anesth Analg* 89:1587, 1999.

POSITIVE PRESSURE VENTILATED PATIENT

↓

(A) Turn on alarm and check operation

↓

(B) Set alarm threshold

↓

Alarm! → Visually check major connections
Check vital signs
(SpO$_2$, HR, end-tidal CO$_2$, etc.)

↓

Switch to manual bag

(C) Manual bag compression → Bag empty → Refill with O$_2$ flush → Unable to refill

Check airway pressure, end-tidal CO$_2$ and patient's chest movement

Check fresh gas flow and connections

(D) Unable to deliver adequate airway pressure and/or ventilation

Adequate ventilation

Check ventilator and connections

Manually ventilate

Check obvious hose disconnects

Check for partial or complete extubation

No leak found → (E) Ventilate patient with resuscitation bag via mask or laryngeal mask airway or endotracheal tube

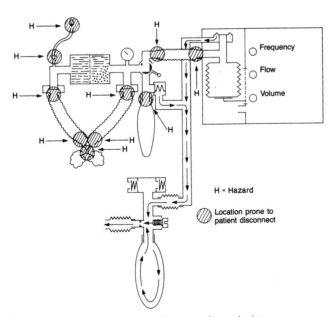

Frequency

Flow

Volume

H = Hazard

⊘ Location prone to patient disconnect

FIGURE 1 Common sites for a disconnection or leak to occur. Standardized connection terminals do not prevent accidental disconnection. Coping with disconnects is considered a routine procedure in many institutions. (From Schreiber P: *Safety guidelines for anesthesia systems*, Telford, PA, 1985, North American Drager.)

6. Sattari R, Reichard P: Temporary malfunction of the Ohmeda Modulus CD series volume monitor caused by the overhead surgical lighting, *Anesthesiology* 91:894–895, 1999.
7. Raphael DT, Weller RS, Doran DJ: A response algorithm for the low-pressure alarm condition, *Anesth Analg* 67:876–883, 1988.
8. Schreiber P: *Safety guidelines for anesthesia systems*, Telford, PA, 1985, North American Drager.

Neuromuscular Blocking Agents

SARA M. METCALF, M.D.

JUERGEN FLEISCH, M.D.

Few classes of drugs carry as much potential for harm as the neuromuscular blockers (NMB). It is critical to be prepared to immediately take over ventilation for a patient whenever NMBs are used.

A. First decide on whether an NMB is indicated. Endotracheal intubation may be accomplished without paralysis; however, adequate neuromuscular blockade improves laryngoscopic conditions and reduces trauma to the vocal cords.[1] Situations in which an NMB might be avoided include predicted difficulty intubating or ventilating or myasthenic syndromes.

B. When RSI is indicated (full stomach or severe reflux) the traditional NMB of choice is succinylcholine (SCCh). The onset of SCCh is 30 to 60 seconds with a dose of 1.5 mg/kg. The duration of action is 5 to 10 minutes with normal plasma pseudocholinesterase levels. With SCCh blockade there is an expected increase in serum potassium of 0.5 to 1 mEq/dl. Other side effects include postoperative myalgias and a transient increase in ICP/IOP/intragastric pressure. Absolute contraindications to SCCh include risk for malignant hyperthermia, extrajunctional receptor proliferation (burn patients, spinal cord injury patients >24 hours after injury, muscular dystrophy, and certain myopathies), preexisting hyperkalemia, or a history of allergic reaction to SCCh. When SCCh is not an option, a nondepolarizing NMB may be used. Rocuronium is the only nondepolarizing NMB that has an indication from the Food and Drug Administration (FDA) to be used as part of an RSI, and the onset time with 1.2 mg/kg is approximately 45 to 60 seconds.

C. If there is no indication for RSI, any NMB may be chosen as part of the induction sequence. The choice of nondepolarizing NMB depends on patient characteristics, surgical requirements, and expected duration of surgery. The most commonly used nondepolarizing NMB agents and their characteristics are listed in Table 1.

TABLE 1
Characteristics of Nondepolarizing Neuromuscular Blocking Agents

Drug	Steroid versus benzylisoquinolinium	2 × ED95 (mg/kg)	Time of onset (mins)	Duration of action (mins)	Primary elimination pathway	Clinically significant metabolites	Nonrelaxant side effects
d-Tubocurare	Benzylisoquinolinium	1	2–4	70–90	Renal	—	Histamine release, ganglion blockade
Mivacurium	Benzylisoquinolinium	0.15–0.3	2–4	10–20	Plasmacholinesterase Hydrolysis	—	Histamine release
Atracurium	Benzylisoquinolinium	0.15–0.2	2–4	20–25	Nonspecific ester Hydrolysis, Hoffman degradation	Laudanosine	Histamine release
Cisatracurium	Benzylisoquinolinium	0.1	2–4	20–25	Hoffman degradation	Laudanosine	—
Vecuronium	Steroid	0.1–0.2	1.5–2.5	20–40	Biliary/renal excretion	3-OH vecuronium accumulation (prolonged blockade)	—
Rocuronium	Steroid	0.6	1–1.5	20–40	Hepatic	—	Mild vagolytic
Pancuronium	Steroid	0.12	5–7	60	Renal excretion	—	Muscarinic blockade, vagolytic

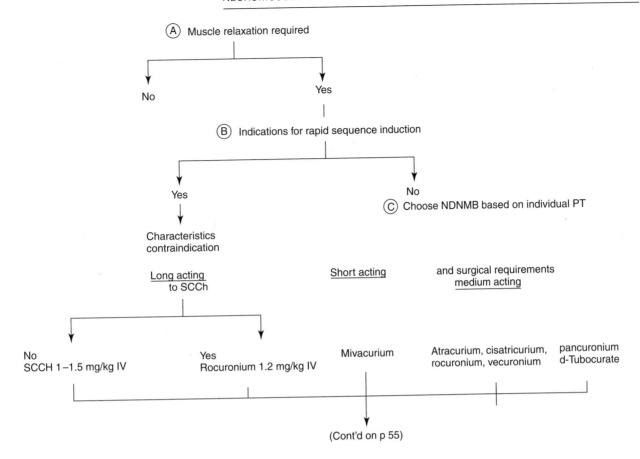

A Muscle relaxation required

No

Yes

B Indications for rapid sequence induction

Yes

No
C Choose NDNMB based on individual PT

Characteristics
contraindication

Long acting
to SCCh

Short acting

and surgical requirements
medium acting

No
SCCH 1−1.5 mg/kg IV

Yes
Rocuronium 1.2 mg/kg IV

Mivacurium

Atracurium, cisatricurium,
rocuronium, vecuronium

pancuronium
d-Tubocurate

(Cont'd on p 55)

D. Monitor NMB and reversal. Choice of muscle monitored is important, as different muscles recover at different rates. The most common muscle monitored for adequacy of neuromuscular recovery for extubation is the adductor pollicus, via ulnar nerve stimulation. Train of four (TOF) ratio, the height of the fourth twitch to that of the first twitch, is a more sensitive indicator than single twitch height, especially when blockade is less than 70%. In most cases it is neither necessary nor desirable to completely paralyze a patient (zero twitches) as this may lead to difficulty with reversal of blockade and residual weakness post-procedure. Other methods of monitoring blockade include double burst stimulation. This involves two short bursts, separated by 750 msec. This correlates well with the TOF response, but its advantage is it provides easier tactile evaluation. Sustained response to tetanic stimulation of 100 Hz for 5 seconds is also more sensitive than TOF for detecting residual blockade.

E. Reverse nondepolarizing NMB with an acetylcholinesterase (ACH) inhibitor. This increases ACH at the neuromuscular junction, antagonizing residual neuromuscular blockade. Factors that may cause residual blockade despite adequate doses of reversal include residual volatile anesthetic, prolonged elimination due to pathological condition, decreased body temperature, interactions with other drugs, and strong neuromuscular blockade when reversal agent is given. It is recommended to reverse all nondepolarizing NMB agents prior to extubation when repeated doses or infusions are used. Patients with a TOF of <90% have been shown to have worsened postoperative outcomes, so extubation should be delayed until recovery if this is noted.[2] Patients with prolonged blockade after SCCh should not be given reversal agents, as they will only slow the metabolism. However, they should be evaluated for abnormal pseudocholinesterase activity postoperatively.

REFERENCES

1. Mencke T, Echternach M, Kleinschmidt S, et al.: Laryngeal morbidity and quality of tracheal Intubation: a randomized controlled trial, *Anesthesiology* 98:1049–1056, 2003.
2. Murphy GS: Residual neuromuscular blockade: incidence, assessment, and relevance in the postoperative period, *Minerva Anestesiol* 72 (3):97–109, 2006.
3. Bevan DR, Donati F: Muscle relaxants. In Barash PG, Cullen BF, Stoelting, RK, editors: *Clinical anesthesia*, ed 4, Philadelphia, 2001, Lippincott-Raven.
4. Savarese JJ, Caldwell JE, Lien CA, et al.: Pharmacology of muscle relaxants and their antagonists. In Miller RD, editor: *Anesthesia*, ed 5, Philadelphia, 2000, Churchill Livingstone.

(Cont'd on p 53)

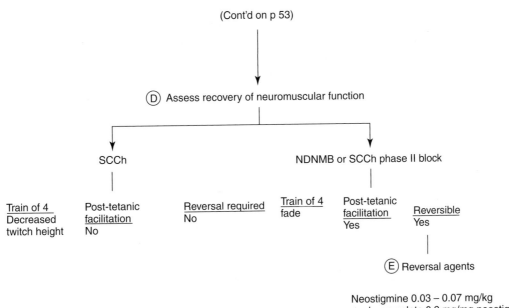

Ⓓ Assess recovery of neuromuscular function

SCCh   NDNMB or SCCh phase II block

Train of 4   Post-tetanic   Reversal required   Train of 4   Post-tetanic   Reversible
Decreased   facilitation   No   fade   facilitation   Yes
twitch height   No   Yes

                                                                      Ⓔ Reversal agents

                                        Neostigmine 0.03 – 0.07 mg/kg
                                        + glycopyrolate 0.2 mg/mg neostigmine
                                        OR
                                        Edrophonium 0.5 – 1 mg/kg
                                        + atropine 0.014 mg/mg edrophonium

The Full Stomach Patient

JOANNE BAUST, M.D.

One of the most feared complications in anesthesia is aspiration. The incidence has been quoted as 1/3,000 for all cases and as low as 0.7 to 10/10,000 in appropriately fasted patients. Even with true aspiration, only one third of patients have symptoms; fewer have significant morbidity or mortality. The death rate of a true aspiration is 3.8% to 4.6%, which has not changed significantly over the past four decades.[1] Recently published large studies have challenged the traditional parameters for at risk patients, much of which have been based on "surrogate markers," such as intragastric volume (>0.4 ml/kg) and pH (<2.5). No controlled study links gastric contents with aspiration. Fasted patients have been shown to exceed these parameters but have not had an increased incidence of aspiration.[2]

A. There is no substitute for proper fasting according to American Society of Anesthesiologists (ASA) guidelines. If possible, delay surgery for 6 to 8 hours after solid food and for 2 hours after clear liquids to allow gastric emptying.[3] Risk factors other than recent oral intake include trauma, emergency surgery, severe illness with an advanced ASA classification, and bowel obstruction or other GI disorders. Delayed gastric emptying (pain or diabetes mellitus), impaired airway reflexes (closed head injury, stroke, or medications/opioids), and certain positions during surgery (lithotomy) add to the risk of aspiration. Patients who have a compromised barrier pressure, the tension of the lower esophageal pressure in relation to intragastric pressure, are thought to be at risk (e.g., obesity or pregnancy). However, as intragastric pressure increases, so does barrier pressure. The presence of a difficult airway, light anesthesia, inexperienced personnel, poor judgment or technique, and poor patient preparation greatly add to the risk.[4]

B. Preoperative medications, which empty the stomach or increase the pH of its contents, have not been shown to affect aspiration risk or outcomes but are routinely used in at risk patients. Passing a nasogastric tube to decompress the stomach does not truly empty the stomach and has been shown to improve outcome only in patients with true bowel obstruction. Passing a nasogastric tube may cause vomiting and compromises the lower esophageal sphincter tone.

C. Use preoperative sedation cautiously so as to maintain laryngeal reflexes. If feasible, consider regional techniques without sedation in place of general anesthesia (GETA). If GETA is necessary, perform intubation with the patient awake if difficulty with intubation is anticipated. This is critically important. One of the most important findings of recent studies is that induction of GETA in a patient with a difficult airway, particularly in the setting of light anesthesia, is a major risk factor for gagging, vomiting, and aspirating.[2] If the airway is deemed an acceptable risk, perform GETA using an RSI with an experienced assistant. For RSI, preoxygenate

and have the assistant apply cricoid pressure. Administer an induction agent followed immediately by a muscle relaxant. Do not mask ventilate. Succinylcholine (1 to 1.5 mg/kg intravenously) offers the most reliable intubating conditions for RSI, but rocuronium (0.8 to 1.2 mg/kg intravenously) provides similar conditions within 60 seconds and is useful when succinylcholine is contraindicated. Properly applied cricoid pressure can decrease passive regurgitation but not activate vomiting and should be released if vomiting occurs. Perform laryngoscopy only when adequate anesthesia and muscle relaxation has been achieved. Place a stylet inside the endotracheal tube (ETT) to allow optimal manipulation. Ask the assistant to release cricoid pressure when placement of the ETT is verified by capnography and auscultation. In the event of a failed intubation, mask ventilate if desaturation occurs; keep peak airway pressure <25 cm of H_2O and maintain cricoid pressure. Follow the ASA difficult airway algorithm during further attempts to secure the airway. (See Chapters 7, 8 and 9.)

D. Extubate the trachea when airway reflexes have returned, muscle relaxation has been reversed, and the patient is awake and meets criteria for extubation. Half of aspirations occur on induction and one quarter on emergence.[4] If vomiting occurs, turn the patient's head or logroll the patient, place the bed in Trendelenburg position, suction the posterior pharynx, and supply 100% oxygen. If necessary, intubate the trachea, suction the ETT, and ventilate with positive pressure. Treat bronchospasm with beta-2 agonists, maintain vigorous pulmonary toilet, and remove solid particles by bronchoscopy. Lavage is not indicated. If problems with oxygenation manifest, admit the patient to an ICU; follow vital signs, chest x-rays, and ABGs. Vigorous fluid resuscitation and inotropes may be necessary. Administer steroids and antibiotics for proven needs. Patients who are asymptomatic for more than 2 hours after vomiting or aspirating are unlikely to manifest serious symptoms and may be discharged.[5]

REFERENCES

1. Ng A, Smith G: Gastroesophageal reflux and aspiration of gastric contents in anesthetic practice, *Anesth Analg* 93 (2):494–513, 2001.
2. Schreiner MS: Gastric fluid volume: is it really a risk factor for pulmonary aspiration? *Anesth Analg* 87 (4):754–756, 1998.
3. ASA Task Force on Preoperative Fasting: *Practice guidelines for preoperative fasting and the use of pharmacologic agents to reduce the risk of pulmonary aspiration: application to healthy patients undergoing elective procedures*, available at: http://www.asahq.org/publicationsandservices/npo.pdf, 1999.
4. Kluger MT, Short TG: Aspiration during anaesthesia: a review of 133 cases from the Australian Anaesthetic Incident Monitoring Study (AIMS), *Anaesthesia* 54:19–26, 1999.
5. Kalinowski CP, Kirsch JR: Strategies for prophylaxis and treatment for aspiration, *Best Pract Res Clin Anaesthesiol* 18 (4):719–737, 2004.

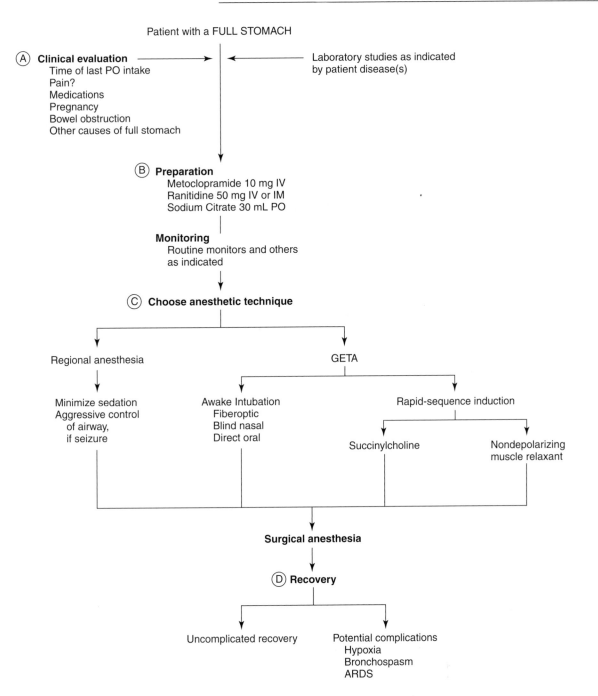

Patient with a FULL STOMACH

Ⓐ **Clinical evaluation**
   Time of last PO intake
   Pain?
   Medications
   Pregnancy
   Bowel obstruction
   Other causes of full stomach

Laboratory studies as indicated
by patient disease(s)

Ⓑ **Preparation**
   Metoclopramide 10 mg IV
   Ranitidine 50 mg IV or IM
   Sodium Citrate 30 mL PO

Monitoring
   Routine monitors and others
   as indicated

Ⓒ **Choose anesthetic technique**

Regional anesthesia

GETA

Minimize sedation
Aggressive control
   of airway,
   if seizure

Awake Intubation
   Fiberoptic
   Blind nasal
   Direct oral

Rapid-sequence induction

Succinylcholine

Nondepolarizing
muscle relaxant

Surgical anesthesia

Ⓓ **Recovery**

Uncomplicated recovery

Potential complications
   Hypoxia
   Bronchospasm
   ARDS

Elderly Patient

ROBERT H. OVERBAUGH, M.D.

Patients over the age of 65 years represent an increasing percentage of those undergoing surgical procedures.[1–3] With increasing age comes significant changes in physiology, pharmacodynamics, and comorbidity. Diligent perioperative management is required to lessen morbidity and mortality.

A. Perform a history and physical examination. Examine airway, lungs, heart and carotids, and neurological system. Look for upper airway obstruction (edentulous or redundant soft tissue) and evaluate aspiration risk (diminished pharyngeal reflexes). Anticipate pulmonary changes (decreased elasticity of small airways, alveolar surface area, responsiveness to hypoxia and hypercarbia, chest wall compliance, cough strength, total lung capacity, and vital capacity; increased closing volume, dead space, and V/Q mismatch).[2] Cardiovascular changes include alterations in rate, rhythm, contractility, and afterload. The resting HR decreases by one beat per minute per year for each year over age 50; atrial fibrillation is common. Fibrosis of ventricular myocardium leads to left ventricular hypertrophy (LVH), stiffening of the ventricles, and diastolic dysfunction. Increases in afterload, SVR, and systolic blood pressure are secondary to increased fibrosis and calcification of the medial layer of the arteries. Decreased elasticity and capacitance of the arterial system may lead to significant intravascular volume reduction with bowel preparations. The resting cardiac output is relatively unchanged; however, reserve is diminished. Evaluate for coronary artery disease (CAD), valvular dysfunction, and dysrhythmias. Assess functional capacity. Evaluate for renal and hepatic disease. Changes include reduced renal blood flow (up to 25% by age 65), glomerular filtration rate (GFR), and creatinine clearance; elderly patients are less able to handle sodium or volume loads (impaired renin-angiotensin response). Serum creatinine usually is unchanged due to decreased muscle mass. Electrolyte derangements occur with diuretic therapy. Hepatic mass, metabolism, and synthetic function diminish. There is also reduced plasma protein binding, resulting in exaggerated clinical effects of highly protein bound drugs. Review current medications and assess preoperative volume status.

B. Obtain an ECG for all patients over age of 50. Consider blood urea nitrogen (BUN), creatinine (Cr) and electrolytes for patients on diuretic or angiotensin-converting enzyme (ACE) inhibitor therapy, and chest x-ray and/or PFTs in patients with pulmonary comorbidity. If exercise tolerance is poor, consider stress testing (e.g., adenosine-thallium scan or dobutamine echocardiography).

C. Premedicate with care; it may be prudent to avoid sedatives or hypnotics in cognitively impaired or demented patients. Anticipate decreased dose requirements of benzodiazepines and opioids, as well as slower onset. Perioperative beta blockers may decrease morbidity and mortality[4] and prevent rebound hypertension. Employ standard monitors, including temperature—elderly patients are less able to regulate body temperature and are thus prone to hypothermia (reduced effectiveness of cutaneous vasoconstriction and decreased basal metabolic rate). Warm the IV fluids and utilize heating blankets when appropriate. Consider noninvasive or invasive cardiac monitors (significant cardiac or cerebral comorbidity or highly invasive operative procedures) and urinary catheter to assess urine output. Ensure proper operative positioning and padding of bony prominences to prevent peripheral nerve and soft tissue injury.

D. Although studies comparing neuraxial block and general anesthesia have failed to reveal significant outcome differences, regional is preferred for transurethral resection of the prostrate (allows continued neurological assessment) and hip procedures (reduced blood loss[5]). Ligamentous calcification and osteophyte formation increase the difficulty of block placement. Decrease the total local anesthetic dose for spinal and epidural anesthesia; higher segmental levels are achieved when compared to younger patients. Consider continuous peripheral nerve catheter techniques for extremity surgery to avoid need for systemic agents. Delayed circulation times slow the response to IV anesthetics. Dose requirements for induction agents are decreased in elderly patients; patients >65 are more sensitive to the hypnotic effects of propofol[6] and are likely to have hypotensive responses to induction doses of thiopental or propofol. Dose requirements of opioids, benzodiazepines, and muscle relaxants are also decreased (volume of distribution, decreased protein binding, and diminished lean body mass), although elimination half-lives are increased. Even small doses of sedative medications, when administered for local cases, may cause significant postoperative cognitive impairment. As patients age, MAC requirements for isoflurane, desflurane, and halothane are reduced, perhaps by as much as 30% when compared with younger adults.

E. Monitor all patients closely in the PACU. Postoperative hypoxemia, hypercarbia, urinary retention, and delirium all are more common in older patients. When appropriate, surgical procedures should be performed on an outpatient basis in elderly patients, as this may be decrease the incidence of postoperative mental dysfunction and confusion.

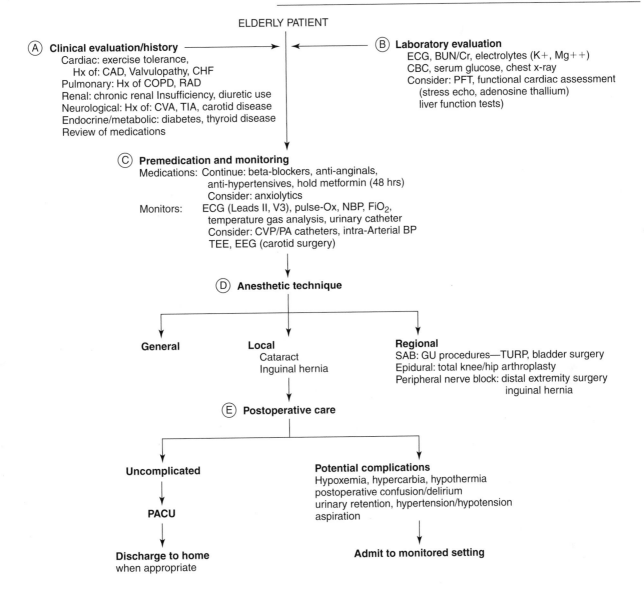

ELDERLY PATIENT

Ⓐ **Clinical evaluation/history**
  Cardiac: exercise tolerance,
    Hx of: CAD, Valvulopathy, CHF
  Pulmonary: Hx of COPD, RAD
  Renal: chronic renal Insufficiency, diuretic use
  Neurological: Hx of: CVA, TIA, carotid disease
  Endocrine/metabolic: diabetes, thyroid disease
  Review of medications

Ⓑ **Laboratory evaluation**
  ECG, BUN/Cr, electrolytes (K+, Mg++)
  CBC, serum glucose, chest x-ray
  Consider: PFT, functional cardiac assessment
    (stress echo, adenosine thallium)
    liver function tests)

Ⓒ **Premedication and monitoring**
  Medications: Continue: beta-blockers, anti-anginals,
      anti-hypertensives, hold metformin (48 hrs)
    Consider: anxiolytics
  Monitors: ECG (Leads II, V3), pulse-Ox, NBP, FiO_2,
      temperature gas analysis, urinary catheter
    Consider: CVP/PA catheters, intra-Arterial BP
    TEE, EEG (carotid surgery)

Ⓓ **Anesthetic technique**

General

Local
  Cataract
  Inguinal hernia

Regional
SAB: GU procedures—TURP, bladder surgery
Epidural: total knee/hip arthroplasty
Peripheral nerve block: distal extremity surgery
      inguinal hernia

Ⓔ **Postoperative care**

Uncomplicated

PACU

Discharge to home
when appropriate

Potential complications
Hypoxemia, hypercarbia, hypothermia
postoperative confusion/delirium
urinary retention, hypertension/hypotension
aspiration

Admit to monitored setting

REFERENCES

1. Liu LL, Wiener-Kronish JP: Perioperative issues in the elderly, *Crit Care Clin* 19 (4):641–656, 2003.
2. Zaugg M, Lucchinetti E: Respiratory function in the elderly, *Anesthesiol Clin North America* 18:47–58, 2000.
3. Cook DJ, Rooke GA: Priorities in perioperative geriatrics, *Anesth Analg* 96:1823–1836, 2003.
4. Wallace A, Layug B, Tateo I, et al.: Prophylactic atenolol reduces postoperative myocardial ischemia. McSPI Research Group, *Anesthesiology* 88:7–17, 1998.
5. Westrich GH, Farrell C, Bono JV, et al.: The incidence of venous thromboembolism after total hip arthroplasty: a specific hypotensive epidural anesthesia protocol, *J Arthroplasty* 14 (4):456–563, 1999.
6. Schnider TW, Minto CF, Shafer SL, et al.: The influence of age on propofol pharmacodynamics, *Anesthesiology* 90:1502–1516, 1999.

Informed Consent for the Anesthesiologist

DAVID B. WAISEL, M.D.

Informed consent is a patient's active, autonomous, knowledgeable authorization to allow a specific anesthetic to be administered or a procedure to be provided by an anesthesiologist. Obtaining informed consent honors a patient's right to self-determination. The following pathway may help anesthesiologists fulfill both the ethical and legal requirements of informed consent.[1,2]

A. *Competence and decision-making capacity.*[1,3] Every adult is assumed to be legally competent to consent to medical procedures unless determined otherwise by a judge. If a patient is considered incompetent to make health care decisions (e.g., children or those who have been declared incompetent), legal consent should be obtained from the surrogate. The patient should be encouraged to participate in decision making to the best of his or her capacity. For example, children may be able to choose between an inhalation or IV anesthetic induction but may be unable to determine whether to have the operation. Decision-making capacity refers to the ability of a person to make a specific decision at a specific time. Decision-making capacity may vary depending on the patient's age, medical situation, current physical condition, and level of risk in the decision. For example, some believe a patient, after receiving sedation, may be able to consent to lower risk procedures but not to higher risk procedures. When the sedation recedes, the patient returns to his or her usual decision-making capacity. Anesthesiologists are obligated to consider the patient's decision-making capacity when obtaining informed consent.

B. *Voluntariness.* An anesthesiologist should perform a procedure only for a patient who voluntarily gives consent. Although this may seem obvious, the anesthesiologist may encounter a patient with questionable decision-making capacity who refuses a procedure. These confusing situations must be approached cautiously, and help should be sought in resolving these dilemmas.

C. *Disclosure.* Most local statutes use the *reasonable person standard* of disclosure, which requires disclosure to be to the extent that would satisfy the hypothetical reasonable person. The difficulty with this standard is that it does not articulate exactly what a patient should be told. One option is to discuss risks that cause a minor and temporary complication 10% of the time and a more permanent complication 0.5% of the time.[4] The anesthesiologist can then ask the patient if he or she wishes to know about the less common but more severe risks. This technique approaches the ideal of informed consent, which is to have the disclosure tailored to each patient's wants and needs.

D. *Recommendation.* The anesthesiologist should offer an opinion about the advantages, disadvantages, and desirability of each acceptable anesthetic option. By explaining the underpinnings of the recommendations, the anesthesiologist gives the patient the benefit of his or her expertise and the opportunity to understand the opinion. The patient may then decide which anesthetic fits best with his or her own priorities.

E. *Decision.* The patient then selects an anesthetic technique. The patient may prefer a technique the anesthesiologist considers unsafe. When faced with this situation, the anesthesiologist should extend the disclosure process to include any information that may be relevant to the patient's choice and the medical opinion. This is the concept of informed refusal. It is appropriate for the anesthesiologist to use information to persuade the patient to change his or her mind. It is inappropriate for the anesthesiologist to manipulate information or coerce the patient into choosing a different technique. If an anesthesiologist believes the technique desired by the patient is inappropriate, he or she is not obligated to administer that anesthetic in a nonemergent situation.[5] The anesthesiologist may best serve the patient by attempting to find a replacement health care provider.

F. *Autonomous authorization.* The process of obtaining informed consent concludes with the patient intentionally authorizing an anesthesiologist to administer a specific anesthetic or perform a particular procedure. Institutional requirements should then be fulfilled.

G. *Get help.* Many of these issues have subtexts that are beyond the scope of this chapter. Anesthesiologists are encouraged to recognize these dilemmas (e.g., the 15-year-old child who will not agree to urgent surgery or the patient with suspect decision-making capacity) and to seek help. Help can usually be obtained from more experienced colleagues or the institutional ethics committee. Anesthesiologists are encouraged to locate appropriate consultants before a crisis situation occurs.

NEED FOR INFORMED CONSENT

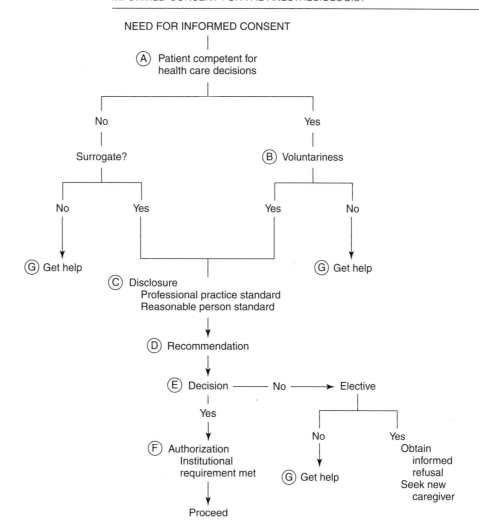

REFERENCES

1. Beauchamp TL, Childress JF: *Principles of biomedical ethics*, ed 5, New York, 2001, Oxford University Press.
2. Waisel DB, Truog RD: Informed consent, *Anesthesiology* 87: 968–978, 1997.
3. Bianco EA, Hirsch H: Consent to and refusal of medical treatment, legal medicine. In Sanbar S, Gibofsky A, Firestone M, et al., editors: St. Louis, 1995, Mosby.
4. Dornette WH: Informed consent and anesthesia, *Anesth Analg* 53:832, 1974.
5. American Society of Anesthesiologists: *Guidelines for the ethical practice of anesthesiology*, available at: http://www.asahq.org/publicationsandservices/standards/10.pdf, 2003.

Advance Directives (AD)

WENDY B. KANG, M.D., J.D.

Patients' autonomous wishes must be respected, and anesthesiologists should understand legal imperatives that impact care. Patients have both the rights to consent and to refuse invasive medical procedures. The Patient Self-Determination Act (PSDA) of 1990 recognizes a patient's right to advance directives (AD).

A. The anesthesiologist must follow the ethical responsibilities of a health care provider. Beginning with the Hippocratic Oath, the anesthesiologist observes the core values of doing no harm (nonmaleficence) and beneficence while respecting patient autonomy. The anesthesiologist's knowledge must be used to recommend the best treatment options for the patient. When treatment options would only be futile (i.e., delaying death), the ethical principle of distributive justice in allocating health resources may come into play—even if counter to the patient's desires.

B. Medicare-funded facilities must inquire of all patients about AD, must provide information about end-of-life decisions, and must recognize the patient's right to draft AD.[1–6] AD exists in different forms; the most common is the living will. The mentally competent patient executes a legal document instructing the world which medical treatments are desired or refused when he or she is unable to express those wishes. Usually in combination with the living will is a durable power of attorney for health care, designating a proxy who will make health care decisions on the patient's behalf. (The circumstances under which the proxy may speak for the mentally incapacitated patient may be limited to terminal care or persistent vegetative state,[1] and *not* to potentially reversible anesthesia-related sequelae.) A values history adds depth to the living will and durable power of attorney by surveying the personal beliefs of the individual. A comprehensive advance medical care directive instructs precisely and rigidly the type of care in different scenarios. Due to differing state laws, health care providers must become familiar with the requirements of the specific state(s) in which they practice and should recommend that patients consult with health care attorneys.

C. Patients have the right to maintain their AD for no resuscitations during their anesthetic and surgical procedures. However, American Society of Anesthesiologists (ASA) policy stipulates that there should be "required reconsideration" of do-not-resuscitate (DNR) status *before* any anesthetic (see www.ASAhq.org/pulications andservices/standards/09.html). Should AD be temporarily suspended, discussion must determine the point of reinstatement (e.g., PACU or the general ward). Technically, DNR orders are written by health care providers rather than by patients. In the past, health care providers based their actions on knowing what was best for the patient on the basis of superior medical knowledge and the ethical principle of beneficence. Anesthesia care providers may have difficulty obeying orders written by other health care providers unfamiliar with the special nature of the OR environment. The anesthesiologist should avoid being the stranger at the bedside. Rather, he or she should meet the patient and explain his or her role in patient care. If the patient has an AD or some form of DNR, the anesthesiologist should try to understand the reasons for such directives to have a more meaningful discussion and allay anxiety. Such communication might result in changing anesthetic and surgical plans to respect all parties' beliefs. Besides ethical duty, anesthesiologists have a legal duty of prudent care. Two jurisdictional standards apply: whether the actions of the health care provider are considered reasonable to other health care providers or reasonable patients. Should a breach of this duty occur which proximately results in the patient sustaining injury, then legal malpractice is defined. Damages can be assessed against the health care provider. If the patient's AD is incompatible with a prudent standard of anesthetic care, the anesthesiologist should explain this to the patient. The patient may be willing to assume the increased risks (e.g., undergoing a regional anesthetic in the presence of a full stomach and difficult airway), in which case documentation of such assumption is paramount. However, patient refusal to have necessary intubation (e.g., laparoscopic cholecystectomy) is grounds for the anesthesiologist to withdraw from the case. The PSDA allows the health care provider to withdraw from the care of a patient whose AD contradicts the health care provider's moral beliefs. Care of the patient must be transferred to another health care provider of equal competence. When the anesthesiologist is the only one available for the true emergency surgery, should the health care provider's moral beliefs be hostage to the patient's autonomy? In the setting of intense production pressures, limited patient contacts until immediately before surgery, and Health Insurance Portability and Accountability Act (HIPAA) issues of confidentiality, AD adds to the anesthetic complexities. Understanding the rights of the patient to self-determination by the use of AD that encompass DNR issues and consent or refusal to treatments, it behooves the ethical perioperative health care provider to ask, listen, dialogue, then document.

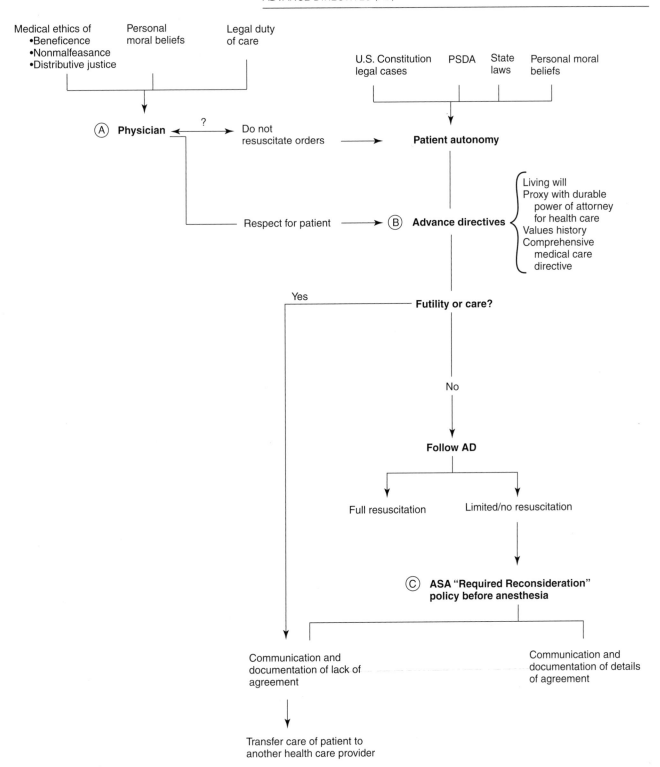

REFERENCES

1. Beauchamp T, Childress J: *Principles of biomedical ethics*, ed 5, New York, 2001, Oxford University Press.
2. ASA Committee on Ethics: *ASA Newsletter* 67 (10), 2003.
3. Szalados J: Do-not resuscitate and end of life care issues: clinical, ethical, and legal principles, *Curr Rev Clin Anesth* 24 (5):45–56, 2003.
4. Boudreaux A: Ethics in anesthesia practice, *Annual Meeting Refresher Course Lectures*, 191:1–7, 2003.
5. Palmer S, Jackson S: What's new in ethics: hot issues in legally sensitive times, *ASA Newsletter* 67 (10):30, 2003.
6. Brown B: The history of advance directives, *J Gerontol Nurs* 4–14, 2003.

Do Not Resuscitate Orders in the OR

DAVID B. WAISEL, M.D.

In 1974 the American Medical Association (AMA) recognized a patient's right to refuse CPR in a policy that stated "cardiopulmonary resuscitation is not indicated in cases of terminal irreversible illness where death is not unexpected."[1] This was soon followed by the development of formal do-not-resuscitate (DNR) policies. However, several problems were identified when patients with such DNR orders required OR surgical procedures. These problems arose from the blurred distinction between incidents that would normally initiate resuscitation on a hospital ward and similar events that occur in the normal course of anesthesia (e.g., respiratory depression, hemodynamic instability, and iatrogenic problems from invasive procedures and drug errors). Although there is an increased incidence of these events in the OR as compared with the ward, there is also an improved outcome following treatment of these events in the OR.[3] Over the past decade, methods of addressing these problems have developed.

A. Unconditionally continuing a DNR order may result in a patient expiring from an easily treated iatrogenic cause, whereas unconditionally rescinding a DNR order may result in a patient undergoing long-term, life-sustaining measures without a significant likelihood of meaningful recovery. Both the American Society of Anesthesiologists (ASA) and the American College of Surgeons (ACS) have proposed guidelines for treating patients who have DNR orders.[4,5] These guidelines recommend that a patient's wishes be reassessed prior to going to the OR. Therefore, an anesthesiologist should arrange a preoperative meeting to discuss the relevant issues involved in the patient's decision to continue, rescind, or modify DNR orders. Most hospitals have also developed guidelines to assist in handling these situations. Be familiar with such institutional policies prior to speaking with the patient so that appropriate mechanisms will be used.

B. If a patient is emergently taken to the OR before proper documentation of a DNR order, assume that the patient would wish to receive all resuscitative measures in the event of a life-threatening complication. Although verbal requests by a patient in extremis or by family members should be considered, it is often prudent to administer full resuscitative treatments with reevaluation of the patient's wishes after medical stabilization.

C. When organizing the meeting to delineate a patient's wishes, include the patient, the anesthesia team, and the surgical team. At times it may also require the presence of the patient's family, the primary care team, the intensive care team, and possibly the ethics consultation service.

D. Two major approaches have been popularized. The first is a procedure-directed approach in which the patient's wishes are determined regarding a list of interventions that might be applied to a life-threatening condition. Typically, a simple checklist of potential interventions is completed by the patient and used for a specified period (usually until discharge from the PACU). This approach may be useful for some patients but is limited by its inflexibility. For example, a patient may wish to receive certain procedures if the cause of the incident is believed to be easily reversible but not if the cause is difficult to reverse or identify.

E. These problems led to the development of a goal-directed approach in which the patient states the overall outcome goals underlying the decision to have a DNR order.[6] Some patients may request that all resuscitative procedures be used if the likelihood of full recovery is high. Others may request only the most minimal and least painful measures regardless of the chance of recovery. The goal-directed approach allows more rational decisions to be made at the time life-threatening events occur. If these goals are understood by all members of the OR team, the actions undertaken will likely be more consistent with the patient's overall wishes. The procedure-directed and goal-directed approaches are not mutually exclusive. Often, the initial procedure-directed approach will stimulate further discussion leading to more goal-directed decisions.

F. Regardless of which approach is used, make plans for the patient who cannot be extubated at the end of the surgical procedure. The patient may request full care postoperatively with withdrawal of care after a specified period of time if improvement has not occurred.

G. At the conclusion of the meeting, restate the patient's wishes so that all involved parties understand and agree to follow them. If a certain party does not believe that he or she can ethically follow the patient's wishes, find a replacement who is comfortable with the decisions made. These decisions need to be clearly documented in the patient's chart before going to the OR.

REFERENCES

1. American Medical Association: Standards for cardiopulmonary resuscitation (CPR) and emergency cardiac care (ECC), *JAMA* 227(suppl): 837, 1974.
2. Truog RD: "Do-not-resuscitate" orders during anesthesia and surgery, *Anesthesiology* 74: 606–608, 1991.
3. Taffet GE, Teasdale TA, Luchi RJ: In-hospital cardiopulmonary resuscitation, *JAMA* 260:2069, 1988.
4. American Society of Anesthesiologists: Ethical guidelines for the anesthesia care of patients with do-not-resuscitate orders or other directives that limit care, *ASA 2003 directory of members*, Park Ridge, IL, 2003, ASA.
5. American College of Surgeons: Statement of the American College of Surgeons on advance directives by patients: "do not resuscitate" in the operating room, *Bull Am Coll Surg* 79:29, 1994.
6. Truog RD, Waisel DB, Burns JP: DNR in the OR: A goal-directed approach, *Anesthesiology* 90:289–295, 1999.

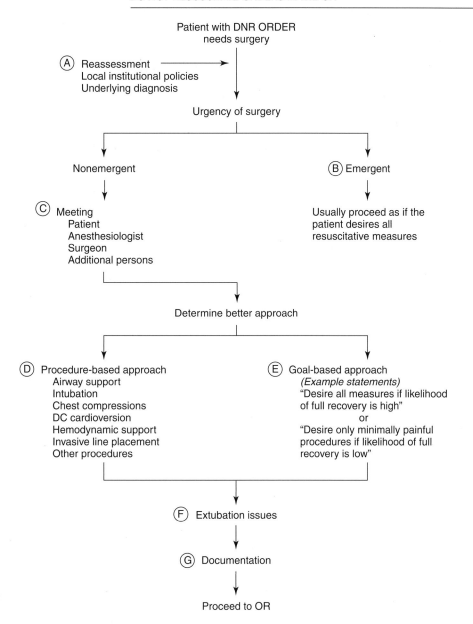

Patient with DNR ORDER
needs surgery

Ⓐ Reassessment
Local institutional policies
Underlying diagnosis

Urgency of surgery

Nonemergent

Ⓑ Emergent

Ⓒ Meeting
Patient
Anesthesiologist
Surgeon
Additional persons

Usually proceed as if the
patient desires all
resuscitative measures

Determine better approach

Ⓓ Procedure-based approach
Airway support
Intubation
Chest compressions
DC cardioversion
Hemodynamic support
Invasive line placement
Other procedures

Ⓔ Goal-based approach
(Example statements)
"Desire all measures if likelihood
of full recovery is high"
or
"Desire only minimally painful
procedures if likelihood of full
recovery is low"

Ⓕ Extubation issues

Ⓖ Documentation

Proceed to OR

CHEMICAL DEPENDENCE IN ANESTHESIOLOGISTS

IDENTIFICATION, INTERVENTION, AND
MANAGEMENT

CHEMICALLY IMPAIRED ANESTHESIOLOGIST:
REENTRY?

Identification, Intervention, and Management

WILLIAM P. ARNOLD III, M.D.

Chemical dependence is a chronic, relapsing disease that has the potential to affect people in all social strata and in all walks of life. It may be defined as *an overwhelming compulsion to use despite adverse consequences*. The disease is particularly conspicuous when it occurs in health care workers, who, by various means, are able to divert medically used drugs for their own use. The impression that the disease is more common in anesthesiologists than all other health care providers has been disproved,[1,2] although for the reasons outlined in this chapter, it may be more evident in this specialty than any other.[3]

Availability and potency of a given drug are two important factors that determine a health care provider's drug of choice and the rapidity of that person's addiction to the drug. Anesthesiologists are unique among health care providers in that they administer drugs to patients, rather than ordering others to manage this task. Thus, drugs are immediately available to anesthesiologists. All practitioners of medicine are vulnerable to drug addiction. The specific drug selected is in large part determined by its availability. For example, internists and psychiatrists may divert drugs for which they write prescriptions (e.g., oxycodone or benzodiazepines), otolaryngologists may select cocaine, and dentists have access to nitrous oxide. For the same reason, anesthesiologists most commonly become addicted to fentanyl and sufentanil, the two most potent mood-altering drugs used in the practice of medicine. Addiction in anesthesiologists becomes apparent to colleagues and others more rapidly than addiction in other medical specialists—perhaps within 6 months of fentanyl use and in as little as a few weeks with sufentanil use, because the rate of onset of addiction is a function of the potency of the drug of choice.

A. A series of behavioral changes usually precedes the overt signs of addiction. For drugs other than fentanyl and sufentanil, the changes may take years to become apparent. They commonly follow an orderly progression with (1) loss of interest in common activities, (2) problems in the home, (3) problems at the work place, and (4) obvious changes in work habits. In contrast, addiction to fentanyl or sufentanil progresses so rapidly that the first three of these stages are bypassed and only the fourth becomes apparent. Some of the changes seen in the final stage include overadministration of opiates, frequent unexplained absences, sloppy records, donning of gowns in the OR (to treat chills from drug withdrawal), inappropriate volunteering for extra work, tremulousness, coma, death, and witnessed self-administration. Only the last is pathognomonic and then only if the drug can be identified.[4]

B. Intervention, an expression of concern from caring friends and colleagues in a formal setting conducted by an expert, is the first step in assisting an addict to seek treatment.[5] Adequate planning is essential for a successful outcome. Requirements include an experienced leader, extensive rehearsing by participants, an unlimited amount of time, irrefutable documentation of the addictive behavior, the willingness of friends and family to describe specific events demonstrating the behavior (in the addict's vernacular, to show tough love), a specific treatment plan, a facility skilled in managing addicted health care providers, and a person willing to accompany the individual to that facility. When all is in order, the addicted person is summoned into the room and is told that his or her friends are concerned and want to share their concerns. The individual will probably deny everything. Success is dependent on persistence, presentation of detailed observations that demonstrate addictive behavior, strong emphasis that the individual has a treatable illness, and insistence that treatment begin immediately. If the individual steadfastly refuses, he or she should be told that the only alternative is to inform the state medical board (i.e., almost certain loss of medical licensure).

C. Treatment for addicted health care providers is best done by those with experience. It commonly requires several months, beginning with a multidisciplinary health evaluation and detoxification (if indicated) and progressing to intensive group therapy and regular 12-step meetings, such as Alcoholics Anonymous (AA), Narcotics Anonymous (NA), and others.[6]

D. Health care providers discharged from formal treatment must avoid all mood-altering drugs, attend regular AA or NA meetings, and understand that recovery is a lifelong process. Because addiction is an incurable, chronic disease, long-term remission is the norm, but relapse may occur.[2,7] Should that happen, the entire process must be repeated. Prolonged monitoring may be indicated in the event of relapse.[2]

CHEMICALLY DEPENDENT ANESTHESIOLOGIST

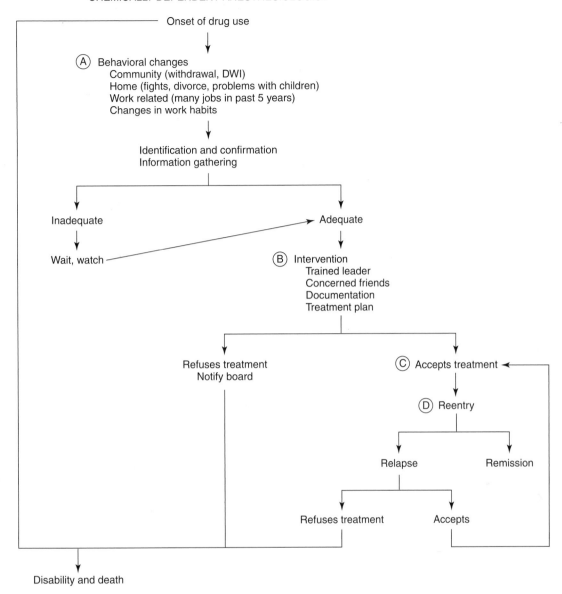

REFERENCES

1. Hughes PH, Brandenburg N, Baldwin DC Jr, et al.: Prevalence of substance use among U.S. physicians, *JAMA* 267:2333-2339, 1992.
2. Domino KB, Hornbein TF, Polissar NL, et al.: Risk factors for relapse in health care professionals with substance use disorders, *JAMA* 293:1453-1460, 2005.
3. Silverstein JH, Silva DA, Ibert TJ: Opioid addiction in anesthesiology, *Anesthesiology* 79:354, 1993.
4. Farley WJ, Arnold WP: Videotape: unmasking addiction: chemical dependency in anesthesiology, Piscataway, NJ, 1991, Janssen Pharmaceutical.
5. Johnson VE: *Intervention: how to help someone who doesn't want help*, Minneapolis, 1986, Johnson Institute Books.
6. Carlson HB, Dilts SL, Radcliff S: Physicians with substance abuse problems and their recovery environment: a survey, *J Subst Abuse Treat* 11:113-119, 1994.
7. Paris RT, Canavan DI: Physician substance abuse impairment: anesthesiologists vs. other specialties, *J Addict Dis* 18:1-7, 1999.

Chemically Impaired Anesthesiologist: Reentry?

WILLIAM P. ARNOLD III, M.D.

When faced with the difficult task of deciding whether a recovering health care provider should be able to return to the practice of anesthesiology, decision makers rely on objective information such as the following. Those who have a history of addiction to potent opioids are statistically more likely to relapse than those who have used less potent drugs.[1,2] Relapse is known to be a function of unalterable modifications in reward pathways in the brain resulting from repeated exposure to addicting drugs.[3,4] If one's decision is based solely on these observations, few individuals with a history of fentanyl or sufentanil abuse would be permitted to return. The Americans with Disabilities Act (ADA) of 1990 defines chemical dependence as a disability. Recovering addicts who have been drug-free for an extended period and who are otherwise capable of practicing medicine may not be refused employment solely on the basis of their disability.[1] Each case must be judged on its own merits, with particular focus on the issues that relate directly to the recovering health care provider and to the environment to which he or she hopes to return.

Several criteria must be satisfied. First, the recovering anesthesiologist should have received top quality treatment at a facility skilled in managing chemically dependent health care providers and positive recommendations from the treating providers concerning the likelihood of good recovery. Second, the recovering health care provider must adhere to a detailed program of recovery specified in a written aftercare contract. Third, the recovering health care provider must be strongly committed to an active, lifelong program of aftercare. Fourth, family, partners, hospital staff, and administration must be accepting of the recovering health care provider's return to work. Finally, the individual must agree to long-term monitoring.

A. Recommendations from the treatment program are usually detailed in a lengthy discharge summary, the release of which must be approved by the recovering health care provider. They will most likely require (1) regular attendance at Alcoholics Anonymous (AA) or Narcotics Anonymous (NA) meetings, (2) random, mandatory urine screens obtained by a monitoring health care provider, (3) a primary care provider who will prescribe *all* drugs for the recovering addict, (4) *no* use of over-the-counter drugs unless they are prescribed, and (5) the use of naltrexone for at least 6 months following discharge from treatment.[5]

B. An aftercare contract, written by the impaired health care provider's program of the medical society in the recovering health care provider's state of residence, will usually mirror the recommendation of the treatment facility. The state program will be responsible for regular monitoring and in many cases, will serve as a buffer between the individual and the licensing agency in that state. The current recommendation of most experts is for 5 years of continuous monitoring. Some state programs are beginning to place less emphasis on the need for urine screens (which only detect relapse after it has occurred) and are substituting weekly, facilitated group meetings of recovering health care providers.[6] Attendees at these meetings (all of whom but the facilitator are recovering) are likely to identify prognostic signs of impending relapse and may prevent relapse. Absence at even a single meeting is usually interpreted as relapse until proven otherwise.

C. Commitment to aftercare is essential to long-term recovery. One of the earliest signs of impending relapse is avoidance of AA or NA meetings.

D. Willingness to allow an impaired colleague who sincerely wants to continue in the specialty to return to anesthesiology is essential for successful reentry. Former colleagues must be ready to accept the individual and to permit him or her gradual reentry (e.g., no call for at least 3 months and no direct contact with the drug of choice for the same period). A caring environment is vital. During this time, some recovering health care providers may conclude that they should leave the specialty whereas others believe they will thrive. The former should be encouraged to enter another specialty. Long-term monitoring (5 years) should be an absolute requirement for credentialing. Some recovering health care providers actually request that it last longer than the recommended period to prove to others that they are maintaining their sobriety.

Chemical dependence is an incurable disease that may remain in long-term remission. Although relapse is not the norm, it may occur.[2,7] In such cases, friends and colleagues should again provide the assistance and advocacy needed to reinstitute treatment, aftercare, and recovery. The same principles should be applied to cases involving recovering health care providers who have returned from treatment after relapse, although more intensive and prolonged monitoring may be indicated.[2]

CHEMICAL DEPENDENCE AND RETURN TO WORK

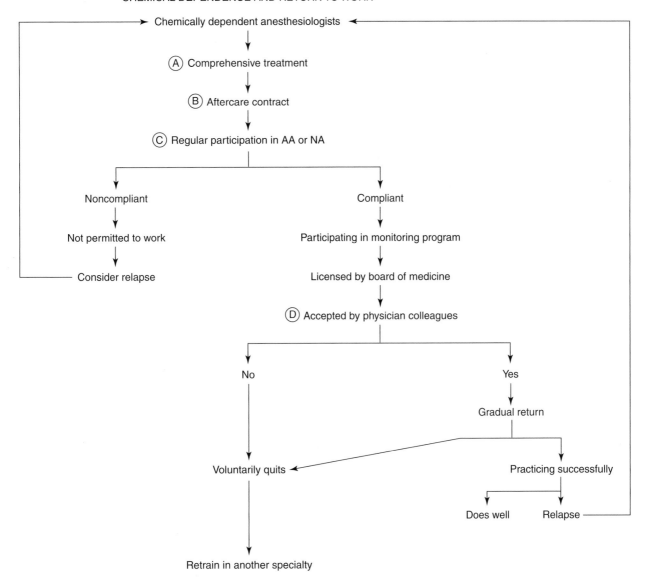

REFERENCES

1. Equal Employment Opportunity Commission: *A technical assistance manual on the employment provisions (Title 1) of the Americans with Disabilities Act*, Washington, DC, 1992, U.S. Government Printing Office.
2. Domino KB, Hornbein TF, Polissar NL, et al.: Risk factors for relapse in health care professionals with substance use disorders, *JAMA* 293:1453-1460, 2005.
3. Nestler EJ, Aghajanian GK: Molecular and cellular basis of addiction, *Science* 278:58-63, 1997.
4. Gold MS, Byars JA, Frost-Pineda K: Occupational exposure and addictions for physicians: case studies and theoretical implications, *Psychiatr Clin N Am* 27:745-753, 2004.
5. Menk EJ, Baumgarten RK, Kingsley CP, et al.: Success of re-entry into anesthesiology training programs by residents with a history of substance abuse, *JAMA* 263:3060-3062, 1990.
6. Talbott GD, Gallegos KV, Wilson PO, et al.: The Medical Association of Georgia's Impaired Physicians Program. Review of the first 1000 physicians: analysis of specialty, *JAMA* 257 (21):2927–2930, 1987.
7. Gallegos KV, Lubin BH, Bowers C, et al.: Relapse and recovery: five to ten year follow-up study of chemically dependent physicians—the Georgia experience, *Md Med J* 41:315-319, 1992.

RESUSCITATION: CARDIAC ARREST

Asystole

Ventricular Fibrillation (VF) and
Pulseless Ventricular Tachycardia
(PVT)

Pulseless Electrical Activity (PEA)

Asystole

ERIK A. BOATMAN, M.D.

Successful pharmacological and electrical treatment of any cardiac arrest depends on definitive identification of the underlying arrhythmia.[1,2] The best survival rates are achieved by early recognition, treatment, and restoration of circulation.[3,4] Asystole is the complete and sustained absence of electrical activity. It is most often irreversible and therefore terminal, but a trial of intervention is warranted in most patients. Paramount in the treatment of this disorder is identification and correction of any underlying etiologies for the arrhythmia; otherwise efforts will likely be futile. Prognosis and survival is generally poor, especially if noted in a prehospital setting. In the OR, asystole is often the result of a strong stimulus, which usually resolves with relief of the stimulus.

A. Check for responsiveness, call for help and a defibrillator, and evaluate the surrounding scene. Perform a primary ABCD survey. Open the airway, check for breathing and provide breaths if necessary, check for a pulse and begin chest compressions if needed. Proper precordial compression can reproduce approximately one third of prearrest stroke volume—evaluate for efficacy by palpating the femoral pulse and observing the end-tidal carbon dioxide (CO_2).[5] Rotate resuscitators when fatigued. On arrival of a defibrillator, immediately apply paddles or pads to evaluate the rhythm. If asystole, ensure that leads are attached properly and asystole exists in more than one lead (to exclude fine ventricular fibrillation).

B. Perform a secondary ABCD survey. Establish and secure a definitive airway (endotracheal tube, laryngeal mask airway [LMA], or Combitube),[6] and ventilate by hand or machine. Significantly higher PaO_2 and delivery of oxygen (O_2) can be provided if pressure support ventilation is enhanced with continuous positive airway pressure or a PEEP valve.[7] Obtain IV access and reevaluate the cardiac rhythm. If asystole is still present, begin administering medications per the advanced cardiac life support (ACLS) algorithm. Flush medications and give chest compressions to facilitate circulation. Develop a differential diagnosis to identify correctable problems. Efficacy of resuscitative efforts are difficult to ascertain; however, bispectral index monitoring (BIS) may offer some reassurance to the resuscitation team if available.[8]

C. Direct therapies at normalization of temperature and correcting deficiencies, overloads, and overdoses. The most frequent etiologies for asystole can be easily remembered as the four "H's" and one "T".[1]

D. At this time, pacing is not recommended for patients with asystolic cardiac arrest as it is rarely effective in unwitnessed arrest and asystole.[2] Use pacing (transcutaneous, transvenous, or transesophageal) to treat conduction disorders or abnormal impulse formation. Institute pacing early. Rarely can fist pacing (repetitive precordial thumps) stimulate ventricular complex formation. However, pacing is extremely effective in bradyasystolic patients with a pulse.

E. Unless a specific etiology is found and treated, the prognosis is poor and therapy is limited. Epinephrine, vasopressin, and atropine (if the underlying rhythm is bradyasystole) are the mainstays of treatment.[2,9] Calcium is recommended only in the treatment of documented hypokalemia, hyperkalemia, or a calcium channel blocker overdose. Bicarbonate is recommended only to treat preexisting metabolic acidosis, hyperkalemia, or to alkalanize the urine. Routine or prophylactic use will rapidly produce high levels of CO_2, which readily crosses cell membranes and the blood-brain barrier, resulting in worsened intracellular acidosis, reduced responsiveness to catecholamines and resuscitation, and alterations in osmolality and the oxygen-hemoglobin dissociation curve. Endogenous adenosine, which is released in response to hypoxia and ischemia, can be competitively reversed with an experimental adenosine antagonist or aminophylline in porcine models.[10] Dextrose, or solutions containing dextrose, may lead to hyperosmotic diuresis, may worsen neurological outcome, and are recommended only in the treatment of hypoglycemia. Free water administration is also not recommended as it may lead to cerebral edema.

F. If asystole persists despite efforts, resuscitation algorithms have been exhausted, and no atypical clinical features are present that have not been addressed, discuss ending the resuscitation. All participants should feel that all efforts have been exhausted prior to termination.

REFERENCES

1. Cummins RO, Field JM, editor: *ACLS Advanced cardiovascular life support provider manual*, The American Heart Association, 2006.
2. AHA in collaboration with ILCOR: Guidelines 2005 American Heart Association guidelines for cardiopulmonary resuscitation and emergency cardiovascular care, *Circulation* 112 (suppl):1–211, 2005.
3. Trappe HJ, Brandts B, Weismueller P: Arrhythmias in the intensive care patient, *Curr Opin Crit Care* 9 (5):345–355, 2003.
4. Gullo A: Cardiac arrest, chain of survival and Utstein style, *Eur J Anaesthesiol* 19 (9):624–633, 2002.
5. Pernat A, Weil MH, Sun S, et al.: Stroke volumes and end-tidal carbon dioxide generated by precordial compression during ventricular fibrillation, *Crit Care Med* 31 (6):1819–1823, 2003.
6. Gabrielli A, Layon AJ, Wenzel V, et al.: Alternative ventilation strategies in cardiopulmonary resuscitation, *Curr Opin Crit Care* 8 (3):199–211, 2002.

Unconscious patient

- Check responsiveness
- Activate emergency response system
- Call for defibrillator
- Rapidly survey the scene: is there any reason that resuscitation should NOT occur (eg, DNR order, signs of death, personal danger)?

Ⓐ **Primary ABCD survey:**
- Airway: open the airway
- Breathing: check for breathing, provide positive-pressure ventilations if indicated
- Circulation: check for pulse, begin chest compressions if indicated
- Defibrillator: identify the rhythm

If VF/PVT—go to VT/PVT algorithm

If PEA—go to PEA algorithm

Asystole

Ⓑ **Secondary ABCD survey:**
- Airway: place airway securing device as soon as possible
- Breathing: confirm airway device placement by exam AND objective confirmation device, demonstrate effective oxygenation and ventilation, secure airway device
- Circulation: establish IV access, identify rhythm on defibrillator monitor, confirm true asystole in two leads, continue chest compressions administer medications appropriate for rhythm and condition
- Differential diagnosis: search for and treat identified reversible causes

Ⓒ **Common etiologies and treatments:**
- Hypoxia—administer 100% F_1O_2
- Hydrogen ion (acidosis)—consider bicarbonate (1 mEq/kg IVP, 0.5 mEq/kg q 10 min) for preexisting metabolic acidosis
- Hyper/hypo-kalemia—consider bicarbonate for hyperkalemia, cautiously assess the need for potassium administration
- Hypothermia—administer warm fluids, warming blanket
- Tablets (drug overdose-tricyclics, barbiturates, digitalis, beta-blockers, calcium channel blockers)—consider bicarbonate for alkalanization of urine, calcium (10 mg/kg slow IVP, repeat as needed) for hyperkalemia and calcium channel blocker overdose

Ⓓ **Pacing–perform immediately if considered:**
- Mode of pacing:
  ° transcutaneous (quick, simple)–negative electrode in the V_2 position, positive electrode on the left posterior chest beneath the scapula and lateral to the spine
  ° transvenous (requires central access, complicated, time-consuming)–negative lead connected to the V lead of the ECG [unipolar electrode], balloon-tipped catheter inflated after it enters the superior vena cava, both the P wave and the QRS complex will be negative, advanced quickly and smoothly, large negative P waves, biphasic and eventually positive, then smaller and QRS larger, contact with RV wall, ST segment elevation
  ° transesophageal (quick, simple)–Tapscope or other esophageal device inserted blindly to the appropriate depth which places it behind the RA
- Current turned up until electrical capture is demonstrated (wide complex QRS complexes)
- Failure to capture may be due to electrode misplacement, poor electrode-to-patient contact, or increased impedance (barrel-chest, pericardial effusion)
- Mechanical capture demonstrated by a palpable pulse

Ⓔ **Other treatments:**
- Epinephrine 1mg IVP, repeat every 3–5 minutes, or
- Vasopressin 40 units IVP, 1 dose, to replace first or second dose of ephinephrine
- Consider Atropine 1 mg IVP, repeat 3-5 minutes up to 3 doses

Return of rhythm with a pulse—
Proceed with cardiovascular support, monitoring, and resuscitation as needed

Return of rhythm without a pulse—
Proceed with appropriate cardiovascular resuscitation algorithm (VF/PVT or PEA)

Ⓕ **Termination of efforts:**
- Asystole persists despite efforts
- Consider quality and duration of resuscitation
- No atypical clinical features unaddressed
- Consider ending resuscitation

7. Kleinsasser A, Lindner K, Schaefer A, et al.: Decompression-triggered positive-pressure ventilation during cardiopulmonary resuscitation improves pulmonary gas exchange and oxygen uptake, *Circulation* 106 (3):373–378, 2002.

8. Szekely B, Saint-Marc T, Degremont AC, et al.: Value of bispectral index monitoring during cardiopulmonary resuscitation, *Br J Anaesth* 88 (3):443–444, 2002.

9. Krismer AC, Wenzel V, Mayr VD, et al.: Arginine vasopressin during cardiopulmonary resuscitation and vasodilatory shock: current experience and future perspectives, *Curr Opin Crit Care* 7 (3): 157–169, 2001.

10. Kelsch T, Kikuchi K, Vahdat S, et al.: Innovative pharmacologic approaches to cardiopulmonary resuscitation, *Heart Dis* 3 (1): 46–54, 2001.

Ventricular Fibrillation (VF) and Pulseless Ventricular Tachycardia (PVT)

ERIK A. BOATMAN, M.D.

Successful pharmacological and electrical treatment of any cardiac arrhythmia depends on definitive identification of the underlying arrhythmia.[1,2] The best survival rates can be achieved by early recognition, treatment, and restoration of circulation.[3,4] Ventricular fibrillation (VF) and pulseless ventricular tachycardia (PVT) are the most common and most treatable and have the best survival rates of all cardiac arrest arrhythmias. The key to survival is early activation of the chain of survival and defibrillation.[1,2] Based on recent studies, the highest survival rates occur when CPR is begun within 4 minutes and advanced cardiac life support (ACLS) is started within 8 minutes. Because of this, automatic external defibrillators (AED) have been widely distributed to locations where large groups of people are commonly found.[1,3]

A. On recognition of an unconscious patient, check for responsiveness, call for help and a defibrillator, and evaluate the surrounding scene. Begin with a primary ABCD survey. Open the airway, check for breathing and provide breaths if necessary, check for a pulse and begin chest compressions if needed. For a witnessed arrest, consider a single precordial thump, but do not delay application of a defibrillator. Proper precordial compression can reproduce approximately one third of prearrest stroke volume—evaluate efficacy by palpating a femoral pulse and measuring end-tidal carbon dioxide (CO_2).[5] Rotate resuscitators when fatigued to maximize efforts. On arrival of a defibrillator, immediately apply paddles or pads to evaluate the rhythm. If VF/PVT, administer shocks up to three times, checking for a change while the defibrillator is recharging one shock and resume CPR. Biphasic electrical countershock may provide better neurological outcomes;[6,7] however, the standard monophasic countershocks are equally effective.

B. After initial assessment, proceed with a secondary ABCD survey, focusing on more advanced assessments and treatments. Place a definitive airway; confirm its location and secure.[1,2] Emphasis is on protecting the airway through any means available (endotracheal tube, laryngeal mask airway [LMA], or Combitube). Ventilate by hand or machine; significantly higher PaO_2 and delivery of oxygen (O_2) can be provided if pressure support ventilation is enhanced with continuous positive airway pressure or a PEEP valve.[8] Obtain IV access if not already available and reevaluate the cardiac rhythm. If VT/PVT, give another and resume CPR.

C. If VT/PVT is persistent, begin administering medications per the ACLS algorithm. Recent studies have changed recommendations quite significantly.

Medications should be flushed into circulation with saline and circulated with chest compressions. Minimize interruptions in chest compressions. There has been no evidence that high-dose epinephrine is any better than standard dose and may produce significant detrimental effects. Vasopressin is now an acceptable first-dose vasopressor[9,10] and may provide better blood flow and gas exchange than epinephrine.[11,12] Amiodarone is now the antiarrhythmic of choice over lidocaine due to much better efficacy and fewer adverse effects.[13,14] Magnesium, lidocaine, and bretylium are no longer recommended in the algorithm for treatment.[6,15] Consider magnesium for torsades de pointes. Dextrose or dextrose-containing solutions may lead to hyperosmotic diuresis, may worsen neurological outcome, and are recommended only in the treatment of hypoglycemia. Free water administration is not recommended as it may lead to cerebral edema. Efficacy of resuscitative efforts are difficult to ascertain, however bispectral index monitoring (BIS) may offer some reassurance to the resuscitation team if available.[15] Continue pharmacological and electrical therapy until the algorithm has been exhausted. If the underlying rhythm on the monitor changes, change the therapy accordingly.

D. Perhaps the most difficult decision to make is termination of efforts. If VF/PVT persists despite efforts and resuscitation algorithms have been exhausted, discuss ending the resuscitation with the team. Participants should feel that all efforts have been exhausted prior to termination.

REFERENCES

1. Cummins RO, editor: *ACLS provider manual*, Dallas, 2001, The American Heart Association. Field JM, editor: Advanced cardiovascular life support provider manual. The American Heart Association, 2006.
2. American Heart Association: 2005 American Heart Association guidelines for cardiopulmonary resuscitation and emergency cardiovascular care.*Circulation* 112(suppl):1-211, 2005.
3. Trappe HJ, Brandts B, Weismueller P: Arrhythmias in the intensive care patient, *Curr Opin Crit Care* 9 (5):345–355, 2003.
4. Gullo A: Cardiac arrest, chain of survival and Utstein style, *Eur J Anaesthesiol* 19 (9):624–633, 2002.
5. Pernat A, Weil MH, Sun S, et al.: Stroke volumes and end-tidal carbon dioxide generated by precordial compression during ventricular fibrillation, *Crit Care Med* 31 (6):1819–1823, 2003.
6. Sarkozy A, Dorian P: Strategies for reversing shock-resistant ventricular fibrillation, *Curr Opin Crit Care* 9 (3):189–193, 2003.
7. Schneider T, Martens P, Paschen H, et al.: Multicenter, randomized, controlled trial of 150-J biphasic shocks compared with 200- to 360-J monophasic shocks in the resuscitation of out-of-hospital cardiac arrest victims, *Circulation* 102 (15):1780–1787, 2000.
8. Kleinsasser A, Lindner K, Schaefer A, et al.: Decompression-triggered positive-pressure ventilation during cardiopulmonary

Unconscious patient

↓

• Check responsiveness
• Activate emergency response system
• Call for defibrillator
• Rapidly survey the scene: is there any reason that resuscitation should
  NOT occur (eg, DNR order, signs of death, personal danger)

↓

Ⓐ **Primary ABCD survey:**
• Airway: open the airway
• Breathing: check for breathing, provide positive-
  pressure ventilations if indicated
• Circulation: check for pulse, begin chest
  compressions if indicated
• Defibrillator: identify the rhythm

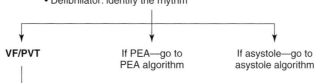

VF/PVT   If PEA—go to   If asystole—go to
                     PEA algorithm   asystole algorithm

↓

Electrical counter shock
• 200 J, 300 J, then 360 J (checking for rhythm changes between shocks) 1 shock and resume
  CPR Manual biphasic: device specific, if unknown use 200 J Monophasic: 360 J
• One paddle should be to the right of the upper sternum, just below the clavicle,
  and the other in the mid axillary line, just to the left of the nipple
• Conductive pads or gel between the paddles and the skin will prevent burns and
  lower thoracic impedance, as will successive shocks
• Paddles should be at least 12 cm away from a pacemaker if present
• Controllable variables for resistance to current flow: proper electrode position,
  firm pressure, optimal electrode-chest wall coupling mechanism such as
  paste or gel

↓

Ⓑ **Secondary ABCD survey:**
• Airway: place airway securing device as soon as possible
• Breathing: confirm airway device placement by exam AND objective confirmation device,
  demonstrate effective oxygenation and ventilation, secure airway device
• Circulation: continue CPR, establish IV access, confirm VF/PVT
• Defibrillate: and resume CPR

↓

Ⓒ **Treatments:**
• Vasopression 40U IVP, one time dose, early
  OR
• Epinephrine 1 mg IVP, repeat every 3–5 minutes, may
  succeed vasopressin
For shock refractory VF/PVT, consider antiarrythmics:
• amiodarone 300 mg IVP, repeat once as 150 mg IVP in 3–5
  minutes, max 2.2 g IV over 24 hours OR
• Procainamide 100 mg IVP, repeat every 5 minutes, max 17 mg/kg
  lidocaine 1-15 mg/kg IVP, repeat as 0.5-0.75 mg/kg IVP, max 3 mg/kg
• Consider magnesium 1-2g IVP for torsades de pointes

**Loss of electrical rhythm and
pulse—** proceed with asystole
algorithm

**Electrical rhythm without a
pulse—** proceed with PEA
algorithm

Ⓓ **Termination of efforts:**
• VF/PVT persists despite efforts
• Consider quality and duration of
  resuscitation
• Consider ending resuscitation

↓

Return of pulse— proceed
with cardiovascular support,
monitoring, and resuscitation as needed

resuscitation improves pulmonary gas exchange and oxygen uptake, *Circulation* 106 (3):373–378, 2002.

9. Nolan JP, de Latorre FJ, Steen PA, et al.: Advanced life support drugs: do they really work? *Curr Opin Crit Care* 8 (3):212–218, 2002.

10. Stiell IG, Hebert PC, Wells GA, et al.: Vasopressin versus epinephrine for in hospital cardiac arrest: a randomised controlled trial, *Lancet* 358:105–109, 2001.

11. Krismer AC, Wenzel V, Mayr VD, et al.: Arginine vasopressin during cardiopulmonary resuscitation and vasodilatory shock: current experience and future perspectives, *Curr Opin Crit Care* 7 (3): 157–169, 2001.

12. Loeckinger A, Kleinsasser A, Wenzel V, et al.: Pulmonary gas exchange after cardiopulmonary resuscitation with either vasopressin or epinephrine, *Crit Care Med* 30 (9):2059–2062, 2002.

13. Taylor SE: Amiodarone: an emergency medicine perspective, *Emerg Med (Fremantle)* 14 (4):422–429, 2002.

14. Somberg JC, Bailin SJ, Haffajee CI, et al.: Intravenous lidocaine versus intravenous amiodarone (in a new aqueous formulation) for incessant ventricular tachycardia, *Am J Cardiol* 90 (8): 853–859, 2002.

15. Szekely B, Saint-Marc T, Degremont AC, et al.: Value of bispectral index monitoring during cardiopulmonary resuscitation, *Br J Anaesth* 88 (3):443–444, 2002.

Pulseless Electrical Activity (PEA)

ERIK A. BOATMAN, M.D.

Successful pharmacological and electrical treatment of any cardiac arrest depends on definitive identification of the underlying arrhythmia.[1,2] The best survival rates can be achieved by early recognition, treatment, and restoration of circulation.[3,4] Pulseless electrical activity (PEA) implies an identifiable organized rhythm other than ventricular fibrillation (VF) or pulseless ventricular tachycardia (PVT) without palpable pulse or effective circulation. Paramount in the treatment of this disorder is effective CPR and identification and correction of any underlying etiologies for the arrhythmia; otherwise efforts will likely be futile. Prognosis and survival is generally poor, especially if noted in a prehospital setting or after blunt trauma.[5] Open cardiac massage may be lifesaving if penetrating cardiac trauma is present.

A. On recognition of an unconscious patient, check for responsiveness, call for help and a defibrillator, and evaluate the surrounding scene. Begin with a primary ABCD survey. Open the airway, check for breathing and provide breaths if necessary, check for a pulse and begin chest compressions if needed. Proper precordial compression can reproduce approximately one third of prearrest stroke volume. Palpate the femoral pulse (evaluate efficacy) and check end-tidal carbon dioxide (CO_2), quantitative measurement.[6] Rotate resuscitators when fatigued to maximize efforts. On arrival of a defibrillator, immediately apply paddles or pads to evaluate the rhythm.

B. After initial assessment, proceed with a secondary ABCD survey, focusing on more advanced assessments and treatments. Place a definitive airway; confirm its location and secure.[7] Emphasis is on protecting the airway through any means available (endotracheal tube, laryngeal mask airway [LMA], or Combitube). Ventilate by hand or machine. One can provide significantly higher PaO_2 and delivery of oxygen (O_2) if pressure support ventilation is enhanced with continuous positive airway pressure or a PEEP valve.[8] Obtain IV access if not already available. Reevaluate the cardiac rhythm. If PEA is still present, begin administering medications per the advanced cardiac life support (ACLS) protocol. Flush medications into circulation with saline and circulate with chest compressions for maximal benefit. Formulate a differential diagnosis to identify potentially correctable etiologies to aid in resuscitation. Efficacy of resuscitative efforts are difficult to ascertain; bispectral index monitoring (BIS) may offer some reassurance to the resuscitation team if available.[9]

C. Direct therapies at normalization of temperature, correcting deficiencies, overloads, and overdoses and relieving blockages and pressures that impede normal blood flow. Pulmonary embolism may be responsible for a large proportion of PEA, which, if diagnosed, may permit wider use of thrombolytic agents to improve survival.[10,11] The most frequent etiologies for PEA can be easily remembered as the five "H's" and five "T's".[1]

D. Unfortunately, unless a specific etiology is found and treated, the prognosis of PEA is poor and therapy is limited. Epinephrine, vasopressin, and atropine (if the underlying rhythm is bradycardic) are the mainstays of treatment. Calcium is recommended only in the treatment of documented hypocalcemia, hyperkalemia, hypermagnesemia, or a calcium channel blocker overdose. Bicarbonate is recommended only in the treatment of preexisting metabolic acidosis, hyperkalemia, or to alkalanize the urine. Routine or prophylactic use will rapidly produce high levels of CO_2, which readily crosses cell membranes and the blood-brain barrier. This results in worsened intracellular acidosis and reduced responsiveness to catecholamines and resuscitation, and detrimentally alters osmolality and the oxygen-hemoglobin dissociation curve. Endogenous adenosine, which is released in response to hypoxia and ischemia, can be competitively reversed with an experimental adenosine antagonist or aminophylline in porcine models.[12] Although it may be effective, data on the usefulness of vasopressin in PEA was insufficient to be recommended in the latest American Heart Association's (AHA) resuscitation guidelines in 2000.[13] Dextrose or dextrose-containing solutions may lead to hyperosmotic diuresis, may worsen neurological outcome, and are recommended only in the treatment of hypoglycemia. Free water administration is also not recommended as it may lead to cerebral edema.

E. Perhaps the most difficult decision to make is termination of efforts. If PEA persists despite efforts, resuscitation algorithms have been exhausted, and no atypical clinical features are present that have not been addressed, discuss ending the resuscitation with the team. All participants should feel that all efforts have been exhausted prior to termination.

REFERENCES

1. Cummins RO, editor: ACLS provider manual. Dallas, 2001, The American Heart Association. Field JM, editor: Advanced cardiovascular life support provider manual. American Heart Association, 2006.
2. American Heart Association: 2005 American Heart Association guidelines for cardiopulmonary resuscitation and emergency cardiovascular care. Circulation 112:1-211, 2005.
3. Trappe HJ, Brandts B, Weismueller P: Arrhythmias in the intensive care patient, Curr Opin Crit Care 9 (5):345–355, 2003.
4. Gullo A: Cardiac arrest, chain of survival and Utstein style, Eur J Anaesthesiol 19 (9):624–633, 2002.
5. Martin SK, Shatney CH, Sherck JP, et al.: Blunt trauma patients with prehospital pulseless electrical activity (PEA): poor ending assured, J Trauma 53 (5):876–881, 2002.

Unconscious patient

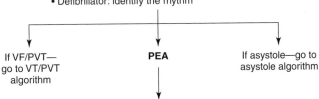

- Check responsiveness
- Activate emergency response system
- Call for defibrillator
- Rapidly survey the scene: is there any reason that resuscitation should NOT occur (eg, DNR order, signs of death, personal danger)

(A) **Primary ABCD survey:**
- Airway: open the airway
- Breathing: check for breathing, provide positive-pressure ventilations if indicated
- Circulation: check for pulse, begin chest compressions if indicated
- Defibrillator: identify the rhythm

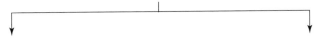

If VF/PVT—
go to VT/PVT
algorithm

PEA

If asystole—go to
asystole algorithm

(B) **Secondary ABCD survey:**
- Airway: place airway securing device as soon as possible
- Breathing: confirm airway device placement by exam AND objective confirmation device, demonstrate effective oxygenation and ventilation, secure airway device
- Circulation: establish IV access, identify rhythm on defibrillator monitor, continue chest compressions, administer medications appropriate for rhythm and condition
- Differential diagnosis: search for and treat identified reversible causes

(C) **Common etiologies and treatments:**
- Hypoxia—administer 100% F_iO_2
- Hypovolemia — administer crystalloid, colloid, or blood products as needed
- Hydrogen ion (acidosis) — consider bicarbonate (1 mEq/kg IVP, 0.5 mEq/kg q10 min) for preexisting metabolic acidosis
- Hyper/hypo-kalemia — consider bicarbonate for hyperkalemia, cautiously assess the need for potassium administration
- Hypothermia — administer warm fluids, warming blanket
- Tension pneumothorax — relieve with needle or tube thoracostomy
- Tamponade (cardiac) — relieve with needle aspiration
- Thrombosis (pulmonary embolism) — consider the use of thrombolytics
- Thrombosis (coronary, massive MI) — consider the use of thrombolytics
- Tablets (drug overdose — tricyclics, barbiturates, digitalis, beta-blockers, calcium channel blockers) — consider bicarbonate for alkalanization of urine, calcium (10 mg/kg slow IVP, repeat as needed) for hyperkalemia and calcium channel blocker overdose

(D) **Other treatments:**
- Epinephrine 1 mg IVP, repeat every 3–5 minutes, or Vasopressin 40 units IVP, 1 dose, to replace first or second dose of epinephrine
- Consider atropine 1 mg IVP for slow PEA, repeat every 3–5 minutes up to 3 doses

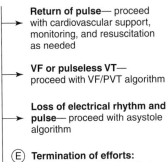

Return of pulse— proceed with cardiovascular support, monitoring, and resuscitation as needed

VF or pulseless VT—
proceed with VF/PVT algorithm

Loss of electrical rhythm and pulse— proceed with asystole algorithm

(E) **Termination of efforts:**
- PEA persists despite efforts
- Consider quality and duration of resuscitation
- No atypical clinical features unaddressed
- Consider ending resuscitation

6. Pernat A, Weil MH, Sun S, et al.: Stroke volumes and end-tidal carbon dioxide generated by precordial compression during ventricular fibrillation, *Crit Care Med* 31 (6):1819–1823, 2003.
7. Gabrielli A, Layon AJ, Wenzel V, et al.: Alternative ventilation strategies in cardiopulmonary resuscitation, *Curr Opin Crit Care* 8 (3):199–211, 2002.
8. Kleinsasser A, Lindner KH, Schaefer A, et al.: Decompression-triggered positive-pressure ventilation during cardiopulmonary resuscitation improves pulmonary gas exchange and oxygen uptake, *Circulation* 106 (3):373–378, 2002.
9. Szekely B, Saint-Marc T, Degremont AC, et al.: Value of bispectral index monitoring during cardiopulmonary resuscitation, *Br J Anaesth* 88 (3):443–444, 2002.

10. Comess KA, DeRook FA, Russell ML, et al.: The incidence of pulmonary embolism in unexplained sudden cardiac arrest with pulseless electrical activity, *Am J Med* 109 (5):351–356, 2000.
11. Newman DH, Greenwald I, Callaway CW: Cardiac arrest and the role of thrombolytic agents, *Ann Emerg Med* 35 (5):472–480, 2000.
12. Kelsch T, Kikuchi K, Vahdat S, et al.: Innovative pharmacologic approaches to cardiopulmonary resuscitation, *Heart Dis* 3 (1): 46–54, 2001.

LIFE-THREATENING DYSRHYTHMIAS WITHOUT CARDIAC ARREST

BRADYCARDIA

VENTRICULAR ECTOPY

TACHYARRHYTHMIAS

Bradycardia

STEPHEN T. ROBINSON, M.D.

Sinus bradycardia in adults occurs when the sinus node discharges less than 60 times per minute. It is considered clinically significant and warrants treatment if there is a decrease in effective cardiac output causing symptomatic hypotension. Sinus bradycardia is the result of a disorder of impulse formation characterized by an inappropriate discharge rate of the normal pacemaker, the sinus node. In humans, the sinus node is less than 1 mm from the epicardial surface. It lies in the right atrial sulcus terminalis at the junction of the superior vena cava and the right atrium. Its arterial supply is from branches of the right coronary artery (55 to 60% of the time) or from the left circumflex (40 to 45% of the time). Sinus node innervation is by both postganglionic adrenergic and cholinergic nerve terminals. Acetylcholine release by vagal stimulation slows the rate of sinus nodal discharge and prolongs intranodal conduction. Adrenergic stimulation increases the rate of sinus nodal discharge.

Treatment of sinus bradycardia is not always necessary, but if symptoms occur because of an inadequate cardiac output or if arrhythmias occur because of the slow rate, atropine is effective in increasing the HR. If atropine is not adequately effective and there are persistent symptoms of congestive heart failure or symptoms of low cardiac output, electrical pacing may be required. In an emergent situation, transcutaneous pacing or insertion of a transvenous pacing wire can be a temporary solution and will act as bridge to placement of a permanent transvenous dual chamber pacemaker.[1]

Sinus node dysfunction (sick sinus syndrome), type II second-degree atrioventricular (AV) block and type III AV block, all have the potential for long sinus pauses or sinus arrest. The decision made regarding the necessity of a pacemaker for these conditions is largely influenced by the presence of symptoms resulting from the bradycardia.

A. Assess vital signs and perform a primary ABCD survey. Apply monitoring. Next perform a secondary ABCD survey. Establish a secured airway if necessary, administer supplemental oxygen (O_2), and gain IV access. Continue to monitor vital signs and obtain a 12-lead ECG and chest x-ray. Attempt a problem-focused history and physical examination.
B. Establish a differential diagnosis and correct possible causes of symptomatic bradycardia. Sinus bradycardia is a result of excessive vagal tone or decreased sympathetic tone. Sinus bradycardia can also be an effect of medications or anatomical changes in the sinus node. In most instances sinus bradycardia is a benign arrhythmia and when it is asymptomatic does not need treatment. Bradycardia in the setting of an acute myocardial infarction (AMI) is common and is usually not harmful.
C. Type II second-degree AV block is usually infranodal, especially when a widened QRS complex is present. Symptoms are frequent, prognosis is poorer, and there is a propensity to progress to third-degree AV block (complete heart block). Bradycardia associated with type II second-degree AV block and complete heart block unresponsive to atropine usually requires temporary pacing.
D. In an unstable patient, treat bradycardia immediately and begin preparations for cardiac pacing. Atropine is effective in increasing the HR by enhancing the rate of discharge of the sinoatrial node and improves AV conduction. Administer atropine for severe sinus bradycardia with hypotension, high-degree AV block, and slow idioventricular rates. Use atropine cautiously in the presence of AMI to correct severe bradycardia that is causing hypotension or ventricular ectopy; a goal heart rate is 60 beats per minute. If the arrhythmia is refractory to atropine, begin cardiac pacing. Start infusions of epinephrine or dopamine during preparations for pacing. Isoproterenol is no longer recommended as a treatment for symptomatic bradycardia.[2]

REFERENCES

1. Gregoratos G, Abrams J, Epstein AE, et al.: ACC/AHA/NASPE 2002 guideline update for implantation of cardiac pacemakers and antiarrhythmia devices: summary article. A report of the American College of Cardiology/American Heart Association Task Force on Practice Guidelines (ACC/AHA/NASPE Committee to Update the 1998 Pacemaker Guidelines), *J Cardiovasc Electrophysiol* 13 (11):1183–1199, 2002.
2. American Heart Association: American Heart Association 2005 guidelines for cardiopulmonary resuscitation and emergency cardiovascular care. Part 7.3: management of symptomatic bradycardia and tachycardia, *Circulation* 112 (24 Suppl): IV-67–77, 2005.

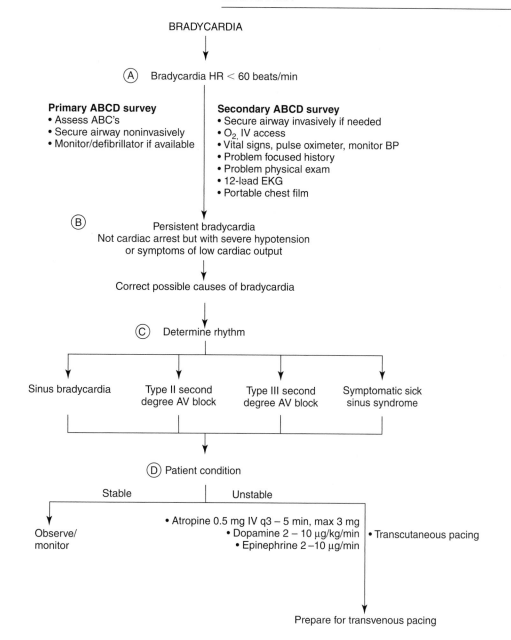

BRADYCARDIA

(A)   Bradycardia HR < 60 beats/min

Primary ABCD survey
• Assess ABC's
• Secure airway noninvasively
• Monitor/defibrillator if available

Secondary ABCD survey
• Secure airway invasively if needed
• O_2, IV access
• Vital signs, pulse oximeter, monitor BP
• Problem focused history
• Problem physical exam
• 12-lead EKG
• Portable chest film

(B)   Persistent bradycardia
Not cardiac arrest but with severe hypotension
or symptoms of low cardiac output

Correct possible causes of bradycardia

(C)   Determine rhythm

| Sinus bradycardia | Type II second degree AV block | Type III second degree AV block | Symptomatic sick sinus syndrome |

(D) Patient condition

Stable

Unstable

Observe/
monitor

• Atropine 0.5 mg IV q3 – 5 min, max 3 mg
• Dopamine 2 – 10 μg/kg/min
• Epinephrine 2 –10 μg/min

• Transcutaneous pacing

Prepare for transvenous pacing

Ventricular Ectopy

KIMBERLY D. MILHOAN, M.D.

Premature ventricular complexes are a common ECG finding and may not signal a risk of more serious dysrhythmia. The need to treat ventricular ectopy is debatable. A stable pattern of ventricular ectopy requires no therapy. New ventricular ectopy requires a search for the inciting cause (see Table 1). Pharmacological suppression of frequent and multifocal ectopy and nonsustained ventricular tachycardia (VT) has become less common in the context of continuous ECG surveillance and immediate defibrillation. Suppressive therapy is indicated on observing an increasing pattern of ectopy, including frequent or multifocal premature complexes or VT outside an ICU and in the absence of an immediate resuscitation capacity. Once ventricular ectopy is suppressed, therapy is maintained by continuous infusion of the effective drug.[1-4]

A. As an alternative to the intermittent bolus technique, lidocaine therapy may be initiated with a loading infusion rate of 15 mg/min until the ectopy resolves or a total loading dose of 3 mg/kg has been given. This dose is reduced by 50% for patients with heart failure, impaired hepatic blood flow or function, or advanced age.

B. Procainamide administration is guided by BP and ECG monitoring. The drug has negative inotropic and vasodilating actions. Adverse ECG effects include widening of the QRS complex by 50% of its original duration and lengthening of the PR and QT intervals. If the premature ventricular contractions (PVCs) occur in the context of bradycardia, speeding up the sinoatrial (SA) node, with drugs such as atropine or isoproterenol or with pacing, may be effective.

REFERENCES

1. Kudenchuk PJ: Advanced cardiac life support antiarrhythmic drugs, *Cardiol Clin* 20:79–87, 2002.
2. Feeley TW: Management of perioperative arrhythmias, *J Cardiothorac Vasc Anesth* 11 (Supp1):10–15, 1997.
3. Miller SM, Mayer RC: Con: antiarrhythmic drugs should not be used to suppress ventricular ectopy in the perioperative period, *J Cardiothorac Vasc Anesth* 8:701–703, 1994.
4. Discher T, Kumar P: Pro: antiarrhythmic drugs should be used to suppress ventricular ectopy in the perioperative period, *J Cardiothorac Vasc Anesth* 8:699–700, 1994.

TABLE 1
Causes of Acute Cardiac Dysrhythmias

Hypoxemia	Major electrolyte abnormalities
Hypercarbia	Hypotension
Drug effects/interactions	Congestive heart failure/fluid overload
Epinephrine-containing local anesthetic solutions	Myocardial ischemia
Local anesthetic toxicity	Intrinsic heart disease
Volatile general anesthetics	Coronary artery disease
High-dose fentanyl and related opioids	Cardiomyopathy
Pancuronium, gallamine, succinylcholine	Wolff-Parkinson-White syndrome
Succinylcholine-induced hyperkalemia	Long QT syndrome
Digitalis toxicity	Mitral valve prolapse
Tricyclic antidepressant drug interaction	Thrombotic/air embolism
Cocaine intoxication	Malignant hyperthermia
Light anesthesia	Pheochromocytoma
Vagal reflexes	Electrocution
Carotid sinus	Extraocular muscles
Abdominal, thoracic viscera	Vasovagal faint
Hypothermia	Hyperthermia

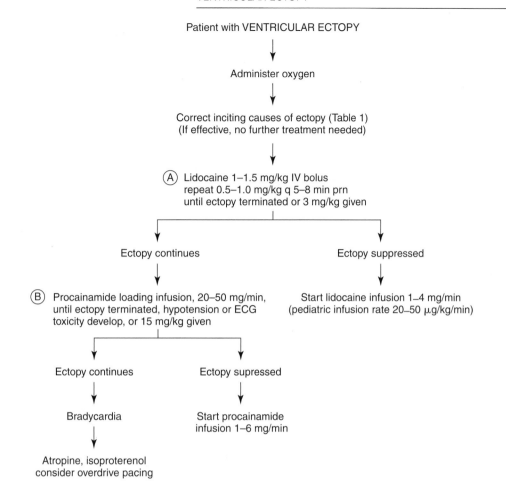

Patient with VENTRICULAR ECTOPY

↓

Administer oxygen

↓

Correct inciting causes of ectopy (Table 1)
(If effective, no further treatment needed)

↓

(A) Lidocaine 1–1.5 mg/kg IV bolus
repeat 0.5–1.0 mg/kg q 5–8 min prn
until ectopy terminated or 3 mg/kg given

Ectopy continues   Ectopy suppressed

(B) Procainamide loading infusion, 20–50 mg/min,   Start lidocaine infusion 1–4 mg/min
until ectopy terminated, hypotension or ECG   (pediatric infusion rate 20–50 μg/kg/min)
toxicity develop, or 15 mg/kg given

Ectopy continues   Ectopy supressed

Bradycardia   Start procainamide
infusion 1–6 mg/min

Atropine, isoproterenol
consider overdrive pacing

Tachyarrhythmias

VIVIAN HOU, M.D.

JORGE PINEDA, M.D.

Arrhythmias are a significant source of perioperative morbidity that may increase the length of hospital stay and surgery.[1] The International Liaison Committee on Resuscitation divides tachycardias into four diagnostic categories.[2] These include atrial fibrillation and atrial flutter, narrow complex tachycardias, wide complex tachycardias of unknown type, and stable monomorphic and polymorphic ventricular tachycardia. Sinus tachycardia will not be addressed.

A. The first critical decision point is whether the patient is hemodynamically stable. If at any point the patient is determined to be unstable, attempt immediate electrical cardioversion. Signs of instability include hypotension, heart failure, shortness of breath, shock, altered consciousness, angina, or acute myocardial infarction. Otherwise, systematic evaluation and medical therapy may be pursued. Obtain cardiology consultation if the time course permits.

B. Examine the ECG rhythm strip closely to determine whether the arrhythmia is wide or narrow complex. Wide complex tachyarrhythmias include narrow complex with aberrancy, antidromic atrioventricular reciprocating tachycardia (AVRT) in patients with WPW, and ventricular tachycardia (monomorphic or polymorphic). Evaluate for treatable causes of ventricular tachycardia (VT) prior to or during the treatment of VT. The most common causes of monomorphic VT include hypoxemia, hypercarbia, hypokalemia, or hypomagnesemia, digitalis toxicity, and acid-base derangements. Polymorphic VT is often rapid, hemodynamically unstable, and life threatening. Polymorphic VT with a prolonged QT interval is known as Torsades de Pointes. This arrhythmia is recognized by its characteristic twisting of the QRS axis around the baseline. Causes include medications (such as quinidine, procainamide, disopyramide, and phenothiazines) and bradycardia, hypokalemia, hypomagnesemia, or acute ischemia or infarction. Polymorphic VT without prolongation of the QT interval is typically caused by ischemia. Treatment of wide complex tachycardias is largely dependent on stable versus unstable hemodynamics. Urgent cardioversion (synchronous for monomorphic VT and asynchronous/defibrillation if synchronous is not possible, delayed, or if patient decompensates) is indicated in the hemodynamically unstable patient, whereas medical management is indicated for the stable patient. The preferred treatment for patients with atrial fibrillation or atrial flutter associated with WPW is electrical cardioversion. Appropriate medications for medical cardioversion include amiodarone, procainamide, flecainide, sotalol, and propafenone. Contraindicated drugs for rate control in this situation include adenosine, beta blockers, calcium channel blockers, and digoxin.

C. Narrow complex tachycardias must be further evaluated for regularity. If regular, vagal maneuvers or adenosine may be used to determine the etiology or terminate the rapid rhythm. Adenosine induces transient block of atrioventricular (AV) nodal conduction. Possible complications of adenosine administration include rate acceleration if administered slowly, or if given to a patient in atrial fibrillation/flutter in association with a preexcitation syndrome. Bronchospasm may result in a patient with reactive airway disease. Patients on methylxanthines (theophylline) are less sensitive to adenosine because methylxanthines have adenosine receptor antagonist activity. Dipyridamole blocks transport of adenosine back into cells and may enhance sensitivity to adenosine. Cardiac transplantation may result in exaggerated bradycardic response to adenosine administration. True junctional tachycardia is rare in adults. It is usually a manifestation of digoxin toxicity or excessive use of exogenous catecholamines or theophylline. If the arrhythmia is unresponsive to vagal maneuvers or adenosine, rate control of the arrhythmia can be accomplished with use of calcium channel blockers or beta blockers. Use caution with primary antiarrhythmic drugs, because their hypotensive effects and potential for proarrhythmia may result in decompensation of the patient.

D. An irregular narrow-complex tachycardia may result from atrial fibrillation or flutter, or multifocal atrial tachycardia (MAT). MAT is usually described as occurring in patients with chronic obstructive pulmonary disease (COPD), especially during exacerbations. Diagnosis requires recognition of at least three morphologically distinct P waves in the same lead with a rate of >100 beats per minute. Misdiagnosis as atrial fibrillation is a concern because it may lead to ineffective and harmful therapy. Digoxin and cardioversion are ineffective in the treatment of MAT. Patients with atrial fibrillation or flutter who are clinically stable can be treated with medications that decrease ventricular rate by inhibiting AV node conduction. If left ventricular function is normal, slow the ventricular rate with a beta blocker or calcium channel blocker. Determine the duration of the arrhythmia. Electric cardioversion is the preferred treatment for conversion to sinus rhythm if duration is <48 hours. If the arrhythmia is present for >48 hours, there is an increased risk of embolism from atrial thrombus, and electrical or pharmacologic cardioversion should be delayed until enough time has passed to allow for anticoagulation.

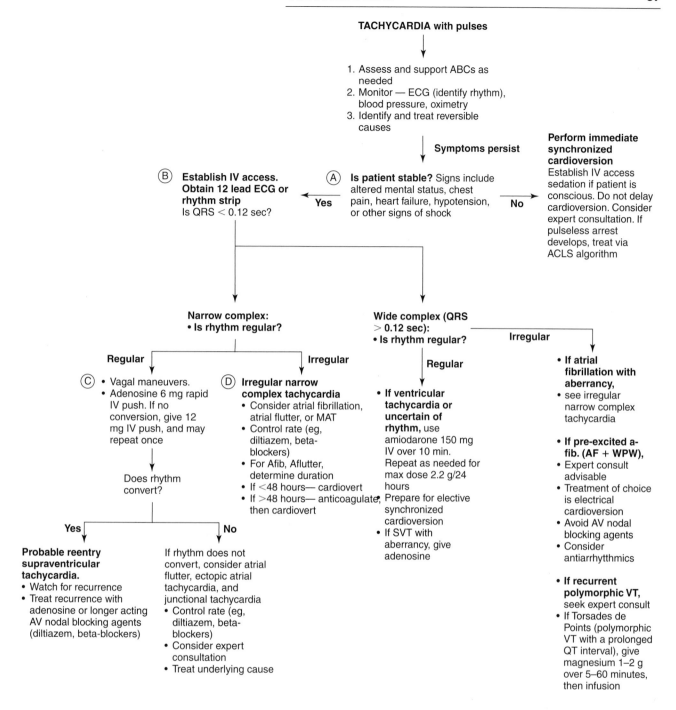

TACHYCARDIA with pulses

1. Assess and support ABCs as needed
2. Monitor — ECG (identify rhythm), blood pressure, oximetry
3. Identify and treat reversible causes

Symptoms persist

(A) **Is patient stable?** Signs include altered mental status, chest pain, heart failure, hypotension, or other signs of shock

Yes →

(B) **Establish IV access. Obtain 12 lead ECG or rhythm strip**
Is QRS < 0.12 sec?

No →

Perform immediate synchronized cardioversion
Establish IV access sedation if patient is conscious. Do not delay cardioversion. Consider expert consultation. If pulseless arrest develops, treat via ACLS algorithm

Narrow complex:
• **Is rhythm regular?**

Wide complex (QRS > 0.12 sec):
• **Is rhythm regular?**

Irregular

Regular

Irregular

Regular

(C)
• Vagal maneuvers.
• Adenosine 6 mg rapid IV push. If no conversion, give 12 mg IV push, and may repeat once

Does rhythm convert?

Yes

No

(D) **Irregular narrow complex tachycardia**
• Consider atrial fibrillation, atrial flutter, or MAT
• Control rate (eg, diltiazem, beta-blockers)
• For Afib, Aflutter, determine duration
• If <48 hours— cardiovert
• If >48 hours— anticoagulate, then cardiovert

• If **ventricular tachycardia or uncertain of rhythm,** use amiodarone 150 mg IV over 10 min. Repeat as needed for max dose 2.2 g/24 hours
• Prepare for elective synchronized cardioversion
• If SVT with aberrancy, give adenosine

• **If atrial fibrillation with aberrancy,**
• see irregular narrow complex tachycardia

• **If pre-excited a-fib. (AF + WPW),**
• Expert consult advisable
• Treatment of choice is electrical cardioversion
• Avoid AV nodal blocking agents
• Consider antiarrhythmics

• **If recurrent polymorphic VT,** seek expert consult
• If Torsades de Points (polymorphic VT with a prolonged QT interval), give magnesium 1–2 g over 5–60 minutes, then infusion

Probable reentry supraventricular tachycardia.
• Watch for recurrence
• Treat recurrence with adenosine or longer acting AV nodal blocking agents (diltiazem, beta-blockers)

If rhythm does not convert, consider atrial flutter, ectopic atrial tachycardia, and junctional tachycardia
• Control rate (eg, diltiazem, beta-blockers)
• Consider expert consultation
• Treat underlying cause

REFERENCES

1. Balser, JR: New concepts in antiarrhythmic therapy, *ASA Refresher Course*, 2000.
2. International Liaison Committee on Resuscitation: 2005 International consensus on cardiopulmonary resuscitation and emergency cardiovascular care science with treatment recommendations,

Circulation 112:III-1–III-136, 2005. American Heart Association guidelines for cardiopulmonary resuscitation and emergency cardiovascular care. Part 7.3: management of symptomatic bradycardia and tachycardia, Circulation 112 (suppl): 67-77, 2005.

PREANESTHESIA ASSESSMENT

PREOPERATIVE LABORATORY TESTING

PERIOPERATIVE ANTICOAGULATION

Preoperative Laboratory Testing

CHRISTOPHER D. NEWELL, M.D.

The purpose of preoperative laboratory testing is to guide clinical decision making and thereby optimize patient outcome. No test is 100% sensitive and specific, and results must be interpreted in the context of the clinical situation. There are costs associated with nonindicated testing—the need to check results and the requirement to follow up on abnormal results. Routine laboratory tests are avoided in favor of those tests that have a reasonable chance of yielding meaningful results, given the particular clinical situation.[1-3]

A. Start with a complete history and physical examination. The patient's medical record is a valuable source of information. In addition, the presenting surgical problem should help guide the preanesthetic evaluation. Before ordering any preoperative laboratory tests, consider how the results will affect the patient's care. A preoperative test is useless if it has no impact on clinical management and may be harmful if it guides interventions that are not appropriate.

B. If the patient's medical condition and treatment have been stable, test results within 6 months of the planned procedure are acceptable.

C. The incidence of abnormal ECGs increases with advancing age. There has been no consensus on the appropriate age when a preoperative ECG is required. Age alone is used by some as an indication for preoperative ECG, and others believe that age is not an important factor. Obtain a preoperative ECG in all patients with cardiovascular disease, uncontrolled hypertension, respiratory disease, or multiple risk factors for coronary artery disease, regardless of age.

D. Obtain a preoperative chest x-ray in patients who have active chest disease or require an intrathoracic procedure. Advanced age, stable pulmonary or cardiac disease, smoking, and resolved upper respiratory infection are generally not indications for a preoperative chest x-ray.

E. Obtain a baseline preoperative hematocrit in patients scheduled for procedures with anticipated large blood loss. Also consider a baseline hematocrit in patients with liver disease, hematologic disorders, extremes of age, or anemia.

F. Obtain coagulation studies (e.g., international normalized ratio [INR], prothrombin time [PT], partial thromboplastin time [PTT], platelet count, other studies as indicated) in patients who have known bleeding disorders, renal disease, or hepatic disease, and in patients taking anticoagulant medications. Always consider the nature of the planned procedure as well as the anesthetic plan.

G. Serum chemistries are most frequently ordered as various panels including electrolytes, glucose, and measures of renal and liver function. Obtain appropriate serum chemistries in patients with a history of renal, hepatic, or endocrine disease and those patients taking medications which may affect chemistries (e.g., diuretics) or be affected by them (e.g., digoxin).

H. The use of routine preoperative pregnancy tests is controversial. History is unreliable for identifying early pregnancy. Consider pregnancy testing for all women of childbearing capability.

REFERENCES

1. Pasternak LR, Arens JF, Caplan RA, et al.: Practice advisory for preanesthesia evaluation: a report by the American Society of Anesthesiologists task force on preanesthesia evaluation, *Anesthesiology* 96:485–496, 2002.
2. Hata TM, Moyers JR: Preoperative evaluation and management. In Barash PG, Cullen BF, Stoelting RK, editors: *Clinical anesthesia,* ed 5 chapter 18: 475-501, 2006. Lippincott Williams and Wilkins.
3. Smetana GW, Macpherson DS: The case against preoperative laboratory testing, *Med Clin North Am* 87:7–40, 2003.

PREOPERATIVE LABORATORY EVALUATION

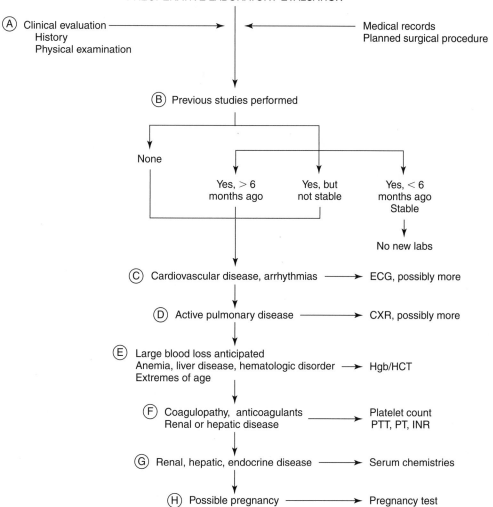

Perioperative Anticoagulation

JAMES C. OPTON, M.D.

THOMAS FRIETSCH, M.D.

Perioperative anticoagulation is indicated in three situations: as thromboprophylaxis, in patients taking chronic oral anticoagulation therapy, and intraoperatively in certain surgical procedures, such as vascular and cardiac surgeries. Intraoperative anticoagulation is usually reversed or allowed to wear off and will not be discussed. The rationale for perioperative prophylactic anticoagulation is based on a high prevalence of venous thromboembolism (VTE) among hospitalized patients and the high morbidity and mortality associated with unprevented thrombi.[1,2]

A. Not all patients need perioperative anticoagulation thromboprophylaxis. Patients having minor surgery, less than 40 years old, and with no additional risk factors (see section C) require only early ambulation.[1]

B. Decisions about anticoagulation weigh the benefit of treatment with the bleeding risk. Absolute Contraindications include active hemorrhage, history of heparin-induced thrombocytopenia (HIT), and indwelling epidural/spinal catheter (depending on timing of placement or removal—see section G). Relative contraindications include history of cerebral hemorrhage, GI/genitourinary hemorrhage within the last 6 months, and active intracranial lesions. Low molecular weight heparin (LMWH) should be used with caution in patients with renal insufficiency.

C. The thromboembolic prophylactic regimen depends on age, surgery type, and risk factors (See Table 1.) Risk factors include prior history of postoperative deep vein thrombosis (DVT), family history of DVT/pulmonary embolism (PE), venous stasis, congestive heart failure (CHF), stroke with paralysis, spinal cord injury, inflammatory bowel disease (IBD), bed immobilization >12 hrs, history of idiopathic DVT, hypercoagulable states, malignancy, trauma, major surgery, and age over 40.[1]

   The specific dosing regimen for LMWH varies depending on the surgical procedure and bleeding risk. New anticoagulants have been developed and clinical trials are ongoing.[1]

D. The most common indications for Coumadin therapy are atrial fibrillation, VTE, and the presence of a mechanical heart valve.[2] Perioperative management is challenging, because medication must be discontinued to prevent excessive bleeding. The perioperative management of patients on chronic Coumadin therapy is challenging. Indications for Coumadin therapy include atrial fibrillation, VTE, and the presence of a mechanical heart valve. If the Coumadin is discontinued temporarily to prevent excessive surgical bleeding, then the risk of a thromboembolic event increases.[3,4] However, interruption of therapy increases the risk of a thromboembolic event.[3,4] Certain minimally invasive procedures carry a low risk of bleeding and oral anticoagulation therapy can continue uninterrupted.[3]

E. Bridging therapy is considered when oral therapy must be interrupted for higher risk surgical procedures. Patients are classified into high, moderate, and low risk groups.[4] (See Table 2.) Bridging anticoagulant therapy is strongly recommended in the high-risk group and should be considered in the moderate risk group. It is optional in the low-risk group and oral anticoagulation can be stopped 5 days before surgery and resumed afterwards.[4] Patients receiving Coumadin with a target international normalized ratio (INR) of 2.0 to 3.0 should stop Coumadin 5 days before surgery. Patients with a target INR of 2.5 to 3.5 should stop Coumadin 6 days before surgery. The INR should be checked the day before surgery and if it is >1.5, 1 mg of vitamin K should be taken. Bridging LMWH is started 36 to 48 hours after discontinuation of Coumadin, with the last dose administered 12 to 24 hours before surgery to minimize the risk of bleeding. If IV unfractionated heparin (UH) is used as bridging therapy, patients are admitted to the hospital 3 to 4 days before surgery with dose adjustments to achieve a therapeutic activated partial thromboplastin time (aPTT). The UH should be discontinued at least 4 hours before surgery.[4]

F. LMWH is typically restarted at full dose 24 hours following the procedure. For patients at high risk of bleeding, a prophylactic dose of LMWH should be started for the first 24 to 72 hours after surgery. Coumadin is resumed at the preoperative dose on the first postoperative day. INR is monitored daily until the patient is discharged and periodically thereafter. When the INR is therapeutic for two consecutive days, LMWH may be discontinued.[5]

   Alternatives to anticoagulant therapy in the setting of poor surgical hemostasis or contraindications to therapy include compression stockings, sequential compression devices (SCDs), and vena cava filters.

G. Neuraxial anesthesia in the setting of perioperative anticoagulation requires caution and health care providers should be familiar with the American Society of Regional Anesthesia guidelines[6] (See Table 3.)

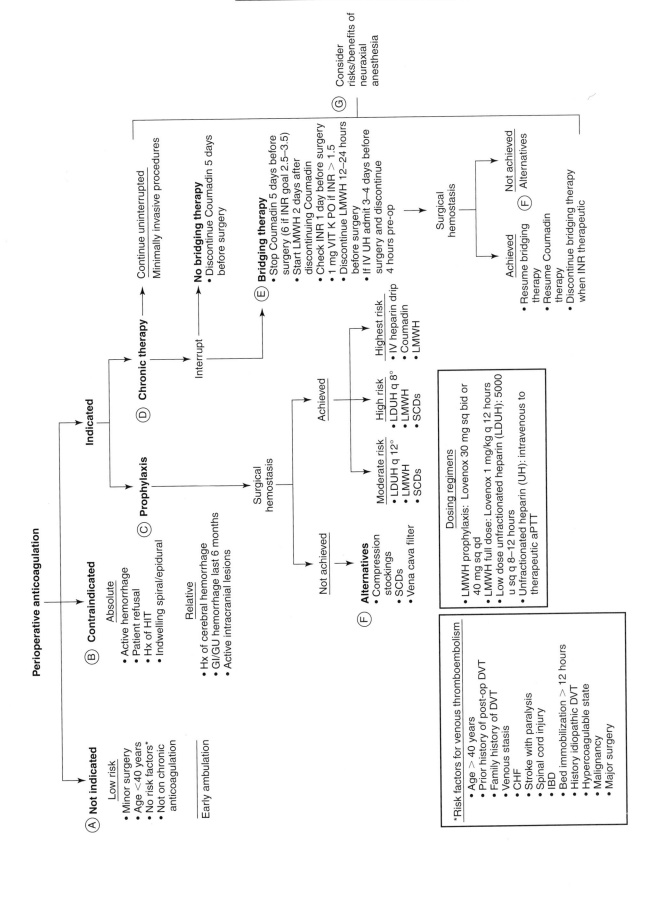

Perioperative anticoagulation

Not indicated (A)

<u>Low risk</u>
• Minor surgery
• Age <40 years
• No risk factors*
• Not on chronic anticoagulation

Early ambulation

(B) **Contraindicated**

<u>Absolute</u>
• Active hemorrhage
• Patient refusal
• Hx of HIT
• Indwelling spiral/epidural

<u>Relative</u>
• Hx of cerebral hemorrhage
• GI/GU hemorrhage last 6 months
• Active intracranial lesions

Indicated

(C) **Prophylaxis**

(D) **Chronic therapy**

Surgical hemostasis

<u>Not achieved</u>

(F) **Alternatives**
• Compression stockings
• SCDs
• Vena cava filter

<u>Achieved</u>

<u>Moderate risk</u>
• LDUH q 12°
• LMWH
• SCDs

<u>High risk</u>
• LDUH q 8°
• LMWH
• SCDs

<u>Highest risk</u>
• IV heparin drip
• Coumadin
• LMWH

Interrupt

Continue uninterrupted

Minimally invasive procedures

No bridging therapy
• Discontinue Coumadin 5 days before surgery

(E) **Bridging therapy**
• Stop Coumadin 5 days before surgery (6 if INR goal 2.5–3.5)
• Start LMWH 2 days after discontinuing Coumadin
• Check INR 1 day before surgery
• 1 mg VIT K PO if INR > 1.5
• Discontinue LMWH 12–24 hours before surgery
• If IV UH admit 3–4 days before surgery and discontinue 4 hours pre-op

(G) Consider risks/benefits of neuraxial anesthesia

Surgical hemostasis

<u>Achieved</u>
• Resume bridging therapy
• Resume Coumadin therapy
• Discontinue bridging therapy when INR therapeutic

<u>Not achieved</u>
(F) Alternatives

<u>Dosing regimens</u>
• LMWH prophylaxis: Lovenox 30 mg sq bid or 40 mg sq qd
• LMWH full dose: Lovenox 1 mg/kg q 12 hours
• Low dose unfractionated heparin (LDUH): 5000 u sq q 8–12 hours
• Unfractionated heparin (UH): intravenous to therapeutic aPTT

---

*Risk factors for venous thromboembolism
• Age > 40 years
• Prior history of post-op DVT
• Family history of DVT
• Venous stasis
• CHF
• Stroke with paralysis
• Spinal cord injury
• IBD
• Bed immobilization > 12 hours
• History idiopathic DVT
• Hypercoagulable state
• Malignancy
• Major surgery

TABLE 1
Prophylaxis regimens determined by risk factors

Low risk	Early ambulation
Moderate risk (1 to 2 risk factors)	Low dose unfractionated heparin (LDUH) SQ every 12 hours or LMWH or SCDs
High risk (3 to 4 risk factors)	LDUH SW every 8 hours or LMWH or SCDs
Highest risk (>4 risk factors)	IV UH or LMWH or warfarin (Coumadin)

TABLE 2
Risk stratification for bridging therapy

	High risk	Moderate risk	Low risk
Atrial fibrillation Mechanical prosthetic heart valve	Previous stroke or TIA Recent stroke or TIA, prosthetic mitral valve, caged-ball valve, or two prosthetic heart valves	Two or more stroke risk factors Prosthetic heart valve and two or more risk factors	Lone AFIB in <65 years old with no risk factors Aortic prosthetic valve and less than two risk factors
History of VTE	Recent VTE, active cancer, antiphospholipid antibody, or major comorbid disease	VTE within last 6 months or in association with interrupted Coumadin therapy	Remote history of VTE with no additional risk factors

TABLE 3
Anticoagulation and regional anesthesia

Heparin	Give at least 1 hour after needle placement; catheter should be removed at least 2 hours after last dose; should be given at least 1 hour after catheter removal
LMWH	Delay at least 24 hours after bloody needle placement; needle placement should occur 12 hours after prophylactic doses and 24 hours after full doses; catheter removal should occur 2 hours before therapy started
Coumadin	Should be discontinued and INR should be within normal limits; catheters should be removed only when INR <1.5
Nonsteroidal antiinflammatory drugs (NSAIDs)	When used alone, do not increase hematoma risk
Other platelet inhibitors—ticlopdine, clopidogrel, or IIb/IIIa inhibitors	Hematoma risk unknown; should be used with caution

REFERENCES

1. Geerts WH, Pineo GF, Heit JA, et al.: Prevention of venous thromboembolism. The seventh ACCP conference on antithrombotic and thrombolytic therapy, *Chest* 126:338S-400S, 2004.
2. Bates SM, Greer IA, Hirsh J, et al.: Use of antithrombotic agents during pregnancy. The seventh ACCP conference on antithrombotic and thrombolytic therapy, *Chest* 126:627S-644S, 2004.
3. Dunn AS, Turpie AG: Perioperative management of patients receiving oral anticoagulants: a systematic review, *Arch Intern Med* 163: 901-908, 2003.
4. Douketis JD: Perioperative anticoagulation management in patients who are receiving oral anticoagulant therapy: a practical guide for clinicians, *Thromb Res* 108 (1):3–13, 2002.
5. Jaffer AK: Issues in anticoagulant therapy: recent trials start to answer the tough questions, *Cleve Clin J Med* 72 (2):157–163, 2005.
6. Horlocker TT, Wedel DJ, Benzon H, et al.: Regional anesthesia in the anticoagulated patient: Defining the Risks (second ASRA consensus conference on neuraxial anesthesia and anticoagulation), *Reg Anesth Pain Med* 28:172–197, 2003.

PREOPERATIVE PROBLEMS: PULMONARY AND THORACIC DISORDERS

ASTHMA

PERIOPERATIVE WHEEZING

CHRONIC OBSTRUCTIVE PULMONARY
DISEASE (COPD)

CIGARETTE SMOKING

OBSTRUCTIVE SLEEP APNEA (OSA)

KNOWN OR SUSPECTED TUBERCULOSIS (TB)

RESTRICTIVE LUNG DISEASE (RLD)

PULMONARY HYPERTENSION (PHTN)

ANTERIOR MEDIASTINAL MASS (AMM)

Asthma

CATHLEEN L. PETERSON-LAYNE, Ph.D, M.D.

WILLIAM R. FURMAN, M.D.

Asthma is a chronic inflammatory disorder that results in recurrent, episodic, reversible lower airway obstruction. Between episodes, asthmatic patients typically have normal or mildly abnormal pulmonary function. Known triggers of airway reactivity include allergens, infectious processes, physical stimuli, and emotional stress. Symptoms vary from patient to patient but generally include cough (with or without sputum), wheezing, shortness of breath, and exertional dyspnea.

A. Estimate baseline airway function between episodes of asthma. Determine the presence or absence of symptoms at baseline and the medication regimen required to achieve this result. If the patient is not largely symptom-free at baseline, consider the possibility that the patient's asthma is undertreated, or that another process (such as emphysema or chronic bronchitis) is also involved. Review any pre- and postbronchodilator results of spirometry.

B. Based on history and physical examination, decide if the patient is presently at or below baseline. If the patient is at baseline, decide whether the baseline is satisfactory or should be improved with more aggressive pharmacotherapy.

C. Determine if the surgery is elective and should be postponed in favor of further evaluation and therapy.

D. If a delay of surgery is warranted, first-line agents are beta-adrenergic agonists and systemic corticosteroids. For example, initiate therapy with albuterol by metered dose inhaler and a 5-day tapering course of oral prednisone. Ipratropium bromide is a second-line inhaled agent that is sometimes added to treatment with albuterol, especially for smokers. Theophylline, cromolyn sodium, and leukotriene receptor antagonists are not used for treatment of acute exacerbations; however, many patients are maintained on them. As a rule, these agents should be continued perioperatively; encourage strict compliance. If bronchial or pulmonary infection is present, administer antibiotics.

E. If the procedure is urgent or emergent, a nebulization of albuterol with or without ipratropium offers the best chance of immediate improvement in respiratory mechanics and gas exchange. Other options are subcutaneous epinephrine or terbutaline. Consider starting IV steroids early.[1] Consider other causes for wheezing and dyspnea, such as pulmonary embolism and heart failure.

F. Favored induction agents for general anesthesia are IV propofol, IV or IM ketamine, and inhalational sevoflurane or halothane.[2,3] Induction, analgesic, and muscle relaxant agents that release histamine are *not* associated with poor outcomes, and all may be used safely. Volatile anesthetics, the primary agents for maintenance of general anesthesia, bronchodilate.

Avoid nitrous oxide (or use in concentrations of 50% or less) if there is reason for concern about air trapping in obstructed areas of the lungs. If muscle relaxants are needed, consider the use of agents that will not require antagonism with anticholinesterase agents, because the muscarinic properties of these antagonist drugs can promote bronchospasm. Analgesics that selectively inhibit the COX-2 receptor appear safe to use in patients with aspirin-induced asthma.[4]

G. Endotracheal intubation is potentially problematic for asthmatics. Inadequate anesthetic depth may lead to worsening bronchospasm, especially when there is physical stimulation of trachea, carina, or bronchi by the endotracheal tube or by cold, dry inhaled gases. Administer IV lidocaine[5] (1.5 mg/kg) while deepening the anesthetic to attenuate coughing after intubation. Inhalational albuterol (4 puffs) 15 minutes prior to induction prevents intubation-induced bronchoconstriction.[6] Combine inhaled lidocaine with a beta-agonist to provide additional protection.[7] Other measures include topical lidocaine spray before intubation and the use of atropinic agents. Hyperventilation is unnecessary and may lead to barotrauma; hypocarbia promotes bronchoconstriction. Consider repeat administration of albuterol or lidocaine during emergence. Deep extubation is an option but usually is not necessary.

H. Avoid tracheal instrumentation with general anesthesia by mask or by laryngeal mask airway (LMA), local anesthesia, and regional anesthesia. Sedation is safe in asthmatic patients, as is the appropriate use of IV and neuraxial narcotic agents to treat pain.

REFERENCES

1. Pien LC, Grammer LC, Patterson R: Minimal complications in a surgical population with severe asthma receiving prophylactic corticosteroids, *J Allergy Clin Immunol* 82:696–700, 1988.
2. Eames WO, Rooke GA, Wu RS, et al.: Comparison of the effects of etomidate, propofol, and thiopental on respiratory resistance after tracheal intubation, *Anesthesiology* 84:1307–1311, 1996.
3. Pizov R, Brown RH, Weiss YS, et al.: Wheezing during induction of general anesthesia in patients with and without asthma. A randomized, blinded trial, *Anesthesiology* 82:1111–1116, 1995.
4. Gyllfors P, Bochenek G, Overholt J, et al.: Biochemical and clinical evidence that aspirin-intolerant asthmatic subjects tolerate the cyclooxygenase 2-selective analgetic drug celecoxib, *J Allergy Clin Immunol* 111:1116–1121, 2003.
5. Yukioka H, Hayashi M, Terai T, et al.: Intravenous lidocaine as a suppressant of coughing during tracheal intubation in elderly patients, *Anesth Analg* 77:309–312, 1993.
6. Maslow AD, Regan MM, Israel E, et al.: Inhaled albuterol, but not intravenous lidocaine, protects against intubation-induced bronchoconstriction in asthma, *Anesthesiology* 93:1198–1204, 2000.
7. Groeben H, Silvanus MT, Beste M, et al.: Combined lidocaine and salbutamol inhalation for airway anesthesia markedly protects against reflex bronchoconstriction, *Chest* 118:509–515, 2000.

Clinical Evaluation of the Patient with ASTHMA

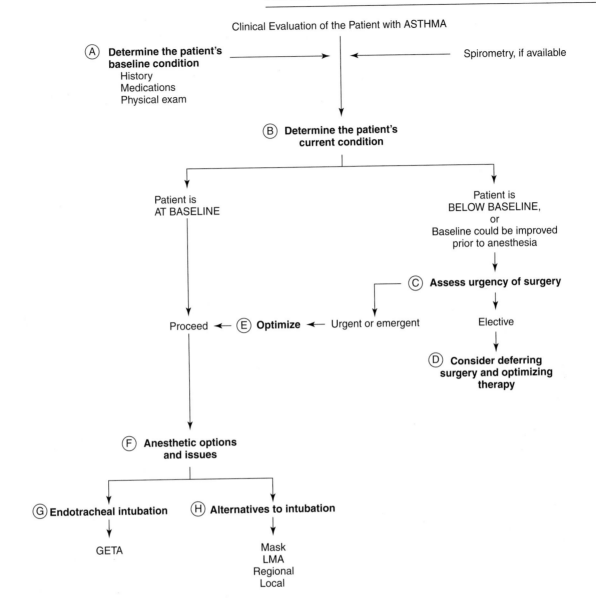

Ⓐ **Determine the patient's baseline condition**
    History
    Medications
    Physical exam

Spirometry, if available

Ⓑ **Determine the patient's current condition**

Patient is AT BASELINE

Patient is BELOW BASELINE, or Baseline could be improved prior to anesthesia

Ⓒ **Assess urgency of surgery**

Proceed ← Ⓔ **Optimize** ← Urgent or emergent

Elective

Ⓓ **Consider deferring surgery and optimizing therapy**

Ⓕ **Anesthetic options and issues**

Ⓖ **Endotracheal intubation**

Ⓗ **Alternatives to intubation**

GETA

Mask
LMA
Regional
Local

Perioperative Wheezing

DEBORAH K. RASCH, M.D.

Wheezing (derived from an Old Norse word meaning "to hiss") is a complex sign encountered during the perioperative care of patients. When bronchospasm occurs, wheezing is accompanied by constriction of the bronchi (and increased distending pressures in the intubated patient). Although predominantly an expiratory sound, there may be a shorter sound during inspiration. Respiratory noises similar to wheezing may be associated with other disorders. Typically, respiratory noises that occur during expiration derive from intrathoracic pathology.

A. Preoperative wheezing may indicate one or more of the following: bronchospastic disease (asthma, chronic obstructive pulmonary disease [COPD], or cystic fibrosis), cardiac disease (congestive heart failure [CHF], congenital heart disease with enlarged pulmonary artery [PA] producing mainstem bronchial compression, or vascular ring surrounding the trachea), aspiration, or inflammatory or infectious disease (chronic bronchitis, pneumonia, or viral infections in children).[1-3] Wheezing may be noted in the patient with laryngeal edema or a foreign body in the bronchus and rarely with pulmonary embolus. Perform a careful history and physical examination (with emphasis on respiratory symptoms, exercise tolerance, response to bronchodilators, cardiac gallop rhythm, improvement with diuretics) to categorize the disorder(s). Further diagnostic studies may be required. Optimize cardiopulmonary function before elective surgery (e.g., bronchodilators and improved pulmonary toilet for bronchospastic disease; management of medications and diuretics for CHF; and postponement of elective procedures until the infectious process has cleared). Consider preoperative steroid treatment in those patients at highest risk for postoperative pulmonary complications.[4]

B. Choose anesthetic drugs that do not promote bronchospasm. All potent inhalational agents are roughly equivalent bronchodilators. Oxybarbiturates may be less likely to cause histamine release than thiobarbiturates in the asthmatic patient. The bronchodilating properties of Ketamine may be helpful. If an endotracheal tube (ETT) is required, intubate (and consider extubation) under a deep plane of anesthesia if possible. Regional anesthetic techniques provide excellent alternatives to general anesthesia.

C. Individualize management of the cardiac patient according to the lesions present. Wheezing, despite appropriate hemodynamic management, may indicate bronchospasm.

D. The patient who had no preoperative wheezing but then begins to have a prolonged expiratory phase and wheezing after intubation presents an acute diagnostic problem. Secretions within the larger airways or ETT may produce expiratory noises that clear with suctioning.

E. Intraoperative bronchospasm may be caused by drug-induced histamine release (thiopental, curare, succinylcholine, or morphine), light anesthesia, parasympathomimetic stimulation (presence of the ETT, surgical stimulation), aspiration, drugs with beta-blocking activity, or anaphylaxis. Anaphylaxis produces hypotension, vasodilation, and periorbital edema and may be caused by certain drugs, latex allergy, blood transfusion, or other administered agents. Treat anaphylaxis with 3 to 5 µg/kg intravenous epinephrine; 2 mg/kg diphenhydramine; and 1 to 2 mg/kg intravenous methylprednisolone.

F. For persistent wheezing, 0.01 mg/kg SQ terbutaline; 0.1 mg/kg inhaled albuterol; 0.1 mg/kg inhaled terbutaline; and inhaled ipratropium bromide have been used with favorable results (ipratropium is not acutely useful in children).[5] If bronchospasm persists, load with methylprednisolone 1 to 2 mg/kg intravenously and consider beginning a terbutaline infusion.

REFERENCES

1. Doherty GM, Chisakuta A, Crean P, et al.: Anesthesia and the child with asthma, *Paediatr Anaesth* 15 (6):446–454, 2005.
2. Tamul PC, Peruzzi WT: Assessment and management of patients with pulmonary disease, *Crit Care Med* 32 (4 Suppl):S137–S145, 2004.
3. Hepner DL, Castells MC: Anaphylaxis during the perioperative period, *Anesth Analg* 97: 1381–1395, 2003.
4. Silvanus MT, Groeben H, Peters J: Corticosteroids and inhaled salbutamol in patients with reversible airway obstruction markedly decrease the incidence of bronchospasm after tracheal intubation, *Anesthesiology* 100:1052–1057, 2004.
5. Kumaratne M, Gunawardane G: Addition of ipratropium to nebulized albuterol in children with acute asthma presenting to a pediatric office, *Clin Pediatr* 42 (2):127–132, 2003.

PERIOPERATIVE WHEEZING

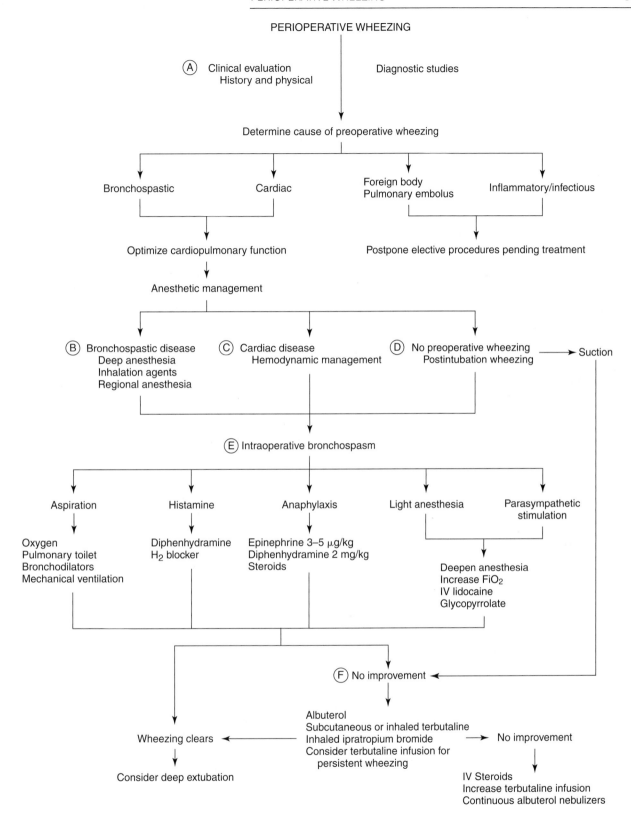

Chronic Obstructive Pulmonary Disease (COPD)

GEORGE A. DUMITRASCU, M.D.

The term "chronic obstructive pulmonary disease" (COPD) describes pathological states characterized by persistent obstruction to expiratory airflow. The severity of COPD in a particular individual (severity of airflow obstruction) is best reflected by the FEV_1/forced vital capacity (FVC) ratio. The most common causes of COPD are chronic bronchitis and emphysema. Chronic bronchitis manifests itself as hypersecretion of mucus and productive cough following prolonged exposure to airway irritants; emphysema is characterized by gradual destruction of lung parenchyma with associated loss of elastic recoil of the lungs and airway collapse during exhalation. Smoking is the major predisposing factor to the development of both chronic bronchitis and emphysema, and many smokers show features of both.[1-7]

A. Preoperative considerations—Focus on determining the severity of disease and elucidate any reversible components (infection or bronchospasm). A history of home oxygen (O_2) use, dyspnea at rest, or worsening sputum production would suggest the need for pulmonary function tests (PFTs) with and without bronchodilators, baseline ABGs, and possible sputum culture. An FEV_1/FVC ratio < 70% of predicted correlates with a higher incidence of perioperative pulmonary complications; a value < 50% of predicted suggests a high likelihood of postoperative respiratory failure (especially if baseline $PaCO_2$ > 50 mm Hg).

B. In the case of elective surgery, optimize pulmonary function: encourage smoking cessation (at least 4 to 6 weeks in advance), adjust bronchodilator and steroid regimens, treat acute respiratory infections, correct malnutrition, and provide supplemental O_2 to improve pulmonary hypertension. Inadequate optimization is directly related to the rate of postoperative pulmonary complications.

C. Intraoperative considerations—Regardless of the anesthetic technique employed, the anesthesiologist should be aware that these patients are susceptible to the development of acute respiratory failure. Consider regional anesthesia as a useful choice for the patient with COPD. Use sedatives sparingly, because these patients can be extremely sensitive to ventilatory depressant drugs. Recent reports have shown that neuraxial blockade to a T4 sensory level can be used safely without increasing the perioperative complication rate, despite initial concerns regarding decreases in expiratory reserve volume and ability to cough. During general anesthesia, focus on minimizing the incidence of bronchospasm during instrumentation of the airway and during emergence; administer prophylactic IV lidocaine (1 mg/kg) and extubate deeply whenever possible. Use volatile anesthetics for maintenance, avoid nitrous oxide, and humidify the inspired gases. If there are no contraindications, use a combination of general anesthesia and regional techniques; this will allow early mobilization, minimize the need for parenteral opioids, and reduce the requirement for neuromuscular blockers. When controlled ventilation is necessary, the anesthesiologist should keep in mind that the gradient between end-tidal carbon dioxide (CO_2) and arterial CO_2 may be increased. Do not attempt to correct arterial CO_2 in a patient with baseline hypercapnia.

D. Postoperative considerations—Postoperative pulmonary complications are often the result of atelectasis followed by pneumonia and hypoxemia; as expected, these occur with a higher incidence after thoracic and upper abdominal procedures. Arterial oxygenation may not return to preoperative levels until 10 to 14 days after surgery, secondary to the persistent decrease in FRC. Focus on treatment regimens which restore FRC. Studies have shown that no single treatment is superior; often, a combination of treatment modalities achieves the best clinical response.

REFERENCES

1. Volta CA, Alvisi V, Petrini S, et al.: The effect of volatile anesthetics on respiratory system resistance in patients with chronic obstructive pulmonary disease, Anesth Analg 100:348–353, 2005.
2. Savas JF, Litwack R, Davis K, et al.: Regional anesthesia as an alternative to general anesthesia for abdominal surgery in patients with severe pulmonary impairment, Am J Surg 188:603–605, 2004.
3. Groeben H: Strategies in the patient with compromised respiratory function. Best Pract Res Clin Anaesthesiol 18:579–594, 2004.
4. Ozdilekcan C, Songur N, Berktas BM, et al.: Risk factors associated with postoperative pulmonary complications following oncological surgery, Tuberk Toraks 52:248–255, 2004.
5. Rock P, Passannante A: Preoperative assessment: pulmonary, Anesthesiol Clin North America 22:77–91, 2004.
6. Smetana GW: Preoperative pulmonary assessment of the older adult, Clin Geriatr Med 19:35–55, 2003.
7. Gruber EM, Tschernko EM: Anaesthesia and postoperative analgesia in older patients with chronic obstructive pulmonary disease: special considerations, Drugs Aging 20:347–360, 2003.

Patient with COPD
PREOPERATIVE CONSIDERATIONS

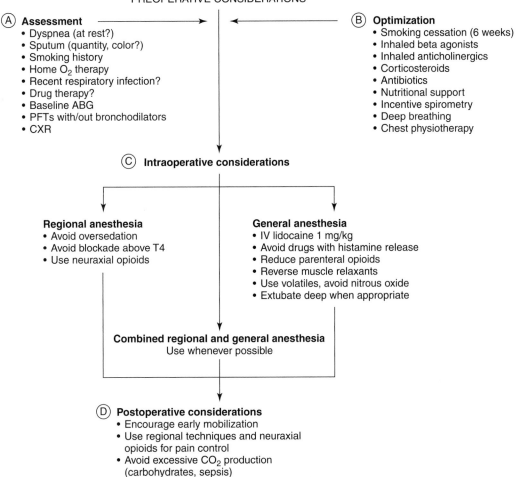

Ⓐ **Assessment**
- Dyspnea (at rest?)
- Sputum (quantity, color?)
- Smoking history
- Home O_2 therapy
- Recent respiratory infection?
- Drug therapy?
- Baseline ABG
- PFTs with/out bronchodilators
- CXR

Ⓑ **Optimization**
- Smoking cessation (6 weeks)
- Inhaled beta agonists
- Inhaled anticholinergics
- Corticosteroids
- Antibiotics
- Nutritional support
- Incentive spirometry
- Deep breathing
- Chest physiotherapy

Ⓒ **Intraoperative considerations**

Regional anesthesia
- Avoid oversedation
- Avoid blockade above T4
- Use neuraxial opioids

General anesthesia
- IV lidocaine 1 mg/kg
- Avoid drugs with histamine release
- Reduce parenteral opioids
- Reverse muscle relaxants
- Use volatiles, avoid nitrous oxide
- Extubate deep when appropriate

Combined regional and general anesthesia
Use whenever possible

Ⓓ **Postoperative considerations**
- Encourage early mobilization
- Use regional techniques and neuraxial opioids for pain control
- Avoid excessive CO_2 production (carbohydrates, sepsis)
- Do not increase FiO_2 in patients dependent on a hypoxic drive for ventilation
- Encourage ventilatory maneuvers (incentive spirometry, deep breathing)
- Chest physiotherapy
- Ventilatory support if necessary

Cigarette Smoking

JUERGEN FLEISCH, M.D.

DAWN DILLMAN, M.D.

Even following a significant decline of smoking in the United States over the last three decades, 25% of Americans consider themselves smokers. Cigarette smoke contains more than 4,000 substances in the gaseous phase and particulate phase. The impact of smoking on key organ systems—even in smokers without clinically apparent disease—influences the likelihood of perioperative complications.[1-6] Cigarette smoking induces liver enzymes, increasing the metabolism of several drugs, for instance, warfarin, imipramine, and theophylline.

A. Important respiratory implications include mucous hypersecretion and impaired tracheal clearance, as well as small airway narrowing with increased closing capacity and a tendency to V/Q mismatching. There is also increased reflex sensitivity of the lower conducting airways and the upper airway, increased permeability of the respiratory epithelium, and some evidence of loss of surfactant. If patients demonstrate signs of acute pulmonary disease (e.g., rhonchi or wheezing), a decision must be made whether to proceed with surgery or attempt to optimize the patient with antibiotics, physiotherapy or beta-agonist, depending on the urgency of surgery. The risk for smokers to develop postoperative pulmonary complications, such as pneumonia, respiratory failure, or atelectasis, is four times higher than for nonsmokers. The question of when to stop smoking preoperatively is much debated. Several observational retrospective studies suggest that there may be a slightly increased risk of complications with short-term abstinence (<8 weeks.) There is evidence that at least 6 months of abstinence is necessary for macrophage function and cytokine levels to return to the level of nonsmokers. However, the increased upper airway sensitivity returns to baseline within a few days of abstinence.

The cardiovascular system is affected by smoking mainly through nicotine and carbon monoxide (CO). Nicotine activation of the adrenergic system increases the oxygen demand of the heart, combined with a decreased oxygen supply because of elevated systemic vascular resistance. In heavy smokers COHb levels can reach 5 to 15% of the hemoglobin content. The left-shift of the oxyhemoglobin dissociation curve impairs oxygen unloading from hemoglobin to tissues. Cessation of smoking the night before surgery will reduce COHb and nicotine levels to that of nonsmokers, normalize the oxyhemoglobin dissociation curve, and should be encouraged by anesthesiologists. However, nicotine replacement therapy (NRT) does not seem to increase the risk of cardiovascular complications.

Smoking impairs the immune response. In addition to global tissue hypoxia and vascular damage, this leads to an increased rate of wound infections in smokers. A combination of smoking cessation counseling and NRT dramatically reduced wound infection in total joint replacement compared to controls. Given these acute and chronic risks of continuing smoking, it seems prudent to recommend cessation of smoking preoperatively regardless of the length of time to surgery and actively support smokers with counseling and NRT if requested.[6]

B. Intraoperatively, oxygen therapy should be actively pursued regardless of type of anesthetic planned. Regional or local anesthesia may allow avoidance of airway instrumentation and potential complications. If general anesthesia is indicated, recognize the increased sensitivity of the upper airway both during induction and emergence. IV lidocaine with induction may reduce airway irritability, and adequate doses of induction agents should be given, especially if supraglottic devices are to be used, to prevent laryngospasm. A humidifier may prevent desiccation and inspissation of secretions. Pulse oximetry may not be accurate with high levels of carboxyhemoglobin, and end-tidal carbon dioxide (CO_2) monitoring may not reflect arterial CO_2 levels secondary to bronchospasm or delayed emptying secondary to secretions. Neuromuscular blockade should be closely monitored as the induction of liver enzymes may alter neuromuscular blocker metabolism. Suctioning of the endotracheal tube prior to extubation may be helpful to reduce secretions in the airway.

C. Postoperatively, smokers should be carefully monitored for the development of pulmonary complications and receive oxygen supplementation as needed in the PACU. Fortunately, the incidence of postoperative nausea and vomiting is less among smokers. Smokers should be encouraged to utilize the perioperative period as a chance to make long-term cessation possible.

REFERENCES

1. Rodrigo C: The effects of cigarette smoking on anesthesia. Review, *Anesth Prog* 47:143–150, 2000.
2. Kumra V, Markoff BA: Who's smoking now? The epidemiology of tobacco use in the United States and abroad, *Clin Chest Med* 21:1–9, vii, 2000.
3. Warner DO, Warner MA, Offord KP, et al.: Airway obstruction and perioperative complications in smokers undergoing abdominal surgery, *Anesthesiology* 90:372–379, 1999.
4. Warner DO: Helping surgical patients quit smoking: why, when, and how, *Anesth Analg* 101 (2):481–487, 2005.
5. Rock P, Passannante A: Preoperative assessment: pulmonary, *Anesthesiol Clin North America* 22 (1):77–91, 2004.
6. Warner DO: Perioperative abstinence from cigarettes: physiologic and clinical consequences, *Anesthesiology* 104:356–367, 2006.

Smoker requiring anesthesia

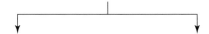

(A) **Stop smoking**
Ideally 8 weeks prior to surgery
Facilitate abstinence of smoking, e.g., by counseling or NRT
If not possible: avoid cigarettes at least 12 hours to negate
effects of nicotine and COHb

Preparation
In symptomatic smokers:
bronchodilators, breathing
exercises, chest physiotherapy

Premedication
Consider nebulizing lidocaine
4% preoperatively to reduce
upper airway sensitivity

(B) **Intraoperative**

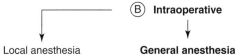

Local anesthesia   **General anesthesia**   Regional anesthesia

Induction
Preoxygenation to decrease CO
Consider IV Lidocaine to decrease
sensitivity of airway reflexes
Manipulation under light anesthesia
may result in coughing, breath holding,
laryngo- or bronchospasm

Maintenance
Consider risk of bronchospasm
Use of humidifier

Monitoring
Pulse oximeter may read higher SpO_2 than actual if COHb present
Peripheral nerve stimulator: various efficacy of NDMR in smokers
In long operations: consider ABG's as $PaCO_2$–$EtCO_2$ may be elevated

Extubation
Do not extubate under light anesthesia: risk of laryngo- or bronchospasm
Consider suctioning the endotracheal tube for secretions

(C) **Postoperative period**
Application of oxygen for transport and in PACU
Be alert for respiratory complications
Encourage permanent smoking cessation

Obstructive Sleep Apnea (OSA)

VERONICA C. SWANSON, M.D.

Obstructive sleep apnea (OSA) is a serious, potentially life-threatening condition that is defined as a repetition of at least 5 to 10 apneic and hypopneic episodes per sleep hour in adults (2 in children) each lasting 10 seconds or longer.[1,2] These apneic and hypopneic episodes occur by complete or partial closure of the pharynx secondary to loss of tone of upper airway musculature. It is a hallmark of increased risk of anesthesia due to intraoperative and postoperative airway concerns.

Incidence of clinically significant OSA among the middle aged is estimated at 15% of men and 5% of women,[1] although 90% of patients with the disease are undiagnosed.[2] Risk factors include obesity, male gender, postmenopause (in females), and hypertension (HTN). Cardiovascular consequences of OSA include HTN, atherosclerosis, stroke, heart failure, pulmonary hypertension, and cardiac arrhythmias.[3] The predominant site of obstruction is the oropharynx, although extensions to the laryngopharynx are frequently observed.[4]

A. Determine history of snoring, excessive daytime sleepiness, and reports of witnessed apneic events. A history of HTN is suggestive of the presence of OSA: one half of patients with essential HTN (EH) have OSA, and about one half of all patients with OSA have EH. Obesity, (primarily central, short neck and increased neck circumference), crowded mouth, large uvula, generalized erythema and swelling of all tissues, large tonsils/adenoids, macroglossia, overbite, retrognathia, micrognathia, and obstructed nasal passages are common physical findings in OSA. In obese subjects, the circumference of the neck is an independent predictor of sleep apnea.[5] The gold standard for an accurate diagnosis of OSA is polysomnography evaluation.

B. Successful treatment of OSA will eliminate apneic and hypopneic breathing episodes, snoring, and the arousal responses caused by these respiratory events. Weight loss is effective in obese patients, but it takes time. Nasal continuous positive airway pressure (CPAP) is the treatment of choice for most patients. The limiting factors that determine patient compliance is noise of the device and discomfort of the mask. Avoiding the supine position is effective in more than half of the patients. Surgical procedures, of which uvulopalatopharyngoplasty is the most common, are effective in 40 to 60% of patients with OSA. However, it is impossible to predict for which patient surgery will work. Tonsillectomy and adenoidectomy are effective techniques in cases of hypertrophy.[2]

C. Commonly used drugs that have been demonstrated to cause pharyngeal collapse are propofol, thiopental, narcotics, benzodiazepines, small doses of neuromuscular blockers, and nitrous oxide.[5] Consider regional anesthesia with minimal or no sedation in patients with OSA, because it may obviate the need for sedative and narcotic drugs both intraoperatively and postoperatively. Tracheal intubation should be undertaken with the expectation that it will be difficult, as OSA and difficult intubation have been shown to be related.[6] If general anesthesia is chosen, consider awake versus asleep intubation. In awake intubation, titrate sedative and analgesic medication judiciously—OSA patients are particularly sensitive to these medications. In asleep intubation, maximum preoxygenation is crucial. Be ready with proper patient positioning, suction, multiple laryngoscope blades and endotracheal tube sizes, stylettes, laryngeal mask airways (LMAs), and other airway adjuncts. Backup help should also be available, as mask ventilation may require two practitioners, or worse, the "cannot ventilate, cannot intubate" pathway of the difficult airway algorithm may be encountered.

D. Patients who were considered a high-risk intubation should also be considered high-risk extubation. This means extubating the patient when he or she is fully awake. Bed position in reverse Trendelenburg helps minimize compression of the diaphragm by the abdominal contents. In addition, the endotracheal tube can be removed over a tube changer, facilitating rapid reintubation if necessary. Besides the risk of an obstructed airway, OSA patients are also at risk for negative pressure pulmonary edema, which can be quite severe. If it develops, reintubate the patient. Patients should bring their CPAP units with them for use in the PACU. Severe OSA patients should spend the night monitored in an ICU.[5]

E. In children, tonsillar and adenoid hypertrophy is the most common cause of OSA. Risk factors for respiratory complications are an associated medical condition and a preoperative saturation nadir less than 80%. Atropine administration may be beneficial as a risk reduction strategy in children with severe OSA.[7]

REFERENCES

1. Silverberg DS, Iaina A: Treating obstructive sleep apnea improves essential hypertension and quality of life, *Am Fam Physician* 65 (2):229–236, 2002.
2. Benumof JL: Obstructive sleep apnea in the adult obese patient: implications for airway management, *Anesthesiol Clin of North America* 20 (4):789–811, 2002.
3. Wolk R, Somers VK: Cardiovascular consequences of obstructive sleep apnea, *Clin Chest Med* 24 (2):195–205, 2003.
4. Rama AN, Tekwani SH: Sites of obstruction in obstructive sleep apnea, *Chest* 122 (4):1139–1147, 2002.
5. Drummond GB: Controlling the airway: Skill and science, *Anesthesiology* 97 (4):771–773, 2002.

Anesthesia in the Patient with OBSTRUCTIVE SLEEP APNEA

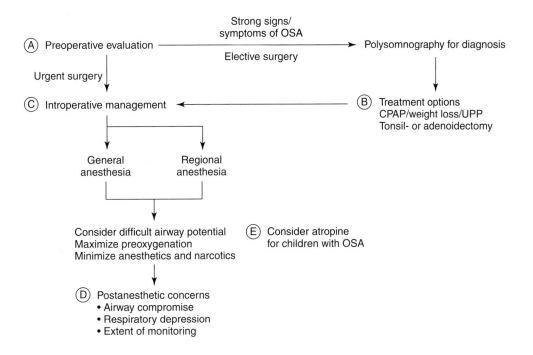

6. Hiremath AS, Hillman DR: Relationship between difficult intubation and obstructive sleep apnea, *Br J Anaesth* 80 (5):606–611, 1998.
7. Brown KA, Morin I: Urgent adenotonsillectomy: An analysis of risk factor associated with postoperative respiratory morbidity, *Anesthesiology* 99 (3):586–595, 2003.

8. American Society of Anesthesiologists Task Force on Management of Difficult Airway: Practice guidelines for management of the difficult airway: an updated report by the American Society of Anesthesiologists Task Force on Management of the Difficult Airway, *Anesthesiology* 98:1269–1277, 2003.

Known or Suspected Tuberculosis (TB)

SUSAN M. RYAN, M.D.

Tuberculosis (TB) may currently infect up to one third of the world's population. In the United States, TB has declined from a recent peak in 1992. Nonetheless, it should remain a public health concern for all. TB is spread by inhalation of droplet nuclei; aerosolized particles dry, remain airborne, and may reach smaller air passages. TB is a particular concern for anesthesiologists because of their exposure to airway secretions during the course of providing care.[1-6]

A. Perform a history and physical examination. TB is primarily a pulmonary disease; 85% of cases involve a pulmonary primary site. Early TB is often asymptomatic or may manifest as nonspecific symptoms that progress to productive cough, hemoptysis, and pleuritic chest pain. On examination, tachypnea, rhonchi, and decreased breath sounds may be present. Lymphadenopathy may suggest extrapulmonary involvement. Obtain a chest x-ray (CXR); findings depend on the stage and chronicity of disease. Review lab tests. A slightly elevated white blood count and anemia may be present. Hyponatremia may occur with pulmonary TB and TB meningitis as a result of the syndrome of inappropriate secretion of antidiuretic hormone (SIADH). Liver function tests (LFTs) may be abnormal because isoniazid can be hepatotoxic.

B. Rule out active, infectious TB in patients with a known history of TB prior to nonemergency surgery. TB is most likely to be infectious in patients who have not been treated for TB and who also have one of the following: pulmonary or laryngeal TB with a cough, a positive acid-fast bacillus (AFB) sputum sample, or a cavitation on CXR. Observe TB precautions if there is any suspicion of active TB. If the CXR suggests active disease or clinical suspicion is high for new or inadequately treated TB, obtain three sputum samples for AFB smears and TB cultures. One positive AFB smear confirms the diagnosis. If the AFB smear is negative but active TB cannot be ruled out until cultures are final (high-risk or symptomatic patient), consider postponing surgery and treating.

C. Suspect TB in symptomatic patients who are HIV-positive, immigrants from high prevalence areas, residents of long-term care facilities, substance abusers, TB contacts, health care workers, homeless, malnourished, or debilitated. Consider the diagnosis when pneumonia occurs in a high-risk patient or when the patient is unresponsive to antibiotic therapy. Also consider TB in any patient with a recent positive screening test by purified protein derivative (PPD) or QuantiFERON (QFT).

D. Adhere to respiratory precautions in patients with suspected active TB. This requires a private room with negative pressure ventilation and a minimum flow rate of six room air changes per hour, a sign warning of respiratory precautions, and masks or respirators for anyone entering the room. During transportation, place a surgical mask on the patient (never a respirator with an exhalation valve, as droplet nuclei may be expulsed into the air). If the patient is intubated and hand ventilated, place a surgical mask over the expiratory orifice of the system during transportation.

E. If the patient is AFB positive or presumed to have active TB, postpone elective surgery until the patient has begun treatment and is considered to be noninfectious. Urgent cases require clinical judgment; treat for as long as possible before surgery and observe TB precautions in the OR.

F. Response to therapy is noted by decreased bacterial load, AFB-negative sputum, and clinical improvement. If the patient is initially AFB-positive, maintain TB precautions until the patient has had a minimum of 2 to 3 weeks of treatment, three AFB-negative sputum samples, and improved clinical condition. If the patient is initially AFB-negative but culture positive or if TB cannot be ruled out in a high-risk, symptomatic patient, continue precautions for a minimum of 1 week of treatment and until the patient's clinical condition is improved.

G. If the patient must undergo a procedure while still infectious, observe TB precautions. First, consider performing the procedure at the bedside. If it is necessary to proceed to the OR, ascertain whether the OR meets ventilation requirements; if not, portable negative-pressure ventilation is acceptable. Keep personnel to a minimum. *Equipment:* Use disposable items. Place a TB approved bacterial filter on the expiratory limb or directly on the endotracheal tube (ETT) to prevent machine contamination (a less desirable alternative is to interrupt gas flow for >1 hour.) Clean the machine components and anesthesia equipment with a tuberculocidal solution and sterilize when possible. *Health Care Workers:* Wear a mask to protect the sterile field. In addition, wear a respirator approved by the National Institute for Occupational Safety and Health (NIOSH) to protect from infectious droplets. One mask may serve both purposes if it meets both standards. Respirators with exhalation valves and positive-pressure respirators do not protect the sterile field. *Surgery:* A high risk of contamination exists during procedures in which infected body fluids are aerosolized (airway or lung procedures, cautery of infected tissue) and during any ETT tube care. Minimize ETT suctioning. *Recovery:* The recovery room location must be private and meet TB precaution standards. If not, recover the patient in the OR or ICU. If possible, designate an OR and recovery room location for these patients away from areas where immunocompromised patients are treated.

Patient with known or suspected TUBERCULOSIS REQUIRING SURGERY

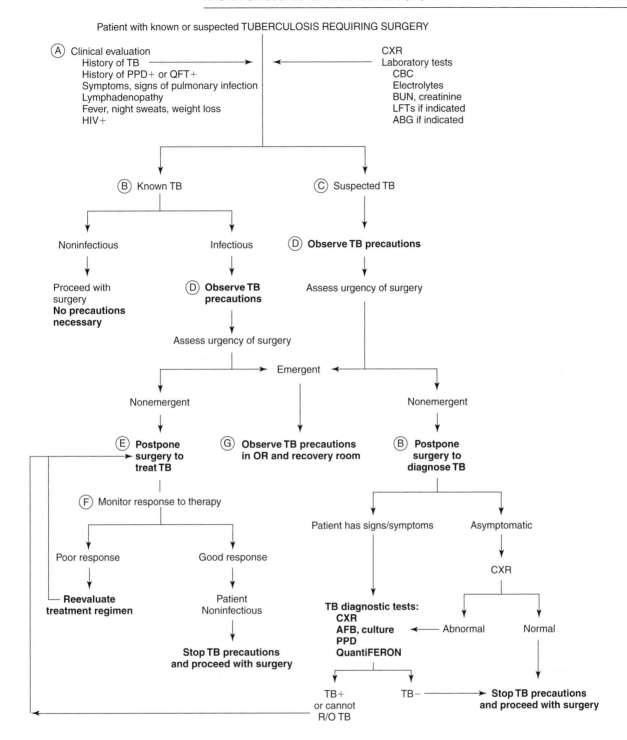

Ⓐ Clinical evaluation
    History of TB
    History of PPD+ or QFT+
    Symptoms, signs of pulmonary infection
    Lymphadenopathy
    Fever, night sweats, weight loss
    HIV+

CXR
Laboratory tests
    CBC
    Electrolytes
    BUN, creatinine
    LFTs if indicated
    ABG if indicated

Ⓑ Known TB

Ⓒ Suspected TB

Noninfectious

Infectious

Ⓓ **Observe TB precautions**

Proceed with surgery
No precautions necessary

Ⓓ **Observe TB precautions**

Assess urgency of surgery

Assess urgency of surgery

Emergent

Nonemergent

Nonemergent

Ⓔ **Postpone surgery to treat TB**

Ⓖ **Observe TB precautions in OR and recovery room**

Ⓑ **Postpone surgery to diagnose TB**

Ⓕ Monitor response to therapy

Patient has signs/symptoms

Asymptomatic

Poor response

Good response

CXR

Reevaluate treatment regimen

Patient Noninfectious

TB diagnostic tests:
CXR
AFB, culture ← Abnormal
PPD
QuantiFERON

Normal

Stop TB precautions and proceed with surgery

TB+ or cannot R/O TB

TB− ⟶ **Stop TB precautions and proceed with surgery**

REFERENCES

1. Small PM and Fujiwara PI: Management of tuberculosis in the United States, *N Engl J Med* 345:189–200, 2001.
2. Centers for Disease Control and Prevention: Guidelines for preventing the transmission of *Mycobacterium tuberculosis* in health-care facilities, *MMWR Recomm Rep* 43(RR-13), 1994.
3. U.S. Department of Health and Human Services, National Institute for Occupational Safety and Health: TB respiratory protection program in healthcare facilities, available at: *http://www.cdc.gov/niosh/99-143.html*, 1999.
4. Guidelines for using the QuantiFERON-TB test for diagnosing latent *Mycobacterium tuberculosis* infection, *MMWR Morb Mortal Wkly Rep* 52 (RR02):15–18, 2003.
5. Langevin PB, Rand KH, Layon AJ: The potential for dissemination of *Mycobacterium tuberculosis* through the anesthesia breathing circuit, *Chest* 115:1107–1114, 1999.
6. Centers for Disease Control: *CDC information on tuberculosis*, available at *http://www.cdc.gov/nchstp/tb/*, 2006.

Restrictive Lung Disease (RLD)

A. SUE CARLISLE, M.D., PH.D.

"Restrictive lung disease" (RLD) is a term used to describe a set of physiological parameters chiefly characterized by a decrease in total lung capacity.[1,2] RLD can be caused by a wide variety of intrinsic conditions that decrease the compliance of the lung parenchyma or by extrinsic conditions affecting the chest wall, pleura, or abdomen. These conditions can individually or collectively produce restrictive physiology. Intrinsic changes can be permanent (e.g., pulmonary fibrosis) or reversible (e.g., pulmonary edema or pneumonia). Extrinsic changes can be secondary to many diverse conditions, including respiratory muscle weakness, pleural thickening, kyphoscoliosis, chest wall scarring, and obesity.[1–5] Additionally, some procedures, such as laparoscopic surgery, which require insufflation of gas into the peritoneal cavity, can temporarily produce restrictive physiology. RLD frequently occurs in the presence of obstructive lung disease (OLD); the combined physiology may complicate the diagnosis and treatment.

A. Perform a history and physical examination. Inquire about symptoms including decreased exercise tolerance, dyspnea on exertion, cough, or difficulty taking a deep breath. Observe the respiratory pattern. These patients tend to have decreased tidal volumes and increased respiratory rates, because this results in less work of breathing than the expansion of a noncompliant system. Examine carefully for skeletal deformities, weakness, rales, and rhonchi. Obesity is an important common cause of severe RLD.

B. Obtain a chest x-ray (CXR) to evaluate many causes of RLD that are treatable, such as pulmonary edema, pneumonia, and some interstitial pneumonitides. Evaluate pulmonary function using simple spirometry to detect reduced lung volumes and mixed obstructive and restrictive physiology. If necessary, obtain other pulmonary function tests (PFTs), including expiratory flow volume curves, total lung capacity, and diffusing capacity to aid in diagnosis and to quantify the severity of the RLD (Figure 1).[3] Obtain a preoperative ABG to help determine if postoperative ventilatory support will be necessary. In severe cases, consider preoperative echocardiography (echo) or right-sided heart catheterization to evaluate the extent of pulmonary hypertension (HTN) or ventricular failure. Treat all reversible components before elective surgery.

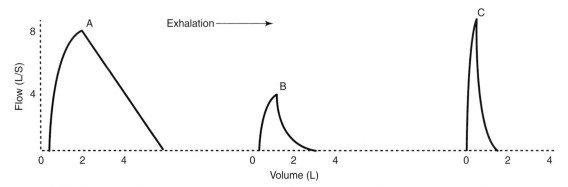

FIGURE 1 Expiratory flow volume curves in **A**, normal, **B**, obstructed, and **C**, restricted spirographic patterns.

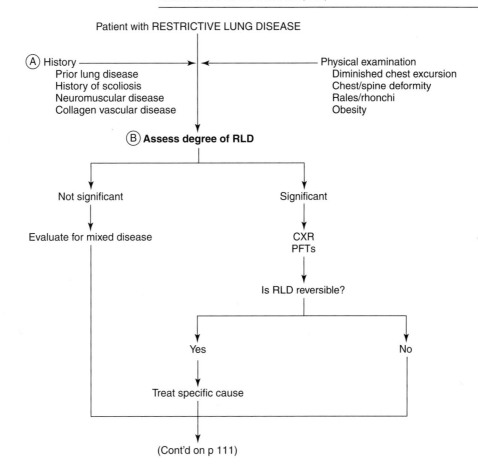

Patient with RESTRICTIVE LUNG DISEASE

(A) History
   Prior lung disease
   History of scoliosis
   Neuromuscular disease
   Collagen vascular disease

Physical examination
   Diminished chest excursion
   Chest/spine deformity
   Rales/rhonchi
   Obesity

(B) **Assess degree of RLD**

Not significant

Evaluate for mixed disease

Significant

CXR
PFTs

Is RLD reversible?

Yes

No

Treat specific cause

(Cont'd on p 111)

C. Whenever possible, choose an anesthetic technique that does not require extensive sedation or mechanical ventilation.[1,4] Regional techniques may be used if they do not compromise the respiratory muscles. In many cases, however, general anesthesia and mechanical ventilation will be necessary. In addition to standard American Society of Anesthesiologists (ASA) monitors, consider placing an arterial line for BP monitoring and blood gas sampling. In severe cases, particularly in the presence of pulmonary HTN or ventricular failure, consider placing a pulmonary artery (PA) catheter or transesophageal echocardiogram (TEE) probe to monitor changes in PA pressure and ventricular function. Many OR ventilators are insufficient in providing pressures and flows necessary for adequate ventilation of patients with poor compliance.[5] An ICU-type ventilator may be required. Set the ventilator to deliver decreased tidal volumes at an increased frequency in patients with poor compliance. This maneuver or the use of pressure control ventilation may avoid problems associated with excessive peak pressures, such as barotrauma and hemodynamic compromise. Hemodynamic compromise can present as decreased cardiac output (CO) and BP or decreased ventilation with increased dead space.

D. Postoperatively, assess the patient's ability to maintain adequate oxygenation and a normal pH. If the trachea can be extubated, pay meticulous attention to pain control. Methods that have minimal effect on respiratory drive (a compensatory mechanism for these patients) are most desirable. If the patient will not tolerate extubation, ventilate, optimize volume status, and provide good pulmonary toilet and nutrition. Consider noninvasive ventilation, such as bilevel positive airway pressure.

REFERENCES

1. Groeben H: Strategies in the patient with compromised respiratory function, *Best Pract Res Clin Anaesthesiol* 18 (4):579–594, 2004.
2. Golden JA: Interstitial (diffuse parenchymal) lung disease: physiology. In Baum GL, Wolinsky E, editors: *Textbook of pulmonary diseases*, ed 5, Boston 1994, Little, Brown & Co.
3. Zanen P, Folgering H, Lammers JW: Flow-volume indices as means to discriminate between intra- and extrapulmonary restrictive disease, *Respir Med* 99 (7):825–829, 2005.
4. Tobin MJ: Advances in mechanical ventilation, *N Engl J Med* 344:1986–1996, 2001.
5. Marks JD, Schapera A, Kraemer RW, et al.: Pressure and flow limitations of anesthesia ventilators, *Anesthesiology* 71:403–408, 1989.

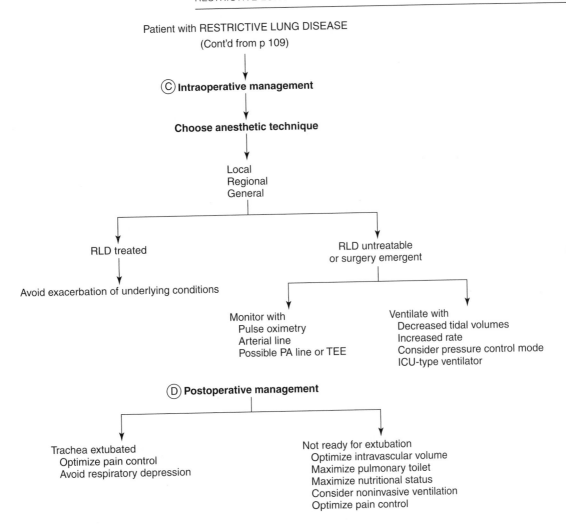

Patient with RESTRICTIVE LUNG DISEASE
(Cont'd from p 109)

Ⓒ **Intraoperative management**

Choose anesthetic technique

Local
Regional
General

RLD treated

Avoid exacerbation of underlying conditions

RLD untreatable
or surgery emergent

Monitor with
   Pulse oximetry
   Arterial line
   Possible PA line or TEE

Ventilate with
   Decreased tidal volumes
   Increased rate
   Consider pressure control mode
   ICU-type ventilator

Ⓓ **Postoperative management**

Trachea extubated
   Optimize pain control
   Avoid respiratory depression

Not ready for extubation
   Optimize intravascular volume
   Maximize pulmonary toilet
   Maximize nutritional status
   Consider noninvasive ventilation
   Optimize pain control

Pulmonary Hypertension (PHTN)

DEBORAH K. RASCH, M.D.

Pulmonary hypertension (PHTN) may be either primary (idiopathic) or secondary to other causes, most commonly cardiac or pulmonary disease. In primary pulmonary hypertension (PPH), autosomal dominant transmission sometimes occurs, and there is a female/male predominance of 3:1. PPH patients are usually asymptomatic until the second to fourth decades of life; worsening of pulmonary function occurs with development of right ventricular (RV) failure (cor pulmonale). Secondary pulmonary hypertension (SPH) is more common and may present in infancy or early childhood. SPH occurs as the result of a variety of conditions including hypoxemia (upper airway obstruction, cystic fibrosis, asthma, or bronchopulmonary dysplasia); obstruction (total anomalous pulmonary venous return, or mitral or aortic stenosis); intracardiac shunt (atrial septal defect, ventricular septal defect, patent ductus arteriosus, or transposition of the great vessels); collagen vascular diseases (rheumatoid arthritis, scleroderma, or systemic lupus erythematosus); thromboembolism (sickle cell disease, fat emboli, or venous emboli); exposure to infection, toxins, or drugs; and persistent fetal circulation.[1,2]

A. Obtain a history and perform a physical examination. Determine the cause of the PHTN. Symptoms are not specific. Look for dyspnea, easy fatigability, syncope, chest pain, or congestive heart failure (CHF). A prominent P_2 heart sound, tricuspid regurgitation murmur, S_3 gallop, and peripheral edema may be apparent. Wheezing can occur in patients with chronic obstructive pulmonary disease (COPD), asthma, and cystic fibrosis. Obtain a chest x-ray (CXR). Review ECG and echocardiogram (echo) to evaluate anatomic and functional parameters. (Cardiac catheterization with angiography has a high mortality rate in patients with PPH but is essential for patients with congenital heart disease [CHD].) Review patient medications. Treatment may include bronchodilators, corticosteroids, and anticoagulants as well as vasodilators, inotropes, and diuretics (Table 1).[3-6] Supplemental oxygen (O_2) may improve both pulmonary and cardiac function. Reduction of pulmonary artery (PA) pressures in response to O_2 carries a better prognosis. Newer therapies include inhaled nitric oxide (NO), phosphodiesterase inhibitors (e.g., sildenafil or dipyridamole), and prostaglandins (e.g., epoprostenol or treprostinil).[1,2,6] Continue chronic medical treatment perioperatively, replacing indirect anticoagulants with heparin. Order pertinent laboratory tests.

B. The extent of invasive monitoring depends on the operative site and severity of the underlying disease. Use caution when inserting central lines, because this may provoke arrhythmia. PA catheters may be technically difficult to position in patients with severe disease. For abdominal and thoracic procedures, place an arterial cannula and PA catheter. For infants with CHD, a CVP is sufficient because a PA catheter may interfere with the procedure. A direct PA monitor can be placed intraoperatively. Monitor the ECG for development of ischemia or acute strain patterns in leads II, III, and AVF. Use bubble precautions if there is a shunt defect. Consider transesophageal echocardiography (TEE) as a valuable tool, if available. In the absence of a PA catheter, use tricuspid valve regurgitation to estimate changes in PA pressures.

(Continued on page 114)

TABLE 1
Medications Useful in the Treatment of Pulmonary Hypertension

Drug	Route of administration	Dose
Digitalis	IV, oral	Total digitalizing dose: Adult 1 mg in 24 hours
		Child 30–50 µg/kg in 24 hours
Furosemide	IV, oral	0.5–1 mg/kg
Hydralazine	IV, oral	Adult 10–50 mg/kg dose
		Child 0.75–3 mg/kg/day
Nifedipine	Sublingual/oral	Adult 10 mg SL
		Child 0.25–0.50 mg/kg to max of 10 mg
Diazoxide	Oral	3–8 mg/kg/day
Albuterol	Nebulized/oral	0.1 mg/kg/dose
Dobutamine	IV continuous infusion	2–10 µg/kg/min
Nitroglycerin	IV continuous infusion	5–50 µg/kg/min
Nitroprusside	IV continuous infusion	2–10 µg/kg/min
Milrinone	IV continuous infusion	0.2–1 µg/kg/min
Adenosine	IV continuous infusion	25–50 µg/kg/min
Epoprostenol (prostacyclin)		Begin with 2 ng/kg/min and titrate
Lisinopril	Oral	0.1–0.5 mg/kg/day
Sildenafil	Oral	25 mg tid for adults
		No pediatric dosing

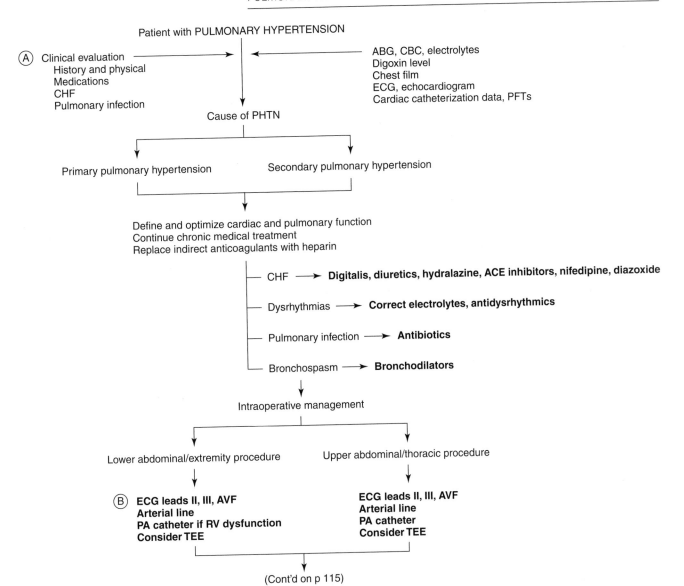

Patient with PULMONARY HYPERTENSION

Ⓐ Clinical evaluation
    History and physical
    Medications
    CHF
    Pulmonary infection

ABG, CBC, electrolytes
Digoxin level
Chest film
ECG, echocardiogram
Cardiac catheterization data, PFTs

Cause of PHTN

Primary pulmonary hypertension   Secondary pulmonary hypertension

Define and optimize cardiac and pulmonary function
Continue chronic medical treatment
Replace indirect anticoagulants with heparin

CHF ⟶ **Digitalis, diuretics, hydralazine, ACE inhibitors, nifedipine, diazoxide**

Dysrhythmias ⟶ **Correct electrolytes, antidysrhythmics**

Pulmonary infection ⟶ **Antibiotics**

Bronchospasm ⟶ **Bronchodilators**

Intraoperative management

Lower abdominal/extremity procedure   Upper abdominal/thoracic procedure

Ⓑ **ECG leads II, III, AVF
Arterial line
PA catheter if RV dysfunction
Consider TEE**

**ECG leads II, III, AVF
Arterial line
PA catheter
Consider TEE**

(Cont'd on p 115)

C. Many anesthetic techniques affect vascular tone. Most agents and techniques have been used safely in patients with PHTN; choose techniques and agents according to personal experience and preference recalling that PHTN is exacerbated by hypoxemia, acidosis, hypercapnia, hypothermia, and sympathetic stimulation. During the anesthetic, optimize preload, afterload, contractility, HR, and rhythm. For extremity procedures and lower abdominal surgery, consider regional anesthesia (peripheral nerve block, epidural) as an excellent option.[1,2] If general anesthesia is required, avoid systemic vasodilating and cardiac depressant agents in patients with CHF and opt for a narcotic/relaxant technique. In the absence of RV failure, select inhalational anesthetics, which bronchodilate and decrease hypoxic pulmonary vasoconstriction.[7] Avoid nitrous oxide, which may increase PA pressures. Monitor intermittent positive-pressure ventilation (IPPV) and PEEP closely; they may reduce RV preload and increase PA pressures.

D. If PHTN worsens in the OR, consider the implications of treatment (e.g., changes in cardiac output [CO]) prior to any intervention. Treatments include the following options: nitroglycerin (5 to 50 mcg/kg/min), dobutamine (2 to 10 mcg/kg/min), milrinone (0.2 to 1 mcg/kg/min), adenosine (25 to 50 mcg/kg/min), and inhaled NO (can be added to the anesthetic circuit, beginning at 20 parts per million). NO provides dramatic reductions in PA pressure, particularly in neonates and children with CHD.[8]

E. Consider postoperative ventilation, especially after repair of CHD. Wean FiO_2 cautiously to reduce the risk of fatal pulmonary hypertensive crisis. Sedation with morphine may be beneficial. In neonates, inhaled NO and extracorporeal membrane oxygenation (ECMO) have proven useful in treating PPH.[8,9]

REFERENCES

1. Blaise G, Langleben D, Hubert B: Pulmonary arterial hypertension. Pathophysiology and anesthetic approach, *Anesthesiology* 99:1415–1432, 2003.
2. Fischer LG, Van Aken H, Burkle H: Management of pulmonary hypertension: physiological and pharmacological considerations for anesthesiologists, *Anesth Analg* 96:1603–1616, 2003.
3. Rich S, Ganz R, Levy PS: Comparative actions of hydralazine, nifedipine, and amrinone in primary pulmonary hypertension, *Am J Cardiol* 52:1104–1107, 1983.
4. Kanthapillai P, Lasserson T, Walters E: Sildenafil for pulmonary hypertension, *Cochrane Database Syst Rev* (4):CD003562, 2004.
5. Konduri GG, Garcia DC, Kazzi NJ, et al.: Adenosine infusion improves oxygenation in term infants with respiratory failure, *Pediatrics* 97:295–300, 1996.
6. Shapiro S: Management of pulmonary hypertension resulting from interstitial lung disease, *Curr Opin Pulm Med* 9:426–430, 2003.
7. Benumof JL, Wahrenbrock EA: Local effects of anesthetics on regional hypoxic pulmonary vasoconstriction, *Anesthesiology* 43:525–532, 1975.
8. Abman SH, Griebel JL, Parker DK, et al.: Acute effects of inhaled nitric oxide in children with severe hypoxemic respiratory failure, *J Pediatr* 124:881–888, 1994.
9. Gorenflo M, Nelle M, Schnabe PA, et al.: Pulmonary hypertension in infancy and childhood, *Cardiol Young* 13:219–227, 2003.

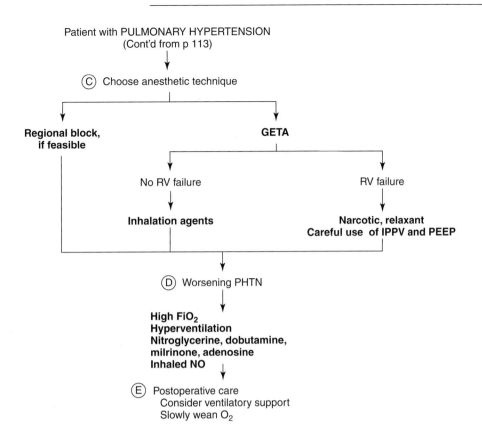

Patient with PULMONARY HYPERTENSION
(Cont'd from p 113)

Ⓒ Choose anesthetic technique

**Regional block,
if feasible**

GETA

No RV failure

RV failure

Inhalation agents

**Narcotic, relaxant
Careful use of IPPV and PEEP**

Ⓓ Worsening PHTN

**High FiO$_2$
Hyperventilation
Nitroglycerine, dobutamine,
milrinone, adenosine
Inhaled NO**

Ⓔ Postoperative care
   Consider ventilatory support
   Slowly wean O$_2$

Anterior Mediastinal Mass (AMM)

VERONICA C. SWANSON, M.D.

ANGELA KENDRICK, M.D.

The anterior mediastinum is bounded by the sternum anteriorly, the heart posteriorly, the thoracic inlet superiorly, and the diaphragm inferiorly. It contains the superior vena cava, tracheal bifurcation, main pulmonary artery, aortic arch, thymus, thyroid, parathyroid, esophagus, and lymphatic tissues. In children, the most common anterior mediastinal tumors are lymphomas, germ cell tumors, and thymic masses. Of these, 80% are malignant.[1] In adults, thymomas account for half of anterior mediastinal tumors; 50% are malignant and 50% are associated with myasthenia gravis.[2] Because of the location, an anterior mediastinal mass (AMM) causes three problems of particular concern to the anesthesiologist: compression of the heart, compression of the large vessels, and compression of the trachea and main bronchi.[3] Risk stratification allows an organized approach to the anesthetic management of these patients.

A. Look for signs and symptoms suggesting compression of the tracheobronchial tree, the great vessels, and the heart, including shortness of breath, orthopnea, wheezing, cough, hoarseness, tachypnea, arterial oxygen desaturation, neck and face edema (SVC syndrome), and syncope. Of these symptoms, orthopnea and SVC syndrome have the greatest prognostic value for complications.[2,4]

B. Review noninvasive diagnostic tests including chest x-ray (CXR), CT/magnetic resonance imaging (MRI), flow-volume loops, and echocardiogram (echo). Although CXR provides reliable information about the location and size of the AMM, it does not adequately assess degree of tracheal compression.[2] CT may be the best tool to evaluate this. When the cross-sectional area of the trachea is less than 50% of normal, there is a high incidence of complications with general anesthesia, which should be avoided whenever possible.[1] Although seated-to-supine spirometry has been recommended to evaluate airway obstruction, little data exist correlating this with complication risk.[5] Intrathoracic obstruction produces marked reduction in maximum expiratory flow rate.[6] Peak expiratory flow rate (PEFR) can be obtained with a hand-held device; a PEFR <50% of predicted indicates a high-risk pediatric patient.[7] Echo is used to evaluate direct compression of the heart (diminishing cardiac output), great vessels (SVC syndrome), and presence of pericardial effusion (tamponade).

C. If the patient does not have significant risk factors based on the results of noninvasive tests, there is no documented increased risk of complications from airway or cardiovascular compression during general anesthesia.

D. If the patient has just one significant finding during preoperative testing, the risk of general anesthetic complications is less clear.[7] Carefully assess symptoms and patient cooperation. Consider the use of awake, fiberoptic bronchoscopy to facilitate tracheal intubation as a safe method in adults.[8] Place IV catheters in the lower extremities (if there is evidence of SVC syndrome), use a semiupright position for induction and maintenance of anesthesia, and allow the patient to breathe spontaneously. Make arrangements to have a rigid bronchoscope and a health care provider skilled in its use, immediately available.

E. A patient with two or more significant abnormal findings in CT, spirometry, or echo is in the highest risk group for complications from general anesthesia. Therefore, choose local anesthetic techniques whenever possible in such cases (e.g., tissue biopsy). If a patient has two positive findings and tissue diagnosis cannot be obtained under local anesthesia, attempt shrinkage of the tumor with steroids or radiation treatment prior to administration of general anesthesia whenever possible. If general anesthesia is required, proceed with the additional precautions of an arterial catheter and CPB standby (machine and team, with groin prepped and draped). If airway or cardiovascular collapse occurs, attempt to reposition the patient to alleviate mediastinal compression prior to the institution of CPB.

F. Airway obstruction can occur at any time in the perioperative period. Selected patients may require prolonged intubation until therapy has begun. Proceed with extubation only in a fully awake, cooperative patient. Consider postoperative care in an ICU setting.

REFERENCES

1. Ricketts RR: Clinical management of anterior mediastinal tumors in children, *Semin Pediatr Surg* 10:161–168, 2001.
2. Pullerits J, Holzman R: Anaesthesia for patients with mediastinal masses, *Can J Anaesth* 36:681–688, 1989.
3. Goh MH, Liu XY, Goh YS: Anterior mediastinal masses: an anaesthetic challenge, *Anaesthesia* 54:670–674, 1999.
4. Anghelescu DL, De Armendi AJ, Sandlund JT, et al.: Anesthetic complications of mediastinal masses associated with childhood malignancies, *Anesthesiology* A1380, 2003.
5. Hnatiuk OW, Corcoran PC, Sierra A: Spirometry in surgery for anterior mediastinal masses, *Chest* 120:1152–1156, 2001.
6. Azizkhan RG, Dudgeon DL, Buck JR, et al.: Life-threatening airway obstruction as a complication to the management of mediastinal masses in children, *J Pediatr Surg* 20:816–822, 1985.
7. Shamberger RC: Preanesthetic evaluation of children with anterior mediastinal masses, *Semin Pediatr Surg* 8:61–68, 1999.
8. Narang S, Harte BH, Body SC: Anesthesia for patients with a mediastinal mass, *Anesthesiol Clin North America* 19:559–579, 2001.

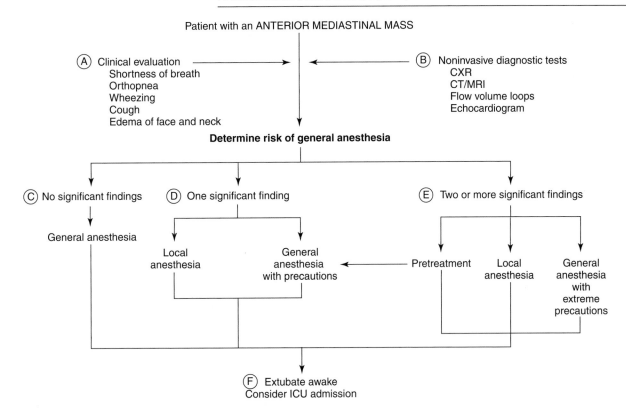

Patient with an ANTERIOR MEDIASTINAL MASS

(A) Clinical evaluation
　　Shortness of breath
　　Orthopnea
　　Wheezing
　　Cough
　　Edema of face and neck

(B) Noninvasive diagnostic tests
　　CXR
　　CT/MRI
　　Flow volume loops
　　Echocardiogram

Determine risk of general anesthesia

(C) No significant findings

General anesthesia

(D) One significant finding

Local anesthesia

General anesthesia with precautions

Pretreatment

(E) Two or more significant findings

Local anesthesia

General anesthesia with extreme precautions

(F) Extubate awake
Consider ICU admission

PREOPERATIVE CARDIOVASCULAR PROBLEMS

Preoperative Cardiac Evaluation for Noncardiac Surgery

STEPHEN T. ROBINSON, M.D.

MICHAEL P. HUTCHENS, M.D., M.A.

Surgery and anesthesia cause significant stress on the cardiovascular system. The relative risk to a patient is determined by the extent of preexisting disease and the invasiveness of the proposed surgical procedure. The goals of preoperative evaluation are to identify patients who would benefit from treatment of heart disease prior to surgery, to provide assessment of cardiac risk prior to surgery (which might alter type of surgery, delay elective surgery, or encourage nonsurgical treatment), to determine the level of perioperative vigilance required, and to initiate health maintenance that will be continued after surgery. When a procedure is delayed, the expected benefit must outweigh the harm of delay. Good communication between the anesthesiologist and surgeon is therefore essential. The American College of Cardiology and the American Heart Association, applying evidenced-based techniques, have established guidelines for the perioperative cardiovascular evaluation.[1,2]

A. Assess the urgency and risk of the proposed surgical procedure. During the history and physical examination, note preexisting cardiac disease (e.g., coronary artery disease [CAD], valvular lesions, arrhythmia, congenital lesions, and peripheral vascular disease). Recent cardiac events present higher risk than remote events. Note prior cardiac evaluation and cardiovascular surgical procedures, including device implementation. Determine if the condition is stable and adequately treated. Document current medications, especially angiotensin-converting enzyme (ACE) inhibitors, anticoagulants, antiplatelet medications, beta-blockers, and statins. Identify other cardiac risk factors (e.g., age, hypertension [HTN], family history, diabetes, hypercholesterolemia, renal dysfunction, tobacco use, obesity, alcohol and other substance abuse, and rheumatic fever).[3]

B. Next, determine the patient's functional capacity. A patient who is unable to generate four METs (metabolic equivalents) has poor functional capacity. Ask about symptoms (e.g., does angina occur with exertion or at rest?). Consider potential anginal equivalents (i.e., shortness of breath, abdominal pain). Diabetics may not have angina, and women are more likely to have atypical symptoms. Complaints of lightheadedness, syncope, or fluttering sensations may indicate arrhythmia or valvular disease. Dyspnea may be a symptom of left-sided ventricular failure. The New York Heart Association (NYHA) classification is useful.[4]

C. Perform a physical examination. Assess general appearance (e.g., cyanosis, clubbing, dyspnea, or generalized distress). Jugular venous distention occurs with hypervolemia, right-sided ventricular failure, and impaired venous blood return. Check the pulse; rate, strength, and character are important. For example, tachycardia is undesirable in patients with CAD, because it increases oxygen consumption and reduces the time for oxygen delivery to the left ventricle (LV). Take the blood pressure. Auscultate heart and lungs to identify valvular lesions, arrhythmias, and other abnormal sounds, such as rubs and crackles. Measure oxygen saturation.

D. Order laboratory studies based on the clinical evaluation and the surgical procedure. Evaluate the ECG for baseline information and compare to prior ECGs, if available. Review the chest x-ray (CXR) for cardiomegaly or pulmonary edema.

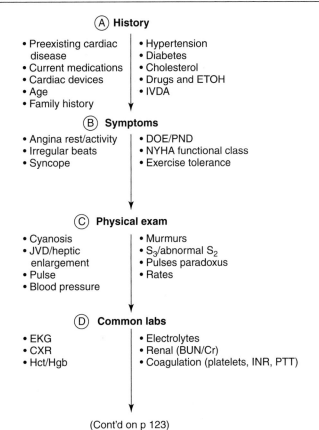

Ⓐ **History**

- Preexisting cardiac disease
- Current medications
- Cardiac devices
- Age
- Family history

- Hypertension
- Diabetes
- Cholesterol
- Drugs and ETOH
- IVDA

Ⓑ **Symptoms**

- Angina rest/activity
- Irregular beats
- Syncope

- DOE/PND
- NYHA functional class
- Exercise tolerance

Ⓒ **Physical exam**

- Cyanosis
- JVD/heptic enlargement
- Pulse
- Blood pressure

- Murmurs
- S_3/abnormal S_2
- Pulses paradoxus
- Rates

Ⓓ **Common labs**

- EKG
- CXR
- Hct/Hgb

- Electrolytes
- Renal (BUN/Cr)
- Coagulation (platelets, INR, PTT)

(Cont'd on p 123)

E. Obtain additional preoperative tests if the results will affect patient management and outcome—e.g., patients with poor functional capacity or those scheduled for high-risk surgical procedures. Consider consultation with a cardiologist. The heart can be imaged using transthoracic (TTE) or transesophageal echocardiography (TEE). These tests reveal valvular abnormalities, wall motion abnormalities, and other anatomic lesions (e.g., IHSS, pericardial effusion, intracardiac tumors). Ejection fraction (EF) can be measured noninvasively using the nuclide technetium-99. High-resolution magnetic resonance imaging (MRI) demonstrates coronary artery calcium, but it is unclear how this information will be used to predict risk or prescribe further treatment. Exercise stress testing is easy to perform but is highly influenced by patient factors and often has low predictive value. Imaging techniques enhance the sensitivity and specificity over ECG interpretation of ischemia. Thallium is taken up only by functioning myocardium and can aid in identifying myocardium at risk. Increased myocardial work can be chemically induced with dobutamine; coronary steal can be induced with dipyridamole or adenosine. TTE can also be used in conjunction with stress testing. Cardiac catheterization is the gold standard for diagnosing CAD. Some lesions can be treated with angioplasty or stenting; others require surgery. Disadvantages include cost, complications, and delay of treatment of the primary problem.

F. Optimize the patient. Attempt to stabilize fluid status, BP, and HR. Consider perioperative beta-blockade to prevent myocardial injury and the addition of statins for additional protection. Regulate anticoagulation. Patients taking warfarin (Coumadin) may benefit from conversion to heparin perioperatively. Have all mechanical devices checked by appropriately trained individuals. Sophisticated devices may require the presence of a specialist in the OR. For some patients, surgical delay will be required pending necessary interventions.

REFERENCES

1. Eagle KA, Berger PB, Calkins H, et al.: ACC/AHA guideline update for perioperative cardiovascular evaluation for noncardiac surgery: a report of the American College of Cardiology/American Heart Association Task Force on Practice Guidelines (Committee to Update the 1996 Guidelines on Perioperative Cardiovascular Evaluation for Noncardiac Surgery), available at: http://www.acc.org/clinical/guidelines/perio/dirIndex.htm, 2002.
2. Eagle KA, Berger PB, Calkins H, et al.: ACC/AHA guideline update for perioperative cardiovascular evaluation for noncardiac surgery: executive summary: a report of the American College of Cardiology/American Heart Association Task Force on Practice Guidelines (Committee to Update the 1996 Guidelines on Perioperative Cardiovascular Evaluation for Noncardiac Surgery), *J Am Coll Cardiol* (39):542–553, 2002.
3. Mangano DT, Kaplan JA, Reich DL, et al.: Preoperative assessment of cardiac risk. In *Cardiac anesthesia*, ed 4, Philadelphia, 1999, W.B. Saunders.
4. The Criteria Committee of the New York Heart Association: *Nomenclature and criteria for diagnosis of diseases of the heart and great vessels*, ed 9, Boston, 1994, Little, Brown & Co.

(Cont'd from p 121)

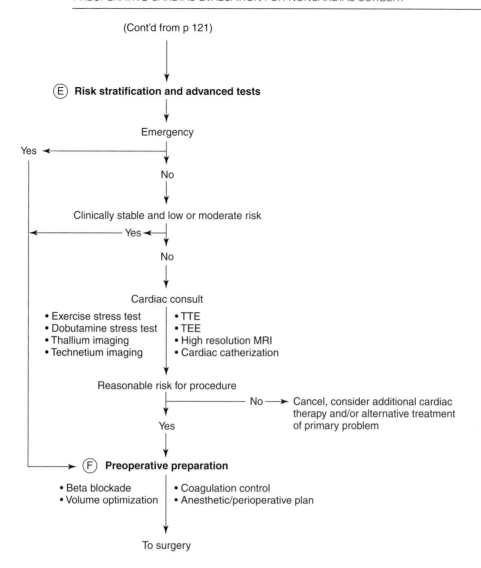

Ⓔ **Risk stratification and advanced tests**

Emergency

Yes ←

No

Clinically stable and low or moderate risk

← Yes ←

No

Cardiac consult

- Exercise stress test
- Dobutamine stress test
- Thallium imaging
- Technetium imaging

- TTE
- TEE
- High resolution MRI
- Cardiac catherization

Reasonable risk for procedure

No → Cancel, consider additional cardiac therapy and/or alternative treatment of primary problem

Yes

Ⓕ **Preoperative preparation**

- Beta blockade
- Volume optimization

- Coagulation control
- Anesthetic/perioperative plan

To surgery

Perioperative Hypertension (HTN)

FRANKLIN L. ANDERSON, M.D.

LAUREN L. SALGADO, M.D.

CHARLES B. HANTLER, M.D.

———

The perioperative management of hypertension (HTN) has varied a great deal over the past 30 years due to the absence of a large-scale, prospective, randomized study on perioperative outcome versus control of blood pressure (BP). However, some clinical patterns have appeared: BP lability is greater in uncontrolled hypertensive patients; poorly controlled hypertensive patients have increased BP after vascular surgery (carotid surgery). HTN is defined by the World Health Organization in levels[1]: *prehypertension* systolic blood pressure (SBP) 120 to 139 or diastolic blood pressure (DBP) 80 to 89; *Stage 1 HTN* SBP 140 to 159 or DBP 90 to 99; and *Stage 2 HTN* SBP >160 or DBP >100 mm Hg. Long-standing HTN increases the risk of renal failure, stroke, congestive heart failure (CHF), and myocardial infarction (MI). The aggressive control of HTN reduces cardiovascular complications, particularly in patients with evidence of cardiovascular disease (i.e., renal insufficiency or cerebral vascular disease), and morbidity can be reduced.[2] New classes of antihypertensive medication are produced each year; the anesthesiologist must be aware of potential anesthetic interactions.[3] For example, angiotensin converting enzyme (ACE) inhibitors and angiotensin-receptor blockers (ARBs) can sometimes lead to postinduction hypotension refractory to conventional treatment. A recent double-blind study demonstrated that the risk of hypotension is reduced if these medications are discontinued >10 hours prior to induction.[4] Further investigation will define optimal management.

A. Evaluate the cause of HTN. Common causes include essential (80 to 90%), chronic renal disease 5 to 10%, renovascular disease 2 to 5%, endocrine (pheochromocytoma, Cushing's syndrome, primary aldosteronism) < 1%, aortic coarctation < 1%, and miscellaneous 1 to 5%. Patients with prehypertension (DBP < 90) or labile HTN are more likely to have elevated cardiac output with normal vascular resistance. In those with Stage 1 or 2 HTN (DBP > 90), vascular resistance is usually elevated and cardiac output (CO) may be normal or reduced. Evaluate for end-organ disease. Renal function, although best assessed by more sophisticated tests, can be evaluated by blood urea nitrogen (BUN) and creatinine (Cr) levels. Collect clinical and laboratory evidence of myocardial ischemia and function. LVH is determined by ECG and, when indicated, by echocardiography (echo). Take a careful history, investigating the occurrence of strokes and reversible ischemic neurological events, and listen for carotid bruits. Review all medications and continue antihypertensive agents perioperatively. Consider withholding ARBs, ACE inhibitors, and diuretics. Beta-blockers and alpha$_2$-agonists must be continued through surgery to avoid withdrawal syndromes; perioperative use has been associated with a reduced risk of in-hospital death among high-risk patients undergoing major noncardiac surgery.[5,6]

B. In the absence of well-controlled studies on perioperative risks in hypertensive patients, clinical judgment is important. Many authors suggest that elective surgery may proceed when DBP is < 110 mm Hg. This recommendation follows from the study by Goldman and Caldera,[7] but randomization of patients in that study has been questioned. The most conservative recommendation is to achieve optimal BP control for several weeks before elective surgery. This approach may be too constraining to be justified in the absence of prospective studies. Most authorities agree that elective surgery should be postponed when the DBP > 110 mm Hg. Careful use of anxiolytics may prove useful in reducing resting BP. Consider the surgical risk, anesthetic risk, and underlying end-organ disease.

C. Monitoring is based on the type of surgery, preoperative BP control, and end-organ damage. Consider direct arterial monitoring in patients with poor BP control preoperatively.

D. During any anesthetic technique, anticipate swings in BP and be aware of potential drug interactions between antihypertensive agents and anesthetics or vasopressors. Determine a perioperative BP profile and set limits of intraoperative deviation (e.g., aggressively treat a 15% decrease in BP for > 10 to 15 minutes).

E. Continue antihypertensive medications postoperatively, particularly beta-blockers and alpha$_2$-agonists. Treat postoperative hypertension to avoid complications, including ischemia, stroke, and bleeding.

REFERENCES

1. Chobanian AV, Bakris GL, Black HR, et al.: The seventh report of the Joint National Committee on prevention, detection, evaluation, and treatment of high blood pressure: the JNC 7 report, *JAMA* 289:2560–2572, 2003.
2. Five-year findings of the hypertension detection and follow-up program. I. Reduction in mortality of persons with high blood pressure, including mild hypertension. Hypertension Detection and Follow-up Program Cooperative Group, 1979, *JAMA* 277:157–166, 1997.
3. Sullivan JM: A 1996 update on antihypertensive agents, *Curr Opin Cardiol* 11:496–500, 1996.
4. Comfere T, Sprung J, Kumar MM, et al.: Angiotensin system inhibitors in a general surgical population, *Anesth Analg* 100:636–644, 2005.
5. Lindenauer PK, Pekow P, Wang K, et al.: Perioperative beta-blocker therapy and mortality after major noncardiac surgery, *N Engl J Med* 353:349–361.
6. Wijeysundera DN, Naik JS, Beattie WS: Alpha-2 adrenergic agonists to prevent perioperative cardiovascular complications: a meta-analysis, *Am J Med* 114 (9):742–752, 2003.
7. Goldman L, Caldera DL: Risks of general anesthesia and elective operations in the hypertensive patient, *Anesthesiology* 50:285–292, 1979.

HYPERTENSIVE PATIENT FOR SURGERY

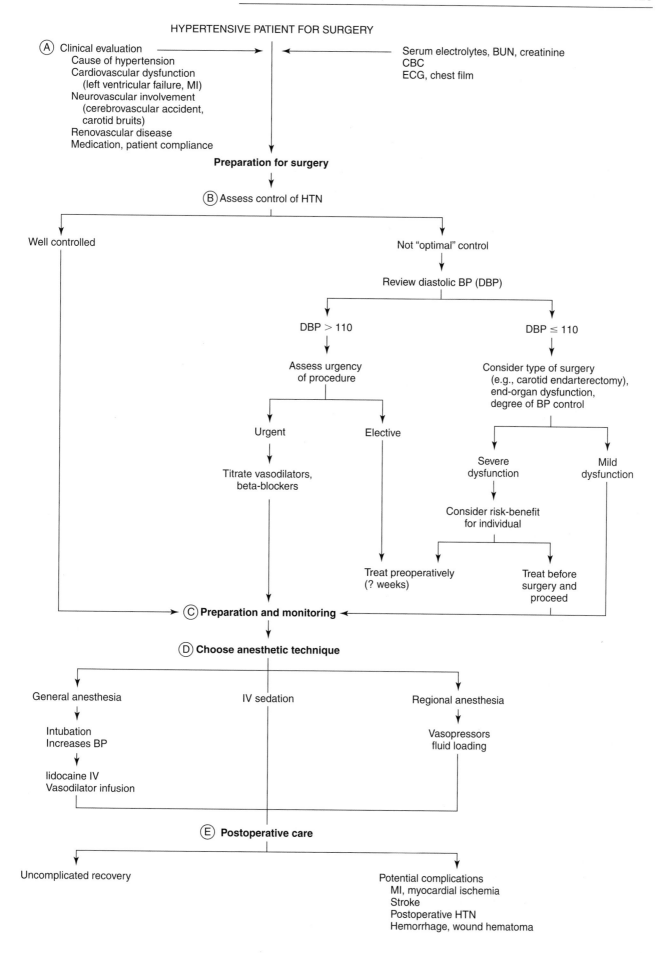

Coronary Artery Disease (CAD)

CHARLES B. HANTLER, M.D.

Preoperative cardiac evaluation is indicated in cases in which perioperative management may be altered by test results. The American College of Cardiology (ACC) and the American Heart Association (AHA) algorithm is depicted.[1] These recommendations have been endorsed by the Society of Cardiovascular Anesthesiologists. Aggressive perioperative beta-blockade may reduce the perioperative cardiac risk such that only a small minority of patients would benefit from cardiac workup. A recent randomized trial in patients undergoing vascular surgery failed to show any benefit (harm was not examined) from randomization to coronary intervention or coronary artery bypass grafting (CABG).[2] These trials suggest that cardiac workup may not be required in most patients in whom the ACC/AHA have recommended further coronary evaluation.

A. Perform a history and physical examination and review laboratory studies. Determine the functional capacity of the patient. Major clinical predictors of increased perioperative cardiovascular risk include unstable or severe angina, recent myocardial infarction (MI), poorly controlled congestive heart failure (CHF), symptomatic arrhythmias, and severe valvular disease. Medically treat and perform cardiac evaluation in all patients in this category before surgery, except in the case of certain emergency procedures. Intermediate clinical predictors include mild angina, prior MI, compensated CHF, and diabetes mellitus. These patients can undergo intermediate and low-risk operations without further testing but should have noninvasive cardiac testing performed before major risk surgery (unless such a patient has excellent exercise tolerance).[2] Patients with poor exercise tolerance (<4 metabolic equivalents [METs]) should be evaluated before intermediate risk surgical procedures (Table 1). Minor clinical predictors of risk include patients aged 65 to 75, who have carotid bruit, abnormal ECG, or poorly controlled hypertension (HTN). Perform cardiac work-up if high-risk surgery is planned and if the patient has low exercise tolerance (<4 METs). Many other patients are considered to be low risk for cardiac events.[3,4] These include patients

TABLE 1
Estimated Energy Requirements for Various Activities*

Energy expenditure	Activity
1–4 METs	Eating, dressing, walking around the house, light housework (e.g., washing dishes)
4–10 METs	Climbing a flight of stairs, walking on level ground at 6.4 km/hr, running a short distance, scrubbing floors, golfing
>10 METs	Swimming, singles tennis, football

*MET indicates metabolic equivalent
Modified from Hlatky MA, Boineau RE, Higginbotham MB, et al: *Am J Cardiol* 64: 651—654, 1989.

who have undergone cardiac workup with favorable findings within 2 years of proposed surgery and have had no change in their symptoms, and patients who have had CABG within 5 years and have had no recurrent symptoms. The effect of angioplasty with or without the placement of intracoronary stents before elective surgery is unknown.

B. Surgery-specific risk depends on the type of procedure and the degree of hemodynamic stress associated with that procedure. High-risk procedures include emergency major surgery, aortic or other major vascular surgery, peripheral vascular surgery (fem-pop), and prolonged intraabdominal or intrathoracic surgery with large fluid shifts. Intermediate risk procedures include carotid endarterectomy, major head and neck surgery, intraabdominal or intrathoracic surgery, major orthopedic surgery, or prostate surgery. Low-risk procedures include endoscopy, cataract extraction, superficial operations, and breast surgery.

C. Cardiac workup may include exercise and pharmacological stress testing, stress echocardiography, other nuclear tests, and coronary angiography. Rarely will CABG be performed before surgery. Noninvasive testing may be unnecessary in patients with intermediate clinical risk scheduled for high-risk surgery if exercise tolerance is excellent (>7 METs).

(Continued on page 128)

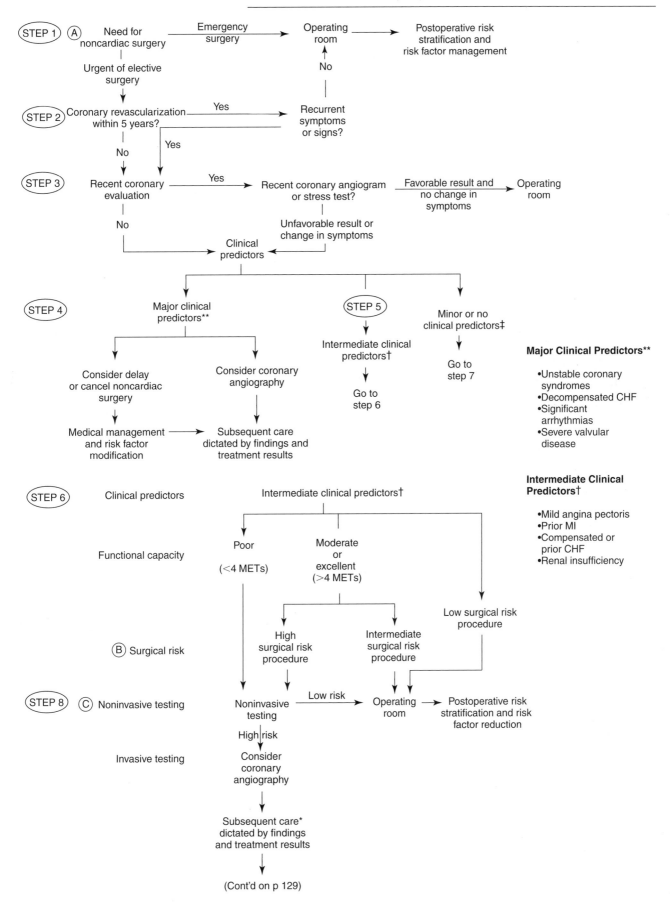

STEP 1 (A) Need for noncardiac surgery — Emergency surgery → Operating room → Postoperative risk stratification and risk factor management

No

Urgent of elective surgery

STEP 2 Coronary revascularization within 5 years? — Yes → Recurrent symptoms or signs?

No   Yes

STEP 3 Recent coronary evaluation — Yes → Recent coronary angiogram or stress test? — Favorable result and no change in symptoms → Operating room

No   Unfavorable result or change in symptoms

Clinical predictors

STEP 4   STEP 5 Minor or no clinical predictors‡

Major clinical predictors**   Intermediate clinical predictors†   Go to step 7

Consider delay or cancel noncardiac surgery   Consider coronary angiography   Go to step 6

Medical management and risk factor modification → Subsequent care dictated by findings and treatment results

Major Clinical Predictors**
•Unstable coronary syndromes
•Decompensated CHF
•Significant arrhythmias
•Severe valvular disease

Intermediate Clinical Predictors†
•Mild angina pectoris
•Prior MI
•Compensated or prior CHF
•Renal insufficiency

STEP 6 Clinical predictors   Intermediate clinical predictors†

Functional capacity   Poor (<4 METs)   Moderate or excellent (>4 METs)   Low surgical risk procedure

(B) Surgical risk   High surgical risk procedure   Intermediate surgical risk procedure

STEP 8 (C) Noninvasive testing   Noninvasive testing — Low risk → Operating room → Postoperative risk stratification and risk factor reduction

High risk

Invasive testing   Consider coronary angiography

Subsequent care* dictated by findings and treatment results

(Cont'd on p 129)

D. Continue the patient's usual cardiac medications (e.g., nitrates, beta-blockers, calcium channel blockers, and antihypertensives) preoperatively. Give adequate sedation. Aggressive beta-blockade is strongly recommended for HR control in the perioperative period.[5,6]

E. Choose intraoperative monitoring based on the expected physiological insult of the procedure and the patient's cardiovascular status. For minor surgical procedures in patients with mild to moderate disability, use basic monitors. When the procedure will compromise cardiovascular function (e.g., large blood loss, fluid shifts), monitor direct arterial and cardiac filling pressures. Note that pulmonary artery (PA) pressure may not be an early indicator of myocardial ischemia and is most useful in patients with significant left ventricular dysfunction and dyspnea as an "angina equivalent." Transesophageal echocardiography (TEE) is becoming a standard for the early detection of intraoperative myocardial ischemia and determination of ventricular function and volume status.

F. Select an anesthetic technique that provides analgesia and sedation adequate for the surgical and emotional stress. Many agents have been used successfully. Maintain the balance between myocardial oxygen (O_2) supply and demand. Treat hemodynamic aberrations promptly. When myocardial ischemia occurs, the pattern reflects the preoperative pattern and is associated with the distribution of postoperative MI; a causal relationship has not been proven. Many anesthetics possess potential for myocardial protection when used intraoperatively. This is particularly true for volatile anesthetics in patients undergoing coronary artery bypass surgery and might apply to noncardiac surgery.[7]

G. The highest incidence of reinfarction occurs 24 to 72 hours after surgery. In the very-high-risk patient, consider continuing invasive monitoring in an ICU for up to 4 days. Control HR with beta-blockers; resume antiplatelet, antilipid, and antiinflammatory.

REFERENCES

1. Eagle KA, Berger PB, Calkins H, et al.: ACC/AHA guideline update for perioperative cardiovascular evaluation for noncardiac surgery: executive summary: a report of the American College of Cardiology/American Heart Association Task Force on Practice Guidelines (Committee to Update the 1996 Guidelines on Perioperative Cardiovascular Evaluation for Noncardiac Surgery), *J Am Coll Cardiol* 39:542–553, 2002.

2. Moscucci M, Eagle KA: Coronary revascularization before noncardiac surgery, *N Engl J Med* 351 (27):2861–2863, 2004.

3. Ashton CM, Petersen NJ, Wray NP, et al.: The incidence of perioperative myocardial infarction in men undergoing noncardiac surgery, *Ann Intern Med* 118:504–510, 1993.

4. Warner MA, Shields SE, Chute CG: Major morbidity and mortality within one month of ambulatory surgery and anesthesia, *JAMA* 270:1437–1441, 1993.

5. Mangano DT, Layug EL, Wallace A, et al.: Effect of atenolol on mortality and cardiovascular morbidity after noncardiac surgery. Multicenter study of perioperative ischemia research group, *N Engl J Med* 335:1713–1720, 1996.

6. Boersma E, Poldermans D, Bax JJ, et al.: Predictors of cardiac events after major vascular surgery: role of clinical characteristics, dobutamine echocardiography, and beta-blocker therapy, *JAMA* 285:1865–1873, 2001.

7. De Hert SG, Turani, F, Mathur S, et al.: Cardioprotection with volatile anesthetics: mechanisms and clinical implications, *Anesth Analg* 100 (6):1584–1593, 2005.

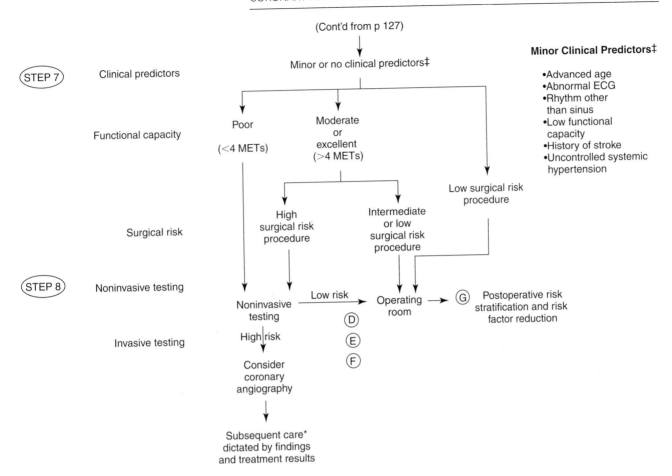

From Eagle KA, Berger PB, Calkins H, et al.: ACC/AHA guideline update for perioperative
cardiovascular evaluation for noncardiac surgery: executive summary: a report of the
American College of Cardiology/AAA/American Heart Association Task Force on Practice
Guidelines (Committee to Update the 1996 Guidelines on Perioperative Cardiovascular
Evaluation for Noncardiac Surgery). *J Am Coll Cardiol* 39:542–53, 2002.

Hypertrophic Cardiomyopathy (HCM)

CHARLES B. HANTLER, M.D.

KIMBERLY D. MILHOAN, M.D.

Hypertrophic cardiomyopathy (HCM) is the most common genetic (autosomal dominant) cardiovascular disease, the incidence is 0.2% in the general adult population but frequently unrecognized, and is the most common cause of sudden cardiac death (SCD) in the young. HCM can present clinically at any phase of life, from infancy to very late adulthood. HCM is a primary disorder of the sarcomere caused by mutations (>400 now identified) in 1 of at least 12 sarcomeric or nonsarcomeric genes. Clinical diagnosis is usually established by two-dimensional echocardiographic demonstration of left ventricular (LV) hypertrophy associated with a nondilated chamber, in the absence of another cardiac or systemic disease capable of producing the magnitude of hypertrophy present. No pattern of LV wall thickening is classic or typical, but the predominant region of hypertrophy is the anterior ventricular septum. Distribution is almost always (99%) asymmetric. Most patients have diffuse involvement of the septum and LV-free wall, but 30% have only localized thickening of a single segment of the LV wall. The disease is characterized histopathologically by cardiac muscle disarray throughout the LV (not just in hypertrophied regions), significant collagen distribution within an expanded interstitial matrix, thickened intramural coronary arterioles with narrow lumen, and primary malformations of the mitral valve apparatus. These characteristics place patients with HCM at risk for (1) dynamic LV outflow obstruction, (2) diastolic dysfunction, (3) myocardial ischemia, and (4) supraventricular and ventricular tachyarrhythmias. The clinical course of symptomatic patients involves a combination of progressive heart failure with exertional dyspnea, sometimes progressing to end-stage disease, fatigue and chest pain, atrial fibrillation (AF), and sudden death.[1-4]

A. Assess symptoms of systolic and diastolic ventricular dysfunction, myocardial ischemia, and serious dysrhythmias, such as exertional dyspnea, fatigue, angina, palpitations, syncope, or near-syncope. When these symptoms, a family history of HCM or SCD, or a systolic ejection murmur at the left lower sternal border and apex (may be present in the supine position or provoked with standing or Valsalva, or diminished with squatting) in previously undiagnosed patients are encountered, initiate referral for full cardiovascular evaluation prior to the administration of anesthesia. (The lack of murmur on preoperative examination does not rule out HCM, as LV outflow tract obstruction does not always accompany HCM, but is usually dynamic in nature if it does.)

B. The 12-lead electrocardiogram is abnormal in 75 to 90% of HCM patients. Abnormalities include tall voltages consistent with LV hypertrophy, ST-segment abnormalities and T-wave inversion, left atrial enlargement, abnormal Q waves, and diminished or absent R waves in the left precordial leads. Chest x-rays (CXR) may reveal a prominent left atrial (LA) shadow, interstitial edema, or prominent pulmonary arteries. Echocardiography (echo) is the noninvasive test of choice—look for LV hypertrophy not associated with ventricular cavity enlargement. Markedly impaired myocardial relaxation is also characteristic. Assess for LV outflow tract obstruction, either at rest or with physiological provocation of exercise conditions, as well as the presence of mitral regurgitation (frequently accompanies outflow obstruction).

C. The most commonly used medications in HCM are beta-blockers and calcium channel blockers. Patients resistant to these agents alone may be treated with the type 1-A antiarrhythmic disopyramide, in combination with a beta-blocker. Some patients will be anticoagulated (systemic emboli secondary to AF). Because of the increased incidence of SCD, a subset of patients may present on antiarrhythmic therapy, such as amiodarone, or with an implantable cardioverter-defibrillator in place. Preoperative sedation is recommended, if it can be tolerated. Consider subacute bacterial endocarditis (SBE) prophylaxis if LV outflow obstruction or mitral regurgitation is present. Avoid anticholinergics.

(Continued on page 132)

Patient with HYPERTROPHIC CARDIOMYOPATHY

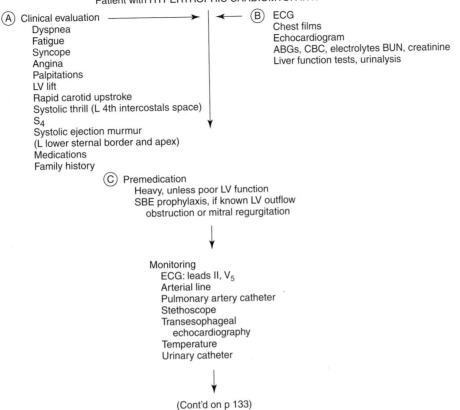

(A) Clinical evaluation ─────────────➤ │ ◀─── (B) ECG
    Dyspnea   Chest films
    Fatigue   Echocardiogram
    Syncope   ABGs, CBC, electrolytes BUN, creatinine
    Angina   Liver function tests, urinalysis
    Palpitations
    LV lift
    Rapid carotid upstroke
    Systolic thrill (L 4th intercostals space)
    S_4
    Systolic ejection murmur
    (L lower sternal border and apex)
    Medications
    Family history

(C) Premedication
    Heavy, unless poor LV function
    SBE prophylaxis, if known LV outflow
      obstruction or mitral regurgitation

Monitoring
    ECG: leads II, V_5
    Arterial line
    Pulmonary artery catheter
    Stethoscope
    Transesophageal
      echocardiography
    Temperature
    Urinary catheter

(Cont'd on p 133)

D. Consider potential for dynamic LV outflow obstruction (Table 1), diastolic dysfunction, myocardial ischemia, and malignant arrhythmias. Maintain normal preload (small ventricles obstruct but diastolically dysfunctional ventricles fail), reduce myocardial oxygen (O_2) demand (by decreasing HR and reducing contractility), maintain afterload (to reduce ventricular emptying and perfuse the myocardium), and maintain normal sinus rhythm (ventricular filling is dependent on LA contraction). Sevoflurane and vecuronium are acceptable agents. Beta-blockers (esmolol, metoprolol) are useful to treat elevations in HR and contractile state, especially during emergence. Vasodilators are not indicated. Treat acute hypotension with volume replacement and alpha$_1$- agonists, not with drugs with beta-adrenergic activity. Ventilation strategies include small tidal volumes and increased respiratory rates to avoid the decrease in venous return associated with high airway pressures.

TABLE 1
Maneuvers Affecting HCM

Increased obstruction to LV outflow	Reduced obstruction to LV outflow
Increased contractility	Increased mean arterial pressure
Exercise, stress	Squatting, leg raising
Decreased LV end-diastolic volume	Hypervolemia
Valsalva, sudden standing	Increased systemic vascular resistance
Nitroglycerin, nitroprusside, amyl nitrate	Isometric exercise
Tachycardia	Decreased contractility
Decreased afterload	Beta-blockers
Isoproterenol, digitalis, dopamine, dobutamine	Phenylephrine

REFERENCES

1. Poliac LC, Barron ME, Maron BJ: Hypertrophic cardiomyopathy, *Anesthesiology* 104:183–192, 2006.
2. Sasson Z, Rakowski H, Wigle ED: Hypertrophic cardiomyopathy, *Cardiol Clin* 6:233, 1988.
3. Thompson RC, Liberthson RR, Lowenstein E: Perioperative anesthetic risk of noncardiac surgery in hypertrophic obstructive cardiomyopathy, *JAMA* 254:2419, 1985.
4. Hreybe H, Zahid M, Sonel A, et al: Noncardiac surgery and the risk of death and other cardiovascular events in patients with hypertrophic cardiomyopathy, *Clin Cardiol* 29 (2):65–68, 2006.

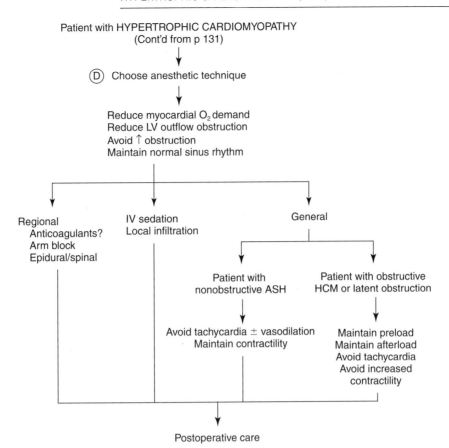

Patient with HYPERTROPHIC CARDIOMYOPATHY
(Cont'd from p 131)

(D)   Choose anesthetic technique

Reduce myocardial O_2 demand
Reduce LV outflow obstruction
Avoid ↑ obstruction
Maintain normal sinus rhythm

Regional
Anticoagulants?
Arm block
Epidural/spinal

IV sedation
Local infiltration

General

Patient with
nonobstructive ASH

Patient with obstructive
HCM or latent obstruction

Avoid tachycardia ± vasodilation
Maintain contractility

Maintain preload
Maintain afterload
Avoid tachycardia
Avoid increased
contractility

Postoperative care

Mitral Valve Prolapse (MVP)

NICHOLAS R. SIMMONS, M.D.

CHARLES B. HANTLER, M.D.

Mitral valve prolapse (MVP) is a condition in which there is excessive billowing of the mitral valve leaflets (most commonly, the posterior leaflet) into the left atrium during systole.[1-3] The incidence of MVP syndrome has been reported to be as high as 10%, however, this is an overestimation with the true incidence being approximately 3%.[4] There may be myxomatous proliferation of the leaflets, annulus, and chordae leading to prolapse and in severe cases, may result in chordae rupture and severe mitral regurgitation (MR). Prolapse and regurgitation are made worse by conditions that reduce left ventricular (LV) size: reduced preload or afterload, tachycardia, or an enhanced contractile state. Subsets of these patients are prone to both atrial and ventricular dysrhythmias; an association with atrioventricular bypass tracks and prolonged QT interval has been described. Asymptomatic patients without evidence of MR or patients with mild, stable MR do not require routine echo surveillance; those with symptomatic MR or LV dysfunction are followed more closely. Patients with a systolic murmur or echocardiographic evidence of MR require antibiotic prophylaxis. Patients with palpitations or syncopelike symptoms are followed with interval Holter monitoring. Recent echocardiographic studies suggest that patients with redundant leaflets are prone to emboli, bacterial endocarditis (BE), and perhaps sudden death. Those with simple billowing of the mitral valve appear to have low risk for cardiac events. Although the long-term prognosis and the perioperative course are usually excellent, patients with MVP have had significant perioperative dysrhythmias, including asystole.[1,2]

A. Perform a history and physical examination. Patients with MVP are usually asymptomatic. Complaints may include palpitations, chest discomfort, and dyspnea. The chest pain may be anginal in quality or sharp and stabbing. When there is significant MR, patients may present with symptoms of cardiac failure. There is frequently a midsystolic click, which may be followed by a middle-to-late systolic murmur: the greater the regurgitation, the longer the murmur. The click occurs earlier and the murmur lasts longer with maneuvers that reduce ventricular chamber size (e.g., Valsalva). Obtain an ECG. Although the ECG is typically normal, there may be nonspecific ST-T wave changes in the inferior or lateral leads. Atrial and ventricular tachydysrhythmias or bradydysrhythmias are more common in older patients with MVP and MR than in those without the disease. Echocardiography (echo) is diagnostic of this syndrome, demonstrating at least 2 mm prolapse of one or both leaflets. MR may also be seen on the echocardiogram. When significant MR is present or when the patient is symptomatic, consider a preoperative transesophageal echocardiography (TEE) to assess LV function and the degree of MR.

B. Prepare the patient psychologically and pharmacologically. Patients with MVP may be anxious and tachycardia exaggerates prolapse. Administer antibiotic coverage to patients with MR for operations known to seed the bloodstream with bacteria.

C. Use standard monitoring in the absence of significant MR. When significant MR is present or when the patient is symptomatic, consider invasive monitoring or TEE as would be appropriate for a patient with MR.

D. Choose the anesthetic technique least likely to cause tachycardia or to alter the hemodynamic status. For peripheral procedures, a nerve/plexus block is appropriate. Spinal and epidural blocks are more likely to cause an abrupt decrease in preload and afterload, which might increase the MVP. Avoid histamine-releasing drugs and choose muscle relaxants with consideration of their cardiovascular effects. Avoid atropine, ketamine, and dehydration (tachycardia); replace fluid and blood loss aggressively. If tachycardia occurs despite euvolemia, treat with beta-blockers after other causes of tachycardia have been ruled out. If vasopressors are needed acutely for relative hypovolemia (e.g., high spinal), choose those with a predominant alpha effect (phenylephrine).

E. Continue monitoring BP, HR, and intravascular volume status postoperatively according to the patient's clinical status and intraoperative hemodynamic stability.

REFERENCES

1. Abraham ZA, Lees DE: Two cardiac arrests after needle punctures in a patient with mitral valve prolapse: psychogenic? *Anesth Analg* 69:126–128, 1989.
2. Twersky RS, Kaplan JA: Junctional rhythm in a patient with mitral valve prolapse, *Anesth Analg* 65:975–978, 1986.
3. Hanson EW, Neerhut RK, Lynch C III: Mitral valve prolapse, *Anesthesiology* 85:178–195, 1996.
4. Hayek E, Gring CN, Griffin BP: Mitral valve prolapse, *Lancet* 365:507–518, 2005.

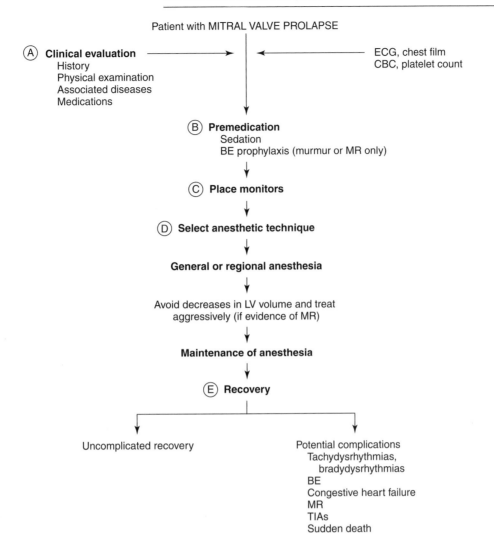

Patient with MITRAL VALVE PROLAPSE

Ⓐ **Clinical evaluation** ⟶   ⟵   ECG, chest film
    History   CBC, platelet count
    Physical examination
    Associated diseases
    Medications

Ⓑ **Premedication**
    Sedation
    BE prophylaxis (murmur or MR only)

Ⓒ **Place monitors**

Ⓓ **Select anesthetic technique**

General or regional anesthesia

Avoid decreases in LV volume and treat
aggressively (if evidence of MR)

Maintenance of anesthesia

Ⓔ **Recovery**

Uncomplicated recovery   Potential complications
                                Tachydysrhythmias,
                                    bradydysrhythmias
                                BE
                                Congestive heart failure
                                MR
                                TIAs
                                Sudden death

Mitral Stenosis (MS)

ANTONIO HERNANDEZ, M.D.

Mitral stenosis (MS) is most commonly rheumatic in origin with clinical disease becoming manifest within three to four decades of initial infection. Of these, 25% have pure MS, and 40% have combined MS with mitral regurgitation (MR).[1] Stenosis results from commissural fusion, calcification and thickening of leaflets, or thickening and contraction of chordae tendineae. MS is characterized by mechanical obstruction to left ventricular (LV) diastolic filling secondary to progressive decrease in the size of the mitral valve orifice. MS is severe when the mitral opening is <1 cm^2. MS prevents filling of the left ventricle, which results in decreased stroke volume and cardiac output (CO). MS prevents emptying of the left atrium, which results in increased left atrial (LA) and pulmonary artery (PA) pressures to maintain CO.[1] Patients are prone to developing pulmonary edema. Pulmonary hypertension (HTN) frequently complicates the course of MS. LV end-diastolic pressure (LVEDP) is usually normal or low. An elevation of LVEDP should suggest the presence of coexisting disease, such as HTN, coronary artery disease (CAD), or aortic valvular disease.[2] In patients with elevated pulmonary vascular resistance (PVR), right ventricular (RV) function is often impaired, and a rise in RV output is impossible. The hemodynamic goals for MS include a low normal HR of approximately 60 to 80 beats per minutes and an adequate perfusion pressure based on the patient's preoperative hemodynamic data.

A. Assess severity of MS. Determine if the patient has exercise-induced symptoms or hemodynamic abnormalities. The principle symptom is dyspnea, largely the result of reduced lung compliance. Orthopnea, paroxysmal nocturnal dyspnea, and dyspnea at rest usually relate to elevated LA pressures, secondary to the diastolic pressure gradient between the left atrium and left ventricle. This gradient can change quickly and dramatically as a result of changes in CO and diastolic filling times.

B. Review preoperative studies. LA enlargement and atrial fibrillation (AF) are the principal ECG features. Right axis deviation and RV hypertrophy occur with pulmonary HTN. Chest x-rays (CXRs) show LA and RV enlargement and Kerley B lines. Echocardiography (echo) is the most useful, noninvasive test. Doppler echo can quantify the severity of MS and estimate the transvalvular gradient. The peak velocity of transmitral flow is increased; the rate of decline of flow during early systole is reduced. Two-dimensional echo is used to determine mitral orifice size. It reveals restricted motion and doming of the valve leaflets. Two-dimensional echo will also recognize LA thrombus and assess mitral valve calcification and LV contractility. An echocardiographic scoring system has been devised to predict the outcome of percutaneous balloon valvuloplasty.[3] It may be useful in certain high-risk patients (elderly or those with pulmonary, renal, or neoplastic disease). Cardiac catheterization can determine transvalvular gradient, mitral valve area, LV function, and right-sided pressures. Obtain cardiac catheterization in patients with suspected CAD.

C. Review medications. Patients with MS often receive medical therapy for heart failure: digitalis to slow ventricular rate in AF, diuretics, and sodium restriction. Discontinue anticoagulants two to three days before the operation.[4] Administer antibiotic prophylaxis for subacute bacterial endocarditis (SBE). Place an arterial line. Consider placing a PA catheter in patients with known pulmonary HTN. Use the pulmonary capillary wedge pressure (PCWP) as an index of LV filling, keeping in mind that it is higher than the true LVEDP, at least by the amount of the pressure gradient. During episodes of tachycardia or increased flow, the wedge pressure continues to reflect LA pressure but is no longer indicative of filling pressure. Transesophageal echocardiography (TEE) is the best method of monitoring and assessing the severity of MS and allowing quantitative analysis.

Choose an appropriate anesthetic technique. Patients are sensitive to respiratory depressants. For general anesthesia, maintain perfusion pressure and avoid hypoxia, hypercarbia, hypothermia, tachycardia, and increases in PVR. Epidural anesthesia is the preferred regional anesthetic technique. Hemodynamic goals remain the same. Avoid rapid hydration. Establish the anesthetic level slowly. Avoid ephedrine, which may increase the HR. Phenylephrine causes increases in ventricular afterload, which can precipitate heart failure; use judiciously to achieve the appropriate hemodynamic goals.

(Continued on page 138)

Patient with MITRAL STENOSIS

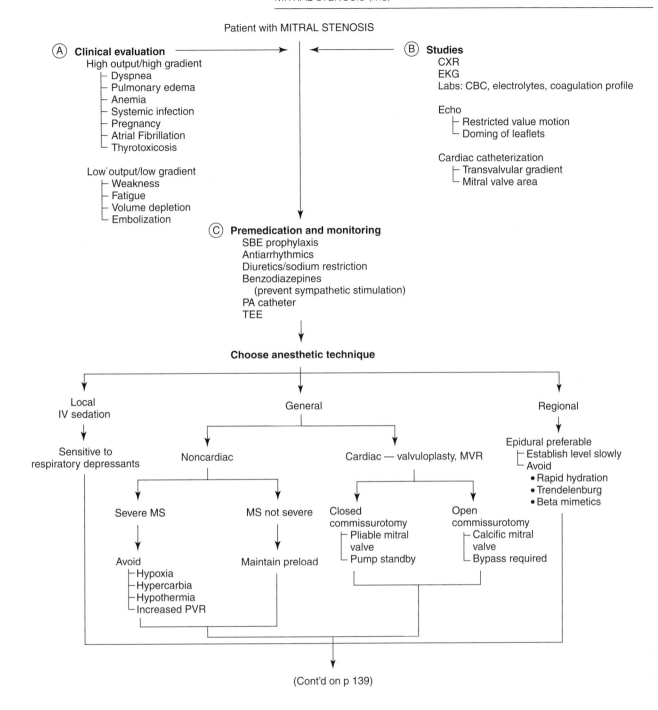

Ⓐ **Clinical evaluation**
   High output/high gradient
      ├ Dyspnea
      ├ Pulmonary edema
      ├ Anemia
      ├ Systemic infection
      ├ Pregnancy
      ├ Atrial Fibrillation
      └ Thyrotoxicosis

   Low output/low gradient
      ├ Weakness
      ├ Fatigue
      ├ Volume depletion
      └ Embolization

Ⓑ **Studies**
   CXR
   EKG
   Labs: CBC, electrolytes, coagulation profile

   Echo
      ├ Restricted value motion
      └ Doming of leaflets

   Cardiac catheterization
      ├ Transvalvular gradient
      └ Mitral valve area

Ⓒ **Premedication and monitoring**
   SBE prophylaxis
   Antiarrhythmics
   Diuretics/sodium restriction
   Benzodiazepines
      (prevent sympathetic stimulation)
   PA catheter
   TEE

Choose anesthetic technique

Local
IV sedation

Sensitive to
respiratory depressants

General

Noncardiac

Cardiac — valvuloplasty, MVR

Regional

Epidural preferable
   ├ Establish level slowly
   └ Avoid
      • Rapid hydration
      • Trendelenburg
      • Beta mimetics

Severe MS

MS not severe

Closed
commissurotomy
   ├ Pliable mitral
   │ valve
   └ Pump standby

Open
commissurotomy
   ├ Calcific mitral
   │ valve
   └ Bypass required

Avoid
   ├ Hypoxia
   ├ Hypercarbia
   ├ Hypothermia
   └ Increased PVR

Maintain preload

(Cont'd on p 139)

D. Treat hemodynamic abnormalities. Tachycardia worsens the hemodynamics by decreasing diastolic time. The reduction in CO during stress is related not only to the severity of stenosis but also to secondary circulatory alterations, such as pulmonary vascular disease and reflex vasoconstriction of the systemic circulation. Sudden marked increases in central blood volume may precipitate edema, right-sided heart failure, or AF. Direct immediate treatment of AF toward reducing the ventricular rate by pharmacological cardioversion and if a LA thrombus has been ruled out, electrical cardioversion. Maintain systemic vascular resistance (SVR); acute afterload reduction or hypotension may decrease CO and coronary perfusion pressure. Hypercarbia, hypoxia, hypothermia, N_2O, alpha-adrenergic agonists, calcium chloride, and positive-pressure ventilation can elevate PA pressures, leading to pulmonary HTN and RV compromise. There are new pharmacological agents for treatment of severe pulmonary hypertension: inhaled prostacyclin and nitric oxide (NO).[5] A single oral dose of sildenafil 75 mg showed similar ability to decrease PVR when compared to NO, but sildenafil was superior to NO by improving CO and reducing LVEDP.[6] (Sildenafil's effect peaks at approximately 50 minutes and lasts approximately 3 hours; redose via nasogastric tube if necessary.)

E. Postoperatively, patients with MS are at risk for developing pulmonary edema and right-sided heart failure. Pain, hypercarbia, respiratory acidosis, and arterial hypoxemia may be responsible for increasing heart rate or PVR. Continue antibiotics and restart anticoagulation.

REFERENCES

1. Braunwald E, Turzi ZG: Pathophysiology of mitral valve disease. In: Wells FC, Shapiro LM, editors: *Mitral valve disease*, ed 2, London, 1996, Butterworth.
2. Wray DL, Hughes CW, Fine R, et al: Anesthesia for cardiac surgery. In: Barash PG, Cullen BF, Stoelting RK, editors: *Clinical anesthesia*, New York, 2005, Lippincott, Williams, & Wilkins.
3. Wilkins GT, Weyman AE, Abascal VM, et al.: Percutaneous balloon dilatation of the mitral valve: an analysis of echocardiographic variables related to outcome and the mechanism of dilatation, *Br Heart J* 60:299–308, 1988.
4. Committee on Management of Patients with Valvular Heart Disease. ACC/AHA guidelines for the management of patients with valvular heart disease. A report of the American College of Cardiology/American Heart Association Task Force on Practice Guidelines, *J Am Coll Cardiol* 32 (5):1486–588, 1998.
5. Girard C, Lehot JJ, Pannetier JC, et al.: Inhaled nitric oxide after mitral valve replacement in patients with chronic pulmonary artery hypertension, *Anesthesiology* 77:880–883, 1992.
6. Michelakis E, Tymchak W, Lien D, et al: Oral sildenafil is an effective and specific pulmonary vasodilator in patients with pulmonary arterial hypertension: comparison with inhaled nitric oxide, *Circulation* 105:2398–2403, 2002.

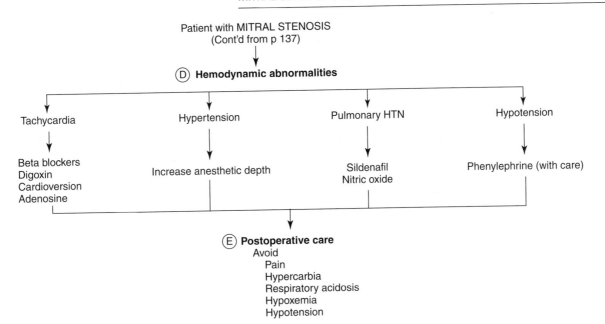

Patient with MITRAL STENOSIS
(Cont'd from p 137)

Ⓓ **Hemodynamic abnormalities**

| Tachycardia | Hypertension | Pulmonary HTN | Hypotension |

Tachycardia

Beta blockers
Digoxin
Cardioversion
Adenosine

Hypertension

Increase anesthetic depth

Pulmonary HTN

Sildenafil
Nitric oxide

Hypotension

Phenylephrine (with care)

Ⓔ **Postoperative care**
Avoid
Pain
Hypercarbia
Respiratory acidosis
Hypoxemia
Hypotension

Mitral Regurgitation (MR)

ANTONIO HERNANDEZ, M.D.

Mitral valve prolapse (MVP) and rheumatic heart disease are the leading causes of chronic mitral regurgitation (MR). Rupture of chordae tendineae and prolapsing mitral valves may result from trauma or endocarditis. Papillary muscle dysfunction secondary to inferior or posterior myocardial infarction (MI) may result in catastrophic acute MR. The severity of regurgitation and the cause of the lesion determines the course of this condition. The prognosis in acute, severe MR, from whatever cause, is poor without surgical intervention. Acute MR may manifest as severe congestive heart failure (CHF) and pulmonary edema. Cardiovascular collapse and hypotension can also occur. Most patients with chronic, mild MR do well for many years without evidence of left ventricular (LV) dysfunction. Fatigue and dyspnea on exertion occur as a consequence of LV dysfunction. Mitral valve replacement should be considered before the onset of significant LV failure; the postoperative and long-term outcomes are better in patients with preserved LV function.

A. Evaluate the patient and look for manifestations of MR. LV volume overload occurs in chronic MR. Eccentric hypertrophy of the LV allows preservation of a relatively normal LV end-diastolic pressure (LVEDP) despite increased LV end-diastolic volume (LVEDV). The left atrium enlarges and becomes distensible, allowing for normal left atrial (LA) pressures in the face of large regurgitant volumes. LV stroke volume increases. The reduced impedance to ejection in chronic MR may lead to overestimation of LV function if ejection fraction (EF) is the index used. Eventually, LV function deteriorates as forward stroke volume is compromised. In acute MR, compliance of the left atrium is limited, and the significant increase in LA pressure leads to pulmonary edema. Compensatory sympathetic stimulation increases contractility and produces tachycardia.

B. Review results of complementary studies. The ECG may reveal LA enlargement, LV hypertrophy, and atrial fibrillation (AF). Transthoracic echocardiography (TTE) may reveal the etiology of valvular disease. However, transesophageal echocardiography (TEE) is superior to TTE due to the close proximity of the TEE probe to the heart and the lack of acoustic interference from adjacent air-occupying lung parenchyma. Doppler echocardiogram in MR shows a high-velocity jet in the left atrium during systole.[1] Both color-flow Doppler and pulsed techniques correlate well with angiographic methods in estimating the severity of MR.[2]

The most reliable method of detecting severe MR is identifying blunting or reversal of the systolic component of the pulsed wave Doppler scan of the pulmonary vein. Radionuclide angiograms are useful for interval follow-up of patients. Progressive increases in LVEDV or LV end-systolic volume (LVESV) suggest the need for surgical treatment. Preoperative end-systolic diameter and EF are important predictors of short- and long-term outcomes for mitral valve replacement.

C. Review the patient's medications. Patients with AF usually take anticoagulants, which need to be discontinued prior to most surgical procedures.[3] (Do not perform electrocardioversion on such patients unless a TEE has ruled out the presence of an atrial thrombus.) Patients are often treated with digitalis and diuretics for CHF. Afterload reduction is beneficial for patients with both acute and chronic MR.[4] Afterload reducers maintain forward stroke volume and by decreasing LV volume, reduce the size of the mitral annulus thus reducing the regurgitant orifice. Administer antibiotics for prophylaxis against subacute bacterial endocarditis (SBE) to all patients with MR.[5] Determine appropriate preoperative sedation, taking into account the degree of LV dysfunction. Select appropriate intraoperative monitors. Pulmonary artery (PA) catheters are useful to assess ventricular filling pressures, cardiac output (CO), and the effect of vasodilator therapy. The size of the regurgitant "giant V wave" does not correlate with the severity of MR. Consider intraoperative TEE, which provides information on anatomy and physiology of the mitral valve and the physiological impact of the regurgitant jet. Keep in mind that with general anesthesia, the resulting physiological changes (i.e., decrease in systemic vascular resistance [SVR], increase in HR) will reveal an improvement in measured parameters, thereby underestimating the severity of the MR.[6] Patients with papillary muscle dysfunction secondary to ischemia are frequently helped by the preoperative insertion of an intraaortic balloon pump.

D. Choose an anesthetic technique. Regional anesthesia is usually well tolerated. Epidural anesthesia may result in a decreased SVR, which promotes forward flow of blood and helps prevent pulmonary congestion. Regardless of the anesthetic technique chosen, prevent pain, hypoxemia, hypercarbia, and acidosis to avoid increases in pulmonary vascular resistance (PVR).

(Continued on page 142)

Patient with MITRAL REGURGITATION

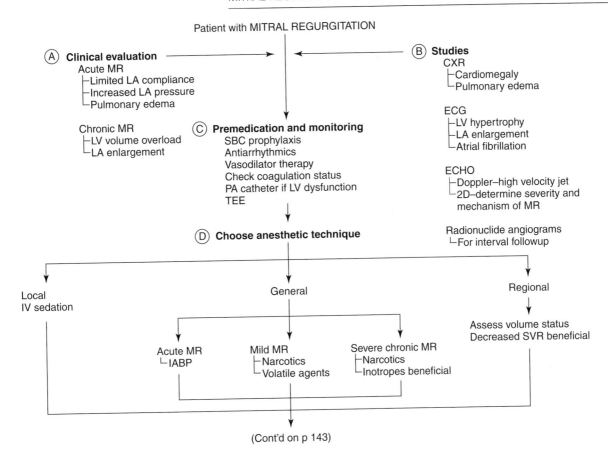

Ⓐ **Clinical evaluation**
   Acute MR
   ├─Limited LA compliance
   ├─Increased LA pressure
   └─Pulmonary edema

   Chronic MR
   ├─LV volume overload
   └─LA enlargement

Ⓒ **Premedication and monitoring**
   SBC prophylaxis
   Antiarrhythmics
   Vasodilator therapy
   Check coagulation status
   PA catheter if LV dysfunction
   TEE

Ⓑ **Studies**
   CXR
   ├─Cardiomegaly
   └─Pulmonary edema

   ECG
   ├─LV hypertrophy
   ├─LA enlargement
   └─Atrial fibrillation

   ECHO
   ├─Doppler–high velocity jet
   └─2D–determine severity and
      mechanism of MR

   Radionuclide angiograms
   └─For interval followup

Ⓓ **Choose anesthetic technique**

Local
IV sedation

General

Acute MR
└─IABP

Mild MR
├─Narcotics
└─Volatile agents

Severe chronic MR
├─Narcotics
└─Inotropes beneficial

Regional

Assess volume status
Decreased SVR beneficial

(Cont'd on p 143)

E. Remember the important hemodynamic goals. Maintain a HR of 80 to 90 bpm, except when the MR is caused by MVP. Bradycardia is harmful, because it increases the regurgitant fraction. In patients with contradictory physiological goals, compare the severity of MR with the severity of coronary artery disease (CAD). For example, if MR is mild and CAD severe, maintain coronary perfusion pressure and a conservative HR. Otherwise, avoid alpha-adrenergic agents, because increases in afterload lead to an increased regurgitant fraction and reduced CO. Consider inotropic support to improve myocardial contractility and decrease the regurgitant fraction. This is also helpful in treating hypotension.

F. During the postoperative period, ensure adequate oxygenation, ventilation, and analgesia. Continue antibiotics and cardiac medications. Restart anticoagulation when appropriate.

REFERENCES

1. Jenni R, Ritter M, Eberli F, et al.: Quantification of mitral regurgitation with amplitude-weighted mean velocity from continuous wave Doppler spectra, *Circulation* 79:1294–1299, 1989.
2. Pu M, Griffin BP, Vandervoot PM, et al.: The value of assessing pulmonary venous flow velocity for predicting severity of mitral regurgitation: A quantitative assessment integrating left ventricular function, *J Am Soc Echocardiogr* 12:736–743, 1999.
3. Committee on Management of Patients with Valvular Heart Disease: ACC/AHA guidelines for the management of patients with valvular heart disease. a report of the American College of Cardiology/American Heart Association Task Force on Practice Guidelines, *J Am Coll Cardiol* 32 (5):1486–1588, 1998.
4. Hoit BD: Medical treatment of valvular heart disease, *Curr Opin Cardiol* 6:207–211, 1991.
5. Dajani AS, Taubert KA, Wilson W, et al: Prevention of bacterial endocarditis. Recommendations by the American Heart Association, *JAMA* 277 (22):1794–1801, 1997.
6. Grewal KS, Malkowski MJ, Piracha AR, et al.: Effect of general anesthesia on the severity of mitral regurgitation by transesophageal echocardiography, *Am J Cardiol* 85 (2):199–203, 2000.

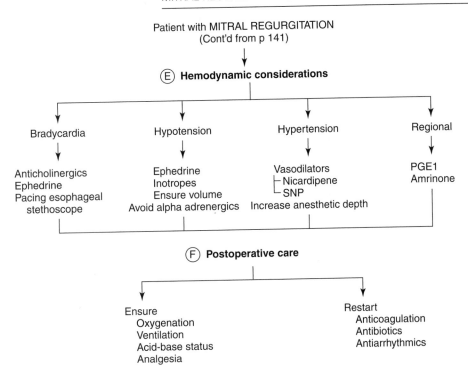

Patient with MITRAL REGURGITATION
(Cont'd from p 141)

Ⓔ **Hemodynamic considerations**

Bradycardia	Hypotension	Hypertension	Regional
Anticholinergics	Ephedrine	Vasodilators	PGE1
Ephedrine	Inotropes	├ Nicardipene	Amrinone
Pacing esophageal	Ensure volume	└ SNP	
stethoscope	Avoid alpha adrenergics	Increase anesthetic depth	

Ⓕ **Postoperative care**

Ensure
    Oxygenation
    Ventilation
    Acid-base status
    Analgesia

Restart
    Anticoagulation
    Antibiotics
    Antiarrhythmics

Aortic Stenosis (AS)

JAYDEEP S. SHAH, M.D.

Aortic stenosis (AS) is the most common cardiac valve lesion in the United States. The end result of AS is obstruction of left ventricular (LV) outflow producing a systolic pressure gradient between the left ventricle and aorta. As the disease progresses and the pressure gradient increases, cardiac output (CO) is maintained by the development of LV hypertrophy. This results in decreased compliance and increased LV end-diastolic pressure (LVEDP). Myocardial oxygen demand increases as a result of the increased muscle mass. Cardiac ischemia may occur from obstruction of coronary artery blood flow due to increased extramural pressure on the coronaries in excess of perfusion pressure, even if CO is normal and there is no significant coronary artery disease (CAD). On average, symptoms develop once the aortic valve area is $<1cm^2$.[1]

A. Perform a history and physical examination. Look for the classic symptoms of AS—angina, syncope, and dyspnea. Angina occurs due to an imbalance of myocardial oxygen demand and supply, secondary to compression of vessels by the hypertrophied LV muscle, impaired relaxation, and increased LVEDP. Peripheral vasodilation in the presence of a fixed CO or sudden decreases in CO can result in a syncope in the AS patient. Dyspnea develops when reduced LV compliance increases LVEDP and left atrial pressure, and subsequently causes pulmonary hypertension (HTN). Auscultate for findings of a high-pitched systolic murmur with the presence of S_3 or S_4 gallop. The presence of carotid bruits or CNS deficits are consistent with reduced cerebral flow reserve.

B. Review the ECG and echocardiogram (echo) results. ECG may show a pattern of LV "strain." Echo provides a comprehensive hemodynamic and morphologic evaluation of AS, including the degree of valvular calcification, the size of the aortic annulus and supravalvular ascending aorta, and the possibility of other subvalvular obstructions.[2] LV function, LV hypertrophy, left atrial enlargement, and the functional integrity of other cardiac valves can be assessed with echo. Consider cardiac catheterization in those patients with severe AS for evaluation of CAD.

C. Management of the asymptomatic patient with severe AS is determined by routine exercise testing.[3] If the patient demonstrates poor exercise tolerance, exercise-induced hypotension, or ventricular arrhythmia, aortic valve replacement (AVR) is probably indicated. The decision to perform AVR in the symptomatic patient with severe AS is obvious given that, after surgery is performed, the age-corrected survival is essentially normal.[4] For symptomatic patients with severe AS and associated depressed LV function, determine whether afterload mismatch is the cause of low ejection fraction (EF). Patients with afterload mismatch have a better response to surgery compared to those with contractile dysfunction.[5] Balloon aortic valvuloplasty in elderly patients with coexisting coronary deficits may be useful to palliate symptoms prior to urgent (nonemergency) noncardiac surgery, especially in those with cardiogenic shock, in whom it may be lifesaving.[6]

D. Patients with symptomatic, severe AS are at significant risk for perioperative cardiac morbidity and should have elective AVR prior to elective, noncardiac surgery. A more common clinical situation is that of the elderly, asymptomatic patient with severe AS who is presenting for elective, noncardiac surgery. In these patients, obtain a preoperative echo, which will assess the severity of the stenosis and cardiac function. Continue preoperative antiarrhythmic medications and antibiotic prophylaxis against infective endocarditis. During the intraoperative period, avoid hypotension, maintain sinus rhythm, maintain preload, and recognize myocardial ischemia. Treat hypotension with alpha-agonists while searching for the primary cause. Consider an arterial line to follow blood pressures. Aggressively treat arrhythmias; the atrial "kick" may account for up to 40% of LV filling. Maintain adequate intravascular volume. Pulmonary capillary wedge pressure (PCWP) poorly estimates LV filling pressures in the presence of decreased LV compliance and elevated LVEDP. Likewise, the use of CVP to guide volume status may be misleading and result in under filling of the LV. Consider intraoperative transesophageal echocardiography [TEE] by an experienced practitioner, the most useful monitoring technique in differentiating systolic from diastolic failure. Do not confuse a baseline LV "strain" pattern on ECG with intraoperative myocardial ischemia. Avoid treatment of suspected myocardial ischemia with vasodilators; even a transient episode of hypotension may be fatal. Instead, maintain perfusion pressure with alpha-agonists and volume. Consider epidural anesthetic techniques but administer slowly and cautiously in accordance with the listed principles.

REFERENCES

1. Otto CM, Burwash IG, Legget ME, et al.: Prospective study of asymptomatic valvular aortic stenosis. Clinical, echocardiographic, and exercise predictors of outcome, Circulation 95:2262–2270, 1997.
2. Currie PJ, Seward JB, Reeder GS, et al.: Continuous-wave Doppler echocardiographic assessment of severity of calcific aortic stenosis: a simultaneous Doppler-catheter correlative study in 100 adult patients, Circulation 71:1162–1169, 1985.
3. Carabello B: Evaluation and management of patients with aortic stenosis, Circulation 105:1746–1750, 2002.
4. Lindblom D, Lindblom U, Qvist J, et al.: Long-term relative survival rates after heart valve replacement, J Am Coll Cardiol 15:566–573, 1990.
5. Connolly HM, Oh JK, Schaff HV, et al.: Severe aortic stenosis with low transvalvular gradient and severe left ventricular dysfunction: result of aortic valve replacement in 52 patients. Circulation 101:1940–1946, 2000.
6. Cribier A, Letac B: Percutaneous balloon aortic valvuloplasty in adults with calcific aortic stenosis, Curr Opin Cardiol 6 (2):212–218, 1991.

AORTIC STENOSIS

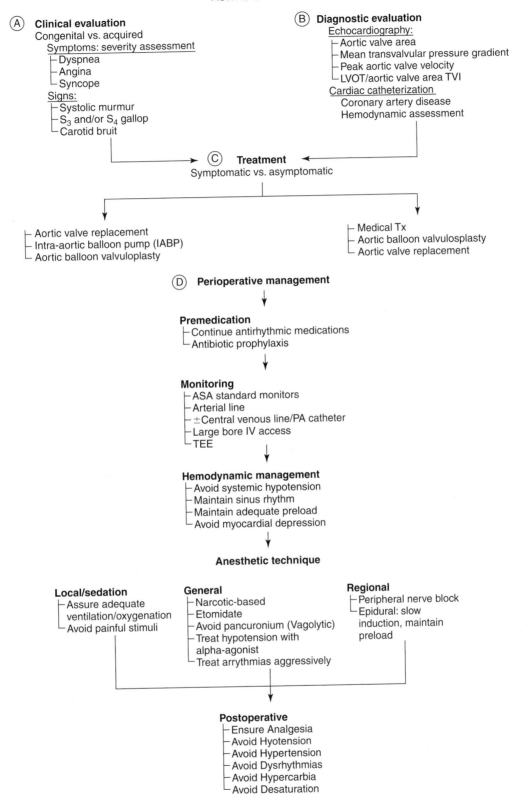

(A) **Clinical evaluation**
Congenital vs. acquired
Symptoms: severity assessment
├─ Dyspnea
├─ Angina
└─ Syncope
Signs:
├─ Systolic murmur
├─ S_3 and/or S_4 gallop
└─ Carotid bruit

(B) **Diagnostic evaluation**
Echocardiography:
├─ Aortic valve area
├─ Mean transvalvular pressure gradient
├─ Peak aortic valve velocity
└─ LVOT/aortic valve area TVI
Cardiac catheterization
Coronary artery disease
Hemodynamic assessment

(C) **Treatment**
Symptomatic vs. asymptomatic

├─ Aortic valve replacement
├─ Intra-aortic balloon pump (IABP)
└─ Aortic balloon valvuloplasty

├─ Medical Tx
├─ Aortic balloon valvulosplasty
└─ Aortic valve replacement

(D) **Perioperative management**

Premedication
├─ Continue antirhythmic medications
└─ Antibiotic prophylaxis

Monitoring
├─ ASA standard monitors
├─ Arterial line
├─ ±Central venous line/PA catheter
├─ Large bore IV access
└─ TEE

Hemodynamic management
├─ Avoid systemic hypotension
├─ Maintain sinus rhythm
├─ Maintain adequate preload
└─ Avoid myocardial depression

Anesthetic technique

Local/sedation
├─ Assure adequate
│   ventilation/oxygenation
└─ Avoid painful stimuli

General
├─ Narcotic-based
├─ Etomidate
├─ Avoid pancuronium (Vagolytic)
├─ Treat hypotension with
│   alpha-agonist
└─ Treat arrhythmias aggressively

Regional
├─ Peripheral nerve block
└─ Epidural: slow
    induction, maintain
    preload

Postoperative
├─ Ensure Analgesia
├─ Avoid Hyotension
├─ Avoid Hypertension
├─ Avoid Dysrhythmias
├─ Avoid Hypercarbia
└─ Avoid Desaturation

Aortic Insufficiency (AI)

JAYDEEP S. SHAH, M.D.

Aortic valve insufficiency (AI) results from abnormalities of the aortic valve (AV) leaflets—infective endocarditis, trauma, systemic diseases (rheumatic fever, systemic lupus erythematosus [SLE]), connective tissue syndromes (Marfan, Turner, and Ehlers-Danlos type IV) or the proximal aortic root (anuloaorticectasia occurs due to aging and chronic hypertension [HTN][1]). AI is also associated with congenital heart defects (bicuspid AV, subvalvular aortic stenosis, dysplasia of valve cusps, and ventricular septal defect [VSD] of the membranous or conal septal types). Regardless of etiology, AI results in volume overload on the left ventricle (LV).

A. In acute AI, the LV end-diastolic and left atrial (LA) pressures increase rapidly (lack of time for compensatory chamber dilation). Pulmonary edema or cardiogenic shock occurs when tachycardia cannot compensate for decrease in forward stroke volume.[2] Echocardiography (echo) is indispensable. Acute AI due to aortic root dissection is a surgical emergency, confirmed by transesophageal echocardiography (TEE) and cardiac catheterization and aortography, typically including coronary angiography. Vasodilators (nicardipine or nitroprusside) or inotropic agents (dopamine or dobutamine), or a combination (milrinone) may be helpful prior to surgical intervention. However, use of vasodilators to increase forward flow may also exacerbate hypotension and potentially lead to LV ischemia and dysfunction. Pressor agents increase systemic vascular resistance (SVR) and worsen AI. Intraaortic balloon counterpulsation increases AI and is contraindicated. Beta-blocker treatment for aortic dissection is beneficial, but blockade of compensatory tachycardia may result in further decreases in cardiac output (CO). Mortality rate for medical management alone is 75%, but surgical intervention for acute AI carries a mortality rate of 25%.[3]

B. Chronic AI results in both volume and pressure overload of the LV. The recruitment of preload reserve and compensatory hypertrophy maintain normal EF in the face of disease progression. Initially, LV dysfunction can be reversed with therapeutic afterload reduction.[4] Over time, dilatation of the LV chamber results in depressed myocardial contractility and EF. Timing for aortic valve replacement (AVR) surgery balances avoiding increased morbidity and mortality from irreversible LV dysfunction with avoiding excess years with a valve prosthesis (and consequent need for anticoagulation). Factors associated with decreased survival and function after AVR in patients with preoperative LV dysfunction and AI include enlarged LV end-systolic size (>50 to 55 mm), severity of LV dysfunction (ejection fraction <0.50), severity of symptoms, and duration of preoperative systolic dysfunction.[2] Eventually the balance between afterload excess, preload reserve, and hypertrophy deteriorates, and chronic AI patients develop dyspnea (declining systolic function or elevated filling pressures). Other symptoms typical of left-sided heart failure (orthopnea, fatigue, or paroxysmal nocturnal dyspnea) may be present. Angina and syncope may be result from reduced diastolic BP. The murmur associated with AI is a diastolic blowing murmur loudest along the left lower sternal border.

C. Echo is the mainstay of chronic AI evaluation. The cause of AI, valve morphology, assessment of LV function and size, estimation of the severity of regurgitation, and aortic root size are determined by echocardiography, and in the asymptomatic patient, the results can serve as a baseline index with which future serial measurements can be gauged. Repeat echocardiograms are performed when there is acute exacerbation or change in symptoms, a progressive decline in exercise tolerance, or worsening regurgitation or progressive LV dilatation. Serial radionuclide ventriculography or serial magnetic resonance imaging (MRI) may serve as an alternative to serial echo. ECG and chest x-ray (CXR) are helpful in evaluating overall heart size and rhythm, evidence of LV hypertrophy, and the presence of conduction disorders (left bundle branch block is common).

D. TEE is the gold standard for intraoperative cardiac monitoring of severe AI. Arterial and right-sided heart catheterizations are useful for optimizing preload and afterload. There is no data available showing the superiority of pulmonary artery (PA) catheterization over that of CVP monitoring for intraoperative fluid management. Follow trends rather than specific pressures. In patients with preserved LV function, a mean pulmonary capillary wedge pressure (PCWP) of 10 to 15 mm Hg ensures adequate LV end-diastolic volume (LVEDV); in the presence of depressed LV function, adequate PCWP may be as high as 20 to 25 mm Hg. Premature closure of the mitral valve results in underestimation of LVEDV, and the presence of mitral regurgitation as a result of LV dilatation will cause an overestimation of LVEDV when referencing to normal PCWP. Maintain systemic BP within 20% of preinduction values. Monitor leads II and V5 and ST-segment analysis for signs of myocardial hypoperfusion.

(Continued on page 148)

Patient with AORTIC INSUFFICIENCY

Clinical presentation

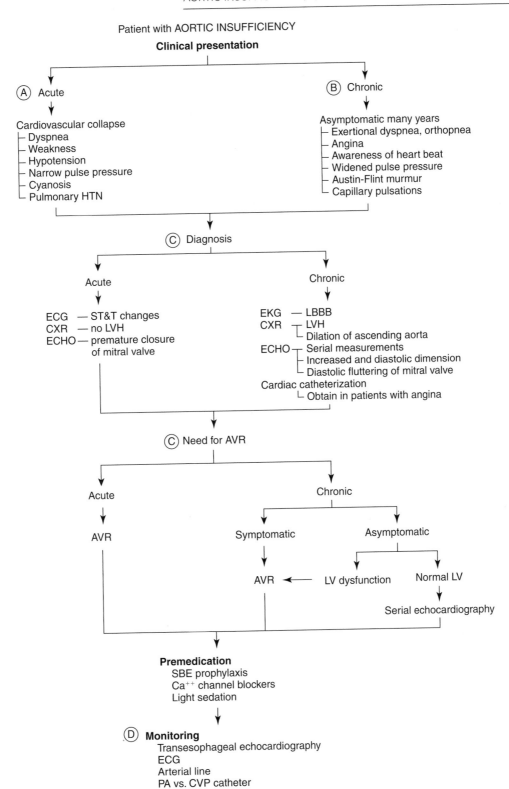

(A) Acute

Cardiovascular collapse
 ├ Dyspnea
 ├ Weakness
 ├ Hypotension
 ├ Narrow pulse pressure
 ├ Cyanosis
 └ Pulmonary HTN

(B) Chronic

Asymptomatic many years
 ├ Exertional dyspnea, orthopnea
 ├ Angina
 ├ Awareness of heart beat
 ├ Widened pulse pressure
 ├ Austin-Flint murmur
 └ Capillary pulsations

(C) Diagnosis

Acute

ECG — ST&T changes
CXR — no LVH
ECHO — premature closure
         of mitral valve

Chronic

EKG — LBBB
CXR ┬ LVH
    └ Dilation of ascending aorta
ECHO ┬ Serial measurements
     ├ Increased and diastolic dimension
     └ Diastolic fluttering of mitral valve
Cardiac catheterization
     └ Obtain in patients with angina

(C) Need for AVR

Acute

AVR

Chronic

Symptomatic

AVR ◄— LV dysfunction

Asymptomatic

Normal LV

Serial echocardiography

Premedication
 SBE prophylaxis
 Ca^{++} channel blockers
 Light sedation

(D) **Monitoring**
 Transesophageal echocardiography
 ECG
 Arterial line
 PA vs. CVP catheter

(Cont'd on p 149)

E. Avoid sudden decreases in HR, increases in SVR, and drug-induced myocardial depression, because each will increase the regurgitant flow. Atrial fibrillation or other supraventricular tachycardias are poorly tolerated and require aggressive treatment. Inotropic agents may be necessary to maintain adequate CO. Maintain normal to increased HR, normal to reduced SVR, and preserve myocardial contractility. Intraoperative administration of inotropic or vasodilating agents may be required. Regional anesthesia, including both epidural and spinal anesthesia can be performed with adequate preloading.

REFERENCES

1. Waller BF, Howear J, Fess S: Pathology of aortic valve stenosis and pure aortic regurgitation: II: a clinical morphological assessment, *Clin Cardiol* 17:150–156, 1994.
2. Bonow RO, Carabello BA, de Leon AC, et al.: Guidelines for the management of patients with valvular heart disease: executive summary. A report of the American College of Cardiology/American Heart Association Task Force on Practice Guidelines (Committee on Management of Patients with Valvular Heart Disease), *Circulation* 98 (18):1949–1984, 1998.
3. Carabello BA: Progress in mitral and aortic regurgitation, *Curr Probl Cardiol* 28:553–582, 2003.
4. Bonow RO, Rosing DR, Maron BJ, et al.: Reversal of left ventricular dysfunction after aortic valve replacement for chronic aortic regurgitation: influence of duration of preoperative left ventricular dysfunction, *Circulation* 70 (4):570–579, 1984.

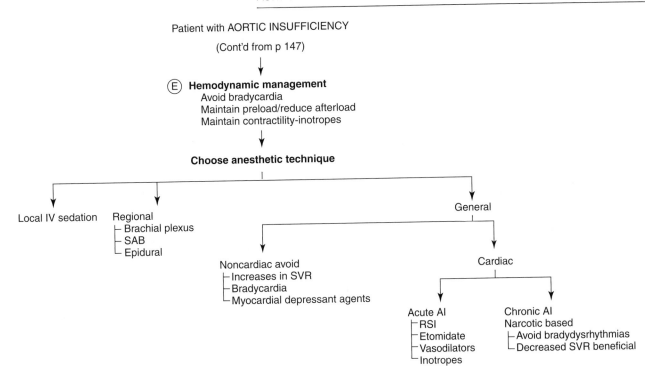

Patient with AORTIC INSUFFICIENCY

(Cont'd from p 147)

(E) **Hemodynamic management**
　　Avoid bradycardia
　　Maintain preload/reduce afterload
　　Maintain contractility-inotropes

Choose anesthetic technique

Local IV sedation

Regional
├ Brachial plexus
├ SAB
└ Epidural

General

Noncardiac avoid
├ Increases in SVR
├ Bradycardia
└ Myocardial depressant agents

Cardiac

Acute AI
├ RSI
├ Etomidate
├ Vasodilators
└ Inotropes

Chronic AI
Narcotic based
├ Avoid bradydysrhythmias
└ Decreased SVR beneficial

Pericardial Tamponade

D.M. ANDERSON, M.D.

Pericardial tamponade results when the cardiac chambers become compressed due to pericardial effusion. This can occur acutely or chronically from multiple etiologies. The treatment of cardiac tamponade is drainage of the effusion. The 30-day mortality of patients with cardiac tamponade was 16% in one recent study.[1] Anesthetizing a patient with cardiac tamponade is a challenging task that requires several important decisions.

A. Look for clinical signs and symptoms of pericardial effusion, which include tachypnea, hypotension, narrow pulse pressure, tachycardia, pulsus paradoxus, and acidosis. The CVP is elevated; CVP and pulmonary artery (PA) diastolic pressures are equalized. Cardiac output (CO) is low. The ECG will have low voltage QRS complexes and electrical alternation. The diagnosis of pericardial effusion and tamponade is usually made with Doppler echocardiography (echo).

B. Stabilize the patient. Consider volume loading in hypovolemic patients and inotropic support. Maintain preload, tachycardia, ventricular contractility, and peripheral vasoconstriction.

C. Place an arterial line and consider other invasive cardiac monitors if not already in place.

D. Discuss the operative plan with the surgeon; the anesthetic challenges depend on which procedure is performed. There are several options for drainage of a pericardial effusion.[2] Many surgeons prefer percutaneous pericardiocentesis for drainage of an acute pericardial tamponade, possibly guided by echo. If needle drainage is not possible or ineffective, surgical drainage is required. The terms subxiphoid drainage, pericardial window, and pericardiostomy are used to describe similar surgical techniques. Chronic pericardial effusion is often drained by subxiphoid pericardiostomy under local anesthesia and has an operative mortality of 5%.[2,3]

E. Choose the anesthetic technique based on the hemodynamic status of the patient; avoid general anesthesia when the status is poor. Most procedures can be performed safely under local anesthesia.[3,4] Consider careful titration of a sedative, such as ketamine. Ketamine is useful because adequate heart rate is maintained and it vasoconstricts without significant myocardial depression. In one report, ketamine 0.5 mg/kg was administered intravenously during opening of the sternum; after initial drainage, general anesthesia was induced and the patient intubated.[5]

F. If general anesthesia is required, consider the following. Prep and drape the surgical site prior to induction of general anesthesia. Positive-pressure ventilation can reduce venous return and may adversely affect CO. Therefore, maintain spontaneous ventilation when possible, perhaps with a laryngeal mask airway (LMA) for airway control. Alternatively, perform awake intubation and maintain spontaneous ventilation.[6,7] General anesthetic induction agents and inhalational anesthetics can reduce HR and cause vasodilatation, resulting in excessive hypotension.[8,9] Manage decreased BP with IV fluids or potent vasoconstrictors, such as norepinephrine. Preload reduction is likely to be detrimental. CO depends on a rapid HR because of impaired ventricular filling and fixed stoke volume. Therefore, medications that lower heart rate (e.g., narcotics) may produce hypotension. Vasodilating techniques (e.g., neuraxial blockade) or medications may be problematic. Bilateral thoracic paravertebral blocks provide analgesia with little change in sympathetic tone, but this has not been well studied.

G. Postoperative low cardiac output syndrome (PLCOS) is a rarely mentioned potential complication that occurs immediately after drainage of a pericardial effusion. This is an unexplained, severe systolic heart dysfunction that has been described in a small number of reports.[10] The incidence of PLCOS was 4.8% and had a mortality of 80% in one recent study.[1]

REFERENCES

1. Dosios T, Theakos N, Angouras D, et al.: Risk factors affecting the survival of patients with pericardial effusion submitted to subxiphoid pericardiostomy, *Chest* 124 (1):242–246, 2003.
2. Campione A, Cacchiarelli M, Ghiribelli C, et al.: Which treatment in pericardial effusion? *J Cardiovasc Surg (Torino)* 43 (5): 735–739, 2002.
3. Figueroa W, Alankar S, Pai N, et al.: Subxiphoid pericardial window for pericardial effusion in end-stage renal disease, *Am J Kidney Dis* 27 (5):664–667, 1996.
4. Kaplan JA, Bland JW Jr, Dunbar RW. The perioperative management of pericardial tamponade, *South Med J* 69:417–429, 1976.
5. Aye T, Milne B: Ketamine anesthesia for pericardial window in a patient with pericardial tamponade and severe COPD, *Can J Anaesth* 49 (3):283–286, 2002.
6. Breen PH, MacVay MA: Pericardial tamponade: a case for awake endotracheal intubation, *Anesth Analg* 83 (3):658, 1996.
7. Webster JA, Self DD: Anesthesia for pericardial window in a pregnant patient with cardiac tamponade and mediastinal mass, *Can J Anaesth* 50 (8):815–818, 2003.
8. Lake CL. Anesthesia and pericardial disease, *Anesth Analg* 62:431–443, 1983.
9. Stanley TH, Weidauer HE: Anesthesia for the patient with cardiac tamponade, *Anesth Analg* 52:110–114, 1973.
10. Sunday R, Robinson LA, Bosek V: Low cardiac output complicating pericardiectomy for pericardial tamponade, *Ann Thorac Surg* 67:228–231, 1999.

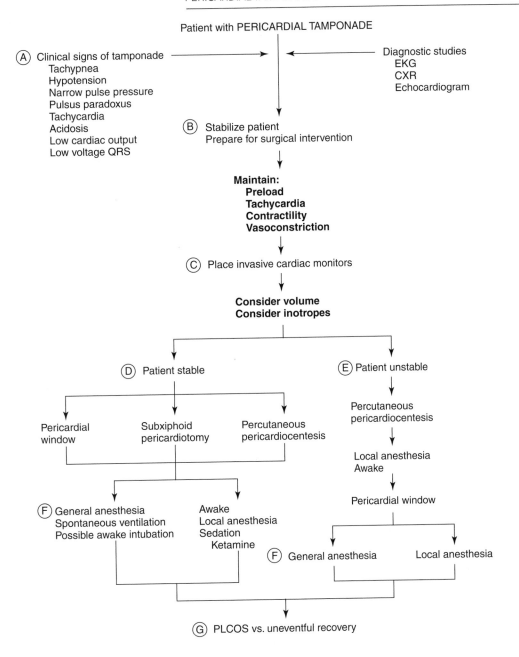

Superior Vena Cava Syndrome (SVCS)

ANTONIO HERNANDEZ, M.D.

Superior vena cava syndrome (SVCS) results from mechanical obstruction (compression, invasion, or thrombosis) of the superior vena cava (SVC) and the ensuing venous hypertension (HTN) in the tissues it drains. SVCS is caused by bronchogenic carcinomas (80%), mediastinal masses (15%), sarcoidosis, fungal infections, aortic aneurysms, and clots around central venous catheters or pacemaker leads.[1]

A. Perform a history and physical examination. Obstruction of venous drainage from the head and upper thorax results in distended veins, edema, and cyanosis in the head, neck, and upper extremities. Venous distension is most prominent in the supine position; however, it usually does not completely disappear in the upright position. Mental status may be altered in severe cases as a result of increased cerebral edema and decreased cerebral perfusion (look for papilledema). Review the chest x-ray (CXR) (for superior mediastinal widening, pleural effusion, or hilar mass), ABG (for hypoxemia), flow-volume loops, and CT scan of the chest (for tumor invasion versus compression). Upper extremity venography may confirm the diagnosis in more subtle presentations and transesophageal echocardiography (TEE) can identify the mechanism for SVC obstruction.[2]

B. SVCS secondary to thrombosis can be treated with thrombolytic therapy, anticoagulation, and removal of the intravascular foreign body.

C. Most patients with SVCS secondary to tumors will require a tissue biopsy under local anesthesia for diagnosis and determination of appropriate therapy.

D. If a tissue diagnosis is not obtained or not possible with local anesthesia and general anesthesia (GETA) is required, determine the risk of airway and vascular compromise. If the risk is present, the patient should be treated prior to GETA with selective radiotherapy, chemotherapy, or angioplasty with intravascular stenting.[3] The goal of these therapies is to reduce venous obstruction, symptoms, and the risk of GETA without interfering with tissue diagnosis. These options may not be possible or successful in some patients; if surgery with GETA is still necessary, proceed with the appropriate precautions.

E. Intubate the awake, seated, topically anesthetized patient with a fiberoptic bronchoscope, and then use the semi-Fowler's position, maintaining spontaneous ventilation (creates negative distending pressure throughout the thoracic compartment, prevents collapse of pulmonary and vascular structures, and promotes venous return to the heart). If airway obstruction or hemodynamic compromise occurs, move the patient into the. left lateral or prone position. Extracorporeal axillary-femoral venous bypass (A-F VBP) has been used successfully before induction to decrease the symptoms from SVC obstruction.[4]

F. Postoperatively, airway edema can result in complete loss of airway patency; do not extubate a patient with swelling of the face or tongue for at least 24 to 36 hours or until the head and facial edema has regressed. Consider assessing for a cuff leak of <15 to 20 cm of water and extubate over an exchange catheter when the patient may require reintubation. Although a size 11 Cook exchange catheter (internal diameter of 3 mm) has been used for reintubation,[5] the use of a size 19 Cook exchange catheter (internal diameter of 7 mm) allows for improved ventilation due to its larger diameter, should reintubation fail. Furthermore, the larger size Cook exchange catheter may enable adequate ventilation without requiring jet ventilation (potential barotrauma and pneumothorax[6]). Some patients may develop pulmonary edema from an increased venous return after relief of the caval obstruction.

REFERENCES

1. Bechard P, Letourneau L, Lacasse Y, et al.: Perioperative cardiorespiratory complications in adults with mediastinal mass: incidence and risk factors, Anesthesiology 100 (4):826–834, 2004.
2. Lin CM, Hsu JC: Anterior mediastinal tumour identified by intraoperative transesophageal echocardiography, Can J Anaesth 48 (1):78–80, 2001.
3. Foley RW, Rodriguez MI: Preoperative irradiation of selected mediastinal masses, J Cardiovasc Surg (Torino) 42 (5):695–697, 2001.
4. Shimokawa S, Yamashita T, Kinjyo T, et al.: Extracorporeal venous bypass: a beneficial device in operation for superior vena caval syndrome, Ann Thorac Surg 62:1863–1864, 1996.
5. Loudermilk EP, Hartmannsgruber M, Stoltzfus DP, et al.: A prospective study of the safety of tracheal extubation using a pediatric airway exchange catheter for patients with a known difficult airway, Chest 111:1660–1665, 1997.
6. Baraka AS: Tension pneumothorax complicating jet ventilation via a cook airway exchange catheter, Anesthesiology 91:557–558, 1999.

Patient with SUPERIOR VENA CAVA SYNDROME

(A) **Clinical evaluation**
  Headaches, dizziness, dyspnea,
    epistaxis, flushed skin,
    increased collar size, inability
    to sleep supine
  Venous distension; cyanosis, swelling
    of head, tongue, airway,
    trunk, upper extremities

Chest film, ECG, ABG, hemoglobin, prothrombin
    time, partial thromboplastin time
Blood cross-matched
±CT/magnetic resonance imaging (MRI), upright
    and supine flow-volume loops, upright
    and supine transthoracic/transesophageal
    echocardiograms

(B) **Thrombosis**
  Remove intravascular foreign body
  Thrombolytic therapy
  Anticoagulation

(C) **Tumor**
  Biopsy under local anesthesia

Success

Failure
Surgery imperative

(D) Selective radiotherapy
  Chemotherapy
  Angioplasty/stent

Repeat work-up
  CT/MRI, upright and supine flow-volume loops,
    upright and supine echocardiograms/TEE

GETA ◄— Success

Failure

Appropriate therapy

(E) GETA and SVCS precautions
  ├─Blood in room
  ├─Upright position
  ├─Arterial line/CVP
  ├─Femoral IV access
  ├─Legs wrapped
  ├─Rigid bronchoscope
  ├─CPB available
  ├─Preinduction (A-F VBP)
  ├─Awake intubation
  ├─Inhalational induction
  ├─Spontaneous ventilation
  └─Change position if necessary
      (lateral, prone)

Intraoperative management

(F) **Postoperative care**
  Airway obstruction
  Bleeding
  Persistent swelling of face, tongue
  Pulmonary edema

Maintain intubation until edema improves
(24–36 hr)

PREOPERATIVE NEUROLOGIC AND NEUROMUSCULAR PROBLEMS

Anesthesia for Dental Surgery in the
Mentally Handicapped Adult

Muscular Dystrophy (MD)

Myotonic Dystrophy
(Myotonia Dystrophica)

Myasthenia Gravis (MG) and
Eaton-Lambert Syndrome (ELS)

Malignant Hyperthermia (MH):
Prophylaxis

Malignant Hyperthermia (MH):
Treatment of Acute Episode

Neuroleptic Malignant Syndrome
(NMS)

Tetraplegia

Multiple Sclerosis (MS)

Parkinson's Disease (PD)

Anesthesia for Dental Surgery in the Mentally Handicapped Adult

TOD B. SLOAN, M.D., PH.D.

Dental rehabilitation in the mentally handicapped adult usually requires general anesthesia because of the patient's inability to cooperate. Many patients have significant comorbidities.[1,2]

A. History of medical disease and past experiences may be difficult to obtain. Note specific syndromes and inborn errors of metabolism. If handicap is mild (MMR) (IQ 50 to 70), associated medical problems are less likely. Individuals with severe handicap (SMR) (IQ <50) have more severe CNS disease with a greater likelihood of associated problems (58 to 71% probably have a defined diagnosis if evaluated fully).[1] Patients often have spasticity, hypotonia, seizures, and aberrant behavior. Down syndrome accounts for 6 to 10% of mentally handicapped patients. Review records and look for cerebral palsy (CP), motor disorders, epilepsy, and neuromuscular disorders (associated with scoliosis; may have respiratory problems). Perform a physical examination if possible; look for signs of difficult intubation. Consider minimal testing: pregnancy testing, or anticonvulsant levels as indicated. Consider cervical spine flexion-extension films in patients with Down syndrome. Look for recent changes in seizure activity or behavior (infection, change in drug levels, or recent head trauma) and foul-smelling breath (rumination or regurgitation). Institutionalized patients are at greater risk for hepatitis B virus and tuberculosis (TB). CP patients may be mentally normal and should be addressed as such.

B. If preoperative antibiotics are indicated, give orally if possible; an IV line may be difficult to acquire.[3–7] Patients with food access may not be NPO (behavior problems or inability to understand surgery). Consider oral sodium citrate preoperatively. Avoid provoking outbursts of uncontrollable behavior. Consult with legal counsel if the patient can legally sign his or her own consent but is unable to understand the dental procedure and anesthesia.

C. Premedication is important. Docile patients tolerate IV line placement (consider EMLA® cream), but others can become violent, give them oral midazolam (0.5 mg/kg to maximum of 20 mg)[4] or oral ketamine (5 to 10 mg/kg)[5] individually or combined (reduced dosages).[6] If a gastrostomy tube is in place, use it to administer sedatives. Intranasal midazolam (0.2 mg/kg) has also been used.[7] Intramuscular ketamine (2 to 4 mg/kg) may be needed for uncooperative patients or those who refuse oral sedation.

D. Perform inhalation induction or IV line placement induction. If an intracardiac shunt defect is present, remove IV air bubbles. Nasal endotracheal tubes (ETTs) are more convenient for dental surgery but may cause bleeding and bacteremia. If a pharyngeal pack is used, be certain it is *removed* before extubation.

E. Positioning may be difficult because of scoliosis and contractures. Watch for dysrhythmias from injected vasoconstrictor. Watch for subcutaneous emphysema from air-powered dental instruments; turn off N_2O if noted. Muscle relaxants are not specifically required but should be monitored if used. Some antiseizure medications (e.g., carbamazepine [Tegretol]) induce hepatic enzymes, increasing drug clearance. CNS stimulants (e.g., methylphenidate [Ritalin]) and amphetamines may increase anesthetic requirements. Use appropriate x-ray shielding for staff and patients.

F. Suction the stomach. Remove the urinary catheter or empty the bladder by straight catheterization to reduce emergence phenomena. Watch for bleeding from extraction sites. Inspect the mouth for swelling and foreign bodies, and *remove* the pharyngeal pack before extubation. Consider long-acting analgesics (e.g., ketorolac) if the patient will awaken with pain. Long-acting neural blockade may predispose patients to oral or lingual trauma. Consider IV fluid loading and IV medications (e.g., antiseizure drugs) if a prolonged time to resumption of oral intake is anticipated. Anticipate uncontrolled behavior on awakening and have a familiar caregiver present at the bedside as the patient awakens. Abbreviated routines for vital sign measurement and early removal of IV lines may be necessary. Consider a shortened stay in the conventional PACU. Adjust discharge criteria as appropriate to the preoperative function level.

REFERENCES

1. Jones, KL: Approaches to categorical problems of growth deficiency, mental efficiency, arthrogryposis, ambiguous genitalia. In Jones KL, editor: *Smith's recognizable patterns of human malformation*, ed 5, Philadelphia, 1997, W.B. Saunders.
2. Butler MG, Hayes BG, Hathaway MM, et al.: Specific genetic diseases at risk for sedation/anesthesia complications, *Anesth Analg* 91:837–855, 2000.
3. Chancellor JW: Is there a need for a specialty in dental anesthesia? *Tex Dent J* 111:15–18, 1994.
4. Silver T, Wilson C, Webb M: Evaluation of two dosages of oral midazolam as a conscious sedation for physically and neurologically compromised pediatric dental patients, *Pediatr Dent* 16:350–359, 1994.
5. Petros AJ: Oral Ketamine. Its use for mentally retarded adults requiring day care dental treatment, *Anaesthesia* 46:646–667, 1991.
6. Warner DL, Cabaret J, Velling D: Ketamine plus midazolam, a most effective paediatric oral premedicant, *Paediatr Anaesth* 5:293–295, 1995.
7. Fukuta O, Braham RL, Yanase H, et.al.: The sedative effect of intranasal midazolam administration in the dental treatment of patients with mental disabilities. Part 1—The effect of a 0.2 mg/kg dose, *J Clin Pediatr Dent* 17:231–237, 1993.

MENTALLY HANDICAPPED ADULT FOR DENTAL REHABILITATION

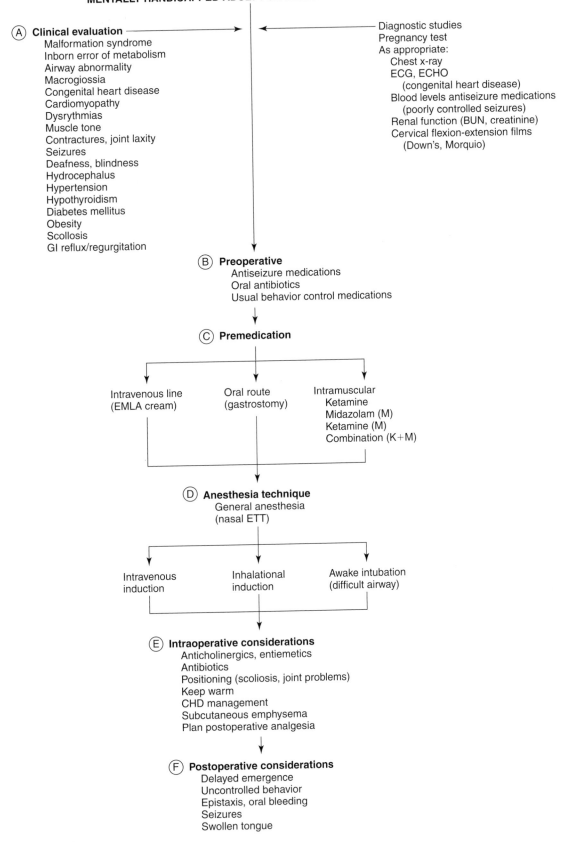

Ⓐ **Clinical evaluation**
  Malformation syndrome
  Inborn error of metabolism
  Airway abnormality
  Macrogiossia
  Congenital heart disease
  Cardiomyopathy
  Dysrythmias
  Muscle tone
  Contractures, joint laxity
  Seizures
  Deafness, blindness
  Hydrocephalus
  Hypertension
  Hypothyroidism
  Diabetes mellitus
  Obesity
  Scollosis
  GI reflux/regurgitation

  Diagnostic studies
  Pregnancy test
  As appropriate:
    Chest x-ray
    ECG, ECHO
      (congenital heart disease)
    Blood levels antiseizure medications
      (poorly controlled seizures)
    Renal function (BUN, creatinine)
    Cervical flexion-extension films
      (Down's, Morquio)

Ⓑ **Preoperative**
  Antiseizure medications
  Oral antibiotics
  Usual behavior control medications

Ⓒ **Premedication**

Intravenous line
(EMLA cream)

Oral route
(gastrostomy)

Intramuscular
Ketamine
Midazolam (M)
Ketamine (M)
Combination (K+M)

Ⓓ **Anesthesia technique**
  General anesthesia
  (nasal ETT)

Intravenous
induction

Inhalational
induction

Awake intubation
(difficult airway)

Ⓔ **Intraoperative considerations**
  Anticholinergics, entiemetics
  Antibiotics
  Positioning (scoliosis, joint problems)
  Keep warm
  CHD management
  Subcutaneous emphysema
  Plan postoperative analgesia

Ⓕ **Postoperative considerations**
  Delayed emergence
  Uncontrolled behavior
  Epistaxis, oral bleeding
  Seizures
  Swollen tongue

Muscular Dystrophy (MD)

JOANNE BAUST, M.D.

Muscular dystrophy (MD) is a group of diseases characterized by these four criteria: (1) primary myopathy, (2) genetic basis, (3) progressive course, and (4) degeneration of muscle fibers. The most common types are pseudotrophic (Duchenne's MD), Becker's MD, Emery-Dreifuss MD (EDMD), limb-girdle, facioscapulohumeral (Landouzy-Dejerine), oculopharyngeal dystrophy, nemaline rod myopathy, and myotonic dystrophy. These patients present for muscle biopsy, dental rehabilitation, contracture release, and kyphoscoliosis instrumentation.[1–5]

A. Perform a preoperative evaluation. Confirm the specific type of MD. Duchenne's muscular dystrophy is the most common and most severe hereditary neuromuscular disease (3 per 10,000 live male births). It is X-linked and most commonly presents in males 2 to 5 years old. All muscle fibers are affected, including skeletal muscle (proximal muscle weakness; kyphoscoliosis; respiratory muscle weakness and restrictive lung disease leading to pulmonary hypertension [HTN]), smooth muscle (impaired swallowing; delayed gastric emptying) and cardiac muscle (decreased contractility with cardiomyopathy; mitral regurgitation from papillary muscle degeneration; sinus tachycardia, heart block, and arrhythmias). These boys typically use their arms to stand (Gower's sign), have a waddling gait, frequently fall down, and have difficulty climbing stairs due to proximal muscle weakness. They may be wheelchair bound by 10 to 12 years of age. Death occurs by age 15 to 25, usually a result of pneumonia and respiratory failure or congestive heart failure (CHF). The diagnosis is confirmed by muscle biopsy. Laboratory findings include markedly elevated serum creatinine phosphokinase (CK), 15,000 to 30,000 international units/Liter, which declines with progressive atrophy. Female carriers may have a modestly elevated CK with some skeletal weakness but rarely have cardiac abnormalities. Obtain ECG, echocardiogram (echo), chest x-ray (CXR), and pulmonary function tests (PFTs). These patients may be at risk for rhabdomyolysis, hyperkalemia, or malignant hyperthermia (MH) when presented with a triggering agent, although volatile agents have been used successfully. Becker's MD is similar to Duchenne's, except that it presents later in life (usually adolescence), has a slower progression, and less mental retardation. It is also X-linked, affecting 1 per 30,000 male births. Death usually results from respiratory complications. EDMD is an X-linked, recessive MD. It presents at age 4 to 5 with humeroperoneal muscle weakness and contractures at the elbows, Achilles tendons (toe walking), and posterior cervical muscles (difficult airway). Cardiac involvement includes atrial conduction defects, bradycardia, heart block, and cardiomyopathy. A pacemaker may be needed perioperatively. Avoid succinylcholine and the risk of hyperkalemia or MH.

B. Facioscapulohumeral (FSHMD), limb-girdle (LGMD), and oculopharyngeal (OPMD) MD all are a collection of multiple variants of slowly progressive, adult onset diseases. These MDs are less severe and primarily involve skeletal muscle. CK levels with these diseases may vary widely. FSHMD presents in the second to third decades of life and is autosomal dominant with an incidence of 1 per 100,000. Facial, shoulder, and hip girdle muscle weakness with kyphosis is characteristic. Respiratory muscle involvement (chronic respiratory infections, risk of aspiration) is common. Rarely, cardiac conduction disturbances require pacing. LGMD is autosomal recessive, presenting in the first to third decades, and involves the shoulder or hip girdle muscles. Cardiac involvement is rare but may result in sinus tachycardias or heart block. Patients with FSHMD and LGMD have normal responses to nondepolarizing muscle relaxant (NDMR); avoid succinylcholine due to risk of rhabdomyolysis and hyperkalemia. OPMD presents with dysphagia and ptosis; these patients are at risk for aspiration from pharyngeal weakness and may be sensitive to the effects of NDMR. Nemaline rod MD (NRMD) involves proximal skeletal muscle, and presents in infancy with hypotonia, dysphagia, bulbar palsy, macroglossia, kyphoscoliosis, and pectus excavatum with restrictive lung disease and respiratory distress. These infants may be difficult to intubate and are sensitive to NDMR but resistant to succinylcholine. There is no correlation between NRMD and MH.

C. Myotonic dystrophy is discussed in a separate chapter.

D. Consider regional anesthesia as an excellent option, although it may be technically challenging. Use MH precautions and avoid succinylcholine. Do not administer prophylactic dantrolene. Premedicate cautiously in the event of respiratory insufficiency. Consider a rapid sequence induction (GI dysmotility) with a NDMR and monitor neuromuscular blockade. Plan postoperative observation, vigorous pulmonary toilet, or mechanical ventilation.

REFERENCES

1. Ames WA, Hayes JA, Crawford MW: The role of corticosteroids in Duchenne muscular dystrophy: a review for the anesthetist, *Paediatr Anaesth* 15:3–8, 2005.
2. Frankowski GA, Johnson JO, Tobias JD: Rapacuronium administration to two children with Duchenne's muscular dystrophy, *Anesth Analg* 91 (1):27–28, 2000.
3. Ririe DG, Shapiro F, Sethna NF: The response of patients with Duchenne's muscular dystrophy to neuromuscular blockade with vecuronium, *Anesthesiology* 88 (2):351–354, 1998.
4. Aldwinckle RJ, Carr AS: The anesthetic management of a patient with Emery-Dreifuss muscular dystrophy for orthopedic surgery, *Can J Anaesth* 49 (5):467–470, 2002.
5. Caron MJ, Girard F, Girard DC, et al.: Cisatracurium pharmacodynamics in patients with oculopharyngeal muscular dystrophy, *Anesth Analg* 100 (2):393–397, 2005.

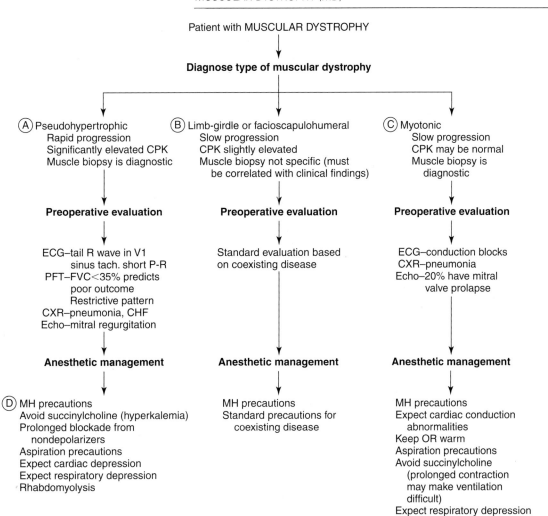

Patient with MUSCULAR DYSTROPHY

Diagnose type of muscular dystrophy

Ⓐ Pseudohypertrophic
Rapid progression
Significantly elevated CPK
Muscle biopsy is diagnostic

Ⓑ Limb-girdle or facioscapulohumeral
Slow progression
CPK slightly elevated
Muscle biopsy not specific (must
be correlated with clinical findings)

Ⓒ Myotonic
Slow progression
CPK may be normal
Muscle biopsy is
diagnostic

Preoperative evaluation

Preoperative evaluation

Preoperative evaluation

ECG–tail R wave in V1
sinus tach. short P-R
PFT–FVC<35% predicts
poor outcome
Restrictive pattern
CXR–pneumonia, CHF
Echo–mitral regurgitation

Standard evaluation based
on coexisting disease

ECG–conduction blocks
CXR–pneumonia
Echo–20% have mitral
valve prolapse

Anesthetic management

Anesthetic management

Anesthetic management

Ⓓ MH precautions
Avoid succinylcholine (hyperkalemia)
Prolonged blockade from
nondepolarizers
Aspiration precautions
Expect cardiac depression
Expect respiratory depression
Rhabdomyolysis

MH precautions
Standard precautions for
coexisting disease

MH precautions
Expect cardiac conduction
abnormalities
Keep OR warm
Aspiration precautions
Avoid succinylcholine
(prolonged contraction
may make ventilation
difficult)
Expect respiratory depression

Myotonic Dystrophy (Myotonia Dystrophica)

JOANNE BAUST, M.D.

Myotonic dystrophy, or Steinert's disease, is a progressive, hereditary neuromuscular disorder characterized by myotonia (difficulty initiating voluntary movement with delayed relaxation) and dystrophy (progressive weakness and muscular atrophy).[1–6] Myotonic contractions are stimulated by voluntary effort, direct muscle stimulation, shivering, or stress. The defect, located on chromosome 19, involves production of an abnormal protein kinase that regulates the skeletal muscle sodium and chloride ion channels (return intracellular calcium into the sarcoplasm reticulum). Inheritance is autosomal dominant with variable expression.

The adult form of myotonic dystrophy typically presents between 15 and 35 years of age and may involve the following systems: skeletal muscle (respiratory muscle weakness with chronic hypoventilation, weak cough, recurrent pneumonias, aspiration, or restrictive lung disease [RLD]), smooth muscle (pharyngeal weakness with obstructive sleep apnea [OSA], GI reflux, or uterine hypotonia), cardiac (atrioventricular [AV] block, atrial tachycardias, mitral valve prolapse [MVP], and cardiomyopathy), CNS (retardation, developmental delay, or abnormal respiratory control), endocrine (diabetes mellitus or infertility), ocular (cataracts), and skin (frontal balding). Cardiac abnormalities may be extensive and progressive, even when skeletal disease is mild. The diagnosis is confirmed by elevated serum creatine (CK) levels and abnormal electromyography findings. Treatment is primarily symptomatic.

Congenital dystrophia myotonica, the most severe but rarest form, presents at birth, often to mothers unaware of their own disease. Pregnancy is complicated by polyhydramnios, premature labor, uterine hypotonus, prolonged labor, and postpartum hemorrhage due to undiagnosed maternal myotonic dystrophy. These infants have a characteristic tent-shaped mouth, require aggressive resuscitation for hypotonia, and experience respiratory insufficiency with poor central ventilatory drive and weak cough, hyporeflexia, cerebral ventricular enlargement, insulin resistance and hyperglycemia, and feeding difficulties from poor suck/swallow coordination and chronic aspiration. Mortality is 25% by 18 months. Survivors have psychomotor and mental retardation. These babies present to the OR for equinovarus correction, myringotomies, feeding tubes, and inguinal hernias.

A. Determine medications, baseline neurological status, and known triggers of the patient's myotonic episodes. Medications for reduction of myotonic episodes include phenytoin, quinine, and procainamide. Look for elevated white count (aspiration pneumonia), anemia, low platelets, low albumin (poor nutrition), hypokalemia (increases the risk of myotonia), and elevated serum creatinine (dehydration, renal impairment). Review chest x-ray (CXR), ECG, pulmonary function tests (PFTs), and echocardiogram (echo). Interrogate pacemaker if present. Neonates may need perioperative antibiotic (aspiration pneumonia) and intensive nutritional support. Provide subacute bacterial endocarditis (SBE) prophylaxis for MVP.

B. Consider the potential for respiratory insufficiency, aspiration, dysrhythmias, and CNS or myocardial depression. Patients are exquisitely sensitive to sedatives, but some sedation is prudent—anxiety plus starvation and dehydration may trigger a myotonic episode. Warm the OR suite, IV fluids, and ventilator circuit. Have an external pacemaker available or consider the preoperative placement of a transvenous pacemaker.

C. Use local or regional anesthesia when possible to lessen risks of postoperative respiratory depression and need for prolonged ventilatory support. Limit sedation and neuraxial narcotics. If a general anesthetic is required, use aspiration precautions and avoid inhalational induction and laryngeal mask airways (LMAs) if possible (risk of aspiration). If rapid sequence induction is indicated, do *not* use succinylcholine (SCC)—the resulting myotonia cannot be overcome by nondepolarizing muscle relaxants (NDMRs) or nerve blocks. Masseter spasm, laryngospasm, and chest wall and diaphragmatic rigidity lead to difficult ventilation. The myotonic episodes associated with SCC have raised the question of an association with malignant hyperthermia (MH). However, this has not been shown; inhalational agents may be used. Anticipate a variable response to NDMRs, including prolonged response even to short-acting agents. Therefore, monitor closely. NDMRs can be avoided with a propofol-based anesthetic with lidocaine and a short-acting narcotic to reduce postoperative respiratory depression.[1] Thiopental may cause postoperative respiratory depression. Neostigmine reversal is unpredictable, may intensify the block, and may stimulate myotonia due to hypersensitivity to acetylcholine. If reversal cannot be avoided, administer agents over *several* minutes with continuous monitoring. Watch for conduction abnormalities and medication-induced myocardial depression. Myotonia may be induced by tourniquet use, IV propofol, local infiltration of anesthetics, electrocautery, nerve stimulator use, surgical manipulation, and shivering (cold or inhalational agents), even in the presence of full neuromuscular blockade. Treatment may include direct infiltration of the affected muscles with a local anesthetic or administration of quinidine 300 to 600 mg intravenously.

(Continued on page 162)

160

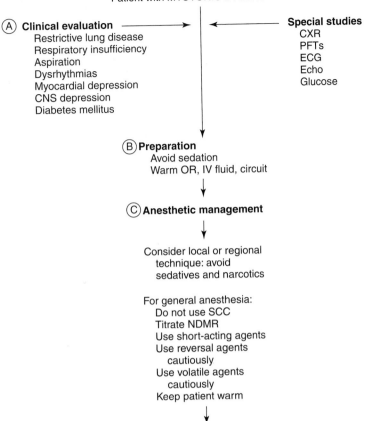

Patient with MYOTONIC DYSTROPHY

Ⓐ **Clinical evaluation**
    Restrictive lung disease
    Respiratory insufficiency
    Aspiration
    Dysrhythmias
    Myocardial depression
    CNS depression
    Diabetes mellitus

Special studies
    CXR
    PFTs
    ECG
    Echo
    Glucose

Ⓑ **Preparation**
    Avoid sedation
    Warm OR, IV fluid, circuit

Ⓒ **Anesthetic management**

Consider local or regional
    technique: avoid
    sedatives and narcotics

For general anesthesia:
    Do not use SCC
    Titrate NDMR
    Use short-acting agents
    Use reversal agents
        cautiously
    Use volatile agents
        cautiously
    Keep patient warm

(Cont'd on p 163)

D. Expect markedly prolonged recovery from anesthetic agents and muscle relaxants. Risk factors predicting the need for postoperative ventilatory support include preoperative proximal muscle weakness, upper abdominal surgery, RLD, poor cough, pharyngeal weakness, and age over 37 years. Have an ICU bed available for observation, aggressive pulmonary toilet, and possible prolonged postoperative ventilation. Avoid postoperative shivering, as this may precipitate myotonia. Manage postoperative pain using regional or local anesthetic techniques to avoid narcotic-induced respiratory depression. nonsteroidal antiinflammatory drugs (NSAIDs) are effective in patients without renal concerns. Transcutaneous electric nerve stimulation (TENS) has proven useful for pain relief and reduction of myotonia.

REFERENCES

1. Bennun M, Goldstein B, Finkelstein Y, et al.: Continuous propofol anaesthesia for patients with myotonic dystrophy, *Br J Anaesth* 85 (3):407–409, 2000.
2. Colovic V, Walker RW: Myotonia dystrophica and spinal surgery. *Pediatr Anaesth* 12 (4):351–355, 2002.
3. Jenkins JA, Facer EK: Anesthetic management of a patient with myotonic dystrophy for a Nissen fundoplication and gastrostomy, *Paediatr Anaesth* 14:693–696, 2004.
4. Mathieu J, Allard P, Gobeil G, et al.: Anesthetic and surgical complications in 219 cases of myotonic dystrophy, *Neurology* 49 (6):1646–1650, 1997.
5. Moxley RT III: The myotonias: their diagnosis and treatment, *Compr Ther* 22:8–21, 1996.
6. White RJ, Bass SP: Myotonic dystrophy and paediatric anaesthesia, *Paediatr Anaesth* 13 (2):94–102, 2003.

Patient with MYOTONIC DYSTROPHY
(Cont'd from p 161)

Ⓓ **Postoperative considerations**
Prolonged recovery
ICU
Local anesthetics for pain
TENS

Myasthenia Gravis (MG) and Eaton-Lambert Syndrome (ELS)

MARCO S. ROBIN, D.O.

JEFFREY R. KIRSCH, M.D.

———

MYASTHENIA GRAVIS (MG)

First described by Thomas Willis in 1672, myasthenia gravis (MG) is an autoimmune disease manifested by muscle weakness and fatigability that improves with rest. Bimodal in distribution, MG favors women in early presentation and men later in life. Incidence ranges from 0.25 to 2 per 100,000, increasing in frequency over age 60. For most, pathology occurs at the postsynaptic terminal of the neuromuscular junction. The nicotinic acetylcholine receptors (AChR) are targeted and bound by circulating autoantibodies. The result is a significant reduction (up to 80%) of functional motor receptors. Thymomas occur with MG 30 to 60% of the time, and 10 to 15% of patients with MG have thymomas.[1]

Respiratory and bulbar compromise are of paramount concern, necessitating intensive monitoring and intervention in the postoperative period. Symptomatology varies according to muscle involvement and tends to exacerbate and remit. Extraocular weakness is most common, usually presenting as ptosis or diplopia. Rheumatoid arthritis (RA), systemic lupus erythematosus (SLE), hypothyroidism, and anemia are associated with MG, each engendering unique anesthetic risks.

First-line pharmacotherapy is with anticholinesterase drugs, commonly pyridostigmine. Immunosuppression, commonly with prednisolone, helps control symptoms. Azathioprine, cyclosporine, methotrexate, and cyclophosphamide are alternatives. Plasmapheresis and IV immunoglobulin G (IgG) produce a rapid but temporary improvement in symptoms and may be helpful in preparing marginal patients for the stress of surgery. Although thymectomy results in reduced rate of deterioration in patients with MG, the exact technique for thymectomy is controversial.

A. Eighty-five percent of patients with generalized MG carries the AChR antibody diagnostic for disease. The edrophonium (Tensilon) test is unreliable and has potential cardiac complications.[2] Diagnosis by single-fiber electromyogram of the orbicularis oculi is 100% sensitive and is considered the gold standard.[2] Evaluate for bulbar and respiratory involvement. Patients with MG typically maintain their respiratory drive and carbon dioxide (CO_2) response, but patients with severe disease may have a reduced vital capacity.[3] Forced vital capacity (FVC) is the most reliable indicator of respiratory function. Large thymomas can lead to airway obstruction; consider obtaining spirometry or computed tomography (CT) studies. Respiratory infections pose a serious postoperative risk; treat prior to surgery. Evaluate cardiac function with a focus on arrhythmias.

B. Osserman and Genkin's original classification by severity of symptoms is still accepted and may be helpful in risk stratification.

C. Continuation of anticholinesterase therapy prior to surgery is debatable. In general, if the patient is reliant on medication, continue the drugs preoperatively. Continue immunosuppressants as well. Plasmapheresis appears to be more effective at improving pulmonary function than pyridostigmine.[3] Consider plasmapheresis for severe disease or in patients with a vital capacity of < 2 L. Avoid preoperative sedation, if possible.

D. Use clinical judgment in selection of anesthetic drugs. IV induction agents are safe. Use potent inhalation agents alone or combined with IV medications for maintenance of anesthesia. Total intravenous anesthesia (TIVA) has been reported as safe.[4] Consider neuraxial or peripheral nerve blockade to avoid the complications linked to general anesthesia. Avoid esters and any drugs reliant on plasma esterase metabolism; enzyme levels may be low after plasmapheresis.

E. The response to nondepolarizing neuromuscular blockers (NDMBs) is unpredictable; avoid these if possible. When necessary, administer in adjusted doses guided by neuromuscular monitoring. Intermediate acting relaxants are best tolerated; most have an ED95 half their normal dose. Be sure to monitor twitch parameters frequently. Consider the risks and benefits of withholding pharmacological reversal agent; there is the potential for residual blockade and respiratory compromise on the one hand and the risk of cholinergic crisis on the other. Patients with MG are resistant to succinylcholine at low doses but have an increased incidence of phase two block at doses higher than the ED95 (0.8 mg/kg).[5]

F. Management of postoperative pain and assessment of ventilatory function are important. To reduce the time to extubation, ensure adequate pain control, avoid opioids and sedatives, and provide pulmonary toilet.[5] Consider the use of epidural analgesia in patients having invasive thoracic or abdominal procedures to help accomplish these goals.

EATON-LAMBERT SYNDROME (ELS)

Eaton-Lambert Syndrome (ELS), or myasthenic syndrome, is a rare neuromuscular disorder in which IgG antibodies attack the presynaptic terminals, inhibiting

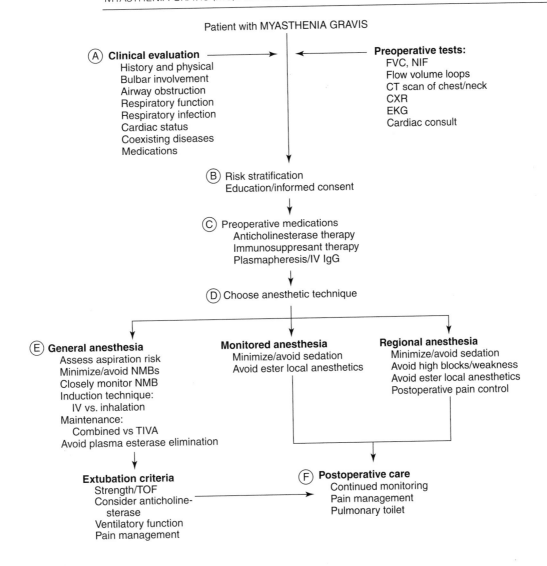

Patient with MYASTHENIA GRAVIS

(A) **Clinical evaluation**
   History and physical
   Bulbar involvement
   Airway obstruction
   Respiratory function
   Respiratory infection
   Cardiac status
   Coexisting diseases
   Medications

Preoperative tests:
   FVC, NIF
   Flow volume loops
   CT scan of chest/neck
   CXR
   EKG
   Cardiac consult

(B) Risk stratification
   Education/informed consent

(C) Preoperative medications
   Anticholinesterase therapy
   Immunosuppressant therapy
   Plasmapheresis/IV IgG

(D) Choose anesthetic technique

(E) **General anesthesia**
   Assess aspiration risk
   Minimize/avoid NMBs
   Closely monitor NMB
   Induction technique:
   IV vs. inhalation
   Maintenance:
      Combined vs TIVA
   Avoid plasma esterase elimination

Monitored anesthesia
   Minimize/avoid sedation
   Avoid ester local anesthetics

Regional anesthesia
   Minimize/avoid sedation
   Avoid high blocks/weakness
   Avoid ester local anesthetics
   Postoperative pain control

Extubation criteria
   Strength/TOF
   Consider anticholine-
      sterase
   Ventilatory function
   Pain management

(F) **Postoperative care**
   Continued monitoring
   Pain management
   Pulmonary toilet

normal release of acetylcholine (ACh). Evident as proximal muscle weakness and hyporeflexia, it differs from MG in that the weakness improves with exertion. Its predilection to males is partly due to its association with small cell lung cancer. Pharmacokinetics of neuromuscular blockers in ELS patients is unpredictable; however most are sensitive to both succinylcholine and NDMBs. Anticholinesterase drugs and steroids are both ineffective in treating ELS but diaminopyridine may be useful.[3]

REFERENCES

1. Vincent A, Palace J, Hilton-Jones D: Myasthenia gravis, *Lancet* 357:2122–2128, 2001.
2. Palace J, Vincent A, Beeson D: Myasthenia gravis: diagnostic and management dilemmas, *Curr Opin Neurol* 14:583–589, 2001.
3. Briggs E, Kirsch J: Anesthetic implications of neuromuscular disease, *J Anesth* 17:177–185, 2003.
4. Lorimer M, Hall R: Remifentanil and propofol total intravenous anaesthesia for thymectomy in myasthenia gravis, *Anaesth Intensive Care* 26:210–212, 1998.
5. Abel M, Eisenkraft J: Anesthetic implications of myasthenia gravis, *Mt Sinai J Med* 69:31–37, 2002.

Malignant Hyperthermia (MH): Prophylaxis

MARILYN GREEN LARACH, M.D., F.A.A.P.

Malignant hyperthermia (MH) susceptibility is an inherited skeletal muscle disorder in which anesthetic medications (Table 1) trigger sustained skeletal muscle hypermetabolism or contracture. To avoid triggering a potentially fatal MH episode in a susceptible patient, the anesthesiologist should (1) carefully evaluate the patient's risk of MH susceptibility, (2) ensure the availability of appropriate personnel and facilities (including adequate dantrolene supply) to diagnose and treat a fulminant MH reaction, (3) choose a regional or general anesthetic without agents that trigger MH, and (4) ensure patient follow-up through referral to the Malignant Hyperthermia Association of the United States (MHAUS).

A. Assess the patient's risk for MH susceptibility. Patients at significantly increased risk for an intraoperative MH episode are those with a personal history of an adverse metabolic or musculoskeletal anesthetic reaction; a first-degree family member with MH susceptibility; or an underlying myopathy associated with MH susceptibility (central-core or King-Denborough syndrome).[1] If the anesthetic is elective, evaluate the patient's MH susceptibility by contacting The North American MH Registry of MHAUS (888-274-7899, http://www.mhreg.org/, or bwb+@pitt.edu) to obtain a one-page summary of the patient's MH history or if the patient is unregistered, review previous anesthesia records. If the patient's MH susceptibility status is unclear, consider consulting an MH Hotline expert and obtaining a diagnostic MH muscle biopsy. Selected members of well-characterized families may be able to have their MH susceptibility determined by molecular genetic analysis.[2] If urgent or emergent, use an MH prophylactic regimen.

B. Check the adequacy of institutional facilities before an elective procedure. Thirty-six vials of dantrolene (and sterile water diluent) should be available within the OR complex. A trained team should be ready to treat an acute MH crisis if it develops. Laboratory facilities must be able to perform blood gas and electrolyte analysis rapidly. Facilities should be available to stabilize a critically ill patient. If facilities are inadequate to treat a fulminant MH episode, the procedure should be rescheduled at an appropriate institution.

C. Prepare an anesthesia machine that is uncontaminated by potent inhalational anesthetics. Empty and inactivate vaporizers, flush with air or oxygen (O_2) at 10 L/min for 10 minutes, and use fresh circuit tubing, gas hose, reservoir bag, and carbon dioxide (CO_2) absorbent. Alternatively, use a freestanding ventilator and an IV anesthetic.

D. Apply monitors, including a capnograph or a dedicated mass spectrometer that continuously displays expired CO_2, a core temperature monitor (do not use a liquid crystal skin probe), ECG, BP monitor, stethoscope, and pulse oximeter. Use new anesthesia masks and airways.

E. Avoid anesthetic agents that trigger MH. An anxiolytic may be desirable if the patient has a history of abnormal temperature regulation, muscle cramps, or myoglobinuria when stressed. Regional anesthesia is preferable for MH-susceptible patients whenever appropriate. All local anesthetic agents, including lidocaine, may safely be administered.[3] For MH-susceptible parturients, an epidural catheter should be placed and tested for appropriate function early in the course of labor. If general anesthesia is required, *avoid* the agents listed in Table 1. Whenever possible, do not allow significant alterations in the patient's temperature. For patients receiving general anesthesia, controlled ventilation may be desirable, because increases in expired CO_2 will be readily appreciated and provide an early warning of a developing MH episode. Be vigilant for the appearance of any MH signs, and initiate rapid treatment for any developing MH episode.

F. Observe the patient postoperatively in your facility for at least 3 hours if the anesthetic course has been unremarkable. If any significant signs of an MH reaction were seen, observe the patient intensively for 12 to 24 hours after resolution of the last MH sign.

G. The patient and family may obtain educational materials from MHAUS (http://www.mhreg.org/) and register their MH susceptibility with the North American MH Registry (http://www.mhreg.org/). The patient should order a medical alert bracelet if the patient does not already have one.

TABLE 1
Malignant Hyperthermia-Triggering Agents

Depolarizing muscle relaxants

Succinylcholine

All volatile inhalational anesthetics including:

Desflurane
Enflurane
Halothane
Isoflurane
Sevoflurane

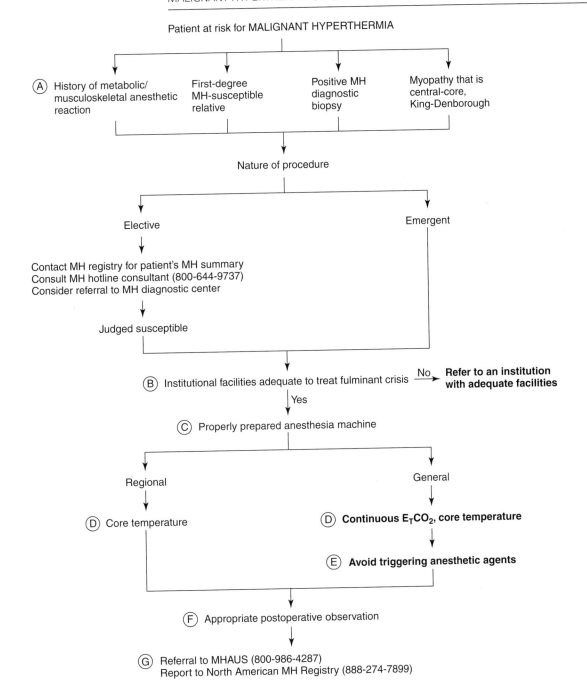

Patient at risk for MALIGNANT HYPERTHERMIA

(A) History of metabolic/ musculoskeletal anesthetic reaction

First-degree MH-susceptible relative

Positive MH diagnostic biopsy

Myopathy that is central-core, King-Denborough

Nature of procedure

Elective

Emergent

Contact MH registry for patient's MH summary
Consult MH hotline consultant (800-644-9737)
Consider referral to MH diagnostic center

Judged susceptible

(B) Institutional facilities adequate to treat fulminant crisis   No → **Refer to an institution with adequate facilities**

Yes

(C) Properly prepared anesthesia machine

Regional

General

(D) Core temperature

(D) **Continuous E_TCO_2, core temperature**

(E) **Avoid triggering anesthetic agents**

(F) Appropriate postoperative observation

(G) Referral to MHAUS (800-986-4287)
Report to North American MH Registry (888-274-7899)

REFERENCES

1. Gronert GA, Pessah IN, Muldoon SM, et al.: Malignant hyperthermia. In Miller RD, editor: *Miller's anesthesia*, ed 6, Philadelphia, 2005, Elsevier.
2. Sambuughin N, Holley H, Muldoon S, et al.: Screening of the entire ryanodine receptor type 1 coding region for sequence variants associated with malignant hyperthermia susceptibility in the North American population, *Anesthesiology* 102:515–521, 2005.
3. Gielen M, Viering W: 3-in-1 lumbar plexus block for muscle biopsy in malignant hyperthermia patients. Amide local anaesthetics may be used safely, *Acta Anaesthesiol Scand* 30:581–583, 1986.

Malignant Hyperthermia (MH): Treatment of Acute Episode

MARILYN GREEN LARACH, M.D., F.A.A.P.

A fulminant malignant hyperthermia (MH) crisis is an uncommon but potentially fatal event. Early diagnosis with rapid, appropriate intervention is necessary to prevent death and reduce the morbidity of this hypermetabolic state. Effective therapy requires termination of anesthetic agents that triggered MH *and* rapid administration of IV dantrolene. All acute MH reactions require dantrolene therapy.

A. The acute MH episode presents during or after exposure to triggering anesthetic agents: succinylcholine (SCC) and all volatile inhalational anesthetics. Signs and laboratory findings may include tachycardia, masseter muscle rigidity, generalized muscle rigidity, skin mottling, cyanosis, tachypnea, dysrhythmias including ventricular tachycardia and fibrillation, cardiac arrest, hypertension, diaphoresis, rapid temperature rise, excessive bleeding, myoglobinuria, increased creatine kinase (CK), hypercarbia, respiratory acidosis, metabolic acidosis, and hyperkalemia.[1]

B. Masseter muscle rigidity (muscle spasm of ≥30-sec duration that significantly interferes with mouth opening despite an appropriate SCC dose) may herald a fulminant MH reaction or may be an isolated adverse anesthetic response. If masseter muscle rigidity occurs without respiratory acidosis, metabolic acidosis, or hyperkalemia, either continue with a nontriggering anesthetic and continuous monitoring of core temperature and end-expiratory carbon dioxide (CO_2) or abort the surgical procedure. Titrate fluids and diuretics to achieve a diuresis of ≥1 to 2 ml/kg/hr (consider insertion of urinary catheter). Send samples of urine and blood for myoglobin analysis and consult a nephrologist if significant myoglobinuria fails to resolve. Measure CK every 6 hours for 24 hours. Refer masseter muscle rigidity patients to an MH diagnostic center for evaluation if no temporomandibular joint dysfunction can be elicited on subsequent physical examination. Report patients to The North American Malignant Hyperthermia Registry (888-274-7899).

C. The differential diagnosis of MH includes insufficient anesthetic depth, hypoxia, hypercarbia, iatrogenic hyperthermia, heat stroke, hyperkalemic cardiac arrest secondary to occult muscular dystrophy, neuroleptic malignant syndrome, sepsis, thyrotoxicosis, pheochromocytoma, recreational drug ingestion (ecstasy, etc.), and radiologic contrast within the CNS. Obtain ABGs and venous blood gas. While blood gases are being analyzed, control the ventilation at an appropriate V_E. Elevated expired CO_2 or expired CO_2 that is increasing rapidly in a nonbronchospastic, paralyzed, and adequately ventilated patient may be an early sign of MH. Turn off external patient warmers, measure core temperatures, and calculate the rate of temperature increase (more than 0.25°C/15 min is suspicious for MH).

D. When fulminant MH is suspected, convert to anesthetic agents that do not trigger MH and initiate the MH treatment regimen. Reconstitute dantrolene with preservative-free sterile water and administer an initial dose of 2.5 mg/kg IV. If the MH reaction does not rapidly resolve, additional dantrolene should be administered until MH signs of rigidity/metabolic or respiratory acidosis have abated. Assign at least one person the job of reconstituting dantrolene. If MH does not recur, give 1 mg/kg of IV dantrolene for three additional doses at 6-hour intervals. *Patients survive fulminant MH reactions only when they receive early and adequate dantrolene therapy.* Side effects of dantrolene include generalized muscle weakness and respiratory failure.[2,3]

E. If not already intubated, intubate the patient (without SCC). Ventilate (FiO_2 1.0) to a PCO_2 of 35; this may require tripling the V_E. Change the anesthesia circuit and reservoir bag. Institute continuous expired CO_2 monitoring and insert urinary and arterial catheters. Because fluid shifts may be significant, consider insertion of a CVP. Monitor temperatures at two sites. Send blood samples for ABGs and venous blood gas, lactate, electrolytes including potassium (K^+), calcium (Ca^{++}), myoglobin, CK, fibrin degradation products, prothrombin time (PT), international normalized ratio (INR), partial thromboplastin time (PTT), platelet count, and fibrinogen analysis. Check urine for myoglobin. Repeat as needed.

F. Cool the patient to 37°C (cooling blankets, iced lavage of body cavities, and cool IV solutions). Promote a diuresis of at least 1 to 2 ml/kg/hr, and treat metabolic acidosis and hyperkalemia. Young children with occult myopathies may experience severe rhabdomyolysis and hyperkalemic cardiac arrest after exposure to SCC or volatile inhalational anesthetics. Treat hyperkalemia with calcium salts (if a child), bicarbonate, glucose, insulin, and epinephrine. Hemodialysis and cardiopulmonary bypass (CPB) may be needed. Give antiarrhythmics as needed.[4] Call the MHAUS MH Hotline Consultant (800-644-9737, press 0) for expert advice in management of the acute crisis. Do not transport the patient until stable unless CPB is required and unavailable within your institution.

(Continued on page 170)

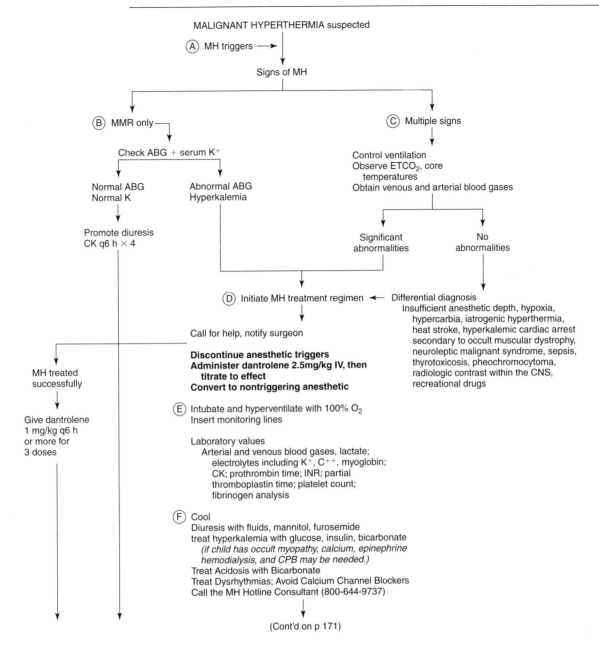

MALIGNANT HYPERTHERMIA suspected

Ⓐ MH triggers ⟶

Signs of MH

Ⓑ MMR only

Ⓒ Multiple signs

Check ABG + serum K^+

Control ventilation
Observe $ETCO_2$, core
  temperatures
Obtain venous and arterial blood gases

Normal ABG
Normal K

Abnormal ABG
Hyperkalemia

Significant
abnormalities

No
abnormalities

Promote diuresis
CK q6 h × 4

Ⓓ Initiate MH treatment regimen ⟵ Differential diagnosis
  Insufficient anesthetic depth, hypoxia,
    hypercarbia, iatrogenic hyperthermia,
    heat stroke, hyperkalemic cardiac arrest
    secondary to occult muscular dystrophy,
    neuroleptic malignant syndrome, sepsis,
    thyrotoxicosis, pheochromocytoma,
    radiologic contrast within the CNS,
    recreational drugs

Call for help, notify surgeon

MH treated
successfully

Discontinue anesthetic triggers
Administer dantrolene 2.5mg/kg IV, then
** titrate to effect**
Convert to nontriggering anesthetic

Give dantrolene
1 mg/kg q6 h
or more for
3 doses

Ⓔ Intubate and hyperventilate with 100% O_2
  Insert monitoring lines

  Laboratory values
    Arterial and venous blood gases, lactate;
      electrolytes including K^+, C^{++}, myoglobin;
      CK; prothrombin time; INR; partial
      thromboplastin time; platelet count;
      fibrinogen analysis

Ⓕ Cool
  Diuresis with fluids, mannitol, furosemide
  treat hyperkalemia with glucose, insulin, bicarbonate
    (if child has occult myopathy, calcium, epinephrine
    hemodialysis, and CPB may be needed.)
  Treat Acidosis with Bicarbonate
  Treat Dysrhythmias; Avoid Calcium Channel Blockers
  Call the MH Hotline Consultant (800-644-9737)

(Cont'd on p 171)

G. If MH signs recur, treat with IV dantrolene (2.5 mg/kg bolus, then titrate to effect). Observe patients intensively for 12 hours after the last dantrolene dose. Patients may develop acute renal failure, acute hepatic failure, CNS dysfunction (seizures, stroke, paraplegia, or quadriplegia), cardiac failure (usually after cardiac arrest from hyperkalemia), and DIC. Report the MH episode to the MH Registry (www.mhreg.org), and refer the patient and family to MHAUS for educational materials (www.mhaus.org or 607-674-7901). Following recovery, refer the patient to an MH diagnostic center to evaluate MH susceptibility. Children suffering a hyperkalemic cardiac arrest should be evaluated by a neurologist for occult myopathy. The patient should request a medical alert bracelet before discharge. The patient or his or her parents should inform first- and second-degree relatives of their possible MH susceptibility.

REFERENCES

1. Larach MG, Localio AR, Allen GC, et al.: A clinical grading scale to predict malignant hyperthermia susceptibility, *Anesthesiology* 80:771–779, 1994.
2. Kolb ME, Horne ML, Martz R: Dantrolene in human malignant hyperthermia, *Anesthesiology* 56:254–262, 1982.
3. Brandom BW, Larach MG: The North American MH Registry, *Anesthesiology* 96:A1199, 2002.
4. Larach MG, Rosenberg H, Gronert GA, Allen GC: Hyperkalemic cardiac arrest during anesthesia in infants and children with occult myopathies, *Clin Pediatr (Phila)* 36:9–16, 1997.

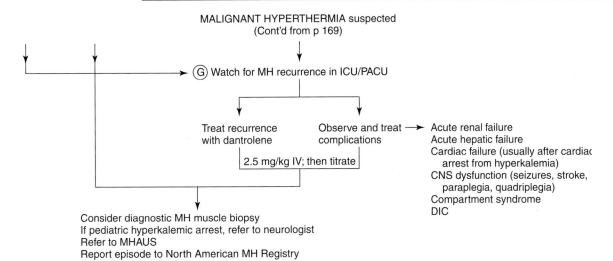

MALIGNANT HYPERTHERMIA suspected
(Cont'd from p 169)

Ⓖ Watch for MH recurrence in ICU/PACU

Treat recurrence
with dantrolene

2.5 mg/kg IV; then titrate

Observe and treat
complications

Acute renal failure
Acute hepatic failure
Cardiac failure (usually after cardiac
   arrest from hyperkalemia)
CNS dysfunction (seizures, stroke,
   paraplegia, quadriplegia)
Compartment syndrome
DIC

Consider diagnostic MH muscle biopsy
If pediatric hyperkalemic arrest, refer to neurologist
Refer to MHAUS
Report episode to North American MH Registry

Neuroleptic Malignant Syndrome (NMS)

MICHAEL P. HUTCHENS, M.D., M.A.

Neuroleptic malignant syndrome (NMS) is a life-threatening metabolic derangement associated with use of multiple classes of antipsychotic agents. Examples of drugs associated with NMS include haloperidol and droperidol, but any patient taking antipsychotic medication (including the novel agents clozapine and risperidone) is at risk. The mechanism of NMS is currently under debate. One hypothesis is alteration of function at hypothalamic dopaminergic neurons; however central dopamine antagonism cannot explain the full syndrome. Recently it has been proposed that dopamine antagonism in the setting of a vulnerable autonomic nervous system leads to a cascade of sympathetic nervous system dysregulation.[1] There are obvious similarities to malignant hyperthermia (MH), because the two entities share aspects of a common final pathway. Although there are obvious parallels, the two entities are distinct. NMS is more common than MH (7/1,000 to 22/1,000 versus 1/15,000 to 1/50,000, respectively).[2] The time course of NMS is more protracted. Individuals who experience NMS are not more likely to experience MH, but it is unclear if MH-susceptible patients are more likely to develop NMS.[3] No genetic abnormality of calcium channels has been found to be associated with NMS. The mortality of NMS is reported to be decreasing, but in the setting of renal failure it may be as high as 50%.[2]

A. There are no accepted formal diagnostic criteria. The sine qua non of NMS is exposure to neuroleptic medication. Symptoms may develop as early as 24 hours after exposure or as late as 20 days after cessation of oral therapy. Look for the classic triad of hyperthermia (98% of cases), lead pipe rigidity (97%), and mental status changes (97%); this triad is the major criteria for diagnosis. Other findings include tachycardia, hypertension (HTN) or hypotension, tachypnea, and diaphoresis. Extrapyramidal symptoms including dyskinesia, opisthotonos, oculogyric crisis, and dysarthria may occur. Order laboratory tests, including a creatine phosphokinase (CPK); elevation of CPK is an important finding which increases the likelihood of NMS and is reported in 95% of cases.[4,5] Leucocytosis is common. Renal failure may ensue from rhabdomyolysis with myoglobinuria. Hypoxia and acidosis may be present if supportive care has not been initiated.

B. The diagnosis of NMS is made after exclusion of a wide differential diagnosis. Fever may be central or peripheral in origin. Consider the following central causes: drug reactions (anticholinergics, amphotericin, or chemotherapeutics), central anticholinergic syndrome, serotonin withdrawal, lethal catatonia, or traumatic brain injury. Peripheral causes include infectious disease, hyperthyroidism, heatstroke, and MH.

C. Do not consider elective surgical procedures in patients with active NMS. Dehydration, hyperpyrexia, autonomic dysfunction, and renal failure all dramatically increase the probability of perioperative morbidity. If NMS presents intraoperatively or if a patient with NMS requires an emergency surgical procedure, initiate supportive care, including volume resuscitation, mechanical ventilation, hemodynamic monitoring, and measurement of urine output. Choose any suitable anesthetic technique; none is specifically contraindicated. Discontinue neuroleptic drugs. Avoid anticholinergic drugs, which can cause hyperthermia. Pharmacotherapy reported to be beneficial includes bromocriptine (a dopamine agonist), dantrolene, benzodiazepines, and muscle relaxants, which facilitate ventilation in patients with rigidity.[3]

D. Plan for postoperative admission to the ICU. Discontinue neuroleptic medications. Administer dantrolene to reduce temperature. (Dantrolene inhibits calcium release from the sarcoplasmic reticulum, thus inhibiting heat generation by skeletal muscle), bromocriptine (a central dopamine agonist), or benzodiazepines. Use nondepolarizing muscle relaxants (NDMRs) to facilitate mechanical ventilation. Continue supportive care to treat hemodynamic instability, impending renal failure, and hypovolemia.

REFERENCES

1. Gurrera RJ: Sympathoadrenal hyperactivity and the etiology of neuroleptic malignant syndrome, *Am J Psychiatry* 156:169, 1999.
2. Adnet P, Lestavel P, Krivosic-Horber R: Neuroleptic malignant syndrome, *Br J Anaesth* 85:129, 2000.
3. Caroff SN, Rosenberg H, Mann SC, et al.: Neuroleptic malignant syndrome in the perioperative period, *Am J Anesthesiol* 28:387, 2001.
4. Caroff SN, Mann SC: Neuroleptic malignant syndrome, *Med Clin North Am* 77 (1):185–202, 1993.
5. Guze BH, Baxter LR Jr: Current concepts. Neuroleptic malignant syndrome, *N Engl J Med* 313:163, 1984.

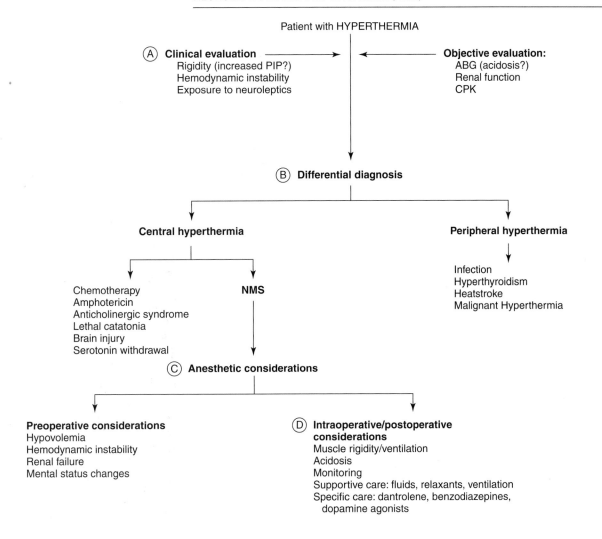

Patient with HYPERTHERMIA

A Clinical evaluation
Rigidity (increased PIP?)
Hemodynamic instability
Exposure to neuroleptics

Objective evaluation:
ABG (acidosis?)
Renal function
CPK

B Differential diagnosis

Central hyperthermia

Chemotherapy
Amphotericin
Anticholinergic syndrome
Lethal catatonia
Brain injury
Serotonin withdrawal

NMS

Peripheral hyperthermia

Infection
Hyperthyroidism
Heatstroke
Malignant Hyperthermia

C Anesthetic considerations

Preoperative considerations
Hypovolemia
Hemodynamic instability
Renal failure
Mental status changes

D Intraoperative/postoperative considerations
Muscle rigidity/ventilation
Acidosis
Monitoring
Supportive care: fluids, relaxants, ventilation
Specific care: dantrolene, benzodiazepines,
　　dopamine agonists

Tetraplegia

TOD B. SLOAN, M.D., PH.D.

The patient with tetraplegia presents a variety of anesthetic challenges.[1-6] Regardless of etiology, the problems are similar to those of chronic spinal cord injury (cSCI). For the purposes of this discussion, acute SCI is differentiated from tetraplegia and cSCI by the resolution of spinal shock, as indicated by the return of spinal cord reflexes below the injury region (usually 4 to 8 weeks after initial injury).

A. Perform a history and physical examination. Pulmonary failure is a major cause of morbidity and death in patients with chronic cervical SCI. Estimate pulmonary reserves by pulmonary function studies; reserves will be limited owing to decreased strength of the chest wall and abdominal muscles. These patients have reduced total lung capacity, expiratory reserve volume, and vital capacity and increased respiratory volume and work of breathing. Vital capacity is a good measure of adequacy. Further, with lesions in C_{3-5}, diaphragmatic control will be reduced, leading to marginal ventilation so that anesthesia or abnormal positions may necessitate ventilatory support. Assess renal function, because renal failure is another major cause of morbidity and death in cSCI; urinary tract infections (UTIs) result in ascending pyelonephritis and amyloidosis, and hypercalciuria or hyperkalemia results in an increased incidence of nephrolithiasis. Check electrolytes to quantitate hypercalcemia and identify whether electrolyte abnormalities have resulted from renal failure or bowel dysfunction (loss of sacral parasympathetics). A variety of other medical problems is usually present in these patients including chronic infections (pulmonary and urinary tract) leading to amyloidosis, anemia of chronic disease, adrenal insufficiency, deep venous thrombosis (DVT) and pulmonary emboli due to leg immobility, gastric erosions, and decubitus ulcers (notably over bony prominences such as the sacrum). Note the presence of autonomic hyperreflexia (65 to 85% of patients with dysfunction above T7). Additional causes of morbidity and death are suicide and drug addiction; the emotional problems and pain syndromes of SCI have a major impact on these patients and their perioperative management.

B. Common surgical procedures include delayed spinal stabilizations for bony nonunion, removal of paraspinal stabilization rods, treatment of decubitus ulcers, release of contractures, and urological procedures. Placement of phrenic pacemakers (in high lesions), spinal stimulators (for chronic pain), and spinal baclofen pumps (to reduce muscle spasms) is also common. Use preoperative medication with caution in patients with limited respiratory reserves. Choose intraoperative monitoring as appropriate to the surgical procedure and patient problems. Pay extra attention to keeping the patient warm, as thermoregulatory responses are reduced with a loss of sympathetic tone. Blood volume is often reduced (60 mL/kg), and patients may have greater orthostatic effects. Choose anesthetic technique based on the surgical procedure and the degree of sensation in the affected area. Surgical procedures in regions of no sensation can often be conducted using local, regional, or no anesthesia. Limitations to success include inability of the patient to assume the required position (owing to contractures) or tolerate this position (e.g., limitations of breathing in the prone position) or the presence of uncontrolled spinal autonomic reflexes. The most important reflex is autonomic-mediated hypertension caused by sensory stimulation (especially manipulation of bowel or bladder), which sends an afferent signal to the spinal cord that results in a sympathetically mediated vasoconstriction uninhibited by the brain. If the lesion includes splanchnic circulation (above T7), hypertension (HTN) results. A reflex bradycardia often ensues but if the efferent sympathetic response includes T1–4, tachycardia may result. This HTN can produce cerebral hemorrhage or cardiac ischemia and can be rapidly treated by removing the stimulus and administering direct-acting vasodilators (e.g., sodium nitroprusside) or drugs producing ganglionic blockade (e.g., trimethaphan). A second reflex arc involves muscle tone and may produce uncontrolled muscle spasms (mass reflex). If anesthesia techniques are required to block autonomic reflexes, neuraxial blockade (spinal or epidural) or general anesthesia can be used unless otherwise contraindicated. Epidural anesthesia has been used successfully to reduce autonomic HTN during labor. If general anesthesia is chosen, evaluate the airway carefully, as difficulty with intubation may occur if neck fusion limits extension. Instability of the spine is uncommon in cSCI, but a failure of fusion may be present if instrumentation has not been performed. Anesthetic agents must be titrated to needs; excessive cardiac depression or vasodilation may not be tolerated because of limited cardiac reserves.

C. Succinylcholine (SCC) may produce lethal hyperkalemia;[6] do not use within 1 year of lesions producing muscle denervation (e.g., SCI). With progressive denervation, SCC may not be advisable at any time (Guillain-Barré and demyelinating disease). Postoperatively, observe patients carefully for ventilatory insufficiency due to residual anesthetic depression and thromboembolic disease.

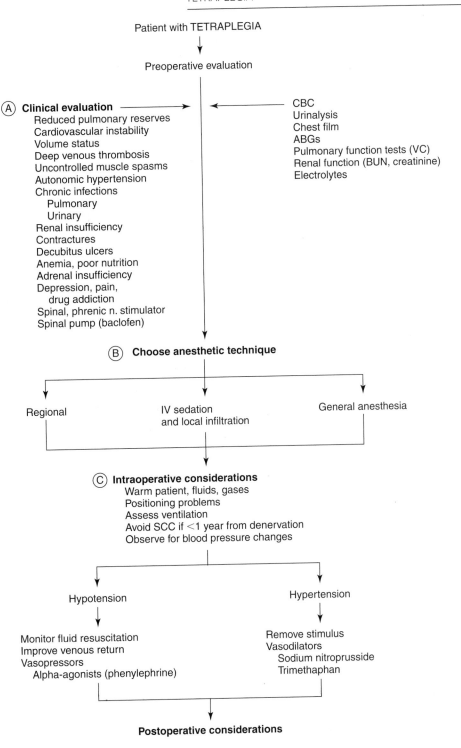

Patient with TETRAPLEGIA

↓

Preoperative evaluation

(A) **Clinical evaluation** ⟶   ⟵ CBC
  Reduced pulmonary reserves   Urinalysis
  Cardiovascular instability   Chest film
  Volume status   ABGs
  Deep venous thrombosis   Pulmonary function tests (VC)
  Uncontrolled muscle spasms   Renal function (BUN, creatinine)
  Autonomic hypertension   Electrolytes
  Chronic infections
      Pulmonary
      Urinary
  Renal insufficiency
  Contractures
  Decubitus ulcers
  Anemia, poor nutrition
  Adrenal insufficiency
  Depression, pain,
      drug addiction
  Spinal, phrenic n. stimulator
  Spinal pump (baclofen)

(B) **Choose anesthetic technique**

Regional   IV sedation   General anesthesia
              and local infiltration

(C) **Intraoperative considerations**
  Warm patient, fluids, gases
  Positioning problems
  Assess ventilation
  Avoid SCC if <1 year from denervation
  Observe for blood pressure changes

Hypotension   Hypertension

Monitor fluid resuscitation   Remove stimulus
Improve venous return   Vasodilators
Vasopressors   Sodium nitroprusside
    Alpha-agonists (phenylephrine)   Trimethaphan

Postoperative considerations

REFERENCES

1. Hambly PR, Martin B: Anaesthesia for chronic spinal cord lesions. *Anaesthesia* 53:273–289, 1998.
2. Mackensie CF, Geisler FH: Management of acute cervical spinal cord injury. In Albin MS, editor: *Textbook of neuroanesthesia with neurosurgical and neuroscience perspectives*, New York, 1996, McGraw-Hill.
3. Gronert GA: Cardiac Arrest after succinylcholine: mortality greater with rhabdomyolysis than receptor upregulation—review article, *Anesthesiology* 94 (3):523–529, 2001.
4. Chiles BW 3rd, Cooper PR: Acute spinal injury, *N Engl J Med* 334:514–520, 1996.
5. Sloan TB, Hickey R, Albin MS: Anesthesia management of the patient with acute spinal cord injury, *Adv Anesth* 8:55, 1991.
6. Martyn JA, Richtsfeld M: Succinylcholine-induced hyperkalemia in acquired pathologic states: Etiologic factors and molecular mechanisms, *Anesthesiology* 104:158–169, 2006.

Multiple Sclerosis (MS)

PATRICK BAKKE, M.D.

JEFFREY R. KIRSCH, M.D.

Multiple sclerosis (MS), affecting 250,000 to 350,000 people in the United States, is a disease characterized by demyelination, axonal injury, and gliosis followed by remyelination. Neurological signs and symptoms correspond to the area of injury in the CNS.[1,2] The cause of MS is elusive, although there is a known autoimmune component. The incidence of MS increases in certain geographical locations, including areas above the 40th parallel; this has led to speculation of an infectious or environmental cause.[1] There are also reports of clusters within families, supported by concordance rates of 30% in monozygotic twins as compared to 5% in dizygotic twins and less than 5% in first-degree family members.[1] The mean age of onset is 30 years, and there is a female to male ratio of 2:1.[1,2] Mean life expectancy is reduced by 6 or 7 years. Approximately 80% of patients have relapsing-remitting MS, in which exacerbation is followed by complete or near complete recovery. Corticosteroids are used to treat relapses; immune modulating drugs (interferon, glatiramer, immunoglobulin, or mitoxantrone) or plasma exchange is used to prevent progression. Eventually half of all MS patients will die from complications related to their disease, such as renal failure secondary to chronic urinary tract infection (UTI), pulmonary embolism related to immobilization, aspiration, suicide, and malnutrition.[2]

A. Obtain an excellent preoperative history and physical examination. Establish rapport to help ease psychological stress and decrease the likelihood of relapse. Relapse can be precipitated by stress, infection, increased ambient temperature, fever, or the postpartum condition.[1-3] Common signs and symptoms include fatigue, cognitive changes, depression, euphoria, dysarthria, internuclear ophthalmoplegia, nystagmus, vertigo, gate disturbances, sensory loss, increased deep tendon reflexes, limb ataxia, spasticity, spasms, amyotrophy, bladder disturbances, GI dysfunction, or platelet dysfunction.[1,2] Identify pain syndromes including trigeminal neuralgia, Lhermitte's sign, dysesthetic pain, optic neuritis, vertebral compression fractures, sacral de cubiti, back pain, leg spasms, bladder spasm, visceral pain, and others.[4,5] Discuss symptoms, duration of disease, treatments, and medications. Baclofen, used to treat spasm, has been implicated in potentiating inhaled and opiate anesthesia secondary to its gamma-aminobutyric acid (GABA) effects.[6,7] Carbamazepine and phenytoin may induce liver enzymes, necessitating increased frequency of dosing neuromuscular blockers and IV anesthetic agents. Plasma exchange can decrease cholinesterase levels, leading to prolonged succinylcholine (SCC) action. Include a careful neurological exam, documenting existing deficiencies. Treat anxiety and spasm prior to induction; diazepam is useful for both conditions.[8,9]

Administer a stress dose of corticosteroids if there was recent or prolonged use of steroids.

B. There have been no reports of increased relapse rates after general anesthesia.[10] In the past, regional anesthesia has been avoided to avoid the possibility that complications could be confused with relapse. To date, there have been no studies examining regional anesthesia and MS. Currently, MS is not thought to be a contraindication to regional anesthesia. There is no statistical increase in relapse rate in women receiving spinal or epidural anesthesia for labor or cesarean section.[3,11] The postpartum period is known to have an increase in relapse rate regardless of anesthetic administration. In one study, however, it was noted that all women who relapsed received bupivacaine in concentrations greater than 0.25%.[3] If general anesthesia is chosen, avoid SCC due to a theoretical risk of hyperkalemic response. Consider modified RSI in the presence of GI dysfunction and dysarthria. Studies have not supported avoidance of any particular medications for maintenance of general anesthesia.[10] Maintain normothermia, sterile technique, and fluid and electrolyte balance. Be vigilant for signs of autonomic hyperreflexia because of the high incidence of spinal cord lesions. Consider a possible increased risk of embolic events due to increased platelet aggregation in MS; there are no studies addressing this issue.

C. During the postoperative period, maintain normothermia, control pain, alleviate stress, and take all reasonable measures to prevent infection. Compare postoperative neurological finding so to results of the preoperative neurological examination.

REFERENCES

1. Noseworthy JH, Lucchinetti C, Rodriguez M, et al.: Multiple sclerosis. N Engl J Med 343 (13):938–952, 2000.
2. O'Connor P, Canadian Multiple Sclerosis Working Group: Key issues in the diagnosis and treatment of multiple sclerosis. An overview, Neurology 59 (6 Suppl 3):S1–S33, 2002.
3. Bader AM, Hunt CO, Datta S, et al.: Anesthesia for the obstetric patient with multiple sclerosis, J Clin Anes 1 (1):21–24, 1988.
4. Ehde DM, Jensen MP, Engel JM, et al.: Chronic pain secondary to disability: a review, Clin J Pain 19 (1):3–17, 2003.
5. Moulin DE: Pain in central and peripheral demyelinating disorders, Neurol Clin 16 (4):889–898, 1998.
6. Panerai AE, Massei R, de Silva E, et al.: Baclofen prolongs the analgesic effect of fentanyl in man, Br J Anaesth 57 (10):954–955, 1985.
7. Sugimura M, Kitayama S, Morita K, et al.: Effects of GABAergic agents on anesthesia induced by halothane, isoflurane and thiamylal in mice, Pharmacol Biochem Behav 72 (1–2):111–116, 2002.
8. Calabresi PA: Considerations in the treatment of relapsing-remitting multiple sclerosis, Neurology 58 (8 Suppl 4): S10–S22, 2002.
9. Clanet MG, Brassat D: The management of multiple sclerosis patients, Curr Opin Neurol 13 (3):263–270, 2000.
10. Bamford C, Sibely W, Laguna J. Anesthesia in multiple sclerosis, Can J Neurol Sci 5 (1):41–44, 1978.
11. Jones RM: Lumbar epidural anesthesia in patients with multiple sclerosis, Anesth Analg 62 (9):856–857, 1983.

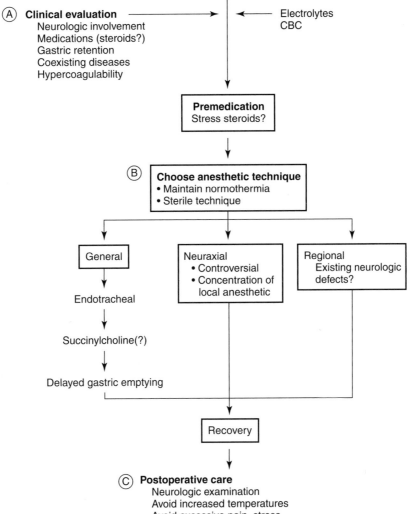

Patient with MULTIPLE SCLEROSIS

(A) **Clinical evaluation**
   Neurologic involvement
   Medications (steroids?)
   Gastric retention
   Coexisting diseases
   Hypercoagulability

Electrolytes
CBC

Premedication
Stress steroids?

(B) **Choose anesthetic technique**
   • Maintain normothermia
   • Sterile technique

General

Endotracheal

Succinylcholine(?)

Delayed gastric emptying

Neuraxial
   • Controversial
   • Concentration of local anesthetic

Regional
   Existing neurologic defects?

Recovery

(C) **Postoperative care**
   Neurologic examination
   Avoid increased temperatures
   Avoid excessive pain, stress
   Wound, respiratory, and urinary care

Parkinson's Disease (PD)

ANSGAR M. BRAMBRINK, M.D, PH.D.

INES P. KOERNER, M.D.

Parkinson's disease (PD) affects about 1 million patients in the United States. The primary biochemical disturbance is thought to be an imbalance in the dopamine/acetylcholine ratio, resulting from a progressive loss of dopaminergic neurons in the substantia nigra of the basal ganglia, which leads to the Parkinson's triad: tremor, muscle rigidity, and bradykinesia. Drug treatment aims to increase the supply of dopamine, affect the biological balance of dopamine or act as a dopamine substitute. The keys to reducing perioperative morbidity are (1) meticulous preoperative assessment; (2) maintenance of anti-parkinsonian drug therapy before, during, and after surgery; and (3) avoidance of agents that may precipitate parkinsonian symptoms.[1-5]

A. Perform careful preoperative evaluation.

B. Muscle rigidity and weakness may cause poor fluid intake and hypovolemia. Severe tremor can interfere with monitoring and may exclude straight regional anesthesia. Depression, confusion, and hallucination may appear during the perioperative period; this is especially uncomfortable for a patient, whose ability to communicate is already impaired by PD.

C. PD is associated with dysfunctional pharyngeal and laryngeal musculature, rendering patients at risk for chronic aspiration. Many patients present with chronic obstructive breathing pattern or chronic obstructive pulmonary disease (COPD). ABG analysis, pulmonary function tests (PFTs), or chest X-ray (CXR) may help to plan for adequate postoperative support.

D. Patients with PD may have cardiac arrhythmias and orthostatic hypotension, both of which may be drug induced (Levodopa [L-DOPA], bromocriptine, tricyclic antidepressants) or disease related (autonomic imbalance, relative hypovolemia).[4] Preoperative electrocardiography rules out acute changes and establishes a baseline.

E. Patients may suffer from sialorrhea, resulting from reduced autonomic swallowing. Antimuscarinic drugs may further exacerbate this by increasing viscosity of secretions. Abnormal esophageal function eventually leads to gastroesophageal reflux disease (GERD). Dysphagia renders patients at risk for malnutrition and dehydration.

F. The most frequently used anti-parkinsonian drug is L-DOPA, which crosses the blood-brain barrier and acts as a dopamine precursor in the CNS. Dopamine agonists (e.g., bromocriptine) are provided to reduce the overall need for L-DOPA. In addition, Monoamine oxidase-B (MAO-B) inhibitors (e.g., selegiline and lazabemide) prolong the action of dopamine in the striatum. Respectively treated patients should not receive indirect-acting sympathomimetic drugs. Anticholinergic drugs (e.g., benztropine or trihexyphenidyl) may be useful to treat tremor in early disease.[4]

G. It is of paramount importance to continue the specific anti-parkinsonian drug therapy throughout the perioperative period. L-DOPA has a short half-life (about 3 hours); therefore, treatment must be continued until surgery and immediately resumed thereafter. L-DOPA can also be provided intraoperatively, using a nasogastral tube.[1] Potent nonsteroidal anti-inflammatory drugs (NSAIDs) may reduce the overall requirement for opioids. It is crucial to avoid drugs which may precipitate parkinsonian symptoms (e.g., phenothiazines, butyrophenones, metoclopramide, and anti-muscarinerics). Meperidine must be avoided in patients receiving selegiline because of the risk of muscle rigidity and hyperthermia.[6]

H. During induction of general anesthesia, use specific means to reduce the risk of aspiration. Opioids may be associated with increased muscle rigidity. Postinduction hypotension may be more pronounced in patients with PD. Among all IV-induction agents, propofol theoretically has the best profile, and it has been described to be beneficial. Succinylcholine (SCC) carries an increased risk for hyperkalemia.[6] General anesthesia may contribute to significant postoperative nausea and vomiting (PONV), and patients may benefit from adequate prophylaxis but avoid metoclopramide.

I. Regional anesthesia may avoid the risks of general anesthesia (e.g., respiratory depression, exaggerated postoperative pain, and PONV). This is countered by increased technical difficulties for both anesthesiologist and surgeon due to involuntary movements of the patient. Diphenhydramine as well as low-dose propofol may reduce these problems. Systemic hypotension may be significant with onset of spinal or epidural blockade. In addition, preexisting difficulties in micturition may be aggravated after regional anesthesia.

J. In some patients, awake functional neurosurgery may be planned. Stereotactic ablation of circumscribed brain areas aims to reduce parkinsonian symptoms. Patients undergo surgery with local anesthesia and little sedation to allow full neurological evaluation throughout the procedure. Propofol may be disadvantageous, because it may abolish tremor; remifentanil and midazolam can provide adequate sedation and analgesia, yet allowing fast recovery for adequate neurological monitoring.[3]

K. Before extubation, ensure that patients are awake, with full recovery of neuromuscular function and baseline airway control.

L. Patients may show increased shivering, pathological reflexes, confusion, and hallucinations postoperatively.[2] Parkinson's patients have an abnormal temperature control, and those receiving selegiline may additionally have an abnormal glucose metabolism requiring serum glucose monitoring.[6]

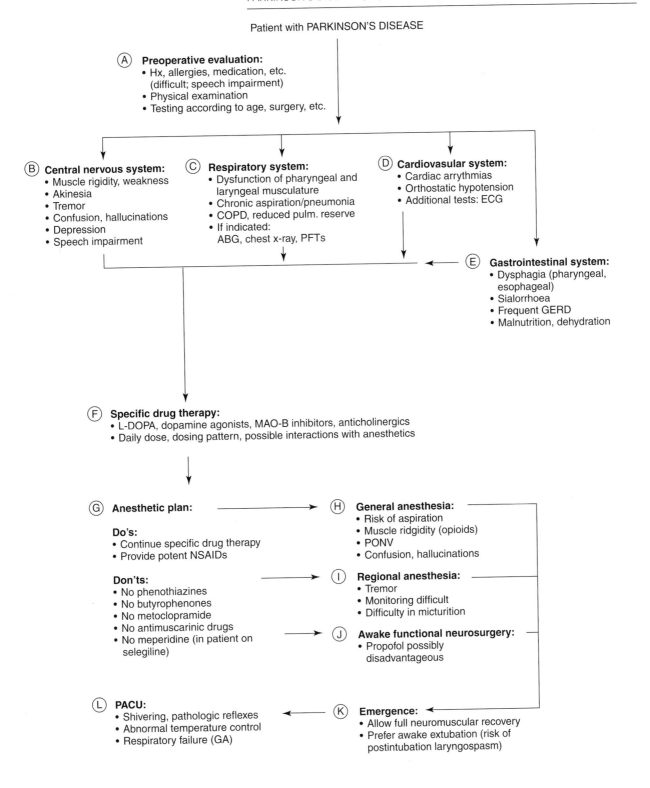

Patient with PARKINSON'S DISEASE

(A) **Preoperative evaluation:**
• Hx, allergies, medication, etc.
  (difficult; speech impairment)
• Physical examination
• Testing according to age, surgery, etc.

(B) **Central nervous system:**
• Muscle rigidity, weakness
• Akinesia
• Tremor
• Confusion, hallucinations
• Depression
• Speech impairment

(C) **Respiratory system:**
• Dysfunction of pharyngeal and
  laryngeal musculature
• Chronic aspiration/pneumonia
• COPD, reduced pulm. reserve
• If indicated:
  ABG, chest x-ray, PFTs

(D) **Cardiovasular system:**
• Cardiac arrythmias
• Orthostatic hypotension
• Additional tests: ECG

(E) **Gastrointestinal system:**
• Dysphagia (pharyngeal,
  esophageal)
• Sialorrhoea
• Frequent GERD
• Malnutrition, dehydration

(F) **Specific drug therapy:**
• L-DOPA, dopamine agonists, MAO-B inhibitors, anticholinergics
• Daily dose, dosing pattern, possible interactions with anesthetics

(G) **Anesthetic plan:**

Do's:
• Continue specific drug therapy
• Provide potent NSAIDs

Don'ts:
• No phenothiazines
• No butyrophenones
• No metoclopramide
• No antimuscarinic drugs
• No meperidine (in patient on
  selegiline)

(H) **General anesthesia:**
• Risk of aspiration
• Muscle ridgidity (opioids)
• PONV
• Confusion, hallucinations

(I) **Regional anesthesia:**
• Tremor
• Monitoring difficult
• Difficulty in micturition

(J) **Awake functional neurosurgery:**
• Propofol possibly
  disadvantageous

(K) **Emergence:**
• Allow full neuromuscular recovery
• Prefer awake extubation (risk of
  postintubation laryngospasm)

(L) **PACU:**
• Shivering, pathologic reflexes
• Abnormal temperature control
• Respiratory failure (GA)

REFERENCES

1. Furuya R, Hirai A, Andoh T, et al.: Successful perioperative management of a patient with Parkinson's disease by enteral levodopa administration under propofol anaesthesia, *Anesthesiology* 89:261–263, 1998.
2. Golden WE, Lavender RC, Metzer WS: Acute postoperative confusion and hallucinations in Parkinson's disease, *Ann Intern Med* 111:218–222, 1989.
3. Gray H, Wilson S, Sidebottom P: Parkinson's disease and anaesthesia, *Br J Anaesth* 90:524, 2003.
4. Lang AE, Lozano AM: Parkinson's disease: first of two parts, *N Engl J Med* 339:1044–1053, 1998.
5. Mason LJ, Cojocaru TT, Cole DJ: Surgical intervention and anesthetic management of the patient with Parkinson's disease, *Int Anesthesiol Clin* 34:133–150, 1996.
6. Nicholson G, Pereira AC, Hall GM: Parkinson's disease and anaesthesia, *Br J Anaesth* 89:904–916, 2002.

PREOPERATIVE ENDOCRINE PROBLEMS

DIABETES MELLITUS (DM)

OBESITY

HYPERTHYROIDISM

HYPOTHYROIDISM

PHEOCHROMOCYTOMA

CARCINOID SYNDROME (CS)

ADRENOCORTICAL HYPOFUNCTION

HYPERPARATHYROIDISM

ACROMEGALY

Diabetes Mellitus (DM)

SAUNDRA E. CURRY, M.D.

Diabetes mellitus (DM) is a disorder of carbohydrate metabolism that causes blood glucose (BG) elevation. Type 1, or juvenile-onset, DM patients lack insulin and are prone to diabetic ketoacidosis (DKA), which is when accelerated lipolysis and excess glucagon cause ketogenesis. Type II, or adult-onset, DM patients are resistant to insulin and less prone to ketosis but may develop hyperosmolar, hyperglycemic, nonketotic coma (HHNKC). Both forms have microangiopathy, accelerated atherogenesis, poor wound healing, and increased perioperative morbidity and mortality. Surgery and anesthesia cause metabolic changes, which can affect DM. There is an increase in the secretion of epinephrine, norepinephrine, cortisol, and growth hormone, all of which are insulin antagonists and cause resistance to insulin at the tissue level. Epinephrine decreases insulin secretion. Stress stimulates gluconeogenesis as well. All of these metabolic changes contribute to hyperglycemia in the perioperative period. The extent of these changes is affected by the type of DM, preoperative DM control, the severity of surgery, and perioperative complications.[1–5]

A. Evaluate the type of DM and history of hypoglycemia, DKA, and HHNKC. The patient who is well controlled on insulin, oral agents, or diet may become hyperglycemic or hypoglycemic when infected, made NPO, or given steroids. Determine the insulin type and dosage or the oral hypoglycemic agent and last dose (the half-life of chlorpropamide is 36 hours). Evaluate for common complications of DM, including renal failure, sensory and autonomic neuropathy (delayed gastric emptying, sick-sinus syndrome, orthostatic hypotension), coronary and peripheral atherosclerosis (silent myocardial infarctions [MIs]), retinal/vitreous hemorrhage and blindness, and stiff joint syndrome, which may make patients hard to intubate.

B. The presence of active infection makes DM resistant to therapy. Begin treatment of DKA before or concurrent with emergency surgery. Hyperglycemia may cause osmotic diuresis, with dehydration and loss of sodium (Na^+) and potassium (K^+). Metabolic acidosis is compensated by hyperventilation when the patient is awake. Treat hyperglycemia by giving enough insulin, by continuous infusion, to reduce BG 10% per hour until well controlled. Monitor fluid resuscitation (CVP or pulmonary artery [PA] catheter, urinary catheter) with saline, and add potassium chloride (KCl) after the urinary output is assured. If hypokalemia is present initially, begin KCl earlier (insulin and glucose administration causes K^+ to move intracellularly, and hypokalemia is worsened). HHNKC usually occurs in older, type II DM patients and carries a high mortality rate. Patients are severely dehydrated (deficit 7 to 8 L) and hyperosmolar. Begin aggressive, monitored fluid resuscitation with enough insulin to reduce BG approximately 10% per hour; too rapid a reduction in BG concentrations may produce cerebral edema and coma. The elective patient who is well controlled may be managed by a variety of regimens.

C. Consider the proposed surgery when planning glucose control. Minor surgery (30 minutes or less) is unlikely to lead to problems with normal diabetic control. Intermediate surgery (30 to 120 minutes) may interfere with diabetic control; major surgery (>120 minutes) will almost certainly affect diabetic control. Emergency surgery has a high risk for loss of glycemic control. Diabetic patients should be scheduled for surgery early in the day, particularly if it is done on an outpatient basis. This allows more time to manage their response to the surgical stress and for evaluation for discharge. For minor and intermediate surgery, noninsulin-dependent diabetes mellitus (NIDDM) patients usually have hypoglycemic agents withheld, and BG is monitored. For major surgery in NIDDM and in all types of surgery for insulin-dependent diabetes mellitus (IDDM), close glucose control is critical throughout the perioperative period. Several regimens are described in the literature, but insulin infusions are the safest way to control glucose. Start an IV of D5W at 1 ml/kg/hr. Then mix an infusion of 50 units regular insulin in 250 ml normal saline (NS) and infuse according to the following formula:

$$\text{Units per hour} = \frac{\text{Plasma glucose (mg/dl)}}{150}$$

(Flush the plastic tubing with 50 to 60 ml of the insulin infusion. Insulin binds to plastic and this saturates the binding sites.) Monitor levels hourly to keep BG in the range of 120 to 180 mg/dl. Infusions should be adjusted in 0.5 unit/hr increments. D50 should be given if BG gets very low (50 mg/dl).

Patient with DIABETES MELLITUS for surgery

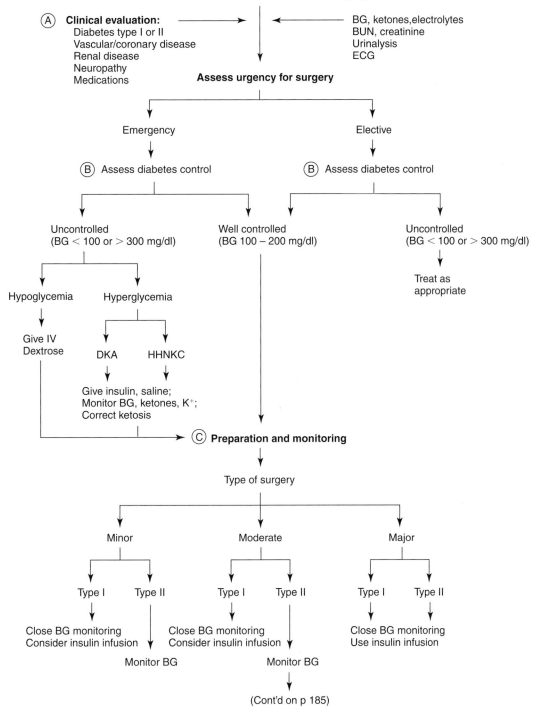

(Cont'd on p 185)

D. Monitor ECG, BP, SpO$_2$, and temperature in all patients. Use more invasive monitors when the general condition of the patient, hemodynamic stability, and duration and extent of surgery warrant their use, because end-organ disease is a greater hazard than diabetes itself. Perform BG assays at hourly intervals. Position carefully to avoid peripheral nerve injuries. Manage BG so as to avoid hyperglycemia (associated with impaired phagocytosis and wound healing) and hypoglycemia (may cause damage to the CNS). Administration of some glucose during the perioperative period is recommended to prevent muscle catabolism and hypoglycemia. Type I patients are usually more brittle and require closer monitoring of BG and serum K$^+$. Symptoms of developing hypoglycemia or hypoperfusion (mental status changes or angina) may be communicated by the awake patient under regional block more readily than if general anesthesia is employed. Under general anesthesia, signs of hypoglycemia mimic "light anesthesia," with tachycardia and hypertension (HTN). By deepening anesthesia in response to these signs without assessing glucose levels, dangerous hypoglycemia can result. Potent inhalational agents, steroids, and surgical stress may lead to increases in BG. Avoid the use of succinylcholine (SCC) in patients with neuropathies. For medicolegal rather than scientific reasons, many anesthesiologists prefer to avoid regional anesthesia in diabetic patients with preexisting neuropathies.

E. Metabolic and hormonal stress changes can continue up to four days postoperatively after major surgery. Patients should be carefully monitored until they can eat and get back on their usual regimen.

REFERENCES

1. Ahmed Z, Lockhart CH, Weiner M, et al.: Advances in diabetic management: implications for anesthesia, *Anesth Analg* 100:666-9, 2005.
2. Schiff RL, Welsh GA: Perioperative evaluation and management of the patient with endocrine dysfunction, *Med Clin North Am* 87: 175-92, 2003.
3. Rhodes ET, Ferrari LR, Wolfsdorf JI: Perioperative management of pediatric surgical patients with diabetes mellitus, *Anesth Analg* 101:986-99, 2005.
4. Tokumine J, Sugahara K, Fuchigami T, et al.: Unanticipated full stomach at anesthesia induction in a type I diabetic patient with asymptomatic gastroparesis, *J Anesth* 19:247-8, 2005.
5. Jellish WS, Kartha V, Fluder E, et al.: Effect of metoclopramide on gastric fluid volumes in diabetic patients who have fasted before elective surgery, *Anesthesiology* 102:904-9, 2005.

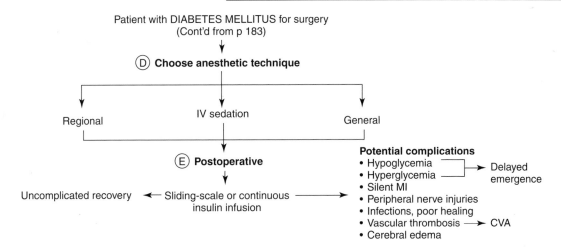

Patient with DIABETES MELLITUS for surgery
(Cont'd from p 183)

Ⓓ **Choose anesthetic technique**

Regional   IV sedation   General

Ⓔ **Postoperative**

Uncomplicated recovery ← Sliding-scale or continuous insulin infusion →

Potential complications
- Hypoglycemia ⎤
- Hyperglycemia ⎦ → Delayed emergence
- Silent MI
- Peripheral nerve injuries
- Infections, poor healing
- Vascular thrombosis → CVA
- Cerebral edema

Obesity

LYNN A. FENTON, M.D.

Patients are considered to be obese if they weigh >20% above their ideal body weight (IBW) or have a body mass index (BMI) > 30 kg/m^2 (see Table 1). Obesity is usually due to overeating. Secondary etiologies include hypothyroidism, Cushing's disease, insulinoma, and hypothalamic disease. Bariatric surgeries are appropriate for patients with BMI > 40 (or BMI > 35 in the presence of significant health complications).[1] Physiologic sequelae of obesity include increased cardiac output (0.1 L/min per kg adipose), hypertension (HTN), coronary artery disease (CAD), pulmonary HTN, type 2 diabetes mellitus (DM), hiatal hernia (HH) with delayed gastric emptying, increased gastric volumes and acid, GERD, fatty infiltration of the liver, venous thrombosis/pulmonary embolism, polycythemia, increased oxygen consumption and carbon dioxide (CO_2) production, V/Q mismatch, pulmonary compromise (decreased vital capacity, FRC, expiratory reserve volume, and inspiratory capacity), obstructive sleep apnea (OSA), and obesity hypoventilation syndrome or Pickwickian syndrome.[2–5]

A. Perform a preoperative evaluation including a thorough history, physical examination, and review of clinical or laboratory data. Determine if further workup is needed for any comorbid conditions. If the patient has OSA or Pickwickian syndrome, evaluate pulmonary function and cardiac function (rule out abnormal ventricular function, pulmonary HTN, and cor pulmonale). If asthma is present, consider pulmonary function tests (PFTs). Examine the airway (AW) carefully to determine the type of intubation required. Discuss anesthetic plans, AW management, and the likely postoperative course with the patient.

B. Premedicate the patient with H$_2$ antagonists, metoclopramide, and nonparticulate antacids. Continue all medications (accepted as safe) used to treat associated morbidities. Use only IV and oral routes to deliver drugs; IM injections usually deposit into adipose tissue resulting in unpredictable absorption. When significant OSA is present, refrain from sedation. Otherwise, titrate sedation carefully to avoid respiratory depression. Vascular access may be difficult. Ultrasound devices may be helpful in locating and assessing blood vessels for cannulation. Patients weighing more than 350 pounds may need a special OR table. Pressure points may require extra padding to avoid decubitus ulcers and neurological injuries.

C. Monitoring the patient can be difficult. To ensure a proper BP cuff fit, use an extra wide BP cuff or select other sites (e.g., leg or forearm). Alternatively, use an arterial catheter to obtain BP. Use a V$_5$ or equivalent ECG on all patients. If cardiac function is compromised, place a CVP or pulmonary artery (PA) catheter.

D. During minimum alveolar concentration (MAC) anesthesia, titrate all drugs to effect. Standard dosing regimens (e.g., mg/kg) risk overdosing and possible loss of the AW.

E. Regional anesthesia reduces the need for respiratory depressants and provides postoperative analgesia. Block placement may be technically difficult—consider using the sitting position to facilitate placement of neuraxial blocks. The response to local anesthetics can be unpredictable—titrate epidural and continuous spinal drugs carefully. Supine and Trendelenburg positions increase V/Q mismatch and may lead to hypoxia in a spontaneously breathing patient.

F. Administration of general anesthesia presents many concerns and challenges—securing and maintaining an AW is paramount. With rare exceptions, deliver GA via endotracheal intubation. If difficulty with intubation is anticipated, perform an awake intubation with continuous supplemental oxygen. Position the patient with the head and shoulders elevated to facilitate preoxygenation and maintain FRC above closing capacity. Ensure complete denitrogenation before induction. Obese patients desaturate rapidly (↓FRC and ↑oxygen consumption). Consider an RSI with cricoid pressure. Intraoperative ventilation of the patient may require high peak airway pressures due to poor chest wall and pulmonary compliance. Consider changes in ventilator type, settings, or the mode of ventilation to maintain adequate oxygenation and ventilation. Obese patients exhibit altered drug pharmacokinetics and pharmacodynamics. Therefore, choose drugs with short half-lives and low blood-fat solubility. As a general rule, calculate drug doses using IBW, except for the water-soluble muscle relaxants, where slightly higher than IBW should be used. Titrate drugs to effect. Before extubation, assure that the patient is awake, cooperative, and fully reversed from neuromuscular blockade.

G. Postoperatively, observe for AW obstruction and hypoxia. Sit the patient upright to improve ventilation. Consider epidural analgesia (particularly after upper, open abdominal surgery) to facilitate early ambulation and decrease postoperative pulmonary thromboembolic complications and length of hospital stay.

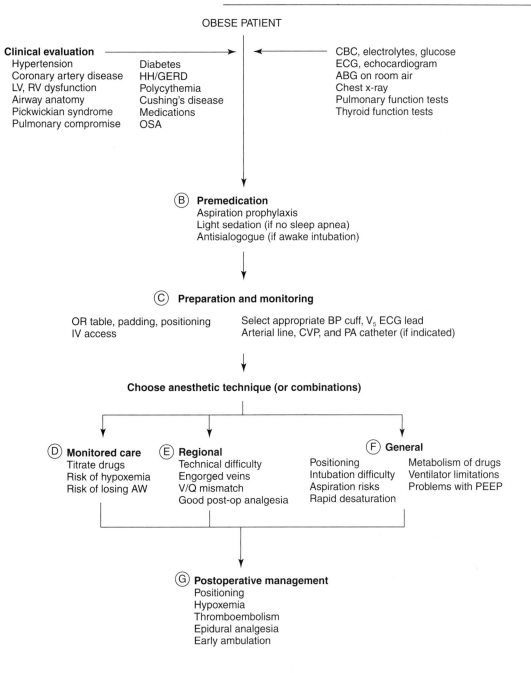

OBESE PATIENT

(A) **Clinical evaluation**
Hypertension   Diabetes
Coronary artery disease HH/GERD
LV, RV dysfunction   Polycythemia
Airway anatomy   Cushing's disease
Pickwickian syndrome   Medications
Pulmonary compromise   OSA

CBC, electrolytes, glucose
ECG, echocardiogram
ABG on room air
Chest x-ray
Pulmonary function tests
Thyroid function tests

(B) **Premedication**
Aspiration prophylaxis
Light sedation (if no sleep apnea)
Antisialogogue (if awake intubation)

(C) **Preparation and monitoring**

OR table, padding, positioning   Select appropriate BP cuff, V_5 ECG lead
IV access   Arterial line, CVP, and PA catheter (if indicated)

Choose anesthetic technique (or combinations)

(D) **Monitored care**   (E) **Regional**   (F) **General**
Titrate drugs   Technical difficulty   Positioning   Metabolism of drugs
Risk of hypoxemia   Engorged veins   Intubation difficulty Ventilator limitations
Risk of losing AW   V/Q mismatch   Aspiration risks   Problems with PEEP
                        Good post-op analgesia   Rapid desaturation

(G) **Postoperative management**
Positioning
Hypoxemia
Thromboembolism
Epidural analgesia
Early ambulation

TABLE 1
Definitions/Formulas for Calculating IBW and BMI

Term	Definition	BMI†
Overweight	20% above IBW*	
Obese	>20% above IBW	>30
Morbidly obese	2 × IBW	>40

*IBW calculation (kg) = height (cm) − 105 (♀) or 100 (♂)
†BMI calculation (weight (kg)/height (meters)^2= [weight (pounds) × 703 / height (inches)]/height (inches)

REFERENCES

1. Foster GD: Principles and practices in the management of obesity, *Am J Respir Crit Care Med* 168:274–280, 2003.
2. Maltby JR, Pytka S, Watson NC, et al.: Drinking 300 mL of clear fluid two hours before surgery has no effect on gastric fluid volume and pH in fasting and non-fasting obese patients, *Can J Anaesth* 51 (2):111–115, 2004.
3. Kessler R, Chaouat A, Schinkewitch P, et al.: The obesity-hypoventilation syndrome revisited: a prospective study of 34 consecutive cases, *Chest* 120 (2):369–376, 2001.
4. Passannante AN, Rock P: Anesthetic management of patients with obesity and sleep apnea, *Anesthesiol Clin North Am* 23 (3): 479–491, vii, 2005.
5. Gander S, Frascarolo P, Suter M, et al.: Positive end-expiratory pressure during induction of general anesthesia increases duration of nonhypoxic apnea in morbidly obese patients, *Anesth Analg* 100 (2):580–584, 2005.

Hyperthyroidism

SUSAN H. NOORILY, M.D.

Hyperthyroidism results from excessive tissue and circulating concentrations of thyroid hormones. Graves' disease is the most common form. Clinical manifestations suggest increased sensitivity to circulating catecholamines, although measured catecholamine levels are within normal limits.[1] These manifestations range from mild symptoms to the extreme symptoms of thyroid storm. Treatments include radioactive iodine (I^{131}), antithyroid drugs, iodides, and thyroidectomy. Thyroidectomy is indicated when medical therapy is contraindicated or fails and with underlying thyroid cancer.

A. Determine whether hyperthyroidism is controlled by looking for signs and symptoms of a hypermetabolic state. Cardiovascular effects include tachycardia, hypertension, arrhythmia, angina, and heart failure. Review thyroid function tests, other pertinent studies, medications, and duration of treatment. Radioablation is the most common therapy for Graves' disease in the United States. Thionamides, such as propylthiouracil (PTU) and methimazole (MMI), are the preferred drugs for preoperative preparation but take weeks to render a patient euthyroid. Iodine is often added to thionamide treatment. Beta-blockers reduce HR and provide symptomatic relief as well as cardiac protection but do not affect thyroxine production or iodine metabolism and do not prevent thyroid storm.[1] If there is a goiter, review the chest x-ray (CXR) and other scans to determine the extent of the mass and the amount of tracheal compression. If the goiter is large, there is a risk of airway obstruction.

B. Avoid elective surgical procedures if thyroid function is abnormal; only emergent procedures preclude waiting for a euthyroid state (which usually requires 1 to 3 months of treatment). Once euthyroid, the thyroid-stimulating hormone (TSH) may remain suppressed despite normal levels of thyroxine (T4) and triiodothyronine (T3); this should not delay surgery. Rapid preparation may be required for emergent procedures: administer a combination of beta-blocker, corticosteroid, thionamide, iodine, and iopanoic acid (contains iodine and blocks release of thyroid hormone).[1] Wait for 2 to 3 hours after giving the thionamide before administering iodines. Pregnant patients require special consideration. Patients undergoing emergent evacuation of hydatidiform mole may be hyperthyroid and are at risk for developing thyroid storm.[2]

C. Monitor ECG, BP, temperature, and neuromuscular blockade (watch for thyrotoxic myopathy). If hyperthyroidism is poorly controlled, place an arterial line for BP monitoring and ABG analysis. Monitor CVP or PA pressure if indicated. Have a cooling blanket and cool fluids available. Titrate beta-blocker to an HR < 90, but be aware that overzealous beta-blockade can precipitate congestive heart failure (CHF), bronchospasm, and hypoglycemia in diabetics. Consider corticosteroids because adrenal reserves may be low.

D. If the patient is euthyroid, choose any appropriate anesthetic technique with attention to manifestations of hyperthyroidism (e.g., goiter, heat intolerance, and eye disease). In the absence of coagulation abnormalities, endoscopic orbital decompression for Graves' disease can be done under local anesthesia to allow monitoring of vision.[3] Regional anesthesia (e.g., cervical plexus blocks or field block) has been used successfully for thyroid surgery and may be useful in certain patients with poor cardiac function.[4,5] Experimental evidence indicates that hyperthyroid animals metabolize inhaled anesthetics to a greater extent than normal. Minimum alveolar concentration (MAC) is not affected. Increased doses of IV anesthetics may be required.[6] For poorly controlled hyperthyroidism, consider deep general anesthesia. Avoid anticholinergics, hyperthermia, hypercarbia, and drugs that stimulate the sympathetic nervous system. Complications of thyroid surgery include postoperative hemorrhage with airway compromise, laryngeal nerve injuries, and hypoparathyroidism.[6]

E. Thyroid storm is rare but is a life-threatening occurrence that must be recognized and treated early to avoid a high mortality rate.[7] It may be associated with severe intercurrent illness or precipitated by surgery, infection, trauma, or withdrawal from treatment. It may occur postoperatively, so consider ICU admission. Signs and symptoms include fever, restlessness, agitation, tachycardia, heart failure, and dehydration. Treat thyroid storm with thionamides; follow with beta-blockers, iodine, corticosteroids, and supportive measures (fluid therapy, cooling blankets, acetaminophen, or sedation), or plasmapheresis.[1] Treat underlying precipitating causes. Thyroid storm can mimic malignant hyperthermia (MH) and due to mistaken diagnosis, has been successfully managed with dantrolene.[8]

REFERENCES

1. Langley RW, Burch HB: Perioperative management of the thyrotoxic patient, *Endocrinol Metab Clin North Am* 32 (2):519–534, 2003.
2. Solak M, Akturk G: Spinal anesthesia in a patient with hyperthyroidism due to hydatidiform mole, *Anesth Analg* 77:851–852, 1993.
3. Metson R, Shore JW, Gliklich RE, et al.: Endoscopic orbital decompression under local anesthesia, *Otolaryngol Head Neck Surg* 113:661–667, 1995.
4. Klein SM, Greengrass RA, Knudsen N, et al.: Regional anesthesia for thyroidectomy in two patients with amiodarone-induced hyperthyroidism, *Anesth Analg* 85:222–224, 1997.
5. Specht MC, Romero M, Barden, CB, Spanknebel K, Chabot JA, DiGiorgi M, et al.: Characteristics of patients having thyroid surgery under regional anesthesia, Thyroidectomy using local anesthesia: a report of 1,025 cases over 16 years, *J Am Coll Surg* 201(3): 375–385, 2005.

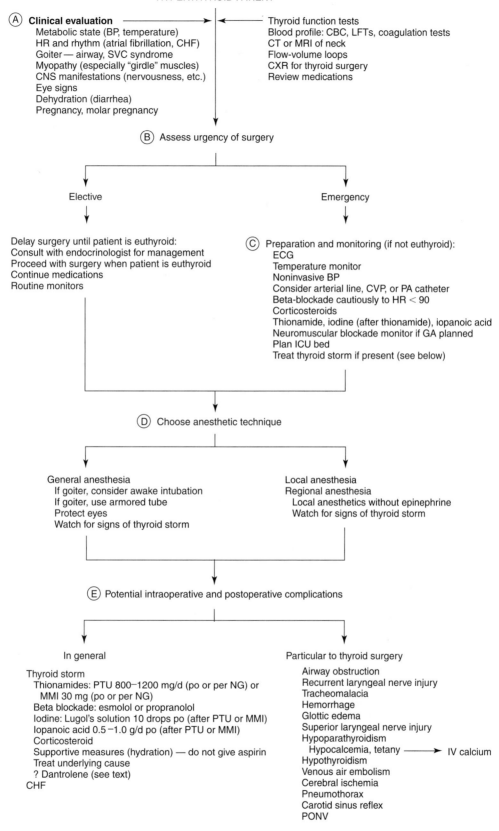

HYPERTHYROID PATIENT

Ⓐ **Clinical evaluation** ——————————→| ←————— Thyroid function tests
Metabolic state (BP, temperature) Blood profile: CBC, LFTs, coagulation tests
HR and rhythm (atrial fibrillation, CHF) CT or MRI of neck
Goiter — airway, SVC syndrome Flow-volume loops
Myopathy (especially "girdle" muscles) CXR for thyroid surgery
CNS manifestations (nervousness, etc.) Review medications
Eye signs
Dehydration (diarrhea)
Pregnancy, molar pregnancy

Ⓑ Assess urgency of surgery

Elective   Emergency

Delay surgery until patient is euthyroid: Ⓒ Preparation and monitoring (if not euthyroid):
Consult with endocrinologist for management   ECG
Proceed with surgery when patient is euthyroid   Temperature monitor
Continue medications   Noninvasive BP
Routine monitors   Consider arterial line, CVP, or PA catheter
                                                 Beta-blockade cautiously to HR < 90
                                                 Corticosteroids
                                                 Thionamide, iodine (after thionamide), iopanoic acid
                                                 Neuromuscular blockade monitor if GA planned
                                                 Plan ICU bed
                                                 Treat thyroid storm if present (see below)

Ⓓ Choose anesthetic technique

General anesthesia   Local anesthesia
If goiter, consider awake intubation   Regional anesthesia
If goiter, use armored tube   Local anesthetics without epinephrine
Protect eyes   Watch for signs of thyroid storm
Watch for signs of thyroid storm

Ⓔ Potential intraoperative and postoperative complications

In general   Particular to thyroid surgery

Thyroid storm   Airway obstruction
  Thionamides: PTU 800–1200 mg/d (po or per NG) or   Recurrent laryngeal nerve injury
    MMI 30 mg (po or per NG)   Tracheomalacia
  Beta blockade: esmolol or propranolol   Hemorrhage
  Iodine: Lugol's solution 10 drops po (after PTU or MMI)   Glottic edema
  Iopanoic acid 0.5 –1.0 g/d po (after PTU or MMI)   Superior laryngeal nerve injury
  Corticosteroid   Hypoparathyroidism
  Supportive measures (hydration) — do not give aspirin   Hypocalcemia, tetany ————→ IV calcium
  Treat underlying cause   Hypothyroidism
  ? Dantrolene (see text)   Venous air embolism
CHF   Cerebral ischemia
                                                 Pneumothorax
                                                 Carotid sinus reflex
                                                 PONV

6. Farling PA: Thyroid disease, *Br J Anaesth* 85:15–28, 2000.
7. Schiff RL, Welsh GA: Perioperative evaluation and management of the patient with endocrine dysfunction, *Med Clin North Am* 87 (1):175–192, 2003.
8. Bennett MH, Wainwright AP: Acute thyroid crisis on induction of anaesthsia, *Anaesthesia* 44:28–30, 1989.

Hypothyroidism

SUSAN H. NOORILY, M.D.

Hypothyroidism is a relatively common disorder (0.5 to 1.5% of adults) in which there is decreased serum thyroxine (T4) or increased thyroid-stimulating hormone (TSH).[1] Many cases occur after surgical thyroidectomy or radioiodine therapy for hyperthyroidism. Other causes are neck irradiation, inadequate dietary iodine, and Hashimoto's thyroiditis. Hypothyroidism may be *subclinical* (TSH elevated, triiodothyronine [T3 and T4] normal; T3 is the active thyroid principle, and its production is via peripheral conversion of T4 to T3), *mild* (T4 low normal and TSH elevated) with nonspecific symptoms of diminished cellular metabolism and oxygen consumption (fatigue, hair loss, or constipation), or *severe/overt* (myxedema coma with lethargy, hypothermia, bradycardia, hypoxia, hypoventilation, hyponatremia, or hypoglycemia). Myocardial contractility may be reduced in overt cases, and patients may have pericardial effusions or congestive heart failure (CHF). There is impaired myocardial and baroreceptor ability to respond to circulatory stresses.[2] Treatment usually consists of replacement of thyroid hormone with oral T4 preparations. T4 has a long half-life (7 days), and initiation of therapy will not result in rapid clearing of hypothyroid manifestations.[1]

A. Determine the severity of hypothyroidism. Look for signs and symptoms of hypometabolism. Review medications, duration of treatment, thyroid function tests, and other pertinent study results. Hypothyroidism affects many organ systems. Tongue enlargement, goiter, and laryngeal myxedema (hoarseness) may interfere with airway control. Hypoxic ventilatory drive may be depressed and sleep apnea may occur. Patients are at risk for cardiac dysfunction, including myocardial depression, cardiomegaly, CHF, and pericardial and pleural effusions. ECG abnormalities have been reported.[2] GI dysfunction (decreased motility) is common; gastric emptying may be slow. Impaired hepatic and renal function may delay drug elimination. The renin-angiotensin-aldosterone system is depressed. Mild anemia is common and platelet and coagulation abnormalities are possible; decreased factor VIII is the most consistent finding and acquired von Willebrand's disease has been reported.[2] If the patient has adequately treated or mild untreated disease, proceed with the planned surgical procedure.[3] Administer thyroid medications preoperatively. Consider treatment with corticosteroids because of an increased incidence of adrenocortical insufficiency and reduced response to stress.[1] Choose an anesthetic technique with attention to potential complications. Hypothyroid patients with coronary artery disease (CAD) present special problems. Balance the need for thyroid hormone replacement against the risk of ischemia and myocardial infarction (MI).

B. If the patient has overt disease, postpone elective surgery until thyroid function is normalized. If coronary revascularization is planned, preoperative thyroid replacement might be omitted.[2]

C. For emergencies in patients with overt hypothyroidism, administer parenteral T4 or T3 (T4, 100 to 500 µg; T3, 10 to 50 µg) and corticosteroids while taking supportive measures and monitoring the patient for dysrhythmias and ischemic changes.[3] The risk of MI in acutely treated patients with CAD is great. The full effect of this treatment is seen in 36 to 72 hours. Premedicate patients minimally, if at all; drugs that depress respiratory function (sedatives, opioids, or general anesthetics) can precipitate respiratory failure.[2,4] Monitor core temperature, ECG, and BP. Place an arterial catheter to monitor ABGs, electrolytes, and serum glucose. Insert a CVP or pulmonary artery (PA) catheter for major surgical procedures and in patients with CAD or CHF. Use a heating blanket and warm fluids and inhaled gases. Hypothyroid patients cannot readily increase core temperature in response to environmental hypothermia.

D. Regional blocks provide excellent anesthesia if local anesthetic doses are minimized and sedatives are used sparingly.[1] If general anesthesia is necessary, intubate the trachea (delayed gastric emptying). Hypothyroid patients are more susceptible to anesthetic medications.[2] Potent inhalational agents contribute to hypotension. Thiobarbiturates may have antithyroid properties.[2] Ensure adequate oxygenation and ventilation and avoid hyperventilation (decreased carbon dioxide production).

E. Postoperative ventilatory failure can occur; consider postoperative ventilatory support and ICU care. Myxedema coma is a rare complication with a high mortality. It may be precipitated by surgery, infection, sedative, drugs, or trauma. Consider this diagnosis in patients with stupor, seizures, coma, hyponatremia, hypoglycemia, hypothermia, hypoventilation, and heart failure. To treat, initiate IV thyroxine therapy with supportive measures used in managing overt disease.[5]

REFERENCES

1. Farling PA: Thyroid disease, *Br J Anaesth* 85 (1):15–28, 2000.
2. Stathatos N, Wartofsky L: Perioperative management of patients with hypothyroidism, *Endocrinol Metab Clin North Am* 32 (2): 503–518, 2003.
3. Schiff RL, Welsh GA: Perioperative evaluation and management of the patient with endocrine dysfunction, *Med Clin North Am* 87 (1):175–192, 2003.
4. Zwillich CW, Pierson DJ, Hofeldt FD, et al.: Ventilatory control in myxedema and hypothyroidism, *N Engl J Med* 292:662–665, 1975.
5. Wall CR: Myxedema coma: diagnosis and treatment, *Am Fam Physician* 62 (11):2485–2490, 2000.

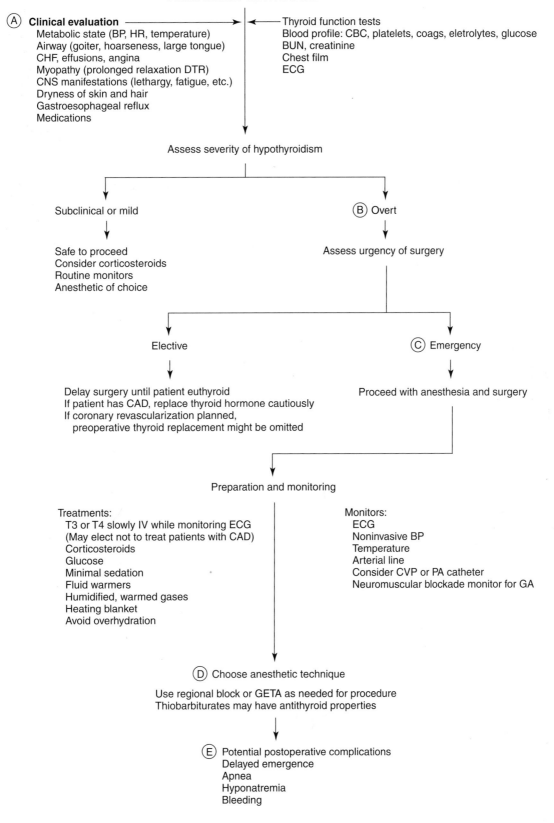

Patient with HYPOTHYROIDISM

(A) **Clinical evaluation** ——————————→ |← — Thyroid function tests
      Metabolic state (BP, HR, temperature)   Blood profile: CBC, platelets, coags, eletrolytes, glucose
      Airway (goiter, hoarseness, large tongue)   BUN, creatinine
      CHF, effusions, angina   Chest film
      Myopathy (prolonged relaxation DTR)   ECG
      CNS manifestations (lethargy, fatigue, etc.)
      Dryness of skin and hair
      Gastroesophageal reflux
      Medications

Assess severity of hypothyroidism

Subclinical or mild   (B) Overt

Safe to proceed   Assess urgency of surgery
Consider corticosteroids
Routine monitors
Anesthetic of choice

Elective   (C) Emergency

Delay surgery until patient euthyroid   Proceed with anesthesia and surgery
If patient has CAD, replace thyroid hormone cautiously
If coronary revascularization planned,
   preoperative thyroid replacement might be omitted

Preparation and monitoring

Treatments: Monitors:
   T3 or T4 slowly IV while monitoring ECG   ECG
   (May elect not to treat patients with CAD)   Noninvasive BP
   Corticosteroids   Temperature
   Glucose   Arterial line
   Minimal sedation   Consider CVP or PA catheter
   Fluid warmers   Neuromuscular blockade monitor for GA
   Humidified, warmed gases
   Heating blanket
   Avoid overhydration

(D) Choose anesthetic technique

Use regional block or GETA as needed for procedure
Thiobarbiturates may have antithyroid properties

(E) Potential postoperative complications
   Delayed emergence
   Apnea
   Hyponatremia
   Bleeding

Pheochromocytoma

VINOD MALHOTRA, M.D.

AARTI SHARMA, M.D.

Epinephrine (E) and norepinephrine (NE) are produced by functioning tumors of chromaffin tissue in the adrenal medulla (90%), sympathetic chain, periaortic areas, aortic bifurcation, bladder, and retroperitoneum. Elevated circulating levels of catecholamines cause clinical manifestations. Preoperative medical stabilization with adrenergic blocking agents has reduced perioperative morbidity. Surgical resection of pheochromocytoma (PHEO) may be technically difficult, and tumor manipulation releases NE and E, causing marked intraoperative hemodynamic instability and significant morbidity.[1]

A. Classic symptoms are headache, sweating, and palpitations; these may be paroxysmal and are often provoked by exercise, anxiety, or positional changes. Hypertension (HTN) and tachydysrhythmias may be constant or episodic, and postural hypotension is common. Commonly employed tests are the measurement of free catecholamines in plasma and urine or of their metabolites, vanillylmandelic acid and total metanephrines. Recent technical advances now allow us to measure plasma-free (unconjugated) metanephrines, thus increasing clinical sensitivity and specificity to close to 100%. Equivocal values are confirmed by a clonidine suppression test. Evaluate the patient for cardiomyopathy and congestive heart failure (CHF). Consider associated disorders (medullary thyroid carcinoma, parathyroid adenoma, neurofibromatosis, or cholelithiasis). Review localizing studies to determine whether the tumor is extraadrenal or multiple to estimate the difficulty of surgery. The most useful localizing procedures are CT, (131)I-MIBG scintiscan, and magnetic resonance imaging (MRI).

B. Adequate preoperative preparation of the patient is the key to reduced morbidity and mortality. Oral phenoxybenzamine for 10 to 14 days is the treatment of choice, starting at 10 mg twice daily and is gradually increased until mild postural hypotension develops. As alpha-blockade develops, increased hydration is necessary. Prazosin proved inadequate to control perioperative hypertensive episodes. Alpha-methyltyrosine is frequently added to the preoperative regimen. Beta-blockers may be given for persistent tachycardia or tachydysrhythmias, always in conjunction with alpha-antagonists (beta-blockade alone allows unopposed alpha activity of E and NE).[5] Labetalol may be preferable to propranolol because it possesses mild alpha-blocking as well as beta-blocking ability.

C. Monitor SpO_2, $ETCO_2$, ECG, arterial BP, CVP or pulmonary artery (PA) pressure, urinary output, and temperature. Have nitroprusside or phentolamine immediately available to treat hypertensive episodes.

Magnesium sulfate has also been used effectively to control hemodynamic changes in the management of PHEO.

D. Many different anesthetic techniques have been successfully employed for intraoperative management.[2-5] It is preferable to induce anesthesia with thiopental or propofol and attain a deep level of anesthesia with inhalational agents. Use IV lidocaine before tracheal intubation. Fentanyl, sufentanil, phentolamine, and nitroprusside are other adjuvants that decrease the pressor response to laryngoscopy. Avoid the use of halothane, ketamine, droperidol, morphine, cocaine, atracurium, pancuronium, ephedrine, and metoclopramide. Nonhistamine-releasing, nondepolarizing relaxants, such as vecuronium, are preferred. Succinylcholine (SCC) causes fasciculations, which may increase intraabdominal pressure and release catecholamines from the tumor. Remifentanil anesthesia has been used successfully. Regional block may be employed for cesarean delivery complicated by PHEO. GETA is preferred for most procedures. Laparoscopic adrenalectomy has emerged as the treatment of choice for most adrenal surgical disorders.[6]

E. Postsynaptic alpha-receptors can still respond to direct effects of increased levels of catecholamines. If hypertension occurs intraoperatively, instruct the surgeons to stop tumor manipulation, and treat with phentolamine or nitroprusside. Atrial or ventricular arrhythmias from excess catecholamines may be treated with lidocaine or beta-blockers if not unstable; electrocardioversion is indicated for unstable arrhythmias. Sympathetic blockade can result in hypotension after tumor removal. Sudden hypotension after removal of the tumor may respond to fluids, but usually pressor support is needed. Use NE, phenylephrine, or dopamine.

REFERENCES

1. Williams DT, Dann S, Wheeler MH: Phaeochromocytoma—views on current management, *Eur J Surg Oncol* 29 (6):483–490, 2003.
2. Prys-Roberts C: Phaeochromocytoma—recent progress in its management, *Br J Anaesth* 85:44–57, 2000.
3. Malhotra V, Artusio JF, Jr: Anesthesia for pheochromocytoma. In *Anesthesia for renal and genito-urologic surgery*, New York, 1996, McGraw-Hill.
4. Breslin DS, Farling PA, Mirakhur RK: The use of remifentanil in the anaesthetic management of patients undergoing adrenalectomy: a report of three cases, *Anaesthesia* 58 (4):358–362, 2003.
5. Kariya N, Nishi S, Hosono Y, et al.: Cesarean section at 28 weeks' gestation with resection of pheochromocytoma: perioperative antihypertensive management, *J Clin Anesth* 17 (4):296–299, 2005.
6. Kebebew E, Siperstein AE, Duh QY: Laparoscopic adrenalectomy: the optimal surgical approach, *J Laparoendosc Adv Surg Tech A* 11 (6):409–413, 2001.

Patient with PHEOCHROMOCYTOMA

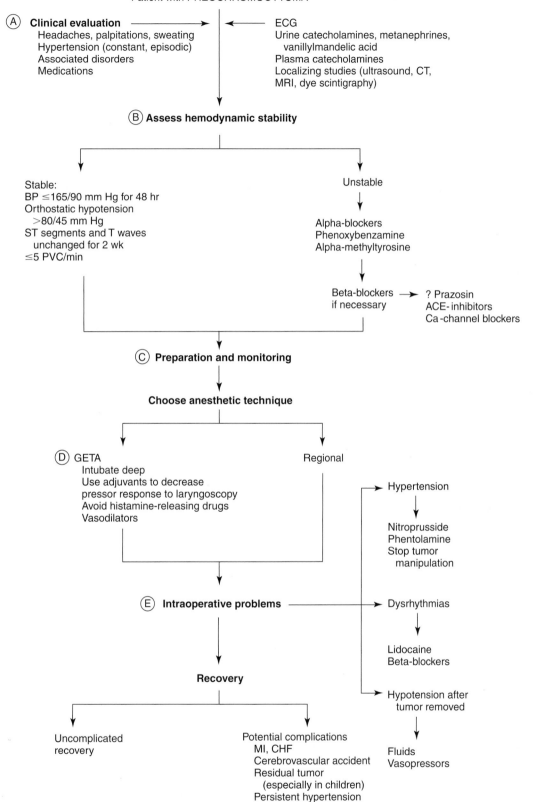

Ⓐ **Clinical evaluation** ⟶   ⟵ ECG
   Headaches, palpitations, sweating   Urine catecholamines, metanephrines,
   Hypertension (constant, episodic)   vanillylmandelic acid
   Associated disorders   Plasma catecholamines
   Medications   Localizing studies (ultrasound, CT,
                 MRI, dye scintigraphy)

Ⓑ **Assess hemodynamic stability**

Stable: Unstable
BP ≤165/90 mm Hg for 48 hr
Orthostatic hypotension   Alpha-blockers
   >80/45 mm Hg   Phenoxybenzamine
ST segments and T waves   Alpha-methyltyrosine
   unchanged for 2 wk
≤5 PVC/min   Beta-blockers ⟶ ? Prazosin
                 if necessary   ACE-inhibitors
                        Ca-channel blockers

Ⓒ **Preparation and monitoring**

Choose anesthetic technique

Ⓓ GETA   Regional
   Intubate deep
   Use adjuvants to decrease   Hypertension
   pressor response to laryngoscopy
   Avoid histamine-releasing drugs   Nitroprusside
   Vasodilators   Phentolamine
                 Stop tumor
                    manipulation

Ⓔ **Intraoperative problems** ⟶   Dysrhythmias

                 Lidocaine
                 Beta-blockers

Recovery   Hypotension after
                    tumor removed

Uncomplicated   Potential complications   Fluids
recovery   MI, CHF   Vasopressors
        Cerebrovascular accident
        Residual tumor
           (especially in children)
        Persistent hypertension

Carcinoid Syndrome (CS)

SUZANNE B. KARAN, M.D.

DENHAM S. WARD, M.D., PH.D.

Carcinoid tumors are slow-growing malignancies arising from enterochromaffin cells of the amine precursor uptake and decarboxylation (APUD) system. The tumors most commonly originate in the midgut (77%), with others from the foregut (lung, thymus, or stomach) and hindgut. U.S. incidence is 1 to 2/100,000/yr; one third has disseminated disease at diagnosis. Carcinoid syndrome (CS) occurs in fewer than 10%—symptoms result from systemic effects of hormones produced by carcinoid tumors. CS occurs when the carcinoid tumors are outside the portal circulation because the liver is effective in clearing the hormones. Rarely, profound flushing and cardiovascular collapse occur. This has been called a "carcinoid crisis" and accounts for 50% of deaths in patients with CS. The severity of preoperative symptoms is a poor predictor of perioperative morbidity; patients with minor symptoms may have a complicated intraoperative course. The release of carcinoid peptides is augmented by stress, surgical manipulation, and beta-adrenergic agents.[1]

A. Serotonin is the most frequently released hormone, but histamine can be secreted from foregut tumors. Many of the common symptoms are related to bradykinin release, which is inhibited by somatostatin.[2] The introduction of a somatostatin analogue, octreotide, has allowed better control of the symptoms of CS.[3] The exception is carcinoid heart disease in which somatostatin therapy has not been shown to delay progression. Review patient medications and their efficacy. Determine the range of BP and HR during symptomatic episodes and if bronchospasm occurs. Evaluate aspiration risk.[4] Note if encephalopathy, dyspnea, or HR variability is present. Long-term secretion of serotonin into the systemic circulation can induce lesions in the tricuspid pulmonary valves leading to regurgitation and right-sided heart failure.[5]

B. The many case reports in the literature of perioperative morbidity related to carcinoid tumors may give a false impression of its frequency. Most patients with carcinoid tumors are successfully anesthetized without any major problems.[6,7] Many anesthetic techniques have been successful. Optimize medications and restore circulating volume and electrolytes (chronic diarrhea is a common symptom). Consider placing an arterial line and a CVP for extensive surgical procedures.

C. Administer prophylactic octreotide at a dosage of 100 µg/hr or as a single dose of 50 µg intravenously, although this might not fully prevent serotonin release.[2] Premedicate with antihistamines (H_1 and H_2) for foregut tumors and cyproheptadine for its antiserotonergic effects.[6] Consider preoperative steroids. Avoid histamine-releasing medications (e.g., morphine or atracurium). Note that ondansetron has been shown to improve GI symptoms, and aprotinin, a kallikrein inhibitor, has been shown to be effective in treating flushing and intraoperative hypotension.[6,8]

D. Select an anesthetic approach appropriate for the planned surgical procedure. Regional techniques have been used successfully.[7] If general anesthesia is chosen, plan the induction to prevent catecholamine release during laryngoscopy or intubation. Epinephrine, through beta-adrenergic action, can stimulate hormone release from carcinoid tumors. Use muscle relaxants that do not release histamine. Avoid succinylcholine if muscle fasciculations could mechanically squeeze the carcinoid tumor. Prepare for the possibility of profuse blood loss; abdominal carcinoid tumors have an abundant vasculature.

E. Prevent or minimize catecholamine release. Maintain adequate hydration. Treat hypotension with an alpha-adrenergic agonist. IV octreotide has been reported to reverse hypotension caused by hormone release. Bronchospasm due to histamine or bradykinin release has been reported to be refractory to inhalational anesthetics or ketamine. Administer inhaled $beta_2$-agonists cautiously to reverse the bronchospasm without increasing hormone release. IV octreotide has been reported to reverse bronchospasm.[3] Hypertension is rarely a significant problem; treat with vasodilators.

F. Emergence should pose no special problems if the carcinoid tumor has been removed; if not, continue measures as outlined previously. Reversal of the muscle relaxants has not been reported to cause a crisis. Prolonged time to recovery from anesthesia has been reported in patients with high serum serotonin concentrations.[3] Provide effective postoperative pain control. Analgesic requirements may be reduced during administration of somatostatin.

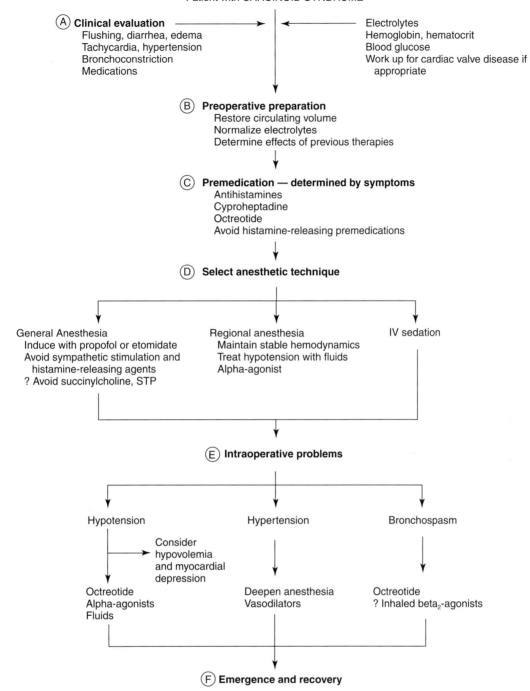

Patient with CARCINOID SYNDROME

(A) **Clinical evaluation**
Flushing, diarrhea, edema
Tachycardia, hypertension
Bronchoconstriction
Medications

Electrolytes
Hemoglobin, hematocrit
Blood glucose
Work up for cardiac valve disease if
    appropriate

(B) **Preoperative preparation**
Restore circulating volume
Normalize electrolytes
Determine effects of previous therapies

(C) **Premedication — determined by symptoms**
Antihistamines
Cyproheptadine
Octreotide
Avoid histamine-releasing premedications

(D) **Select anesthetic technique**

General Anesthesia
Induce with propofol or etomidate
Avoid sympathetic stimulation and
    histamine-releasing agents
? Avoid succinylcholine, STP

Regional anesthesia
Maintain stable hemodynamics
Treat hypotension with fluids
Alpha-agonist

IV sedation

(E) **Intraoperative problems**

Hypotension

Consider
hypovolemia
and myocardial
depression

Octreotide
Alpha-agonists
Fluids

Hypertension

Deepen anesthesia
Vasodilators

Bronchospasm

Octreotide
? Inhaled beta$_2$-agonists

(F) **Emergence and recovery**

REFERENCES

1. Ganim RB, Norton JA: Recent advances in carcinoid pathogenesis, diagnosis and management, *Surg Oncol* 9:173–179, 2000.
2. Zimmer C, Kienbaum P, Wiesemes R, et al.: Somatostatin does not prevent serotonin release and flushing during chemoembolization of carcinoid liver metastases, *Anesthesiology* 98:1007–1011, 2003.
3. Quinlivan JK, Roberts WA: Intraoperative octreotide for refractory carcinoid-induced bronchospasm, *Anesth Analg* 78:400–402, 1994.
4. Pandharipande PP, Reichard PS, Vallee MF: High gastric output as a perioperative sign of carcinoid syndrome, *Anesthesiology* 96:755–756, 2002.
5. Moller JE, Connolly HM, Rubin J, et al.: Factors associated with progression of carcinoid heart disease, *N Engl J Med* 348:1005–1015, 2003.
6. Vaughan DJ, Brunner MD: Anesthesia for patients with carcinoid syndrome, *Int Anesthesiol Clin* 35:129–142, 1997.
7. Orbach-Zinger S, Lombroso R, Eidelman LA: Uneventful spinal anesthesia for a patient with carcinoid syndrome managed with long-acting octreotide, *Can J Anaesth* 49:678–681, 2002.
8. Wymenga AN, de Vries EG, Leijsma MK, et al.: Effects of ondansetron on gastrointestinal symptoms in carcinoid syndrome, *Eur J Cancer* 34:1293–1294, 1998.

Adrenocortical Hypofunction

MICHAEL P. HUTCHENS, M.D., M.A.

Adrenocortical hypofunction refers to a deficiency of one or more hormones produced by the adrenal cortex, glucocorticoids (cortisol) or mineralocorticoids (aldosterone). Cortisol is responsible for the metabolic regulation of proteins, carbohydrates, and fats as well as the maintenance of glucose homeostasis, BP, and free-water clearance. Aldosterone regulates sodium (Na) and potassium (K) balance. Aldosterone secretion is mainly controlled by the renin-angiotensin system, potassium levels, and to a lesser extent, adrenocorticotropic hormone (ACTH). Primary adrenal insufficiency (Addison's disease) results from destruction of the adrenal cortex resulting in deficiencies of cortisol and aldosterone. Common causes are listed in Table 1.[1–3] Secondary adrenal insufficiency is a failure of the signaling mechanism for cortisol secretion, either due to hypothalamic-pituitary axis disease or, most commonly, suppression of ACTH secretion by exogenously administered steroids. In this setting, the important support functions of cortisol in conditions of biological stress are absent, and lethal circulatory shock may be the response to significant stressors such as anesthetic induction or surgery.[4,5] Isolated hypoaldosteronism is rare but should be considered if hyperkalemia is noted in a patient without renal failure. Causes include angiotensin-converting enzyme (ACE) inhibitor and nonsteroidal anti-inflammatory drug (NSAID) administration, as well as congenital disease.

A. Although the presentation of adrenal insufficiency is insidious in outpatients, the presentation in perioperative patients is that of circulatory collapse refractory to pressors. Maintain a high index of suspicion in patients with medical history associated with adrenal disease. Patients who have been on corticosteroid therapy for more than a week within the previous year are at high risk.[3] Patients with hypoaldosteronism present with hyperkalemia and hyponatremia. If not found on laboratory studies, this diagnosis may be suggested by the electrocardiographic changes of hyperkalemia.

B. Ideally, the diagnosis of adrenal insufficiency is made with a provocative test of hypothalamic-pituitary-adrenal axis function. The most commonly used is the short corticotropin stimulation test. Early in the morning, a baseline cortisol level is drawn and then 250 μg of synthetic ACTH is given intravenously. A second cortisol level is drawn 30 to 60 minutes after the ACTH is given. Normal function is indicated by a preprovocation or postprovocation cortisol concentration of >18 μg/dl.[1,5] If the cause of adrenal insufficiency is unknown, a search for diagnosis should be undertaken. Chronicity is a factor in the need for therapy, and patients with acute adrenal failure should be differentiated from those with chronic disease.

C. Determine the need for surgery. Patients with untreated, acute adrenal insufficiency should not be operated unless there is a dire surgical emergency. Patients with treated, acute adrenal insufficiency and those with chronic adrenal insufficiency may have their increased need for corticosteroid managed safely during surgical stress and in the perioperative period.

D. Patients with acute untreated, acute adrenal insufficiency must be managed aggressively. Place two large-bore IVs, as rapid volume expansion is necessary to counteract the loss of cortisol-regulated vascular tone. A central venous catheter is necessary to monitor filling pressures and deliver infusions. In patients with concomitant cardiac disease, place a pulmonary artery (PA) catheter or transesophageal echocardiogram (TEE). An arterial line is necessary for monitoring BP, electrolytes, and blood glucose. Etomidate is specifically contraindicated for induction as it suppresses adrenocortical function even when used as a single dose for induction, and has been shown to increase mortality in critically ill patients.[5] Recommendations for specific intraoperative "stress dose steroids" vary but two common regimens are (1) hydrocortisone 100 mg IV followed by an infusion of 10 mg/hr and (2) hydrocortisone 100 mg IV every 8 hours. If using a different corticosteroid, dose conversion can be made based on relative glucocorticoid activity (Table 2). Vasopressin may be indicated for the hypotension associated with adrenal insufficiency.[1] Patients with treated, acute adrenal insufficiency should be managed similarly. Patients with chronic adrenal insufficiency do not require invasive monitors unless other clinical conditions mandate their use. They should also be given stress dose steroids, though 100 mg of hydrocortisone may be excessive for minor surgical stress. Patients undergoing major surgical stress, however, should be given the full dose. Patients with isolated hypoaldosteronism are not known to be at higher risk perioperatively, but intraoperative monitoring of sodium and potassium is indicated.

E. Postoperatively, monitor BP and electrolytes closely. Patients with intraoperative hypotension and those with acute adrenal insufficiency should be monitored in the ICU. Taper steroid doses slowly to preoperative maintenance levels. Monitor glucose—recipients of high dose steroids may require insulin for hyperglycemia.

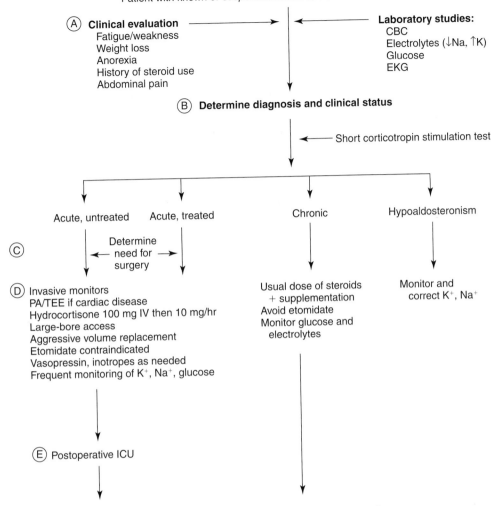

Patient with *known* or *suspected* ADRENOCORTICAL HYPOFUNCTION

Ⓐ **Clinical evaluation**
  Fatigue/weakness
  Weight loss
  Anorexia
  History of steroid use
  Abdominal pain

Laboratory studies:
  CBC
  Electrolytes ($\downarrow$Na, $\uparrow$K)
  Glucose
  EKG

Ⓑ **Determine diagnosis and clinical status**

Short corticotropin stimulation test

Acute, untreated   Acute, treated   Chronic   Hypoaldosteronism

Ⓒ Determine need for surgery

Ⓓ Invasive monitors
  PA/TEE if cardiac disease
  Hydrocortisone 100 mg IV then 10 mg/hr
  Large-bore access
  Aggressive volume replacement
  Etomidate contraindicated
  Vasopressin, inotropes as needed
  Frequent monitoring of K⁺, Na⁺, glucose

Usual dose of steroids + supplementation
Avoid etomidate
Monitor glucose and electrolytes

Monitor and correct K⁺, Na⁺

Ⓔ Postoperative ICU

Taper steroids to maintenance dose, control hyperglycemia, monitor electrolytes

TABLE 1
Causes of Adrenocortical Hypofunction

Causes	Associations
Exogenous steroid therapy	Human immunodeficiency virus (HIV) disease
Autoimmune disease	Lymphoma
Tuberculosis	Hodgkin's disease
Surgical adrenalectomy	Antiphospholipid antibody syndrome
Congenital adrenal hypoplasia	Polyglandular syndrome (with hypothyroidism, hypoparathyroidism, and diabetes mellitus)
Metastasis	
Hemorrhage	
Severe sepsis	
Noncorticosteroid drugs (ketoconazole, etomidate, rifampin, phenytoin, phenobarbital, or anticoagulants)	
Hypothalamic/pituitary tumor	
Sheehan's syndrome	
Adrenoleukodystrophy	

TABLE 2
Glucocorticoid Conversions

Drug	Equivalent dose
Hydrocortisone	100 mg
Cortisone	125 mg
Prednisone	25 mg
Methylprednisolone	20 mg
Dexamethasone	3.75 mg

REFERENCES

1. Oelkers W: Adrenal insufficiency, *N Engl J Med* 335 (16):1206–1212, 1996.
2. Stoelting RK, Dierdorf SF: *Anesthesia and co-existing disease*, ed 4, Philadelphia, 2002, Churchill Livingstone.
3. Jabbour SA: Steroids and the surgical patient, *Med Clin North Am* 85 (5):1311–1317, 2001.
4. White PC: Disorders of aldosterone biosynthesis and action, *N Engl J Med* 331 (4):250–258, 1994.
5. Absalom A, Pledger D, Kong A: Adrenocortical function in critically ill patients 24 h after a single dose of etomidate, *Anaesthesia* 54 (9):861–867, 1999.

Hyperparathyroidism

GEORGE A. DUMITRASCU, M.D.

Patients with hyperparathyroidism have abnormal levels of parathyroid hormone (PTH) released into the circulation.[1] This polypeptide hormone is normally produced by the four parathyroid glands through a process regulated by a negative feedback mechanism dependent on the plasma calcium concentration. The metabolic function of PTH in supporting the serum calcium level is complex. In summary, PTH increases the resorption of bone, releasing calcium and phosphorus; increases renal tubular reabsorption of calcium, thereby conserving it; promotes renal production of vitamin D; and increases renal elimination of phosphorus. Hyperparathyroidism is classified as primary, secondary, or ectopic according to the etiology. *Primary* hyperparathyroidism results from excessive secretion of PTH by a benign parathyroid adenoma (85% of cases), a carcinoma of a parathyroid gland (5% of cases), or a hyperplastic gland (10% of cases). *Secondary* reflects a normal compensatory response to counteract a disease process that produces hypocalcemia (e.g., chronic renal dysfunction). *Ectopic* (pseudohyperparathyroidism) implies production of PTH by tissues other than the parathyroid glands; most likely sites include carcinomas of the lung, pancreas, kidney, and breast as well as lymphoproliferative diseases. Definitive treatment of primary hyperparathyroidism is surgical removal of the involved parathyroid glands. Successful attempt is followed by normalization of the plasma calcium concentration within 3 to 4 days.

A. In a patient with hyperparathyroidism, the plasma calcium concentration may be increased, decreased, or unchanged. Therefore, assess the serum calcium level; hypercalcemia is responsible for the signs and symptoms accompanying hyperparathyroidism (muscle weakness, renal stones, anemia, short QT interval, hypertension, abdominal pain, somnolence, psychosis). If hypercalcemia is symptomatic, treat aggressively, aiming at lowering the serum calcium below 12 mg/dl. Because interventions include vigorous hydration, place invasive monitors in patients with cardiac disease.

B. Parathyroidectomy may be successfully performed under local, regional, or general anesthesia. Recently developed minimally invasive surgical techniques are perfectly suited for local/regional anesthesia;[2,3] more involved cases require general endotracheal anesthesia with controlled ventilation. Propofol does not interfere with PTH testing as was previously thought.[4] On the other hand, previous reports of resistance to nondepolarizing muscle relaxants (NDMRs) have been substantiated by new case reports; therefore, monitor closely the response produced at the neuromuscular junction.[5] Position the patient carefully because of the common presence of osteoporosis (vulnerability to pathological fractures). To avoid possible hemostatic disruption during emergence prevent patient coughing at emergence and consider deep extubation; in addition, on extubation, some practitioners evaluate vocal cord movement under direct visualization.

C. The most important complication after parathyroidectomy is hypocalcemic tetany, a direct manifestation of hypoparathyroidism. Hypomagnesemia, which frequently occurs postoperatively, can worsen the manifestations of hypocalcemia and render it refractory to treatment. Other clinical presentations of hypocalcemia include irritability, sensory disturbances, organic brain syndrome, and cataracts. Recurrent laryngeal nerve injury occurs infrequently but may result in vocal cord paralysis. Postoperative edema or hematoma can also rapidly compromise the airway.

REFERENCES

1. Stoelting RK, Dierdorf SF: *Anesthesia and co-existing disease*, ed 4, New York, 2002. Churchill Livingstone.
2. Monchik JM, Barellini L, Langer P, et al.: Minimally invasive parathyroid surgery in 103 patients with local/regional anesthesia, without exclusion criteria, *Surgery* 131 (5):502–508, 2002.
3. Palazzo FF, Delbridge LW: Minimal-access/minimally invasive parathyroidectomy for primary hyperparathyroidism, *Surg Clin North Am* 84 (3):717–734, 2004.
4. Sippel RS, Becker YT, Odorico JS, et al.: Does propofol anesthesia affect intraoperative parathyroid hormone levels? A randomized, prospective trial, *Surgery* 136 (6):1138–1142, 2004.
5. Munir MA, Jaffar M, Arshad M, et al: Reduced duration of muscle relaxation with rocuronium in a normocalcemic hyperparathyroid patient, *Can J Anaesth* 50 (6):558–561, 2003.

Patient with HYPERPARATHYROIDISM

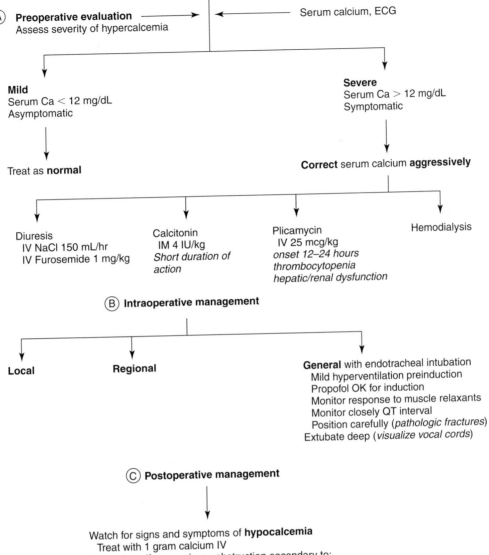

Ⓐ **Preoperative evaluation** ———→   ←——— Serum calcium, ECG
   Assess severity of hypercalcemia

Mild   **Severe**
Serum Ca < 12 mg/dL   Serum Ca > 12 mg/dL
Asymptomatic   Symptomatic

Treat as **normal**   **Correct** serum calcium **aggressively**

Diuresis   Calcitonin   Plicamycin   Hemodialysis
IV NaCl 150 mL/hr   IM 4 IU/kg   IV 25 mcg/kg
IV Furosemide 1 mg/kg *Short duration of *onset 12–24 hours*
                      action*   *thrombocytopenia*
                                          hepatic/renal dysfunction

Ⓑ **Intraoperative management**

Local   **Regional**   **General** with endotracheal intubation
                                         Mild hyperventilation preinduction
                                         Propofol OK for induction
                                         Monitor response to muscle relaxants
                                         Monitor closely QT interval
                                         Position carefully (*pathologic fractures*)
                                      Extubate deep (*visualize vocal cords*)

Ⓒ **Postoperative management**

Watch for signs and symptoms of **hypocalcemia**
   Treat with 1 gram calcium IV
Reintubate if upper airway obstruction secondary to:
   Expanding hematoma, laryngeal edema, recurrent laryngeal nerve injury

Acromegaly

TESSA L. WALTERS, M.D.

Acromegaly is a rare chronic disease caused by excessive secretion of growth hormone (GH), most often from an adenoma of the anterior pituitary gland. Excess GH leads to an overgrowth in bone, connective tissue, and viscera. Clinical features include coarse facial features, enlarged hands and feet, and hoarseness. Extension of the tumor outside the sella turcica can lead to visual field defects, headache, and papilledema caused by increased intracranial pressure.[1] Surgery is the first-line treatment; radiotherapy may follow. A few patients may be treated with dopamine agonists, long-acting analogues of somatostatin, and, recently, the GH-receptor antagonist, pegvisomant.[2]

A. Perform a history and physical examination. Airway abnormalities associated with acromegaly are of particular concern. Upper airway obstruction can arise from an enlarged tongue and epiglottis or collapse of the hypopharynx into the laryngeal inlet. Sleep apnea indicates a potentially high risk of respiratory depression or obstruction. The risk of death from respiratory failure is three times higher in acromegalic patients.[3-4] Overgrowth of the mandible increases the distance from lips to vocal cords and results in a poor mask fit. Enlargement of the nasal turbinates may preclude passage of nasopharyngeal or nasotracheal airways. Enlargement of the vocal cords causes narrowing of the glottic opening, which, along with subglottic narrowing, necessitates the use of a smaller endotracheal tube. Cricoarytenoid joint involvement or stretching of the recurrent laryngeal nerve may lead to vocal cord dysfunction with hoarseness, stridor, or dyspnea. An enlarged thyroid is present in about one fourth of acromegalic patients and may compress the trachea.[3] Indirect laryngoscopy and radiographs of the neck help define the extent of vocal cord dysfunction and laryngeal involvement. Fortunately, vocal cord dysfunction reverts to normal within 10 days of surgical treatment.[3] Acromegaly is associated with increased cardiac morbidity and mortality. One third of patients have hypertension (HTN), and two thirds of patients have concentric hypertrophy at diagnosis. Myocardial hypertrophy and interstitial fibrosis contribute to diastolic dysfunction and eventually systolic compromise.[5] Proposed etiological factors for cardiomegaly include HTN, coronary artery disease, valvular heart disease, compensatory hypertrophy secondary to increased workload induced by generalized splanchnomegaly and somatomegaly, and direct effects of GH and insulin-like growth factor 1 (IGF-1).[6] Be vigilant for potential coexistence of adrenal pheochromocytoma, given overlap or variants of multiple endocrine neoplasia (MEN) syndromes.[7] Insulin-resistance is common, and diabetes occurs in 25% of acromegalic patients. Signs of hypopituitarism may also be present (pallor, scanty hair, and hypogonadism); consider perioperative corticosteroid coverage in such cases. Examine for peripheral neuropathy, especially of the median nerve, caused by trapping of nerves by tissue overgrowth.

B. Categorize acromegalic patients by the extent of airway involvement: (1) normal airway; (2) hypertrophy of nasal and pharyngeal mucosa, normal vocal cords, and glottis; (3) glottic abnormalities, including glottic stenosis or vocal cord paresis; and (4) both glottic and soft tissue abnormalities. In the past, preoperative tracheostomy had been recommended for patients in groups 3 and 4;[8] however, many series suggest that fiberoptic laryngoscopy or intubating laryngeal mask airways (LMAs) may be reasonable alternatives. At a minimum, have large face masks and long-bladed laryngoscopes available.[3]

C. Select monitors appropriate for the planned surgical procedure. Concern has been expressed regarding tissue compression of and decreased flow through the ulnar artery in acromegalic patients,[9] but a retrospective series of acromegalics who were monitored with radial arterial catheters did not show any ischemic complications.[10]

D. Select an anesthetic technique appropriate for the planned surgical procedure, with attention to possible problems of airway management, peripheral neuropathy, positioning, skeletal muscle weakness, and risk of respiratory depression.

E. Observe the patient closely for airway-related complications. Postoperative vocal cord edema after traumatic intubation in the presence of soft tissue hypertrophy may lead to laryngeal obstruction and necessitate a tracheostomy. The risk of respiratory depression is heightened by residual effects of muscle relaxants and centrally depressant drugs. Monitor acromegalic patients closely during the first postoperative night when hypoventilation and airway obstruction may occur; acute pulmonary edema is a risk of airway obstruction previously reported in this patient population.[3]

REFERENCES

1. Melmed S: Acromegaly, N Engl J Med 322:966–977, 1990.
2. Trainer PJ: Lessons from 6 years of GH receptor antagonist therapy for acromegaly, J Endocrinol Invest 26:44–52, 2003.
3. Smith M, Hirsch NP: Pituitary disease and anaesthesia, Br J Anaesth 85:3–14, 2000.
4. Goldhill DR, Dalgleish JG, Lake RH: Respiratory problems and acromegaly. An acromegalic with hypersomia, acute upper airway obstruction and pulmonary oedema, Anaesthesia 37: 1200–1203, 1982.

Patient with ACROMEGALY

(A) **Clinical evaluation**
   History and physical examination
   Airway
   Hypertension
   Cardiac dysfunction
   Increased ICP?
   Peripheral neuropathy
   Skeletal muscle weakness
   Osteoarthritis, osteoporosis
   Hypopituitarism: steroids needed?
   Glucose intolerance
   Indirect laryngoscopy

Skull radiograph and CT
Neck radiography
Other laboratory values as
   indicated for patient's diseases

(B) Categorize by airway involvement

Normal	Normal glottis and vocal cords; soft tissue hypertrophy (nasal, pharyngeal mucosa)	Abnormal glottis, (glottic stenosis, vocal cord paresis)	Abnormal glottis, hypertrophied soft tissue

Airway
management
as for normal
patient

Avoid nasal
instrumentation

Consider tracheostomy awake or before
extubation (see (D))

(C) **Preparation and management**
   Routine monitors and
   any others appropriate for
   planned surgical procedure
   ? Ulnar artery collateral flow

Correct anesthetic technique

Regional anesthesia

(D) General anesthesia

Elective
tracheostomy

Intubate
awake
(fiberoptic)

Intubate
asleep

Difficult or traumatic intubation

Tracheostomy
preextubation

Extubate awake

(E) **Recovery**

Uncomplicated recovery

Potential complications
Respiratory depression
   (if sleep apnea, residual
   depressants)
Airway edema

5. Vitale G, Pivonello R, Lombardi G, et al.: Cardiac abnormalities in acromegaly. Pathophysiology and implications for management, *Treat Endocrinol* 3:309–318, 2004.
6. Rodrigues EA, Caruana MP, Lahiri A, et al.: Subclinical cardiac dysfunction in acromegaly: evidence for a specific disease of heart muscle, *Br Heart J* 62:185–194, 1989.
7. Breckenridge SM, Hamrahian AH, Faiman C, et al.: Coexistence of a pituitary macroadenoma and pheochromocytoma-a case report and review of the literature, *Pituitary* 6:221–225, 2003.
8. Southwick JP, Katz J: Unusual airway difficulty in the acromegalic patient-indications for tracheostomy, *Anesthesiology* 51:72–73, 1979.
9. Campkin TV: Radial artery cannulation. Potential hazard in patients with acromegaly, *Anaesthesia* 35:1008–1009, 1980.
10. Losasso T, Dietz NM, Muzzi DA: Acromegaly and radial artery cannulation, *Anesth Analg* 71:204, 1990.

PREOPERATIVE GI PROBLEMS

Hepatic Dysfunction

Hepatic Dysfunction

LOIS L. BREADY, M.D.

Hepatic dysfunction may manifest as an acute or chronic subclinical cellular disturbance but can progress to life-threatening hepatic failure with multiple organ system compromise. Perioperative morbidity and mortality can be significant; the risk is increased in patients with clinical symptoms, cirrhosis, acute disease, and emergency nature of the surgery.[1] Hepatic function (glucose homeostasis, protein and procoagulant synthesis, bilirubin metabolism, and biotransformation of drugs and endogenous toxins) may all be impaired. The degree of impairment and the severity of extrahepatic involvement can be variable. Clinical manifestations are usually associated with mid- to late-stage disease.[1–6] Liver disease is increasingly being recognized in patients with diabetes—nonalcoholic steatohepatitis.[2]

A. Determine the cause of the hepatic dysfunction. Postpone elective surgery in patients with acute hepatitis (viral, toxic, or drug-related) or undiagnosed hepatic dysfunction to avoid further hepatic insult. A hyperdynamic cardiovascular state ($\uparrow$ cardiac output [CO], HR, and $\downarrow$ systemic vascular resistance [SVR]) may exist because of systemic venous collaterals and humoral mediators. Cardiomyopathy may be present despite an elevated CO. Dysrhythmias are not uncommon. There is a high incidence of arterial hypoxemia (intrapulmonary shunting, hepatopulmonary disease, pulmonary hypertension [HTN], impaired hypoxic pulmonary vasoconstriction). Pleural effusions and ascites contribute to atelectasis and ventilatory compromise. Cirrhotic patients have impaired sodium and water excretion and a decreased glomerular filtration rate (GFR), resulting in hyponatremia and increased total body fluid. Aggressive diuresis or removal of ascitic fluid may render the patient hypovolemic. The hepatorenal syndrome (functional renal failure) and acute tubular necrosis can be precipitated by volume depletion (gastrointestinal [GI] bleeding, paracentesis, diuresis, or surgery). Serum creatinine often overestimates renal function. Hypoglycemia may be present (diabetes, altered glucose homeostasis, and inadequate hepatic glycogen stores). Encephalopathy occurs with advanced hepatic disease and can be exacerbated by volume depletion, sedation, hypokalemia, metabolic acidosis, infection, upper GI (UGI) bleeding, and dietary protein indiscretion. Severe encephalopathy is usually associated with cerebral edema and elevated intracranial pressure (ICP), especially in the setting of fulminant hepatic failure. Coagulopathy may be present and is multifactorial (diminished clotting factor synthesis, thrombocytopenia, vitamin K deficiency, dysfibrinogenemia, accelerated fibrinolysis, and DIC). Anemia is also common.

B. If time permits, optimize the patient's nutritional status and medical management. Restore euvolemia. Correct electrolyte and glucose abnormalities. Administer thiamine to patients experiencing acute ethanol withdrawal and provide prophylaxis for delirium tremens. Treat coagulopathy with FFP, platelets, or vitamin K as directed by the laboratory tests (prothrombin time [PT], complete blood count [CBC], and thromboelastogram [TEG]). TEG assesses the qualitative status of the clotting process.[6] Vitamin K is effective when there is vitamin K deficiency (cholestasis or malabsorption) but must be started early. Other therapies for coagulopathy include DDAVP and aminocaproic acid.

C. Choose an anesthetic technique based on the surgical procedure, patient preference, and medical condition. Drug responses are often unpredictable. Generally, more profound and prolonged effects can be anticipated. Titration is paramount. Expect an increased sensitivity to centrally acting drugs and diminished responses to adrenergic agonists. Drug disposition is affected by decreased hepatic blood flow, decreased intrinsic hepatocellular function, altered volumes of distribution, and changes in the ratio of protein-bound drug to free drug. Assess coagulation status before administration of regional anesthesia. For general anesthesia, consider aspiration prophylaxis and rapid sequence induction (aspiration risk from ascites and altered GI motility). Be cautious during esophageal instrumentation in patients with varices. Avoid hypotension. Maintain adequate splanchnic blood flow and hepatic oxygen delivery. Use vasopressors and inotropes when indicated. Maintain adequate renal perfusion and urine output; consider the use of diuretics (furosemide or mannitol) and low-dose dopamine. Isoflurane, fentanyl, and cisatracurium are appropriate choices for general anesthesia. Succinylcholine may have a prolonged effect. Halothane should be avoided. Patients with severe encephalopathy may have elevated ICP and may benefit from hyperventilation and mannitol administration.

D. Observe for evidence of encephalopathy, renal dysfunction, congestive heart failure (CHF), hypoglycemia, UGI bleeding, and worsened hepatic function. The differential diagnosis of postoperative jaundice and hepatic dysfunction is broad; its appearance should prompt a thorough evaluation.

Patient with PREOPERATIVE HEPATIC DYSFUNCTION

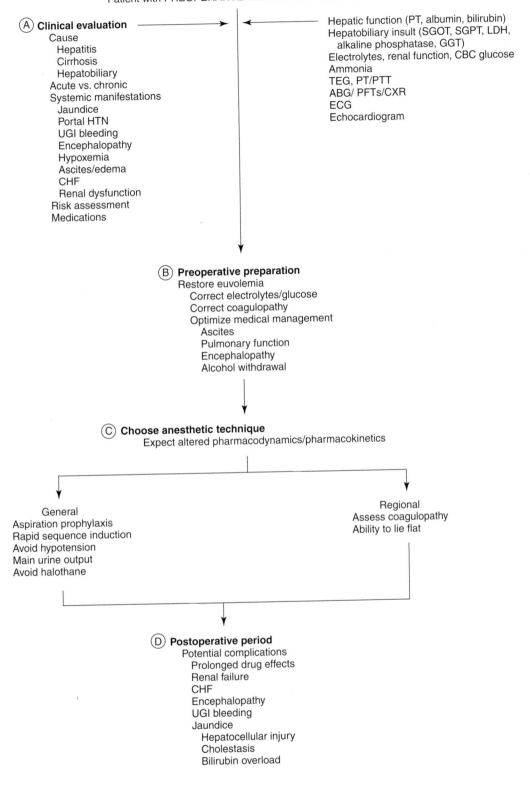

Ⓐ **Clinical evaluation**
 Cause
  Hepatitis
  Cirrhosis
  Hepatobiliary
 Acute vs. chronic
 Systemic manifestations
  Jaundice
  Portal HTN
  UGI bleeding
  Encephalopathy
  Hypoxemia
  Ascites/edema
  CHF
  Renal dysfunction
 Risk assessment
 Medications

Hepatic function (PT, albumin, bilirubin)
Hepatobiliary insult (SGOT, SGPT, LDH,
 alkaline phosphatase, GGT)
Electrolytes, renal function, CBC glucose
Ammonia
TEG, PT/PTT
ABG/ PFTs/CXR
ECG
Echocardiogram

Ⓑ **Preoperative preparation**
Restore euvolemia
 Correct electrolytes/glucose
 Correct coagulopathy
 Optimize medical management
  Ascites
  Pulmonary function
  Encephalopathy
  Alcohol withdrawal

Ⓒ **Choose anesthetic technique**
 Expect altered pharmacodynamics/pharmacokinetics

General
Aspiration prophylaxis
Rapid sequence induction
Avoid hypotension
Main urine output
Avoid halothane

Regional
Assess coagulopathy
Ability to lie flat

Ⓓ **Postoperative period**
 Potential complications
 Prolonged drug effects
 Renal failure
 CHF
 Encephalopathy
 UGI bleeding
 Jaundice
  Hepatocellular injury
  Cholestasis
  Bilirubin overload

REFERENCES

1. Kamath PS, Wiesner RH, Malinchoc M, et al.: A model to predict survival in patients with end-stage liver disease, *Hepatology* 33 (2):464–470, 2001.
2. Harrison SA: Liver disease in patients with diabetes mellitus, *J Clin Gastroenterol* 40 (1):68–76, 2006.
3. Suman A, Carey WD: Assessing the risk of surgery in patients with liver disease, *Cleve Clin J Med* 73 (4):398–404, 2006.
4. Head HW, Dodd GD III: Thermal ablation for hepatocellular carcinoma, *Gastroenterology* 127 (5 Suppl 1):S167–S178, 2004.
5. Garg RK: Anesthetic considerations in patients with hepatic failure, *Int Anesthesiol Clin* 43 (4):45–63, 2005.
6. Whitten CW, Greilich PE: Thromboelastography: past, present, and future, *Anesthesiology* 92 (5):1223–1225, 2000.

PREOPERATIVE HEMATOLOGICAL FUNCTIONS

PROTEIN C AND PROTEIN S DEFICIENCY

ANEMIAS

HEMOGLOBINOPATHIES

COAGULOPATHIES

POLYCYTHEMIA VERA (PV)

PORPHYRIA

COLD AUTOIMMUNE DISEASE (CAID)

HEPARIN-INDUCED THROMBOCYTOPENIA
(HIT)

Protein C and Protein S Deficiency

VERONICA C. SWANSON, M.D.

Protein C and protein S are vitamin K–dependent plasma proteins whose deficiencies result in a hypercoagulable state. Protein C is a serine protease that inhibits activated clotting factors V and VIII and stimulates fibrinolysis.[1–3] It is inhibited by antithrombin and enhanced by protein S. It has a half-life of 6 hours and is produced in the liver. Protein C deficiency can be either inherited or acquired. Inheritance is by autosomal dominant pattern, with variable penetrance. Two types of heterozygous deficiencies exist: type 1 (low levels) and type II (normal levels but functional impairment). Acquired protein C deficiency is seen in liver disease, DIC, acute respiratory distress syndrome (ARDS), postoperatively, postpartum, and in association with hemodialysis.

Protein S is a cofactor for protein C–induced inactivation of factors V and VIII and for protein C acceleration of fibrinolysis.[2,3] It also seems to have anticoagulation function independent of protein C by direct inhibition of procoagulant enzyme complexes. Like protein C, protein S deficiency is also inherited via autosomal dominant transmission with variable penetrance and two types of heterozygous deficiencies. Acquired protein S deficiency has been documented in a variety of conditions, including DIC, type 1 and type II diabetes mellitus, pregnancy, oral contraceptive use, nephrotic syndrome, liver disease, and essential thrombocythemia.[2]

The clinical picture for both protein C and S deficiency is similar. Prevalence is 0.2 to 0.5%. Of persons with these deficiencies, 75% will experience a venous thrombosis (VT), 50% by age 50.[3]

Anesthetic management is of particular importance because the perioperative conditions increase the risk of thrombosis, while surgery increases the risk of bleeding if anticoagulated. The anesthesiologist will be called on to balance the risk of anticoagulation during surgery with the risk of thrombosis in these patients preoperatively, intraoperatively, and postoperatively.

A. Obtain appropriate preoperative tests. It is important to have a high index of suspicion in patients with a personal or family history of the deficiency, a history of thrombotic events beginning in adolescence, or a history of warfarin-induced skin necrosis.[2] If a hypercoagulable condition is suspected, protein C and S levels should be obtained as part of the workup. Protein C and S deficiencies do not cause abnormalities in routine coagulation screening tests (prothrombin time [PT]/international normalized ratio [INR], partial thromboplastin time [PTT], and bleeding time.) Levels are expected to be lowered and are unnecessary if patient is already on anticoagulation. If this is the case, obtain INR and PTT.

B. Therapy of acute thrombotic events in protein C deficiency includes FFP, and plasma-derived factor IX concentrates (containing large amounts of protein C and S), and heparin. Therapy of acute thrombotic events in protein S deficiency is the same as for protein C deficiency.[2]

C. Operative management of anticoagulants[4]:
1. No change is necessary for surgeries with a *low risk of bleeding* (simple dental and ophthalmology procedures) if the INR is low therapeutic.[2] No data exist on cutaneous surgeries, but it is thought to be safe for anticoagulated patients. Transurethral resections of the prostate (TURPs) have also been reported to be performed safely in anticoagulated patients.
2. For surgeries with a *high risk of bleeding and low risk of thrombosis* (patients with hypercoagulable state without a recent thrombotic complication, recurrent thrombosis, or history of a life-threatening thrombosis) discontinue warfarin 4 to 5 days before surgery, heparin 2 to 3 hours before surgery, and low-molecular weight heparin (LMWH) 12 hours before. Check INR morning of surgery: goal is 1.5. More caution is required is neurosurgery; most neurosurgeons recommend a normal INR before surgery. If surgery is urgent, give vitamin K, either orally or subcutaneously, and FFP to reverse the warfarin.
3. For patients with a *high thrombosis risk* (patients with a hypercoagulable state with recurrent thrombosis, recent thrombosis, or life-threatening thrombosis) undergoing procedures *with a high bleeding risk*, anticoagulation should be continued as close as possible to the procedure and started soon after the procedure to help minimize any thrombotic complications. This may require preoperative hospitalization for better control with heparinization.

If regional anesthesia is indicated, patient should be off all anticoagulation with a normal INR when a catheter is placed and removed.[4]

D. Postoperatively, patients may develop a prothrombotic state. Thrombosis may be initiated by the events associated with the perioperative period, including endothelial damage, immobility, and stasis of blood flow.[1] Elevated levels of fibrin degradation products indicating increased fibrin formation have been shown in trauma patients undergoing elective hip surgery. Restart anticoagulation (beginning with heparin) postoperatively when contraindications no longer outweigh the risk of thrombosis.

PROTEIN C AND S DEFICIENCIES

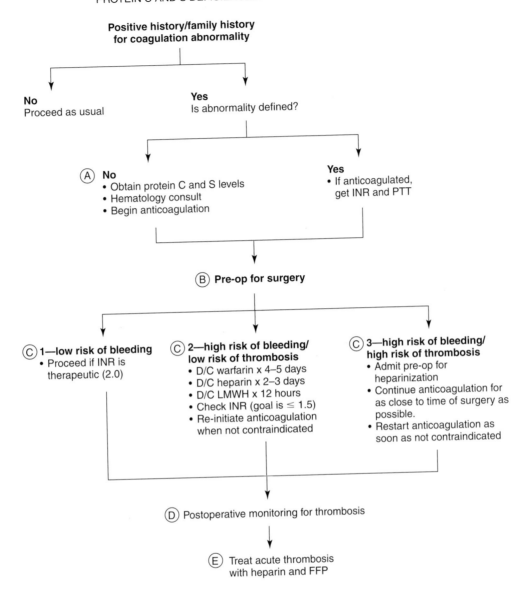

E. Pediatric response to anticoagulation and thrombotic therapy will differ as compared to adults.[3] Protein C and S levels are approximately 50% of adult values at birth and reach adult levels in the late teenage years.[5] These differences reflect changes in the hemostatic system during development and require age- and weight-dependent dosing of anticoagulants.

REFERENCES

1. Stoelting RK, Dierdorf SF: Coagulopathies. In *Anesthesia and co-existing disease*, ed 4, Philadelphia, 2002, Churchill Livingstone.

2. Bick RL: Prothrombin G20210A mutation, antithrombin, heparin cofactor II, protein C, and protein S defects, *Hematol Oncol Clin North Am* 17:9–36, 2003.

3. Hoppe C, Matsunaga A: Pediatric thrombosis, *Pediatr Clin North Am* 49 (6):1257–1283, 2002.

4. Spandorfer J: The management of anticoagulation before and after procedures, *Med Clin North Am* 85 (5):1109–1116, v, 2001.

5. Monagle P, Chan A, Massicotte P, et al.: Antithrombotic therapy in children: the Seventh ACCP Conference on Antithrombotic and thrombolytic therapy, *Chest* 126 (3 Suppl):645S–687S, 2004.

Anemias

JOSEPH R. HOLAHAN, M.D.

Quantitative assessment of oxygen-carrying capacity requires knowledge of hemoglobin (Hb) concentration and P_{50} (PaO_2 at which Hb is 50% saturated). Hb carries 1.39 ml oxygen (O_2) per 100 ml blood. Plasma dissolves only 0.003 ml O_2 per 100 ml blood, yet it is the dissolved O_2 that is reflected by the PaO_2.[1] Normal P_{50} is 27 mm Hg, but variant Hbs may have significantly different P_{50}s.[2] Tissue delivery of O_2 may be maintained if 2,3 diphosphoglycerate (2,3-DPG) is elevated (lesser affinity of Hb for O_2), if there is no increased O_2 demand (manifested by exercise intolerance), or if the cardiac output (CO) increases.[1] There is a greater acceptance of lower Hb levels in patients presenting for elective surgery; concern about blood-borne diseases and observation that stable patients tolerate low Hb have prompted this change.[3] Consult with the patient's hematologist, particularly in complicated cases.

A. Determine the cause of anemia (defective production, excessive red cell destruction, blood loss, or combinations). Primary hematological disease may involve platelets and granulocytes, making coagulopathy and infection more likely. Antibodies in hemolytic disease may make blood transfusion difficult. Many surgical patients have obvious blood loss (trauma, the lesion necessitating repair, repeated operative procedures, or multiple blood samples [7 to 10 ml per tube]). Other common causes of anemia include renal disease, GI malignancy, infections, or toxicities. Postbariatric surgery patients can have deficiencies of iron, B_{12}, or other nutrients.[4] Pernicious anemia is not uncommon in elderly patients, who may have coexistent neurological abnormalities. Chronic anemia is usually better tolerated, in part, because of increased 2,3-DPG. Premature infants and neonates have lower P_{50}s and thus require a higher Hb. In infants and children, consider iron deficiency (milk-fed infants through preschool) and the physiological anemia of infancy (2 to 5 months of age).[5]

B. Preoperative transfusion may be necessary when the cause of anemia is active bleeding, which will continue until surgical correction, and when ischemic symptoms of insufficient delivery are present (angina, congestive heart failure [CHF], TIAs, or claudication). If it is clear that transfusion will be needed, give the transfusion preoperatively if possible, because the signs and symptoms of transfusion reaction are subtle and may be masked by anesthesia. Transfusion is not without risk, and blood-borne infections still occur. Hepatitis caused by hepatitis A, B, or C virus has decreased; the risk of hepatitis is now <0.001% per unit.[3] Directed donation of blood from friends and relatives has become more common but is not necessarily safer. Autologous banking (preoperative donation and banking of patient's own blood) avoids risk of infection but may not be practical in the patient who is already anemic. Rheology is optimized when the hematocrit (Hct) is approximately 30%. The patient who presents for elective surgery and is found to be unexpectedly anemic should be evaluated before transfusion is considered. A preoperative regimen of erythropoietin may improve the Hb or Hct level in some chronic anemias.[6]

C. Choose an anesthetic technique appropriate for the surgical procedure. Anticipate whether there is likely to be extensive blood loss and whether transfusion will be required intraoperatively. An arterial or central venous catheter facilitates intermittent sampling of Hb. Recall that major regional anesthetics may be of shorter duration in the anemic patient (probably because of increased CO and more rapid absorption of local anesthetic).[7]

D. Avoid maneuvers that shift the O_2-Hb dissociation curve to the left, increasing affinity of Hb for O_2, thus reducing tissue delivery (hypothermia, respiratory alkalosis, acute metabolic alkalosis, or chronic acidosis).

REFERENCES

1. Hébert PC, Van der Linden P, Biro G, et al.: Physiologic aspects of anemia, *Crit Care Clin* 20:187–212, 2004.
2. Larson PJ, Friedman DF, Reilly MP, et al.: The presurgical management with erythrocytapheresis of a patient with a high-oxygen-affinity, unstable Hb variant (Hb Bryn Mawr), *Transfusion* 37 (7): 703–707, 1997.
3. Madjdpour C, Spahn DR, Weiskopf RB: Anemia and perioperative red blood cell transfusion, *Crit Care Med* 34 (5 Suppl):S102–S108, 2006.
4. Parkes E: Nutritional management of patients after bariatric surgery, *Am J Med Sci* 331 (4):207–213, 2006.
5. Weldon BC: Blood conservation in pediatric anesthesia, *Anesthesiol Clin North Am* 23 (2):347–361, 2005.
6. Napolitano LM: Perioperative anemia, *Surg Clin North Am* 85: 1215–1227, 2005.
7. Guay J: The effect of neuraxial blocks on surgical blood loss and blood transfusion requirements: a meta-analysis, *J Clin Anesth* 18 (2):124–128, 2006.

Patient with ANEMIA

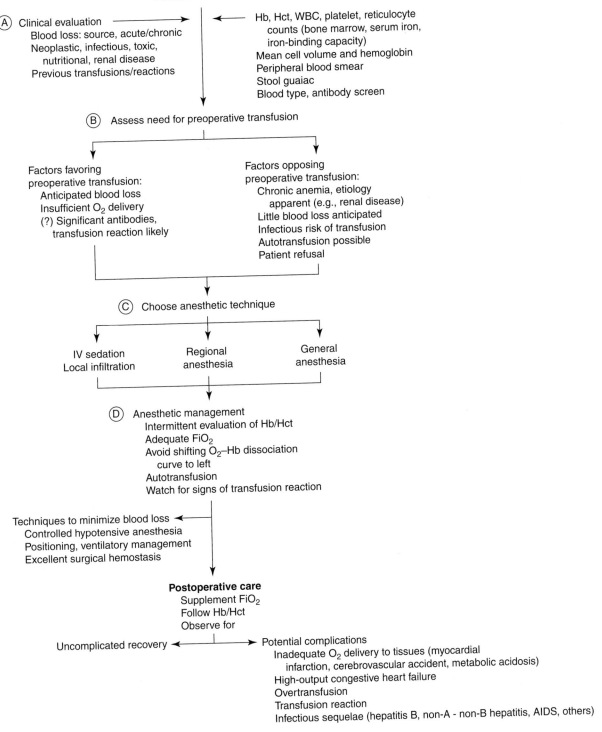

Ⓐ Clinical evaluation
    Blood loss: source, acute/chronic
    Neoplastic, infectious, toxic,
       nutritional, renal disease
    Previous transfusions/reactions

Hb, Hct, WBC, platelet, reticulocyte
   counts (bone marrow, serum iron,
   iron-binding capacity)
Mean cell volume and hemoglobin
Peripheral blood smear
Stool guaiac
Blood type, antibody screen

Ⓑ Assess need for preoperative transfusion

Factors favoring
preoperative transfusion:
   Anticipated blood loss
   Insufficient O_2 delivery
   (?) Significant antibodies,
      transfusion reaction likely

Factors opposing
preoperative transfusion:
   Chronic anemia, etiology
      apparent (e.g., renal disease)
   Little blood loss anticipated
   Infectious risk of transfusion
   Autotransfusion possible
   Patient refusal

Ⓒ Choose anesthetic technique

IV sedation
Local infiltration

Regional
anesthesia

General
anesthesia

Ⓓ Anesthetic management
    Intermittent evaluation of Hb/Hct
    Adequate FiO_2
    Avoid shifting O_2–Hb dissociation
       curve to left
    Autotransfusion
    Watch for signs of transfusion reaction

Techniques to minimize blood loss
   Controlled hypotensive anesthesia
   Positioning, ventilatory management
   Excellent surgical hemostasis

Postoperative care
   Supplement FiO_2
   Follow Hb/Hct
   Observe for

Uncomplicated recovery

Potential complications
   Inadequate O_2 delivery to tissues (myocardial
      infarction, cerebrovascular accident, metabolic acidosis)
   High-output congestive heart failure
   Overtransfusion
   Transfusion reaction
   Infectious sequelae (hepatitis B, non-A - non-B hepatitis, AIDS, others)

Hemoglobinopathies

JOSEPH R. HOLAHAN, M.D.

There are a large variety of hemoglobin (Hb) variants, not all of which are harmful. Hemoglobinopathies result from molecular substitutions within the Hb chain (e.g., HbS or HbC) or from the presence of abnormal chains or abnormal amounts of Hb chains (e.g., thalassemias). Clinical disorders include sickling, anemia, hemolysis, drug-induced hemolysis, and alterations in oxygen (O_2) affinity (both increased and decreased). Perioperative transfusion (or exchange transfusion) can be beneficial in preventing postoperative complications in patients with sickle cell disease.[1] Consider preoperative consultation with a hematologist. In the patient who is heavily transfused, multiple alloantibodies are likely to be present; preoperative type and screen can be performed to identify alloantibodies and to facilitate the procurement of red cells.

A. Determine the nature of the hemoglobinopathy. Be aware that the patient with sickle disease (HbSS) may present with various crises that resemble surgical conditions: bone infarcts may be confused with osteomyelitis; acute hemolytic or sequestration episodes resemble acute hemorrhage; and splenic or pulmonary infarction or lobar pneumonia may mimic an acute abdomen. The chronically anemic patient depends on an increased cardiac output (CO) for normal tissue oxygenation. HbSS is both an inflammatory and pro-thrombotic disease. The routine use of Hydrea has decreased sickling episodes by 50%.[2] Sickling or inflammation in the coronary microvasculature leads to myocardial fibrosis, and cardiopulmonary dysfunction (e.g., pulmonary infarcts, shunting, decreased pulmonary vascular bed, pulmonary hypertension [HTN], or congestive heart failure [CHF]) is progressive. Neurological abnormalities are common, ranging from hemiplegia to visual impairment. Renal problems include reduced ability to concentrate urine and papillary necrosis. Pigment gallstones are common in patients with hemolytic disorders.

B. If sickling is likely, pay meticulous attention to maintenance of adequate circulating blood volume. Prevent intraoperative sickling by providing supplemental O_2, keep the patient warm (heated and humidified gases, forced warm air heating blanket, warmed IV fluids, and warm OR), do not allow venous stasis as a result of positioning or the use of tourniquets (i.e., slowed flow, low PvO_2, and acidotic pH make sickling more likely), and maintain CO. Tailor monitoring to the health of the patient and likelihood of major blood losses and fluid shifts. Transfusion to an adequate Hb is as beneficial as exchange transfusions.[3] Partial exchange transfusion before cardiopulmonary bypass (CPB) may allow the safe use of hypothermia, but it is controversial. Sickling may occur in sickle trait patients (HbAS) under conditions of severe hypoxemia (e.g., cyanotic heart disease, acute ethanol intoxication, hypoxemia, or peripheral venous stasis). Advances in supportive care have made pregnancy in the HbSS patient safer, but it is still associated with excess morbidity and mortality for both the mother and the fetus. Transfusions are indicated for the same reasons as in nonpregnant patients.[4] Psychiatric consultation may be of help as the patient may have problems with pain medications, neurocognitive impairment, and coping strategies.[5]

C. Thalassemia patients may require chronic transfusion therapy and are thus at risk for blood-borne diseases. Frontal bossing and maxillary overgrowth can contribute to difficulty with intubation. Iron overload causes a variety of clinical problems, usually beginning during the second decade. Sulfhemoglobinemia and methemoglobinemia may be congenital or acquired (as in benzocaine topical spray overdose[6]) and cause apparent cyanosis despite adequate O_2 content. Maintain adequate oxygenation, recalling that high-affinity Hbs may not release O_2 normally at the tissue level.

REFERENCES

1. Koshy M, Weiner SJ, Miller ST, et al.: Surgery and anesthesia in sickle cell disease: cooperative study of sickle cell diseases, *Blood* 86:3676–84, 1995.
2. Firth PG. Anaesthesia for peculiar cells—a century of sickle cell disease, *Br J Anaesth* 95:287–99, 2005.
3. Vichinsky EP, Haberkern CM, Neumayr L, et al.: A comparison of conservative and aggressive transfusion regimens in the perioperative management of sickle cell disease. The Preoperative Transfusion in Sickle Cell Disease Study Group, *N Engl J Med* 333:206–13, 1995.
4. ACOG Committee on Obstetrics, ACOG Practice Bulletin No. 78: hemoglobinopathies in pregnancy, *Obstet Gynecol* 109:229–237, 2007.
5. Anie KA: Psychological complications in sickle cell disease, *Br J Haematol* 129:723–9, 2005.
6. LeClaire AC, Mullett TW, Jahania MS, et al.: Methemoglobinemia secondary to topical benzocaine use in a lung transplant patient, *Ann Pharmacother* 39:373–6, 2005.

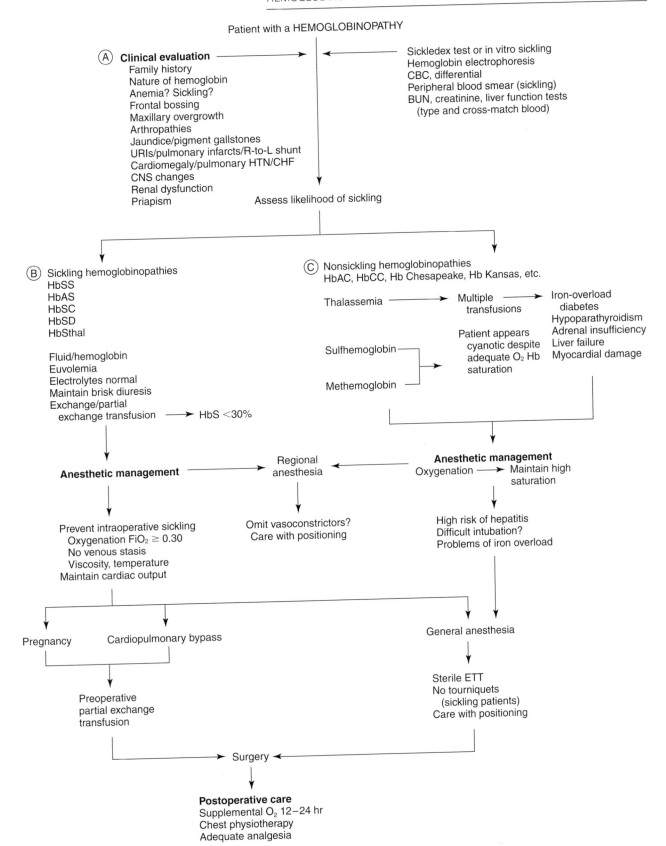

Patient with a HEMOGLOBINOPATHY

Ⓐ **Clinical evaluation**
    Family history
    Nature of hemoglobin
    Anemia? Sickling?
    Frontal bossing
    Maxillary overgrowth
    Arthropathies
    Jaundice/pigment gallstones
    URIs/pulmonary infarcts/R-to-L shunt
    Cardiomegaly/pulmonary HTN/CHF
    CNS changes
    Renal dysfunction
    Priapism

Sickledex test or in vitro sickling
Hemoglobin electrophoresis
CBC, differential
Peripheral blood smear (sickling)
BUN, creatinine, liver function tests
    (type and cross-match blood)

Assess likelihood of sickling

Ⓑ Sickling hemoglobinopathies
HbSS
HbAS
HbSC
HbSD
HbSthal

Fluid/hemoglobin
Euvolemia
Electrolytes normal
Maintain brisk diuresis
Exchange/partial
    exchange transfusion → HbS <30%

Ⓒ Nonsickling hemoglobinopathies
HbAC, HbCC, Hb Chesapeake, Hb Kansas, etc.

Thalassemia → Multiple transfusions → Iron-overload
                                                                diabetes
                                                                Hypoparathyroidism
Sulfhemoglobin ─┐   Adrenal insufficiency
                        Patient appears   Liver failure
                        cyanotic despite   Myocardial damage
                        adequate O₂ Hb
Methemoglobin ─┘   saturation

Anesthetic management

Regional anesthesia

Anesthetic management
Oxygenation → Maintain high saturation

Prevent intraoperative sickling
Oxygenation FiO₂ ≥ 0.30
No venous stasis
Viscosity, temperature
Maintain cardiac output

Omit vasoconstrictors?
Care with positioning

High risk of hepatitis
Difficult intubation?
Problems of iron overload

Pregnancy   Cardiopulmonary bypass

General anesthesia

Preoperative
partial exchange
transfusion

Sterile ETT
No tourniquets
    (sickling patients)
Care with positioning

Surgery

Postoperative care
Supplemental O₂ 12–24 hr
Chest physiotherapy
Adequate analgesia

Coagulopathies

JOSEPH R. HOLAHAN, M.D.

Successful surgery depends, in part, on adequate hemostatic ability of the patient. Hemostasis depends on vascular integrity, platelet function, and coagulation (Figure 1).[1]

A. Hereditary disorders are associated with a lifelong history of bleeding, but von Willebrand's disease (vWD), factor VIII deficiency, and factor XI deficiency may first present in adulthood. Avoid regional anesthesia in the presence of a suspected coagulopathy. The patient who has received thrombolytic therapy may have a severe, refractory coagulopathy.[2] Some herbs (e.g., garlic, ginkgo, or ginseng) may cause bleeding; have the patient stop these before surgery.[3] Bleeding may occur after injury to the brain (defibrination) and after transurethral surgery (fibrinolysis). With massive transfusion, anticipate hypothermia, dilutional thrombocytopenia, and deficiencies of factors V and VIII unless the patient is kept warm and adequate platelets and FFP are given.[4]

B. Evaluate the history of bleeding with procedures. Obtain the prothrombin time (PT), partial thromboplastin time (PTT), platelet count, bleeding time (BT), and fibrinogen level. Obtain blood from a peripheral arterial or venipuncture, from a CVP catheter, or (most subject to error) from the heparinized arterial catheter (after first withdrawing 10 to 15 ml of blood). If abnormalities are identified before elective surgery, consider obtaining assays for the more commonly deficient factors (VIII, IX, and XI); ensure adequate factor levels preoperatively.[5] vWD patients who have increased BT or decreased factor VIII require preoperative treatment with either DDAVP or purified factor concentrate.

C. If a prolonged PT is caused by a deficiency of coagulation factors, consider vitamin K and the judicious use of FFP to correct the problem. PT is generally prolonged secondary to warfarin (Coumadin), thrombin inhibitors (Argatroban and hirudin),[6] vitamin K deficiency, liver disease, or DIC.

D. When PTT is prolonged, look for a specific cause. Hereditary factor deficiencies (e.g., VIII, IX, or XI), vWD, or a lupus anticoagulant are possible causes. Use specific purified clotting factors for specific deficiencies (factor VIII or IX).[7] For the other specific deficiencies, use FFP. Recombinant factor VII is used for patients with coagulation inhibitors but also may be lifesaving in uncontrollable bleeding from overwhelming coagulopathies.[8]

E. Look for a cause of thrombocytopenia. If platelets are not being produced in adequate numbers or dilution is occurring (massive transfusion), give a platelet infusion. If the platelets are being prematurely destroyed (e.g., immune thrombocytopenia, DIC, or sepsis), platelet infusion may not reliably raise the circulating platelet count. Rather, give a specific treatment for the peripheral destruction (e.g., steroids, WinRho, gamma globulin, plasmapheresis, or antibiotics).

F. Causes of increased bleeding time (BT) are a low platelet count ($<100,000/mm^3$) or dysfunctional platelets. Platelet infusion corrects the bleeding time in dysfunctional platelet syndromes but not in vWD. Antiplatelet drugs (e.g., aspirin, Plavix, or abciximab) may require platelet infusions to correct the BT. Uremia prolongs the BT; correct this with dialysis, cryoprecipitate, DDAVP, or RBC transfusion.[9] DIC syndrome also prolongs BT (and may be accompanied by low plasma fibrinogen and increased fibrin degradative products). IV nitroglycerin may produce a prolongation of BT related to vasodilation (without alteration of platelet function tests).[10]

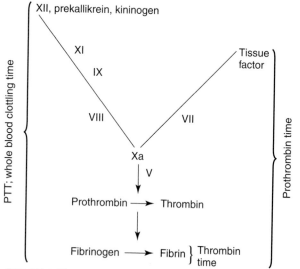

FIGURE 1 The coagulation cascade and tests of coagulation.

REFERENCES

1. Beers MH, Berkow R, editors: *The Merck manual of diagnosis and therapy*, ed 17, Section 11. Hematology and oncology, Chapter 131. Hemostasis and coagulation disorders, available at: www.merck.com/mrkshared/mmanual/home.jsp.
2. Karmanoukian H, Attuwabi B, Nader ND: Antithrombotic controversies in off-pump coronary bypass, *Semin Thorac Cardiovasc Surg* 17 (1):59–65, 2005.
3. Kohler S, Funk P, Kieser M: Influence of a 7-day treatment with Ginkgo biloba special extract EGb 761 on bleeding time and coagulation: a randomized, placebo-controlled, double-blind study in healthy volunteers, *Blood Coagul Fibrinolysis* 15 (4):303–309, 2004.
4. Levy JH: Massive transfusion coagulopathy, *Semin Hematol* 43 (1 Suppl 1):S59–S63, 2006.
5. Ingerslev J, Hvid I: Surgery in hemophilia. The general view: patient selection, timing, and preoperative assessment, *Semin Hematol* 43 (1 Suppl 1):S23–S26, 2006.

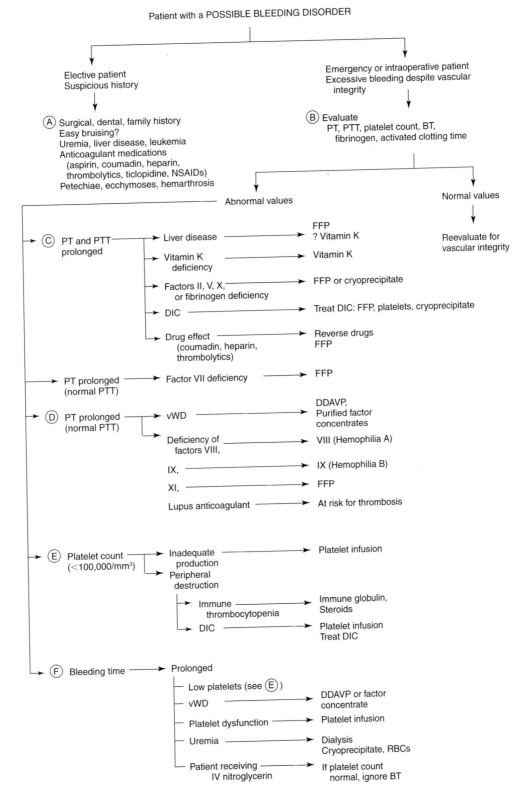

Patient with a POSSIBLE BLEEDING DISORDER

Elective patient
Suspicious history

Emergency or intraoperative patient
Excessive bleeding despite vascular
integrity

(A) Surgical, dental, family history
Easy bruising?
Uremia, liver disease, leukemia
Anticoagulant medications
(aspirin, coumadin, heparin,
thrombolytics, ticlopidine, NSAIDs)
Petechiae, ecchymoses, hemarthrosis

(B) Evaluate
PT, PTT, platelet count, BT,
fibrinogen, activated clotting time

Abnormal values

Normal values

Reevaluate for
vascular integrity

(C) PT and PTT
prolonged

Liver disease ⟶ FFP
? Vitamin K

Vitamin K
deficiency ⟶ Vitamin K

Factors II, V, X,
or fibrinogen deficiency ⟶ FFP or cryoprecipitate

DIC ⟶ Treat DIC: FFP, platelets, cryoprecipitate

Drug effect ⟶ Reverse drugs
(coumadin, heparin,   FFP
thrombolytics)

PT prolonged ⟶ Factor VII deficiency ⟶ FFP
(normal PTT)

(D) PT prolonged ⟶ vWD ⟶ DDAVP,
(normal PTT)   Purified factor
                                        concentrates

Deficiency of ⟶ VIII (Hemophilia A)
factors VIII,

IX, ⟶ IX (Hemophilia B)

XI, ⟶ FFP

Lupus anticoagulant ⟶ At risk for thrombosis

(E) Platelet count ⟶ Inadequate ⟶ Platelet infusion
(<100,000/mm³)   production
                      Peripheral
                      destruction

Immune ⟶ Immune globulin,
thrombocytopenia   Steroids

DIC ⟶ Platelet infusion
      Treat DIC

(F) Bleeding time ⟶ Prolonged

Low platelets (see (E))
vWD ⟶ DDAVP or factor
       concentrate
Platelet dysfunction ⟶ Platelet infusion
Uremia ⟶ Dialysis
          Cryoprecipitate, RBCs
Patient receiving ⟶ If platelet count
IV nitroglycerin   normal, ignore BT

6. Linkins LA, Weitz JI: Pharmacology and clinical potential of direct thrombin inhibitors, *Curr Pharm Des* 11 (30):3877–3884, 2005.

7. Zakarija A: Factor IX replacement in surgery and prophylaxis, *Blood Coagul Fibrinolysis* 15 Suppl 2:S5–S7, 2004.

8. Grounds M: Recombinant factor VIIa (rFVIIa) and its use in severe bleeding in surgery and trauma: a review, *Blood Rev* 17 (Suppl 1):S11–S21, 2003.

9. Fernandez F, Goudable C, Sie P, et al.: Low haematocrit and prolonged bleeding time in uraemic patients: effect of red cell transfusions, *Br J Haematol* 59:139–148, 1985.

10. Lichtenthal PR, Rossi EC, Louis G, et al.: Dose-related prolongation of the bleeding time by intravenous nitroglycerin, *Anesth Analg* 64:30–33, 1985.

Polycythemia Vera (PV)

JOSEPH R. HOLAHAN, M.D.

Polycythemia vera (PV) is a myeloproliferative disorder highly associated with the JAK2 tyrosine kinase mutation and characterized by increased production of erythrocytes, granulocytes, and platelets.[1] Erythrocytosis is an elevation of the RBC count alone. Primary problems are hyperviscosity (leading to RBC sludging and thrombosis) and hemorrhage. Emergency surgery in unprepared PV patients may be associated with perioperative morbidity and mortality four to five times greater than if they are treated with phlebotomy.[1] Secondary polycythemia, or erythrocytosis associated with chronic obstructive pulmonary disease, may not carry such a high perioperative risk.[2]

A. Most PV patients are >60 years of age.[3] Other patients with higher than normal hemoglobin (Hb) may have secondary erythrocytosis, usually associated with chronic hypoxemia (high altitude, chronic cardiac, or pulmonary disease; right to left shunts; sleep apnea; methemoglobin or sulfhemoglobinemia).[1] Use of hormones, such as testosterone, DHEA, or growth hormone, is an increasing cause of erythrocytosis.[4] Tumors of the kidney, liver, or cerebellum that secrete erythropoietin are rare causes of erythrocytosis. Postrenal transplant erythrocytosis may respond to angiotensin-converting enzyme (ACE) inhibitors. "Pseudoerythrocytosis" (hemoconcentration) can be seen with dehydration. Higher than normal RBC concentration in PV (hemoglobin > 18 g/dl) leads to hyperviscosity, commonly manifested by plethoric facies, dilated capillaries, retinal vascular changes, peripheral cyanosis, and cerebral or coronary symptoms. Splenomegaly is common. Spontaneous hemorrhage occurs, particularly from peptic ulcers and nosebleeds. (Even though there is thrombocytosis and abnormal thrombosis, bleeding may occur, probably as a result of platelet dysfunction).[5] Severe thrombocytosis (platelets > 800,000/mm^3) may be associated with hypercoagulability or bleeding from pseudo von Willebrand's disease). Increased nucleic acid turnover leads to elevated uric acid levels and gout in some patients. Therapy is directed toward reducing blood viscosity by removing RBCs (phlebotomy and use of myelosuppressive agents). Aspirin may not decrease thrombotic events and will increase the risk of bleeding.[5]

B. If the proposed surgery is elective and there has been no preoperative preparation of the PV patient, delay surgery while hematological consultation is obtained and reduction of Hb and platelets is undertaken. The primary therapy is phlebotomy to reduce the RBC mass and to deplete iron stores. In an emergency, therapy is directed toward reducing viscosity (give crystalloid and low-molecular-weight [LMW] dextran, phlebotomize, and employ deep vein thrombosis [DVT] prophylaxis). Depending on the cardiopulmonary status of the patient, extensive monitoring may be required. Address comorbid factors, such as diabetes, hypertension (HTN), smoking, and cardiovascular disease, which contribute to increased morbidity.[6]

C. During the surgical procedure, minimize venostasis (limb tourniquets, positioning consideration) and avoid extremes of HTN or hypotension. Maintain slight hypervolemia and anticipate greater than normal bleeding. Transfusion of RBCs may not be necessary as long as circulating blood volume is maintained with crystalloids or colloids. Choose an anesthetic technique appropriate for the surgical procedure, with consideration of possible anticoagulation or platelet dysfunction.

REFERENCES

1. Tefferi A, Spivak JL: Polycythemia vera: scientific advances and current practice, Semin Hematol 42 (4):206–220, 2005.
2. Lubarsky DA, Gallagher CJ, Berend JL: Secondary polycythemia does not increase the risk of perioperative hemorrhagic or thrombotic complications, J Clin Anesth 3:99–103, 1991.
3. Stoelting RK, Dierdorf SF: Anesthesia and co-existing diseases, ed 4, Philadelphia, 2002, Churchill Livingstone.
4. Kwong YL, Lam CC: Polycythemia in a physician secondary to self-administered growth hormone, testosterone, and dehydroepiandrosterone to prevent aging, J Am Geriatr Soc 52 (6):1031–1032, 2004.
5. Michiels JJ, Berneman ZN, Schroyens W, et al.: Pathophysiology and treatment of platelet-mediated microvascular disturbances, major thrombosis and bleeding complications in essential thrombocythaemia and polycythaemia vera, Platelets 15 (2):67–84, 2004.
6. Landolfi R, Marchioli R, Kutti J, et al.: Efficacy and safety of low-dose aspirin in polycythemia vera, N Engl J Med 350:114–124, 2004.

Patient with POLYCYTHEMIA VERA

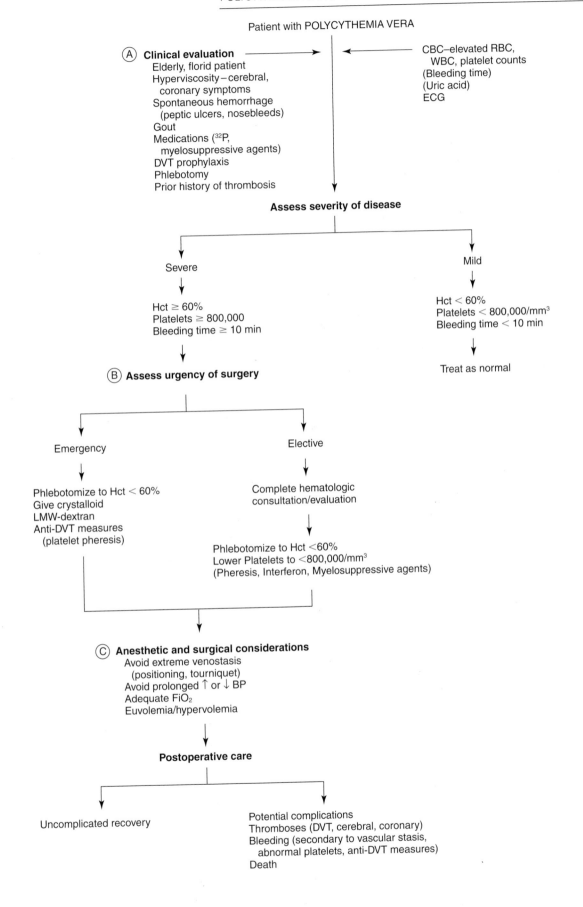

Ⓐ **Clinical evaluation**
    Elderly, florid patient
    Hyperviscosity – cerebral,
      coronary symptoms
    Spontaneous hemorrhage
      (peptic ulcers, nosebleeds)
    Gout
    Medications (^{32}P,
      myelosuppressive agents)
    DVT prophylaxis
    Phlebotomy
    Prior history of thrombosis

CBC – elevated RBC,
    WBC, platelet counts
(Bleeding time)
(Uric acid)
ECG

Assess severity of disease

Severe

Hct $\geq$ 60%
Platelets $\geq$ 800,000
Bleeding time $\geq$ 10 min

Ⓑ **Assess urgency of surgery**

Mild

Hct < 60%
Platelets < 800,000/mm^3
Bleeding time < 10 min

Treat as normal

Emergency

Phlebotomize to Hct < 60%
Give crystalloid
LMW-dextran
Anti-DVT measures
    (platelet pheresis)

Elective

Complete hematologic
consultation/evaluation

Phlebotomize to Hct <60%
Lower Platelets to <800,000/mm^3
(Pheresis, Interferon, Myelosuppressive agents)

Ⓒ **Anesthetic and surgical considerations**
    Avoid extreme venostasis
      (positioning, tourniquet)
    Avoid prolonged ↑ or ↓ BP
    Adequate FiO$_2$
    Euvolemia/hypervolemia

Postoperative care

Uncomplicated recovery

Potential complications
Thromboses (DVT, cerebral, coronary)
Bleeding (secondary to vascular stasis,
    abnormal platelets, anti-DVT measures)
Death

Porphyria

JOSEPH R. HOLAHAN, M.D.

Patients with hereditary hepatic porphyrias (e.g., acute intermittent porphyria [AIP], hereditary coproporphyria [HC], or variegate porphyria [VP]) have abnormal enzymes in the heme synthesis pathway (Figure 1) that cause buildup of porphyrin precursors thought to cause demyelinization centrally and peripherally. Attacks may be precipitated by a variety of lipid-soluble and cytochrome P-450-inducing drugs (Table 1) and are characterized by abdominal pain, mania, coma, or paralysis.[1–4]

A. Porphyria should be quiescent before elective surgery. Pregnancy or menses may exacerbate porphyria. Some patients may be receiving hematin in an attempt to repress induction of ALA-S, the rate-limiting enzyme of the heme pathway. Perform baseline neurological examination which may reveal peripheral neuropathies, extremity weakness, paraplegia or quadriplegia, respiratory insufficiency, autonomic instability, or seizures. Dehydration or carbohydrate limitation may predispose to an attack, so minimize both. Tachycardia and electrolyte abnormalities from the syndrome of inappropriate antidiuretic hormone secretion (SIADH) and vomiting (hyponatremia, hypokalemia, and hypochloremia) may be signs of activity of porphyria.

B. Consider measures for attack prophylaxis including hydration, glucose infusion, and avoidance of drugs associated with attack induction. VP patients who have skin bullae require skin protection. Use monitors appropriate to the patient's degree of autonomic instability, which can be associated with marked hemodynamic lability.

TABLE 1
Drugs Thought to Precipitate Acute Intermittent Porphyria

Barbiturates	Pentazocine
Benzodiazepines?	Althesin
Ethyl alcohol	Etomidate
Phenytoin	Meprobamate
Glutethimide	Ketamine?

C. Choose the anesthetic technique according to surgical requirements. Provide accurate, complete documentation of preexisting neurological deficits to reduce medicolegal risks of regional anesthesia. Select premedication and IV sedation drugs from "safe" drugs (Table 2), and refer to a current reference for a list of drugs in the safe and unsafe category.[5] Barbiturates are most frequently cited as causing attacks. Safe general anesthesia may be given, provided known inducing drugs are omitted. Beta-blockers increase heme synthesis and modfiy the tachycardia and hypertension (HTN) of the porphyria attack.

D. Precipitation of attacks is somewhat unpredictable. Porphyria may become active after safe anesthetics or may not trigger even after thiopental. The attack precipitated in a previously unknown porphyric patient may manifest as paralysis after anesthesia. Death may occur secondary to bulbar involvement and respiratory failure.

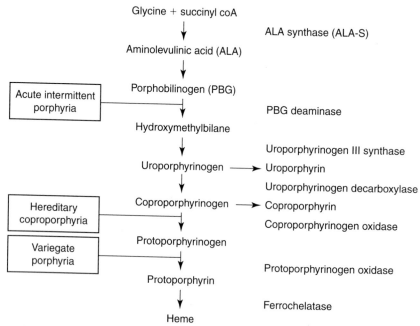

FIGURE 1 Pathway of heme biosynthesis. Shown in boxes are points at which specific enzymatic deficiency is associated with the three types of porphyria susceptible to drug-induced systemic attacks.

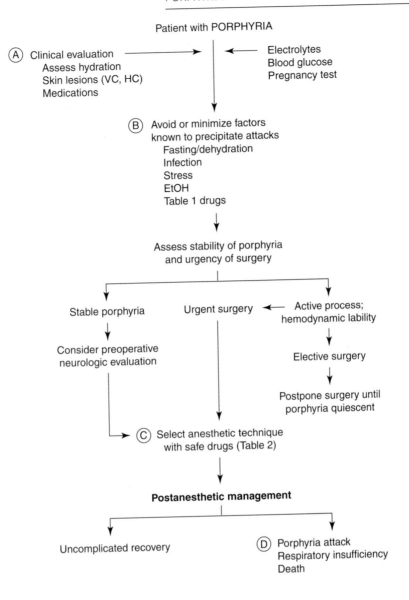

Patient with PORPHYRIA

(A) Clinical evaluation → ← Electrolytes
    Assess hydration   Blood glucose
    Skin lesions (VC, HC)   Pregnancy test
    Medications

(B) Avoid or minimize factors
    known to precipitate attacks
      Fasting/dehydration
      Infection
      Stress
      EtOH
      Table 1 drugs

Assess stability of porphyria
and urgency of surgery

Stable porphyria   Urgent surgery ← Active process;
                                          hemodynamic lability

Consider preoperative   Elective surgery
neurologic evaluation

                                         Postpone surgery until
                                         porphyria quiescent

(C) Select anesthetic technique
    with safe drugs (Table 2)

Postanesthetic management

Uncomplicated recovery   (D) Porphyria attack
                                  Respiratory insufficiency
                                  Death

TABLE 2
**Drugs Thought to Be Safe for Patients with
Acute Intermittent Porphyria**

Propofol	Muscle relaxants, including
Potent inhalational	succinylcholine
anesthetics, N2O	Local anesthetics
Narcotics	Phenothiazines
Phenothiazines	Meperidine
Chlorpromazine	Anticholinergics
Droperidol	

REFERENCES

1. James MF, Hift RJ: Porphyrias, *Br J Anaesth* 85:143–153, 2000.
2. Anderson KE, Bloomer JR, Bonkovsky HL, et al.: Recommendations for the diagnosis and treatment of the acute porphyria, *Ann Intern Med* 142:439–450, 2005.
3. Fleisher LA, editor: *Anesthesia and uncommon diseases*, ed 5, Philadelphia, 2005, Elsevier.
4. Harrison GG, Meissner PN, Hift RJ: Anaesthesia for the porphyric patient, *Anaesthesia* 48:417–421, 1993.
5. University of Cape Town Porphyria Service website, available at: http://web.uct.ac.za/depts/porphyria/professional/prof%20index.htm.

Cold Autoimmune Disease (CAID)

LOIS L. BREADY, M.D.

CHRISTOPHER A. BRACKEN, M.D., PH.D.

MARY ANN GURKOWSKI, M.D.

The cold autoimmune diseases (CAIDs) include cryoglobulinemia, cold agglutinins (idiopathic or secondary), and paroxysmal cold hemoglobinuria (PCH).[1-6] Cryoglobulinemia (Table 1) is an immune complex (IC) disease in which organ dysfunction and palpable petechiae may result. Cold agglutinins are IgM antibodies to RBCs that cause hemolysis. PCH was a more common hemolytic disorder when syphilis was more prevalent.

A. Patients presenting for surgery with an established diagnosis of CAID require recent complete blood count (CBC) and IC determination or antibody titer.

Determine associated diseases (pneumonia, lymphocytic leukemia, or lymphoma) and the severity or degree of organ involvement by the disease. Preoperative plasma exchange or apheresis may be indicated to reduce circulating levels of IC or antibody and thus decrease risks associated with cooling during the perioperative period. Close collaboration with the hematologist is recommended. It may be helpful to know the critical temperature and "thermal amplitude" of the antibody (temperature range of concern) to gauge warming requirements. These patients may be hepatitis B-antigen positive.

TABLE 1
Cold Autoimmune Diseases

	Cryoglobulinemia	Cold agglutinins	Paroxysmal cold hemoglobinuria (PCH)
Pathophysiology	Immune complexes (IgG, IgM) Immune complex disease Hyperviscosity	Anti-RBC antibodies (IgM)	Donath-Landsteiner antibody
Clinical manifestations	Immune complex disease Vascular wall damage Glomerulitis, nephrotic syndrome Neuropathies Pulmonary, GI Palpable petechiae	Hemolytic anemia	Hemolytic anemia
Clinical course	More severe	Milder (occasionally severe)	Self-limited
Associated disease	Idiopathic Myeloma Lymphoma Chronic infection Hepatitis B virus	Pneumonias Infectious mononucleosis Chronic lymphocytic leukemia Lymphoma	Tertiary or secondary syphilis Measles, mumps Idiopathic
Therapy	Plasmapheresis Steroids Cytotoxic agents	Plasmapheresis Steroids Cytotoxic agents	Treat underlying disease

Patient with COLD AUTOIMMUNE DISEASE

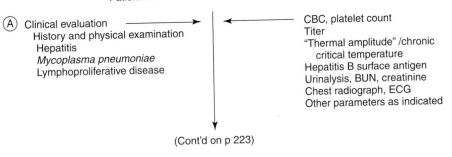

Ⓐ Clinical evaluation
    History and physical examination
    Hepatitis
    Mycoplasma pneumoniae
    Lymphoproliferative disease

CBC, platelet count
Titer
"Thermal amplitude" /chronic
    critical temperature
Hepatitis B surface antigen
Urinalysis, BUN, creatinine
Chest radiograph, ECG
Other parameters as indicated

(Cont'd on p 223)

B. Maintain perioperative patient temperature above 35°C. Adjust the ambient temperature of the OR (watch for cold drafts directed at the patient). Use forced air warming blankets, wrapped extremities, heated humidified gases, and fluid warmers. Multiple temperature probes (skin, esophageal, or rectal) can identify thermal gradients. Because of hemolysis, blood transfusion may be required, even for surgical procedures that do not ordinarily require blood. If blood is needed, give warmed, washed RBCs. Consider placing a urinary catheter to evaluate hemoglobinuria and diminished urinary output that may result from hemolysis. Acute renal failure may occur, even with near-normal body temperature. Use other special preparations and monitors and choose an anesthetic as dictated by the general condition of the patient and the requirements of the surgical procedure.

C. *Cardiopulmonary bypass* (CPB). Screening for CAIDs includes cross-matching at 20°C and testing for RBC agglutination at 10°C in saline and 20°C in albumin. If this is detected, quantify the thermal range of activity and titer. Depending on the thermal amplitude and titer, a decision is made regarding plasmapheresis. All authors agree that systemic cooling needs to be several degrees above critical temperature. Myocardial protection may be provided via several approaches (warm blood potassium cardioplegia; warm crystalloid cardioplegic washout followed by cold crystalloid cardioplegia; cold crystalloid cardioplegia; none). All of these techniques have been used successfully, but use of cold cardioplegia is intellectually less appealing because of concern about noncoronary collateral myocardial blood flow and consequent agglutination.

D. Potential complications, in addition to those of the surgical procedure and anesthetic technique, include perioperative myocardial infarction (MI), hemolytic anemia with cardiac failure, IC nephritis with azotemia, and thrombotic sequelae, typically in cooler areas of the body (digits, ears, or nose). Postoperative laboratory evaluation of organ function is recommended.

REFERENCES

1. Linz WJ, Tauscher C, Winters JL, et al.: Transfusion medicine illustrated: cold agglutinin disease, *Transfusion* 43 (9):1185, 2003.
2. Carloss HW, Tavassoli M: Acute renal failure from precipitation of cryoglobulins in a cool operating room, *JAMA* 244:1472–3, 1980.
3. Kypson AP, Warner JJ, Telen MJ, et al.: Paroxysmal cold hemoglobinuria and cardiopulmonary bypass, *Ann Thorac Surg* 75 (2): 579–581, 2003.
4. Ko W, Isom OW: Cardiopulmonary bypass procedures in patients with cold-reactive hemagglutination. A case report and a literature review, *J Cardiovasc Surg* (Torino) 37 (6):623–626, 1996.
5. Bracken CA, Gurkowski MA, Naples JJ, et al.: Case conference. Case 6–1993. Cardiopulmonary bypass in two patients with previously undetected cold agglutinins, *J Cardiothorac Vasc Anesth* 7:743–9, 1993.
6. Siami FS, Siami GA: A last resort modality using cryofiltration apheresis for the treatment of cold hemagglutinin disease in a Veterans Administration hospital, *Ther Apher Dial* 8 (5): 398–403, 2004.

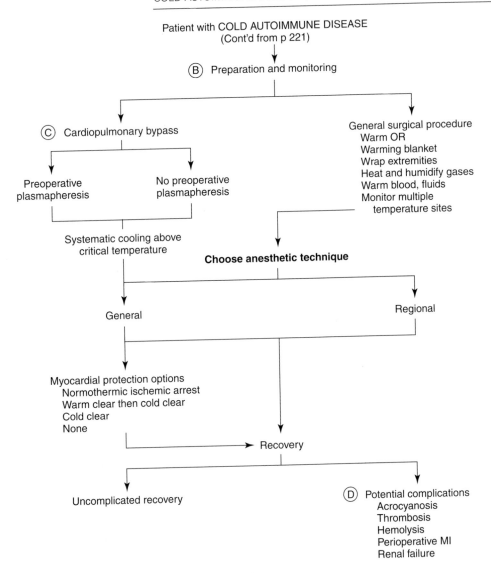

Patient with COLD AUTOIMMUNE DISEASE
(Cont'd from p 221)

Ⓑ Preparation and monitoring

Ⓒ Cardiopulmonary bypass

General surgical procedure
Warm OR
Warming blanket
Wrap extremities
Heat and humidify gases
Warm blood, fluids
Monitor multiple
    temperature sites

Preoperative
plasmapheresis

No preoperative
plasmapheresis

Systematic cooling above
critical temperature

Choose anesthetic technique

General

Regional

Myocardial protection options
Normothermic ischemic arrest
Warm clear then cold clear
Cold clear
None

Recovery

Uncomplicated recovery

Ⓓ Potential complications
Acrocyanosis
Thrombosis
Hemolysis
Perioperative MI
Renal failure

Heparin-Induced Thrombocytopenia (HIT)

SUSAN H. NOORILY, M.D.

CHARLES B. HANTLER, M.D.

Heparin-induced thrombocytopenia (HIT) is a transient, potentially life-threatening complication of heparin therapy. It is an immunogenic-induced hypercoagulable state. HIT occurs in approximately 2% of cardiac surgical patients exposed to heparin, although 27 to 50% of this group will form HIT antibodies.[1] The onset of thrombocytopenia typically begins 5 to 10 days after the initiation of heparin but can begin abruptly after the initiation of heparin (in patients who have received heparin within the past 100 days) or be delayed for several days or weeks after the last dose. HIT presents with arterial or venous thrombosis, leading to major complications including stroke, heart attack, and death.[2] The risk for thrombosis in patients with HIT after discontinuation of heparin is 18.6 to 51.6%.[3] Thrombi are a result of uncontrolled thrombin generation. An IgG heparin-dependent antibody binds to platelets resulting in platelet activation. The antibody is thought to react with heparin or platelet factor 4 (PF4) to form an immune complex which binds to receptors on the platelet membrane or endothelial cells.[2]

A. When a patient receiving heparin develops thrombocytopenia (fall in platelet count of to at least 50%) or thrombosis, consider the diagnosis of HIT.[4] Diagnosis is based on the following criteria: occurrence of one or more HIT-associated clinical events (e.g., thrombocytopenia, thrombosis, skin lesions at the site of the heparin injection, or acute systemic reaction to heparin bolus) and detection of HIT antibodies.[4]

B. No test reliably predicts HIT; thus it is not practical to screen all patients treated with heparin. Testing is performed when HIT is suspected clinically. The two types of tests include platelet activation assays and PF4-dependent antigen assays, and both are highly sensitive.[2] A negative test rules out HIT, but a positive assay does not prove a diagnosis of HIT.

C. In patients with a high clinical suspicion of HIT, stop heparin (and low-molecular weight heparin [LMWH]) and substitute an alternative non-heparin anticoagulant (e.g., argatroban, lepirudin, or bivalirudin), even when there is no evidence of thrombosis.[2] Choose the particular agent based on availability, presence of hepatic or renal disease, and personal experience. Avoid prophylactic platelet transfusions [4]. Avoid warfarin (can cause venous gangrene from reduction in protein C).[4] Screen lower extremities for venous thrombosis.

D. Management of cardiopulmonary bypass (CPB) and major vascular surgery in patients known to have HIT is challenging.[5] If the surgery is not urgent, postpone the procedure for several weeks to allow recovery of platelets and disappearance of antibodies; HIT antibodies are transient and usually are not detectable for more than 100 days.[1] If the antibodies are no longer detectable, administer heparin for anticoagulation during CPB. Avoid preoperative heparin completely, and give alternative anticoagulants postoperatively.[1] For urgent situations in patients with a history of HIT, when there is no opportunity for antibody testing, consider the use of unfractionated heparin (UFH) for CPB only if HIT occurred more than 100 days prior.[1] In patients with current HIT who require urgent cardiac surgery, delay the procedure until HIT antibodies are negative if possible.[4] If not, consider off-pump surgical technique and use alternative anticoagulants (requirements are decreased). If CPB is required, there are two basic approaches. First, consider use of alternative anticoagulants. The ideal agent remains uncertain.[6] Options include a hirudin preparation (lepirudin, or bivalirudin, a synthetic hirudin analog with a short half-life) or argatroban (a direct thrombin inhibitor).[6–8] Choose the particular agent based on availability, presence of hepatic or renal disease, and personal experience. Adjust the dose by intraoperative laboratory testing (ecarin clotting time [ECT] or ACT for argatroban.[1,6] As a second approach, administer heparin along with antiplatelet agents. Options include epoprostenol (a prostacyclin analogue) or tirofiban (glycoprotein IIb/IIIa antagonist; use is discouraged by manufacturer for this indication).[1,4] All of the anticoagulation alternative approaches pose risks including postoperative hemorrhagic complications (hirudin, argatroban, or tirofiban) and severe hypotension requiring vasopressor infusions to maintain hemodynamic stability (epoprostenol). Bivalirudin is currently approved in the United States for use in acute coronary syndromes and is used off-label in HIT; clinical reports suggest that the use of the ECT allows safe titration of this compound.[8] Due to its short half-life, there might be less postoperative bleeding than with other direct thrombin inhibitors.

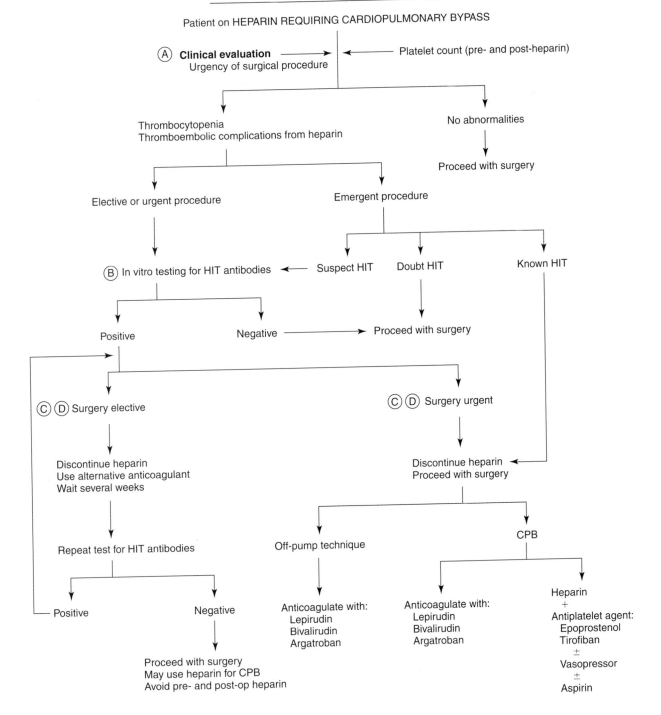

REFERENCES

1. Warkentin TE, Greinacher A: Heparin-induced thrombocytopenia and cardiac surgery, *Ann Thorac Surg* 76:638–648, 2003.
2. Warkentin TE: Heparin-induced thrombocytopenia: pathogenesis and management, *Br J Haematol* 121:535–555, 2003.
3. Hirsh J, Heddle N, Kelton JG: Treatment of heparin-induced thrombocytopenia. A critical review, *Arch Intern Med* 164:361–369, 2004.
4. Warkentin TE, Greinacher A: Heparin-induced thrombocytopenia: recognition, treatment, and prevention: the Seventh ACCP Conference on Antithrombotic and Thrombolytic Therapy, *Chest* 126 (3 Suppl):311S–337S, 2004.
5. Nuttall GA, Oliver WC Jr, Santrach PJ, et al.: Patients with a history of type II heparin-induced thrombocytopenia with thrombosis requiring cardiac surgery with cardiopulmonary bypass: a prospective observational case series, *Anesth Anesth* 96: 344–350, 2003.
6. Hassell K: The management of patients with heparin-induced thrombocytopenia who require anticoagulant therapy, *Chest* 127:1S–8S, 2005.
7. Edwards JT, Hamby JK, Worrall NK: Successful use of Argatroban as a heparin substitute during cardiopulmonary bypass: heparin-induced thrombocytopenia in a high-risk cardiac surgical patient, *Ann Thorac Surg* 75:1622–1624, 2003.
8. Koster A, Chew D, Grundel M, et al.: Bivalirudin monitored with the ecarin clotting time for anticoagulation during cardiopulmonary bypass, *Anesth Analg* 96:383–386, 2003.

PREOPERATIVE RENAL PROBLEMS

RENAL INSUFFICIENCY

ANESTHESIA FOR DIALYSIS-DEPENDENT
PATIENT

Renal Insufficiency

PER-OLOF JARNBERG, M.D., PH.D.

LOIS L. BREADY, M.D.

Patients with renal insufficiency span a wide spectrum of dysfunction, from mild subclinical reduction of creatinine clearance (C_{cr}) to chronic renal failure (CRF) and end-stage renal disease (ESRD). There are multiple causes of CRF, for instance: Ig-A nephropathy, systemic lupus erythematosus (SLE), diabetes, hypertension (HTN), and polycystic kidney disease, some of which carry implications of multisystem involvement and dysfunction. One of the biggest challenges for the anesthesiologist is to avoid worsening of renal failure (RF) in non-ESRD patients undergoing surgery. Preexisting renal dysfunction, diabetes, type of procedure (cardiopulmonary bypass, aortic cross-clamp), nephrotoxin exposure (contrast media, nonsteroidal antiinflammatory drugs, aminoglycoside and other antibiotics), and unstable hemodynamics are all known risk factors for development or worsening of RF perioperatively.

A. Pathophysiologic effects of CRF-induced uremia include:

- Anemia due to depressed erythropoietin production. Treatment with recombinant human erythropoietin normalizes the hematocrit and avoids repetitive transfusions.
- Coagulopathy due to abnormal platelet function, secondary to defective release of von Willebrand factor and factor VIII from capillary endothelium. The thrombocytopathy is improved by dialysis but can, for emergent surgeries, be treated with DDAVP (0.3 μg/kg IV) and cryoprecipitate.
- Peripheral neuropathy and autonomic nervous system dysfunction, decreasing or abolishing cardiac response to hypotension.
- Electrolyte abnormalities including hyperkalemia, hypermagnesemia, hyperphosphatemia, and hypocalcemia. Postpone elective surgery if potassium (K+) levels are above 5.5 to 6 mEq/L. Temporary treatments for hyperkalemia include glucose/insulin infusion, correction of metabolic acidosis with HCO_3^-, terbutaline infusion, and $CaCl_2$.
- HTN, coronary artery disease (CAD), congestive heart failure (CHF), left ventricular hypertrophy, and pericardial effusion.
- Increased susceptibility to infections, exacerbated by the use of steroids and immunosuppressive agents in renal transplant patients.
- Impaired gastric emptying, increasing the risk for aspiration.
- Changed pharmacokinetics and pharmacodynamics of anesthetic agents due to impaired renal excretion, increased volume of distribution, and decreased plasma-protein binding.

B. Glomerular filtration rate (GFR), measured by C_{cr}, is usually evaluated by serum creatinine. A 50% reduction of GFR is necessary before serum creatinine starts to rise. At a GFR of 10 to 30 ml/min, patients develop uremia, metabolic acidosis, anemia, hyperkalemia, and coagulopathy, which all become more severe in ESRD (GFR of 10 to 0 ml/min).

Ⓐ Patient with RENAL INSUFFICIENCY

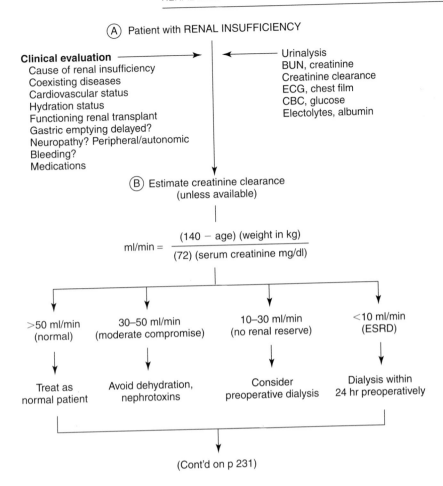

Clinical evaluation
 Cause of renal insufficiency
 Coexisting diseases
 Cardiovascular status
 Hydration status
 Functioning renal transplant
 Gastric emptying delayed?
 Neuropathy? Peripheral/autonomic
 Bleeding?
 Medications

Urinalysis
BUN, creatinine
Creatinine clearance
ECG, chest film
CBC, glucose
Electolytes, albumin

Ⓑ Estimate creatinine clearance
   (unless available)

$$\text{ml/min} = \frac{(140 - \text{age}) \, (\text{weight in kg})}{(72) \, (\text{serum creatinine mg/dl})}$$

>50 ml/min (normal)	30–50 ml/min (moderate compromise)	10–30 ml/min (no renal reserve)	<10 ml/min (ESRD)
Treat as normal patient	Avoid dehydration, nephrotoxins	Consider preoperative dialysis	Dialysis within 24 hr preoperatively

(Cont'd on p 231)

C. Preoperative evaluation should focus on the degree of renal function impairment, cardiac function/HTN, neurological dysfunction, location of shunts/fistulas, and frequency and date of last dialysis (intravascular volume, K+ level, and bleeding status). If extensive blood loss or volume shifts are anticipated or if there is significant cardiac or pulmonary disease, monitor central hemodynamics. Consider evaluating platelet function, by measuring bleeding time or use of thromboelastography, if invasive monitoring or regional anesthesia is planned. Keep in mind that peripheral arteries may be needed for future vascular access to dialysis.

D. Potent inhalational anesthetics cause significant, reversible decreases of GFR, electrolyte secretion, and urine output. These changes are mediated either directly, by changes in renal blood flow (RBF), renal vascular resistance (RVR), GFR, and tubular function, or indirectly, by changes in cardiovascular function and neuroendocrine activity. RBF is maintained during clinical levels of anesthesia through decreases is RVF in PVR, offsetting the effects of a lowered perfusion pressure.[1] Of the modern anesthetics desflurane, isoflurane, and sevoflurane, only the latter produces moderately high plasma levels of inorganic fluoride (F-).[2-6] Despite F- levels sometimes reaching the nephrotoxic threshold of 50 µM, deterioration of renal function has not been demonstrated by soda lime and barium hydroxide lime to a substance known as compound A, which is nephrotoxic in rats at an exposure rate of 180 ppm/hour to occur.[5] Compound A generation does not seem to constitute a significant clinical problem.[5] Sevoflurane has been given to tens of millions of patients in the United States without a single report of nephrotoxicity.[6] Avoid giving succinylcholine to neuropathic or hyperkalemic (K+ > 5.5 mEq/L) patients. Instead, choose a nondepolarizing relaxant that is not primarily renally excreted.

REFERENCES

1. Hysing ES, Chelly JE, Doursout MF, et al.: Comparative effects of halothane, enflurane and isoflurane at equihypotensive doses on cardiac performance and coronary and renal blood flows in chronically instrumented dogs, *Anesthesiology* 76:979–984, 1992.
2. Frink EJ Jr, Malan TP Jr, Isner J, et al.: Renal concentrating function with prolonged sevoflurane or enflurane anesthesia in volunteers, *Anesthesiology* 80:1019–1025, 1994.
3. Nishiyama T, Hirasaki A: Effects of sevoflurane anaesthesia on renal function—duration of administration and area under the curve and rate of decrease of serum inorganic fluoride, *Eur J Anaesthesiol* 12: 477–482, 1995.
4. Conzen PF, Nuscheler M, Melotte A, et al.: Renal function and serum fluoride concentrations in patients with stable renal insufficiency after anesthesia with sevoflurane or enflurane, *Anesth Analg* 81:569–575, 1995.
5. Gonsowski CT, Laster MJ, Eger EI, et al.: Toxicity of compound A in rats: Effect of a 3-hour administration, *Anesthesiology* 80: 556–565, 1994.
6. Bedford RF, Ives HE: The renal safety of sevoflurane, *Anesth Analg* 90:505–508, 2000.

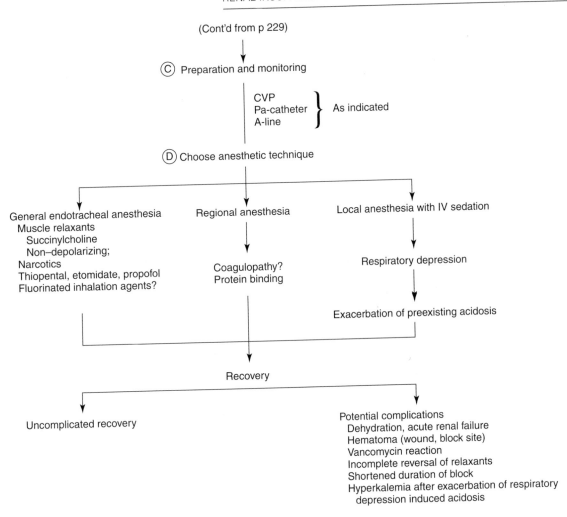

(Cont'd from p 229)

C Preparation and monitoring

CVP
Pa-catheter } As indicated
A-line

D Choose anesthetic technique

General endotracheal anesthesia   Regional anesthesia   Local anesthesia with IV sedation
  Muscle relaxants
    Succinylcholine
    Non–depolarizing;
  Narcotics   Respiratory depression
  Thiopental, etomidate, propofol   Coagulopathy?
  Fluorinated inhalation agents?   Protein binding

                                                                  Exacerbation of preexisting acidosis

                              Recovery

Uncomplicated recovery   Potential complications
                                                 Dehydration, acute renal failure
                                                 Hematoma (wound, block site)
                                                 Vancomycin reaction
                                                 Incomplete reversal of relaxants
                                                 Shortened duration of block
                                                 Hyperkalemia after exacerbation of respiratory
                                                   depression induced acidosis

Anesthesia for Dialysis-Dependent Patient

PER-OLOF JARNBERG, M.D., PH.D.

LOIS L. BREADY, M.D.

Patients on dialysis are in a precarious state of homeostasis and vulnerable to even small errors of omission or lack of detail in their care. Perioperatively, significant morbidity in these chronically ill patients may result from hyperkalemia, hypervolemia or hypovolemia, cardiac decompensation, pneumonia, atelectasis, shunt or fistula occlusion, bleeding, and wound infection. Hemodialysis and peritoneal dialysis correct some of the abnormalities of uremia (water and electrolyte imbalances, neurological abnormalities, or uremic coagulopathy) but do not correct others (renin-induced hypertension [HTN], anemia, and immunodeficiency). Hemodialysis also introduces the problems of hypovolemia and additional bleeding from heparinization. Administer fluids and electrolytes to the patients judiciously, because urine output and pharmacodynamic changes include reduced excretion of drugs and metabolites (prolonged effect), decreased protein binding (increased pharmacological effect due to increased amount of free drug), increased total body water (larger volume of distribution than normal), and potentiation of muscle relaxants by hypokalemia or hypermagnesemia. Common operative procedures include creation or revision of vascular or peritoneal access, as well as other routine surgical procedures.

A. Determine the patient's usual dialysis schedule and the time of the most recent dialysis. Estimate volume status by usual clinical findings and from predialysis and postdialysis weights. Unless the clinical evaluation indicates otherwise, a volume of IV fluid equivalent to one-half of the weight removed may usually be given safely, in addition to replacement of operative losses. Continue medication as needed for concomitant diseases (HTN or cardiac illness) and manage diabetic agents as required for glucose homeostasis. Dialysis patients may be hepatitis B or hepatitis C positive. Use universal precautions and be mindful that these patients may have liver function impairment as well.

B. Employ standard American Society of Anesthesiologists (ASA) monitors, and add invasive monitors as needed.

C. Do not use meperidine as a premedication drug because of its potential for prolonged effect as well as its metabolism to normeperidine, which may lower the seizure threshold.[1] Single doses of morphine do not show any alteration in disposition. Chronic administration results in accumulation of its 6-glucuronide metabolite, which is more potent than morphine itself.[1,2] Fentanyl, which lacks active metabolites, has unchanged free drug fraction, and unchanged redistribution, seems to be an excellent choice. Intermediate duration nondepolarizing muscle relaxants have distinct advantages in end-stage renal disease (ESRD) patients because of reduced risks for prolonged block. The pharmacokinetics of cis-atracurium, which is eliminated by Hoffman degradation in plasma, is unaffected in ESRD, making it an attractive choice.[3]

D. Use anesthetic agents that are not primarily excreted renally. If a regional technique is planned, evaluate for residual heparinization (partial thromboplastin time [PTT], international normalized ratio [INR]). Comparison of different anesthesia techniques (local infiltration, brachial plexus blockade, and general anesthesia) for forearm fistula surgery has not revealed any differences in outcome.[4] Do not use succinylcholine if potassium (K^+) > 5.5 mEq/L.

E. During the perioperative period, patients may be hypercoagulable. In addition, platelets adhere to graft material, contributing to the potential of clotting the vascular access. Position the well-padded extremity with vascular access so that periodic palpitation of the thrill is possible. Document presence on the chart. The access extremity should not be used for BP monitoring during anesthesia because of the risk of thrombosis.

REFERENCES

1. Chan GLC, Matzke GR: Effects of renal insufficiency on the pharmacokinetics and pharmacodynamics of opioid analgesics, *Drug Intell Clin Pharm* 21:773–783, 1987.
2. Kurella M, Bennett WM, Chertow GM: Analgesia in patients with ESRD: a review of available evidence, *Am J Kidney Dis* 42: 217–228, 2003.
3. Boyd AH, Eastwood NB, Parker CJ, et al.: Pharmacodynamics of the 1R cis-1'R cis isomer of atracurium (51W89) in health and chronic renal failure, *Br J Anaesth* 74:400–404, 1995.
4. Solomonson MD, Johnson ME, Ilstrup D: Risk factors in patients having surgery to create an arteriovenous fistula, *Anesth Analg* 79:694–700, 1994.

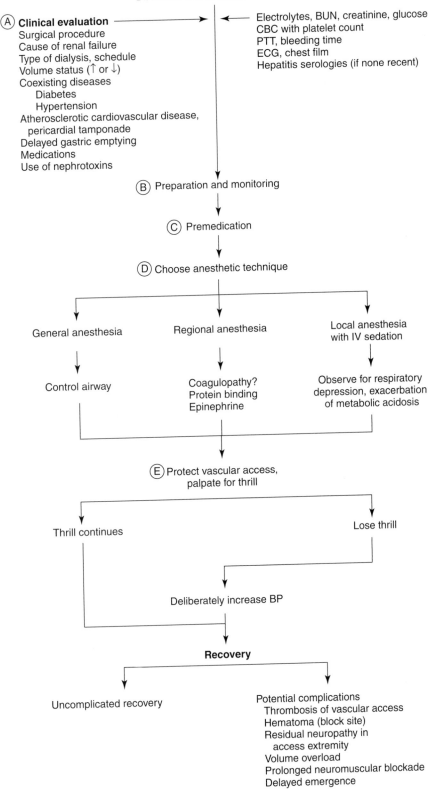

DIALYSIS-DEPENDENT PATIENT

Ⓐ **Clinical evaluation**
Surgical procedure
Cause of renal failure
Type of dialysis, schedule
Volume status (↑ or ↓)
Coexisting diseases
    Diabetes
    Hypertension
Atherosclerotic cardiovascular disease,
  pericardial tamponade
Delayed gastric emptying
Medications
Use of nephrotoxins

Electrolytes, BUN, creatinine, glucose
CBC with platelet count
PTT, bleeding time
ECG, chest film
Hepatitis serologies (if none recent)

Ⓑ Preparation and monitoring

Ⓒ Premedication

Ⓓ Choose anesthetic technique

General anesthesia   Regional anesthesia   Local anesthesia
                                                         with IV sedation

Control airway   Coagulopathy?   Observe for respiratory
                            Protein binding   depression, exacerbation
                            Epinephrine   of metabolic acidosis

Ⓔ Protect vascular access,
  palpate for thrill

Thrill continues   Lose thrill

                    Deliberately increase BP

Recovery

Uncomplicated recovery   Potential complications
                                    Thrombosis of vascular access
                                    Hematoma (block site)
                                    Residual neuropathy in
                                      access extremity
                                    Volume overload
                                    Prolonged neuromuscular blockade
                                    Delayed emergence

OTHER PREOPERATIVE PROBLEMS

HIV AND ACQUIRED IMMUNODEFICIENCY
SYNDROME (AIDS)

NEUROFIBROMATOSIS

MARFAN SYNDROME (MFS)

MUCOPOLYSACCHARIDOSES (MPS)

EPIDERMOLYSIS BULLOSA (EB)

RHEUMATOID ARTHRITIS (RA)

ANKYLOSING SPONDYLITIS (AS)

CANCER PATIENT

EATING DISORDERS

MUNCHAUSEN'S SYNDROME

THERMAL INJURY

JEHOVAH'S WITNESS PATIENT

ALLERGIC REACTIONS

LATEX ALLERGY

SYSTEMIC LUPUS ERYTHEMATOSUS (SLE)

HIV and Acquired Immunodeficiency Syndrome (AIDS)

MALCOLM D. ORR, M.D., Ph.D.

Acquired immunodeficiency syndrome (AIDS) was identified clinically in 1981, although analyses of stored sera show that some patients who died in 1969 had antibodies to the human T cell leukemia virus III (HTLV III), now called human immunodeficiency virus (HIV). The immune deficiency allows normal commensal organisms (e.g., *Pneumocystis carinii, Candida*) to produce overwhelming infections. Tuberculosis (TB) is an additional problem in patients infected with HIV. Kaposi's sarcoma, usually a disease of the elderly, afflicts AIDS patients 30 to 40 years of age. The syndrome represents the end stage of this disease; it is likely that healthy carriers without stigmata are the most infectious to health care workers. Transmission occurs from contact with body fluids of an infected individual—this can be by venereal contact, by shared injection needles, and through blood and blood products. Risk of infection with AIDS from a transfusion is now 1:1,000,000. There is one reported case of a dentist who appears to have transmitted HIV to several of his patients. However, he was also a patient in his own office, so these cases potentially involve patient-to-patient transmission. Health care workers are at risk from patients, and deaths are reported from occupation-acquired HIV. Malnutrition and poor sanitation may be related to some cases of disease transmission. At present, there is no known cure. However, in the United States, HIV and AIDS deaths are decreasing due to antiretroviral therapy, and the disease has become a long-term chronic disorder in many patients.[1-6]

A. Perform a thorough history and physical examination. Review all medications; note possible drug interactions. The incubation period is thought to be 2 to 5 years. There are two serologic tests for HIV: the enzyme-linked immunosorbent assay (ELISA) and an electrophoretic technique (Western blot). The presence of antibody to HIV indicates exposure to the virus and is not a test for the presence of disease. The latent period between infection and disease can be as long as 11 years.

B. Use Centers for Disease Control (CDC) universal, recommended barrier precautions for all patients. Glove or double-glove when coming into contact with mucous membranes or fluids. Use disposable supplies, including breathing circuits. Select appropriate monitors as determined by the physical status of the patient and the requirements of the surgical and anesthetic procedures. Recall that the AIDS patient is immunocompromised; use sterile techniques during placement of invasive monitors. Avoid needle sticks by disposing of used needles before recapping them.

C. Choose an anesthetic technique appropriate for the procedure and acceptable to the patient. Follow blood-borne pathogens recommendations. It is suggested that pregnant health care workers not give direct care to AIDS patients because of the potential for teratogenic effects of viruses (e.g., cytomegalovirus) that commonly infect AIDS patients. Wear gloves, particularly when intubating and inserting IV catheters. There is some controversy over the need to wear eye protection routinely, but other viruses are transmissible via "conjunctival splash." Use of goggles by anesthetists, surgeons, and others working near an open wound is probably wise. Treat blood samples sent intraoperatively (e.g., ABGs) as potentially infectious.

D. In the recovery period use CDC universal blood and body fluid precautions. Wash hands with soap and water before and after contact with known or suspected HIV patients. Clean the anesthesia machine and reusable anesthesia equipment with a dilute solution of sodium hypochlorite (bleach, 1:80 with water). Sterilize lensed optical instruments with ethylene oxide or glutaraldehyde. Label and incinerate disposable supplies. Refer needle stick injuries as soon as possible to the employee health service for the potential implementation of multiple agent therapy.

REFERENCES

1. Hughes SC: HIV and anesthesia, *Anesthesiology Clin North Am* 22:379–404, 2004.
2. Centers for Disease Control: Update: universal precautions for prevention of transmission of human immunodeficiency virus, hepatitis B virus, and other blood-borne pathogens in health-care settings, *MMWR* 37:377, 1988, available at: http://www.cdc.gov/mmwr/preview/mmwrhtml/00000039.htm.
3. Cordero AS, Bonner JT, Brynes RK: AIDS and the anaesthetist, *Can Anaesth Soc J* 32:45–48, 1985.
4. Kelen GD, DiGiovanna T, Bisson L, et al.: Human immunodeficiency virus infection in emergency department patients: Epidemiology, clinical presentations, and risk to health care workers: the Johns Hopkins experience, *JAMA* 262:516–522, 1989.
5. Evron S, Glezerman M, Harow E, et al.: Human immunodeficiency virus: anesthetic and obstetric considerations, *Anesth Analg* 98 (2):503–511, 2004.
6. Avidan MS, Jones N, Pozniak AL: The implications of HIV for the anaesthetist and the intensivist, *Anaesthesia* 55 (4):344–354, 2000.

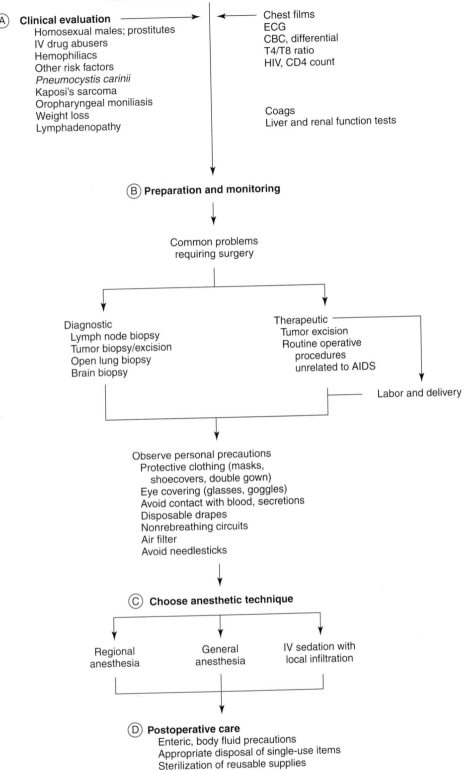

Patient with KNOWN OR SUSPECTED AIDS

(A) **Clinical evaluation**
  Homosexual males; prostitutes
  IV drug abusers
  Hemophiliacs
  Other risk factors
  Pneumocystis carinii
  Kaposi's sarcoma
  Oropharyngeal moniliasis
  Weight loss
  Lymphadenopathy

Chest films
ECG
CBC, differential
T4/T8 ratio
HIV, CD4 count

Coags
Liver and renal function tests

(B) **Preparation and monitoring**

Common problems
requiring surgery

Diagnostic
  Lymph node biopsy
  Tumor biopsy/excision
  Open lung biopsy
  Brain biopsy

Therapeutic
  Tumor excision
  Routine operative
    procedures
    unrelated to AIDS

Labor and delivery

Observe personal precautions
  Protective clothing (masks,
    shoecovers, double gown)
  Eye covering (glasses, goggles)
  Avoid contact with blood, secretions
  Disposable drapes
  Nonrebreathing circuits
  Air filter
  Avoid needlesticks

(C) **Choose anesthetic technique**

Regional
anesthesia

General
anesthesia

IV sedation with
local infiltration

(D) **Postoperative care**
  Enteric, body fluid precautions
  Appropriate disposal of single-use items
  Sterilization of reusable supplies

Neurofibromatosis

CELIA I. KAYE, M.D., PH.D.

TOD B. SLOAN, M.D., PH.D.

Of the several forms of neurofibromatosis, Von Recklinghausen disease (NF1) and NF2 are the best delineated. NF1 is an autosomal dominant neurocutaneous syndrome occurring at a frequency of 1 in 3000 (50% are new mutations). For clinical diagnosis of NF1, patients must exhibit two of the following: six café au lait macules; two neurofibromas or one plexiform neurofibroma; freckling in the axillary or inguinal regions; a tumor of the optic pathway; two or more Lisch nodules (iris hamartomas); a distinctive bony lesion, such as thinning of a long bone cortex, with or without pseudarthrosis; or a first-degree relative who meets the above criteria for NF1.[1] Clinical manifestations range in severity and usually progress with time, but these criteria identify >90% of children with NF1 under age 6 years.[2] Neurofibromas are uncommon at birth put proliferate in adolescence. Of patients with NF1, 50% have neurological manifestations from nerve or spinal compression, and one third have debilitating symptoms.[3] Patients with NF1 occasionally have pheochromocytoma, meningioma, glioma, renal artery dysplasia with hypertension (HTN), and hypoglycemia, and 10% have diffuse interstitial pulmonary fibrosis. Using a protein truncation assay, NF1 can be confirmed in two thirds of familial and sporadic cases.[4] Presymptomatic diagnosis is possible in some familial cases by the use of linkage analysis or direct gene mutation analysis.

NF2, a rare disorder affecting approximately 1 in 40,000, is caused by mutations of the NF2 gene on chromosome 22q12. These patients have bilateral vestibular schwannomas and may also have meningiomas, schwannomas of the dorsal roots of the spinal cord, or gliomas. Café au lait spots, cutaneous neurofibromas, and many of the other associated problems of NF1 are rare in NF2.

A. Preoperatively, identify problems resulting from critically located fibromas or associated disorders.[5,6] Look for kyphoscoliosis, renal artery dysplasia with HTN, bone cysts, pulsating exophthalmos, sarcomatous change, spinal nerve compression, laryngeal stenosis, hydrocephalus, diffuse interstitial pulmonary fibrosis, pulmonary stenosis, epilepsy, deafness, and glaucoma (all reported complications of NF1). Up to 5% of patients with NF1 have intraoral lesions (tongue or larynx) or cervical lesions leading to intubation or airway difficulty. If there is dyspnea or dysphonia, perform indirect laryngoscopy preoperatively. The most dangerous unrecognized conditions are pheochromocytoma, obstructed outflow of the RV, hydrocephalus (aqueductal stenosis), and laryngeal obstruction.[6] Scoliosis is the most common bony manifestation of NF1; up to 60% of patients have a spinal abnormality. Spinal deformity resulting from subperiosteal fibromas, fractures, and bone cyst formation can result in structural deformities, spinal cord compression, and paralysis. Cervical abnormalities (stiff neck or limited range of motion) are increasingly common with increased degrees of spinal curvature (short, kyphotic thoracic or lumbar curves measuring >65E degrees). In these patients, the cervical cord is prone to damage with manipulation; obtain preoperative neck films. Assess pulmonary function if clinically indicated. HTN associated with NF1 (6% patients) is probably caused by renal artery stenosis or aortic coarctation in children and pheochromocytoma in adults (1 to 13%). Intracranial tumors occur in 5 to 50% of patients and account for most disease-related problems. Identify intracranial pathology and any associated reduction in intracranial compliance preoperatively. Look for endocrine dysfunction: pituitary or hypothalamic growths, hyperparathyroidism. Intestinal tumors are commonly seen in NF1, especially in the duodenum or ampulla of Vater. Malignant progression occurs in 2 to 16% of neurofibromas in NF1.

B. Patients may present for nerve decompression, excision of pheochromocytoma, repair of renal artery stenosis, obstructive uropathy, or pathological fractures, in addition to surgical procedures unrelated to NF. Select monitors according to the severity of the disease and extent of planned surgical procedure. Recall that undiagnosed pheochromocytoma may become apparent, and be prepared to treat perioperative hypertensive crisis.

Patient with NEUROFIBROMATOSIS

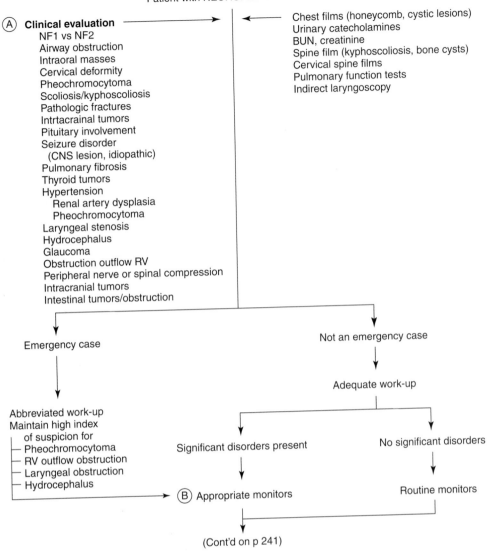

(A) **Clinical evaluation**
NF1 vs NF2
Airway obstruction
Intraoral masses
Cervical deformity
Pheochromocytoma
Scoliosis/kyphoscoliosis
Pathologic fractures
Intrtacrainal tumors
Pituitary involvement
Seizure disorder
  (CNS lesion, idiopathic)
Pulmonary fibrosis
Thyroid tumors
Hypertension
  Renal artery dysplasia
  Pheochromocytoma
Laryngeal stenosis
Hydrocephalus
Glaucoma
Obstruction outflow RV
Peripheral nerve or spinal compression
Intracranial tumors
Intestinal tumors/obstruction

Chest films (honeycomb, cystic lesions)
Urinary catecholamines
BUN, creatinine
Spine film (kyphoscoliosis, bone cysts)
Cervical spine films
Pulmonary function tests
Indirect laryngoscopy

Emergency case

Not an emergency case

Adequate work-up

Abbreviated work-up
Maintain high index
  of suspicion for
— Pheochromocytoma
— RV outflow obstruction
— Laryngeal obstruction
— Hydrocephalus

Significant disorders present

No significant disorders

(B) Appropriate monitors

Routine monitors

(Cont'd on p 241)

C. The anesthetic technique generally can be chosen with regard to the proposed operative procedure, the disease involvement, and the patient's wishes. Spinal anesthesia has been used successfully,[7] but spinal deformities may make spinal or epidural blockade difficult in some patients. Neurofibromas may make peripheral nerve block difficult. A variety of general anesthetics have been used successfully. Effects of succinylcholine (SCC), D-tubocurarine, and pancuronium may be prolonged; monitor neuromuscular blockade. Hypersensitivity, as well as resistance to SCC has been reported,[8] and hyperkalemia is possible if muscle denervation has occurred. If there is laryngeal involvement, anticipate a difficult mask airway and intubation with possible need for tracheostomy. Intraoperative arrhythmias have been reported in patients with renal artery stenosis. This may be due to an activated renin-angiotensin system, to angiotensin-mediated sympathetic effects, or to catecholamines from the adrenal medulla (pheochromocytoma).

REFERENCES

1. Neurofibromatosis. Conference statement. National Institutes of Health Consensus Development Conference, *Arch Neurol* 45:575–578, 1988.
2. Listernick R, Charrow J: Neurofibromatosis type 1 in childhood, *J Pediatr* 116:845–53, 1990.
3. Weinberg GL, editor: Genetics in anesthesiology: Syndromes and science, Boston, 1996, Butterworth-Heinemann.
4. Heim RA, Kam-Morgan LN, Binnie CG, et al.: Distribution of 13 truncating mutations in the neurofibromatosis 1 gene, *Hum Mol Genet* 4:975–81, 1995.
5. Delgado JM, de la Matta Martin MM: Anaesthetic implications of von Recklinghausen's neurofibromatosis, *Paediatr Anaesth* 12:374–379, 2002.
6. Hirsch NP, Murphy A, Radcliffe JJ: Neurofibromatosis: clinical presentations and anaesthetic implications, *Br J Anaesth* 86: 555–564, 2001.
7. Chang-Lo M: Laryngeal involvement in von Recklinghausen's disease: A case report and review of the literature. *Laryngoscope*; 87:435–42, 1977.
8. Fisher MM: Anaesthetic difficulties in neurofibromatosis, *Anaesthesia* 30:648–50, 1975.

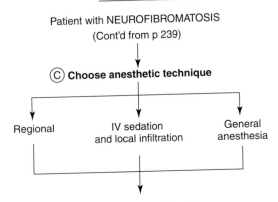

Patient with NEUROFIBROMATOSIS
(Cont'd from p 239)

Ⓒ **Choose anesthetic technique**

Regional   IV sedation   General
                  and local infiltration   anesthesia

Intraoperative considerations
   Difficult airway?
   Hydrocephalus?
   Airway obstruction?
   Hypertensive crisis (pheochromocytoma)
   Monitor ABG
   Decreased respiratory reserve (kyphoscoliosis)
   Positioning problems (kyphoscoliosis)
   Peripheral nerve compression from neurofibroma
   Dysrhythmias (increased with catecholamines
      and renal artery stenosis)
   Abnormal neuromuscular blockade

Postoperative considerations

Marfan Syndrome (MFS)

CELIA I. KAYE, M.D., PH.D.

TOD B. SLOAN, M.D., PH.D.

Marfan syndrome (MFS) is a hereditary disorder of connective tissue (autosomal dominant with a high degree of penetrance) caused by mutation of the fibrillin-1 gene on chromosome 15. The most conspicuous characteristic of MFS is increased length of the long bones (arm span exceeds height). Other abnormalities include arachnodactyly, joint laxity, decreased muscle tone, scant subcutaneous fat, high arched palate, pectus carinatum or excavatum, and pes planus. Scoliosis is common (40 to 70% of patients) but is severe in approximately 10% of patients, resulting in pulmonary dysfunction. Ocular findings include lens dislocation (usually upward), myopia, and retinal detachment. Cardiovascular (CV) complications (>95% of adults) include aortic disease (swelling and fragmentation of elastic fibers), leading to dissection and circulatory collapse, mitral valve prolapse (MVP) and mitral regurgitation (MR), aortic regurgitation (AR), aortic aneurysms, and dilation of the pulmonary artery (PA). The median age of death in MFS was 32 +/− 16 years in 1972 but was 41 +/− 18 years in a cohort studied in 1993, due primarily to better survival after cardiovascular surgery and early, prophylactic surgical intervention. More than 95% of deaths result from CV complications. The utility of beta-adrenergic blockade to delay or prevent severe aortic complications has been shown.[1-5]

A. Identify CV abnormalities preoperatively, particularly in children, in whom manifestations are often subtle (or less severe) but account for most perioperative mortality. Look for AR, MVP, MR, and aortic dissection or dilation. Although MR is the most common valvular abnormality, AR is the most severe. As many as 60% of patients have auscultatory evidence of valvular regurgitation or systolic clicks; however, as many as 80% have prolapse of the posterior mitral leaflet on echocardiography (echo). Because of the high incidence of valvular disease, administer prophylactic antibiotics to almost all patients. Echo or magnetic resonance imaging (MRI) helps to identify dilation of the aortic root, the first indication of dilation of the ascending aorta. The chest x-ray (CXR) is far less sensitive but may show normal vascular shadows with significant disease. Type II dilation of the ascending aorta is most common; rupture is often the cause of death. Treat preoperative hypertension (HTN) because of the aortic disease. Coronary insufficiency (medial necrosis of coronary arteries leads to progressive luminal narrowing) affects the vascular supply of the sinoatrial and atrioventricular nodes, leading to conduction defects and dysrhythmias. The ECG may show left atrial enlargement, left ventricular strain, bundle branch blocks, and axis shifts from pectus excavatum. Chest wall abnormalities (scoliosis, kyphoscoliosis, and pectus excavatum) are usually identified on the CXR; they may cause reduced pulmonary function with decreased forced vital capacity ([FVC] mean 52% of normal) and %FEV$_1$/FVC (mean 83% of normal). Reduced elastic tissue support causes early airway closure, emphysematous bronchogenic cysts, honeycomb lungs, and a tendency toward spontaneous pneumothorax.

B. Common operations for these patients include eye procedures (cataract extraction, repair of retinal detachment, or glaucoma), musculoskeletal repairs (hernias, scoliosis, joint dislocations, or correction of pectus carinatum), and CV corrections (aortic aneurysms, aortic valvular replacement, spontaneous pneumothorax, or pericardial tamponade).

C. The major intraoperative concern is management of CV disease. Optimize AR or MR appropriately. Intraoperative dysrhythmias are not uncommon. Be vigilant regarding potential dissection and dilation of the aorta. Institute measures to treat HTN, decrease the contractile force of the left ventricle, and blunt pulsatile flow and sudden increases in contractility. Consider beta-blockers or inhalational cardiac depressants for this purpose. During pregnancy, aortic dilation is associated with a marked increased risk of aortic rupture.[6] Temporomandibular joint (TMJ) laxity may make these patients susceptible to TMJ injury or dislocation during intubation, although such problems have not been reported. Position for surgery carefully; intraoperative ventilation may be difficult (scoliosis or joint laxity/dislocation). Because spontaneous pneumothorax is common, perform positive-pressure ventilation cautiously. Pectus excavatum may also make cannulation for extracorporeal bypass difficult or cause cardiac compression at sternal closure. Spinal or epidural anesthesia may be technically difficult to perform depending on the degree of scoliosis. Owing to the increased length or diameter of the spine, the CSF volume may be increased, necessitating larger than normal doses of local anesthetics.[7] Airway obstruction and difficult intubation have been reported, possibly due to structural changes, such as cleft palate.[8]

REFERENCES

1. De Paepe A, Devereux RB, Dietz HC, et al.: Revised diagnostic criteria for the Marfan syndrome, Am J Med Genet 62:417–426, 1996.
2. Coselli JS, LeMaire SA, Büket S: Marfan syndrome: The variability and outcome of operative management, J Vasc Surg 21:432–443, 1995.

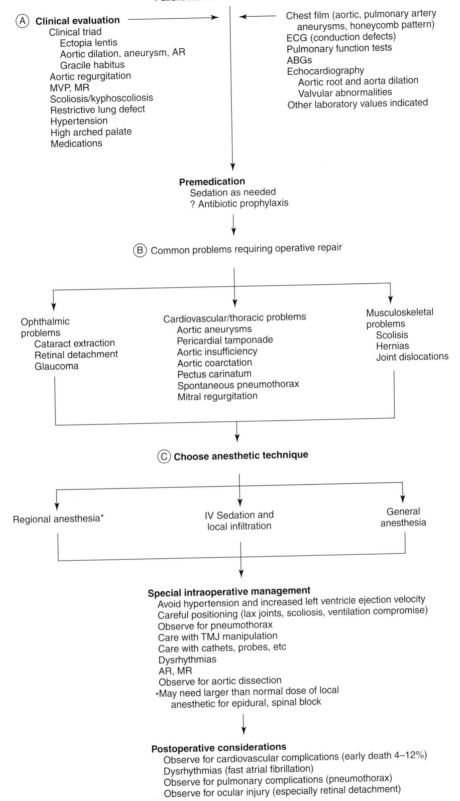

Patient with MARFAN SYNDROME

(A) Clinical evaluation
Clinical triad
Ectopia lentis
Aortic dilation, aneurysm, AR
Gracile habitus
Aortic regurgitation
MVP, MR
Scoliosis/kyphoscoliosis
Restrictive lung defect
Hypertension
High arched palate
Medications

Chest film (aortic, pulmonary artery
aneurysms, honeycomb pattern)
ECG (conduction defects)
Pulmonary function tests
ABGs
Echocardiography
Aortic root and aorta dilation
Valvular abnormalities
Other laboratory values indicated

Premedication
Sedation as needed
? Antibiotic prophylaxis

(B) Common problems requiring operative repair

Ophthalmic
problems
Cataract extraction
Retinal detachment
Glaucoma

Cardiovascular/thoracic problems
Aortic aneurysms
Pericardial tamponade
Aortic insufficiency
Aortic coarctation
Pectus carinatum
Spontaneous pneumothorax
Mitral regurgitation

Musculoskeletal
problems
Scolisis
Hernias
Joint dislocations

(C) **Choose anesthetic technique**

Regional anesthesia*

IV Sedation and
local infiltration

General
anesthesia

Special intraoperative management
Avoid hypertension and increased left ventricle ejection velocity
Careful positioning (lax joints, scoliosis, ventilation compromise)
Observe for pneumothorax
Care with TMJ manipulation
Care with cathets, probes, etc
Dysrhythmias
AR, MR
Observe for aortic dissection
*May need larger than normal dose of local
anesthetic for epidural, spinal block

Postoperative considerations
Observe for cardiovascular complications (early death 4–12%)
Dysrhythmias (fast atrial fibrillation)
Observe for pulmonary complications (pneumothorax)
Observe for ocular injury (especially retinal detachment)

3. Silverman DI, Burton KJ, Gray J, et al.: Life expectancy in the Marfan Syndrome, *Am J Cardiol* 75:157–160, 1995.
4. Zehr KJ, Orszulak TA, Mullany CJ, et al.: Surgery for aneurysms of the aortic root: a 30-year experience, *Circulation* 110 (11): 1364–1367, 2004.
5. Rossi-Foulkes R, Roman MJ, Rosen SE, et al.: Phenotypic features and impact of beta blocker or calcium antagonist therapy on aortic lumen size in the Marfan syndrome. *Am J Cardiol* 83: 1364–1368, 1999.
6. Elkayam U, Ostrzega E, Shotan A, et al.: Cardiovascular problems in pregnant women with the Marfan syndrome. *Ann Intern Med* 123:117–122, 1995.
7. Wells DG, Podolakin W: Anaesthesia and Marfan's syndrome: case report. *Can J Anaesth* 34:311–314, 1987.
8. Butler MG, Hayes BG, Hathaway MM, et al.: Specific genetic diseases at risk for sedation/anesthesia complications. *Anesth Analg* 91:837–855, 2000.

Mucopolysaccharidoses (MPS)

CELIA I. KAYE, M.D., PH.D.

TOD B. SLOAN, M.D., PH.D.

Mucopolysaccharidoses (MPS)[1] are hereditary diseases (mostly autosomal recessive) caused by enzyme deficiencies resulting in accumulation of complex carbohydrates called MPS or glycosaminoglycans. The specific disease depends on the specific enzyme defect (Table 1); severity varies with disorders and among patients with the same enzyme deficiency. The liver, spleen, and bones are among the sites of MPS storage. Hearing, vision, cardiac function, and intelligence may be affected. Hurler syndrome (I-H) is the prototypic form of the disease, in which manifestations are more severe.

A. Hurler patients are normal at birth but develop coarse facial features, hepatosplenomegaly, skeletal deformities, and developmental delay by 6 to 24 months. Patients with types I-S, II (mild), IV, and VII may have normal intelligence and life span. As newer forms of therapy have become available for some of these disorders (recombinant enzyme therapy,[2] hematopoietic stem cell transplantation[3]), the physical findings are modified, and cognitive functioning and life span have shown improvement. Patients with types I, II, IV, and VI are at highest risk during surgery (overall operative mortality 20%). Common preoperative problems are hypertension (pulmonary and systemic) and hepatic dysfunction secondary to hepatic MPS accumulation or right-sided heart failure. Mental status may be abnormal; determine the patient's ability to cooperate.

B. Assess the airway (the most common intraoperative problem). Hurler syndrome has been described as the *worst airway problem in pediatric anesthesia*[4], with MPS infiltration of soft tissues; micrognathia; decreased temporomandibular joint (TMJ) motion; anterior and cephalad larynx; narrowed nasopharynx; and copious, viscous secretions. The lower airway may also be abnormal owing to tracheomalacia. Spine films may assist examination of the airway and are needed to rule out atlantoaxial instability of the odontoid (seen in types IV, VI, and occasionally I-H) that will require neck stabilization during intubation.

C. Assess pulmonary function (chest x-ray, pulmonary function tests [PFTs], ABG). Pulmonary failure is the most common cause of perioperative death. Forced vital capacity, functional residual capacity, total lung capacity, and flow rates are decreased owing to tracheal pathology, restrictive disease (due to pectus excavatum or carinatum or kyphoscoliosis), and intrinsic pulmonary disease (from pulmonary hypoplasia, interstitial diffusion defects, microatelectasis, recurrent airway infections, and aspiration). Aggressive preoperative physiotherapy is important to optimize function.

D. Optimize preoperative cardiac function (digitalis, diuretics). Cardiac failure is the second most common cause of death (thickened valves and shortened chordae, abnormal myocardium and endocardium, and fatty streaks and fibrous plaques in the aorta and larger systemic arteries). Ischemia may also occur owing to narrowed coronary arteries from MPS deposition. Cardiac failure and valvular dysfunction require ECG, echocardiography (echo), and coronary angiography for complete evaluation.

E. Premedicate with anticholinergics (to reduce excessive secretions) and antibiotic prophylaxis when valvular defects are present. Give preoperative sedation cautiously; there are reports of resistance to drug effects as well as excessive respiratory depression (caution in patients with severe respiratory dysfunction).

Patient with MUCOPOLYSACCHARIDOSIS

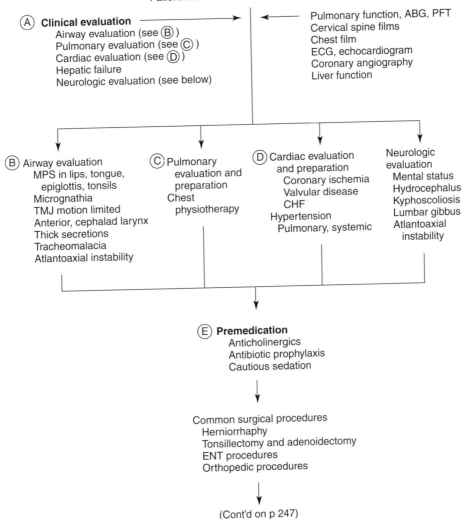

Ⓐ **Clinical evaluation**
   Airway evaluation (see Ⓑ)
   Pulmonary evaluation (see Ⓒ)
   Cardiac evaluation (see Ⓓ)
   Hepatic failure
   Neurologic evaluation (see below)

Pulmonary function, ABG, PFT
Cervical spine films
Chest film
ECG, echocardiogram
Coronary angiography
Liver function

Ⓑ Airway evaluation
   MPS in lips, tongue,
      epiglottis, tonsils
   Micrognathia
   TMJ motion limited
   Anterior, cephalad larynx
   Thick secretions
   Tracheomalacia
   Atlantoaxial instability

Ⓒ Pulmonary
   evaluation and
   preparation
   Chest
   physiotherapy

Ⓓ Cardiac evaluation
   and preparation
      Coronary ischemia
      Valvular disease
      CHF
   Hypertension
      Pulmonary, systemic

Neurologic
evaluation
   Mental status
   Hydrocephalus
   Kyphoscoliosis
   Lumbar gibbus
   Atlantoaxial
      instability

Ⓔ **Premedication**
   Anticholinergics
   Antibiotic prophylaxis
   Cautious sedation

Common surgical procedures
   Herniorrhaphy
   Tonsillectomy and adenoidectomy
   ENT procedures
   Orthopedic procedures

(Cont'd on p 247)

TABLE 1
Mucopolysaccharidoses

Type	Name	Organ involvement and features
I-H	Hurler	Heart, liver, spleen, bones, cornea, mental retardation, communicating hydrocephalus, death in childhood
I-S	Scheie	Aortic valve, cornea, retina, joint stiffness
I-HS	Hurler-Scheie	Intermediate I-H and I-S; normal intelligence
II	Hunter (severe)	Similar to I-H, without corneal clouding
II	Hunter (mild)	Slow progression, normal intelligence
III	Sanfilippo A, B, C, and D	Severe retardation, mild somatic changes
IV	Morquio A, B	Spondyloepiphyseal dysplasia, odontoid hypoplasia, cervical aortic valves, cornea, deafness, normal intelligence
VI	Maroteaux-Lamy	Bone, joints, cornea, liver, heart, cervical myelopathy, normal intelligence
VII	Sly	Liver, bone, cornea, decreased intelligence
IX		Periarticular masses, normal joint movement, normal intelligence

F. Because airway and pulmonary problems are common, local and regional techniques should be considered strongly. General anesthesia has been conducted successfully with inhalational induction, maintaining spontaneous ventilation, or IV induction with rapid acquisition of the airway. Intubation may be difficult in as many as 50% of patients; consider awake intubation with blind or fiberoptic techniques. Maintenance of mask airway may be difficult and an oral airway may not help. Tracheal patency may require neck extension if malacia is present. Oral intubation is generally preferred because of large adenoids and tonsils and friable nasal mucosa. Smaller than usual endotracheal tubes may be required due to narrowing of the laryngeal and tracheobronchial cartilages.[5–6] Emergent tracheostomy has also been reported as difficult.

G. Recovery from anesthesia is often slow and complicated by episodes of apnea, bronchospasm, cyanosis, and respiratory arrest.[4] Copious oral secretions, a rigid rib cage, and altered cardiorespiratory function can contribute to postoperative complications. Postoperative hypoglycemia has also been reported.

REFERENCES

1. Neufeld E, Muenzer J: The mucopolysaccharidoses. In: Scriver C, et al., editors: *The metabolic and molecular basis of inherited disease*, New York, 2001, McGraw-Hill.
2. Muenzer J, Lamsa JC, Garcia A, et al.: Enzyme replacement therapy in mucopolysaccharidosis type II (Hunter syndrome): a preliminary report, *Acta Paediatr Suppl* 439:98–99, 2002.
3. Krivit W: Stem cell bone marrow transplantation in patients with metabolic storage diseases, *Adv Pediatr* 49:359–378, 2002.
4. Sjögren P, Pedersen T, Steinmetz H: Mucopolysaccharidoses and anaesthetic risks, *Acta Anaesthesiol Scand* 31:214–218, 1987.
5. Butler MG, Hayes BG, Hathaway MM, et al.: Specific genetic diseases at risk for sedation/anesthesia complications, *Anesth Analg* 91:837–855, 2000.
6. Ard JK, Bekker A, Frempong-Boadu AK: Anesthesia for an adult with mucopolysaccharidosis I, *J Clin Anesth* 17:624-6, 2005.

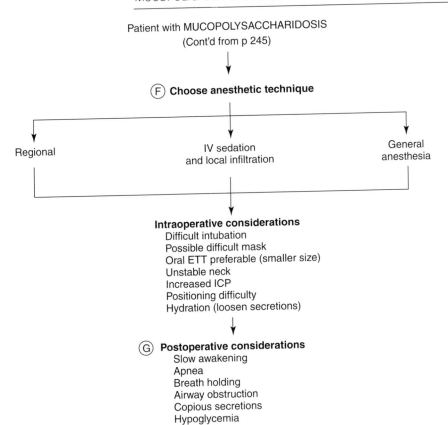

Patient with MUCOPOLYSACCHARIDOSIS
(Cont'd from p 245)

(F) **Choose anesthetic technique**

Regional   IV sedation   General
                  and local infiltration   anesthesia

Intraoperative considerations
    Difficult intubation
    Possible difficult mask
    Oral ETT preferable (smaller size)
    Unstable neck
    Increased ICP
    Positioning difficulty
    Hydration (loosen secretions)

(G) **Postoperative considerations**
    Slow awakening
    Apnea
    Breath holding
    Airway obstruction
    Copious secretions
    Hypoglycemia

Epidermolysis Bullosa (EB)

FRED J. SPIELMAN, M.D.

DAVID C. MAYER, M.D.

Epidermolysis bullosa (EB), first described in 1879, comprises a group of rare, genetically determined diseases characterized by cutaneous formation of skin and mucous membrane bullae and subsequent scarring after lateral shearing forces are applied to the affected skin (Table 1). EB mainly affects stratified squamous keratinizing epithelium of the skin. Severity of disease is determined more by the extent of the bullous lesions and subsequent complications than by the presence of scarring.[1]

A. Encourage frequent communication between the anesthesia care team, primary care providers, and surgeons. Carefully assess each patient; patients with EB often have associated diseases (Table 2). Patients suffer from oral and esophageal ulcers that result in a poor nutritional state, electrolyte imbalance, anemia, and secondary infection. As healing occurs, scarring can result in fixation of the tongue, microstomia, and esophageal strictures, which increase the risk of aspiration. Flexion contractures are common and affect hands, elbows, knees, and feet.[2] Chronic antibiotic therapy is common. Phenytoin and steroids may reduce bullae formation; consider "stress doses" for patients on chronic steroid therapy. Screen patients with dystrophic EB for evidence of dilated cardiomyopathy. Obtain echocardiographic studies prior to surgery in patients with cardiovascular symptoms. Although unclear, high carnitine concentrations may be a factor causing cardiac dysfunction.[3]

B. Patients with EB may present with any surgical condition, although the indications for surgery are often related to the complications of the disease. The most common operations include excision of skin tumors, dressing changes, insertion and revision of gastrostomy tubes, esophageal dilation, dental extractions and restorations, and hand surgery.[4]

C. Patients with EB are often self-conscious and apprehensive; establish good rapport with each patient. Take special care to prevent trauma to the skin and mucosa; even touching the skin can be painful. Allow the patient to move to and from the operating table. Apply hydrocortisone cream prophylactically to all sites where pressure or friction is likely to occur. Pad all equipment that touches the patient's skin with cotton. Remove creases from sheets. Avoid tape or any other adhesive (use nonadhesive ECG leads and pulse oximetry monitor). Do not use indwelling temperature probes, esophageal stethoscopes, and nasal or oral airways unless absolutely necessary. Secure IV and arterial catheters with gauze or sutures. Protect the skin from the BP cuff with cotton padding. Minimize heat loss from damaged skin by warming IV fluids, increasing OR temperature, and applying warm blankets.

D. No anesthetic technique has been shown to have an advantage over another; however, monitored anesthesia care is a suitable technique for many minor peripheral procedures. Ketamine provides rapid-onset analgesia and maintenance of pharyngeal-laryngeal reflexes. Potential deficiencies of this technique include a tendency to increased muscle tone, lack of analgesia to visceral stimulation, and postoperative dysphoria.[5] Venous access is invariably difficult and therefore inhalation induction is common. Succinylcholine-induced fasciculations leading to trauma and hyperkalemic responses in patients with dystrophic muscle are not confirmed.[6] Avoidance of thiopental because of an association of EB with porphyria is not substantiated by published data. Hypoalbuminemia and decreased protein binding may dictate decreased doses of drugs that are protein bound, such as muscle relaxants.

TABLE 1
Types of Epidermolysis Bullosa

Epidermolysis bullosa simplex
Usually autosomal dominant
Benign course, normal development, no mucosal involvement, onset sometimes later in life

Epidermolysis bullosa dystrophica (hyperdysplastic, polydysplastic)
Involves skin and mucosal surfaces
Severe scarring, fusion of digits
Survival past second decade rare

Junctional epidermolysis bullosa
Autosomal recessive
Survival beyond childhood rare
Death from sepsis

TABLE 2
Coexisting Problems in Epidermolysis Bullosa

Chronic infections
Hypercoagulable states
Hypoalbuminemia
Amyloidosis
Multiple myeloma
Diabetes mellitus
Electrolyte abnormalities
Malnutrition
Chronic pain
Dilated cardiomyopathy
Renal dysfunction

Patient with EPIDERMOLYSIS BULLOSA

(A) **Clinical evaluation**
  Coexisting problems
  Review old anesthesia records
  Steroid, phenytoin therapy?
  Contractions of hands, feet
  Careful airway examination
  Microstomia, ankyloglossia,
    esophageal strictures
  Dystrophic changes in teeth,
    hair, nails

Urinalysis
Chest film
Other laboratory values and
  procedures as indicated by
  coexisting problems

(B) **Common operative procedures**
  • Esophageal dilation
  • Dental extractions and restorations
  • Release of contractures, correction
    of pseudosyndactyly, amputations
  • Excision of skin tumors
  • Dressing change

Preparation
  • Communication between
    perioperative team
  • Chronic steroid therapy—"stress"
    steroid coverage
  • Adequate padding
  • Antibiotics
  • Medication for aspiration prophylaxis

(C) **Monitoring: safe minimum**
  • No tape or adhesives
  • Gentle skin preparation
  • Gauze or sutures to secure IV line
  • No esophageal stethoscope or
    temperature probes

(D) **Choose anesthetic technique**

(Cont'd on p 251)

E. Airway management for general anesthesia can pose formidable problems. Patients may have microstomia, poor dentition, esophageal stenosis, and distorted pharyngeal and laryngeal anatomy. Contractures may limit neck flexion and head extension. Tongue mobility may be limited by its adhesion to the floor of the mouth. Choose between intubation and mask anesthesia based on factors such as estimated surgical time and the pressure required to maintain a mask fit. If a tight mask fit is necessary, lubricate the mask to protect the face.[7] If intubating, use a smaller-than-predicted endotracheal tube (ETT); lubricate the shaft and cuff with a water-based gel. Inflate the cuff to maintain its shape but ensure a leak. For laryngeal mask airway (LMA) use, be sure to lubricate the LMA and insert it with extreme care.[8] Gently extubate the patient and note any presence of stridor, which may indicate airway swelling or bullae formation.

F. Regional anesthesia has the advantages of avoidance of airway manipulation and the potential for prolonged postoperative analgesia.[9] Fear of infection and tissue sloughing after skin preparation and local anesthetic infiltration is no longer a concern for most anesthesiologists. Safety and success have been achieved with various regional blocks, including axillary, digital, caudal, lateral cutaneous nerve blocks, spinal, and epidural. Clean the skin by soaking, spraying, or pouring the antiseptic solution over the skin. Avoid subcutaneous infiltration of local anesthetic.

REFERENCES

1. Tamayo L: Epidermolysis bullosa. In: Ruiz-Maldonado R, Parish LC, Beare JM, editors: *Textbook of pediatric dermatology*, Philadelphia, 1989, Grune & Stratton.
2. Boughton R, Crawford MR, Vonwiller JB: Epidermolysis bullosa: a review of 15 years' experience, including experience with combined general and regional anaesthetic techniques, *Anaesth Intensive Care* 16:260–264, 1988.
3. Sidwell RU, Yates R, Atherton D: Dilated cardiomyopathy in dystrophic epidermolysis bullosam, *Arch Dis Child* 83:59–63, 2000.
4. Iohom G, Lyons B: Anaesthesia for children with epidermolysis bullosa: a review of 20 years' experience, *Eur J Anaesthesiol* 18: 745–754, 2001.
5. Lin AN, Lateef F, Kelly R, et al.: Anesthetic management in epidermolysis bullosa: review of 129 anesthetic episodes in 32 patients, *J Am Acad Dermatol* 30:412–416, 1994.
6. Ames WA, Mayou BJ, Williams KN: Anaesthetic management of epidermolysis bullosa, *Br J Anaesth* 82:746–751, 1999.
7. Partridge BL: Skin and bone disorders. In Katz J, Benumof JL, Kadis LB, editors: *Anesthesia and uncommon diseases*, Philadelphia, 1990, W.B. Saunders.
8. Griffin RP, Mayou BJ: The anaesthetic management of patients with dystrophic epidermolysis bullosa. A review of 44 patients over a 10-year period. *Anaesthesia* 48:810–815, 1993.
9. Patch MR, Woodey RD: Spinal anaesthesia in a patient with epidermolysis bullosa dystrophica, *Anaesth Intensive Care* 28: 446–448, 2000.

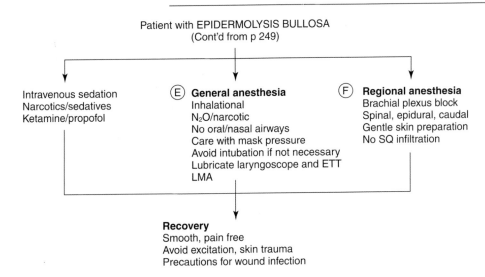

Patient with EPIDERMOLYSIS BULLOSA
(Cont'd from p 249)

Intravenous sedation
Narcotics/sedatives
Ketamine/propofol

(E) **General anesthesia**
Inhalational
N$_2$O/narcotic
No oral/nasal airways
Care with mask pressure
Avoid intubation if not necessary
Lubricate laryngoscope and ETT
LMA

(F) **Regional anesthesia**
Brachial plexus block
Spinal, epidural, caudal
Gentle skin preparation
No SQ infiltration

Recovery
Smooth, pain free
Avoid excitation, skin trauma
Precautions for wound infection

Rheumatoid Arthritis (RA)

MARY ANN GURKOWSKI, M.D.

CHRISTOPHER A. BRACKEN, M.D., Ph.D.

Rheumatoid arthritis (RA) is a systemic, autoimmune, chronic inflammatory disease marked by genetic predisposition and exacerbations and remissions.[1] It most often starts between the ages of 25 and 55 and affects women three times as often as men.[2] The prevalence of RA in the United States is estimated to be between 0.3 to 1.5% Patients suffer from a chronic polyarthritis involving the temporomandibular joint (TMJ), cricoarytenoid, costochondral junction, cervical spine, shoulders, elbows, hips, knees, feet, and hands.[3,4] This disease also involves the heart, lungs, blood vessels, eyes, skin, and kidneys.

A. Evaluate the patient's history for comorbidities and medications, physical examination, and pertinent lab results. Carefully evaluate the airway. Patients with throat fullness, tightness or foreign body sensation, hoarseness, stridor, dysphagia, pain with swallowing, dyspnea, or pain radiating to the ears are most likely to have TMJ or cricoarytenoid joint involvement or both. Evaluate the neck for range of motion, symptoms of vertebral insufficiency or neurological deficit on extension or flexion and subluxation. Patients may complain of occipital headaches caused by entrapment of the C1–C2 roots, dysphagia, dysphonia, or diplopia caused by cranial nerve compression with vertical atlantoaxial subluxation (AAS—a distance of < 3 mm from the anterior arch of the atlas to the odontoid process on lateral neck films), persistent pain in the neck and arms caused by radicular entrapment at the subaxial level, involuntary movements of the extremities, and attacks of dizziness and numbness of the upper extremities caused by long tract compression or vertebral artery insufficiency.[5] With AAS, minor manipulation of the head may cause the odontoid process to compress the cervical cord, medulla, or vertebral arteries, thus producing pyramidal signs, tetraplegia, or death.[4] Consider a radiologic neck evaluation (lateral flexion-extension films) before elective anesthesia in adult patients with RA because cervical involvement in the adult form of RA is common (15 to 86%) and may be present in the absence of signs or symptoms.[2] Pulmonary problems may include pleural effusion, pulmonary vasculitis, interstitial pulmonary fibrosis, rheumatoid nodules in the parenchyma and pleura, and restrictive lung disease. There is a 25% incidence of bronchiectasis.[6]

Cardiac complications include pericardial thickening or effusion, pericarditis, myocarditis, coronary arteritis, cardiac valve fibrosis, rheumatoid nodules in the conduction system, and aortic regurgitation. Neurological complications include peripheral nerve compression (carpal tunnel syndrome) and cervical nerve root compression.

B. Premedicate the patient with an antisialagogue, unless there is salivary gland disease. Sedate the patient if he or she is without pulmonary compromise. Give steroid coverage to those on chronic steroid therapy. Ensure adequate padding of the operating table. Have a variety of sizes of endotracheal tubes (ETTs) available as cricoarytenoid disease may limit the glottic opening.

C. In the emergent situation requiring general anesthesia, assume that the patient has subluxation and plan an approach to intubation that permits immobilization of the head and cervical spine. For elective procedures, choose anesthetic agents and technique based on the surgery planned, the patient's medical status, and the anesthesiologist's skills. For surgery on the extremities, consider regional or local[7] anesthesia which avoids instrumentation of the airway; have a plan for airway management. For other surgery, general anesthesia may be required. If there is TMJ involvement, the larynx may be difficult to visualize with a laryngoscope. Bilateral TMJ involvement can result in acquired micrognathia.[8] Consider fiberoptic laryngoscopy with topical anesthesia.[9] Blind nasal intubation may be unsuccessful because of the anterior position of the larynx and predisposition to bleeding (thin mucosa; aspirin therapy). In patients with cervical subluxation, perform awake fiberoptic intubation followed by verification of intact extremity movement. Alternatively, consider placing a supraglottic airway (e.g., laryngeal mask airway [LMA]), or facemask. Have a tracheostomy tray and a surgeon readily available. Once the airway is secured and ventilation of the lungs verified, administer other anesthetic agents. Titrate drugs, recalling the potential for cardiovascular depression (hypovolemia, hypoproteinemia), reduced ability to handle stress, altered drug response,[3] and possibly impaired renal excretion.

Patient with RHEUMATOID ARTHRITIS

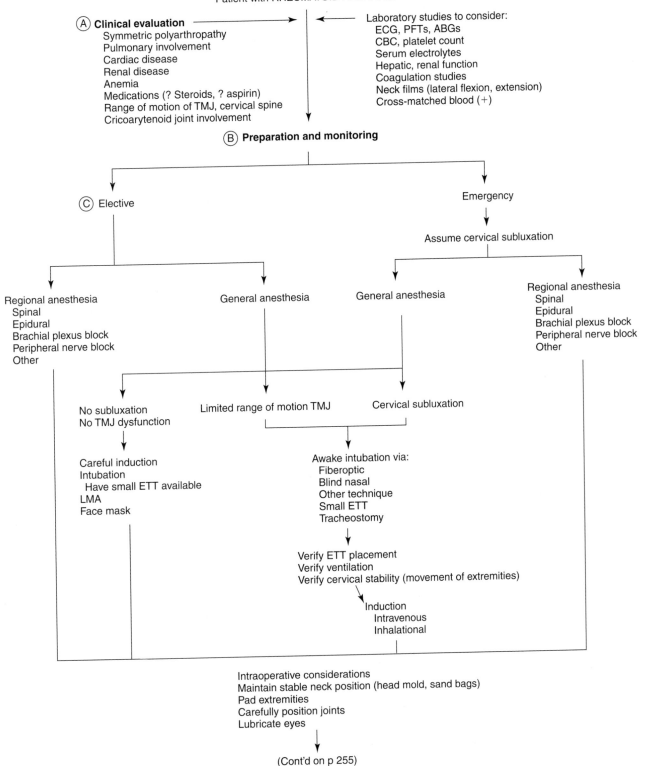

Ⓐ **Clinical evaluation**
    Symmetric polyarthropathy
    Pulmonary involvement
    Cardiac disease
    Renal disease
    Anemia
    Medications (? Steroids, ? aspirin)
    Range of motion of TMJ, cervical spine
    Cricoarytenoid joint involvement

Laboratory studies to consider:
    ECG, PFTs, ABGs
    CBC, platelet count
    Serum electrolytes
    Hepatic, renal function
    Coagulation studies
    Neck films (lateral flexion, extension)
    Cross-matched blood (+)

Ⓑ **Preparation and monitoring**

Ⓒ Elective

Emergency

Assume cervical subluxation

Regional anesthesia
    Spinal
    Epidural
    Brachial plexus block
    Peripheral nerve block
    Other

General anesthesia

General anesthesia

Regional anesthesia
    Spinal
    Epidural
    Brachial plexus block
    Peripheral nerve block
    Other

No subluxation
No TMJ dysfunction

Limited range of motion TMJ

Cervical subluxation

Careful induction
Intubation
    Have small ETT available
LMA
Face mask

Awake intubation via:
    Fiberoptic
    Blind nasal
    Other technique
    Small ETT
    Tracheostomy

Verify ETT placement
Verify ventilation
Verify cervical stability (movement of extremities)

Induction
    Intravenous
    Inhalational

Intraoperative considerations
Maintain stable neck position (head mold, sand bags)
Pad extremities
Carefully position joints
Lubricate eyes

(Cont'd on p 255)

D. Patients with RA are more sensitive to drugs that depress respiratory function,[10] possibly because of reduced inspiratory muscle strength and increased compensatory respiratory drive.

REFERENCES

1. Brooker DS: Rheumatoid arthritis: otorhinolaryngological manifestations, *Clin Otolaryngol Allied Sci* 13:239–246, 1988.
2. Kwek TK, Lew TW, Thoo FL: The role of preoperative cervical spine X-rays in rheumatoid arthritis, *Anaesth Intensive Care* 26 (6): 636–641, 1998.
3. Gorini M, Ginanni R, Spinelli A, et al.: Inspiratory muscle strength and respiratory drive in patients with rheumatoid arthritis, *Am Rev Respir Dis* 142:289–294, 1990.
4. Macarthur A, Kleiman S. Rheumatoid cervical joint disease: a challenge to the anaesthetist, *Can J Anaesth* 40:154–159, 1993.
5. Eisele JH, Jr: Connective tissue diseases. In: Katz J, Benumof J, Kadis LB, editors: *Anesthesia and uncommon diseases*, ed 3, Philadelphia, 1998, W.B. Saunders.
6. Matti MV, Sharrock NE: Anesthesia on the rheumatoid patient [Review], *Rheum Dis Clin North Am* 24 (1):19–34, 1998.
7. Wei N, Delauter SK, Beard S, et al.: Office-based arthroscopic synovectomy of the wrist in rheumatoid arthritis, *Arthroscopy* 17 (8): 884–887, 2001.
8. Kohjitani A, Miyawaki T, Kasuya K, et al.: Anesthetic management for advanced rheumatoid arthritis patients with acquired micrognathia undergoing temporomandibular joint replacement, *J Oral Maxillofac Surg* 60:559–566, 2002.
9. MacKenzie CR, Sharrock NE: Perioperative medical considerations in patients with rheumatoid arthritis. [Review], *Rheum Dis Clin North Am* 24 (1):1–17, 1998.
10. Skues MA, Welchew EA: Anaesthesia and rheumatoid arthritis, *Anaesthesia* 48:989–997, 1993.

Patient with RHEUMATOID ARTHRITIS
(Cont'd from p 253)

↓

Extubate awake

↓

 Postoperative care
    Monitor respiratory function
    Effective analgesia
       Regional analgesia/local anesthesia via catheter
    Restart rheumatoid arthritis medications
    Steroid coverage ($\pm$)
    Minimize immobilization

Ankylosing Spondylitis (AS)

ANDREW S. RUSHTON, M.D.

JEFFREY R. KIRSCH, M.D.

Ankylosing spondylitis (AS) is an inflammatory arthritis that typically affects the axial skeleton. AS clinically manifests as progressive neck, back, and hip pain and stiffness in the second or third decade of life. AS has a prevalence of 0 to 1.4% (higher in northern European population), is more common in men than women (3:1), and is often associated with human leukocyte antigen B-27 (up to 95% of Caucasians with AS).[1]

A. Vertebral ankylosis leads to the radiologic "bamboo spine." Disease severity ranges from simple low back pain and sacroiliitis to full cervical, thoracic, and lumbar flexion and kyphosis. There may be complete inability to extend or rotate the axial skeleton. Fixed cervical flexion deformities lead to obvious airway management difficulties. Severe cervical AS can also predispose patients to vertebrobasilar insufficiency, atlantoaxial subluxation and spine fractures (most often C5–C6) from minor trauma or neck extension.[2] Both fractures and subluxations may lead to spinal cord compression. More rare neurological complaints may be related to cauda equina syndrome. Osteotomy, vertebrectomy, and any spine corrections require monitoring somatosensory evoked potentials.[3,4] The neuraxis can also be monitored by performing wake-up tests or transcranial evoked potentials.[5] Airway management may be complicated by temporomandibular dysfunction and cricoarytenoid involvement. Cricoarytenoid disease may be assessed preoperatively by eliciting a history of hoarseness or dyspnea or by indirect laryngoscopy.[2] Cardiovascular disease from AS is usually from aortitis, aortic insufficiency, or conduction defects.[3] An ECG or echocardiogram (echo) may be prudent if suspected clinically. Pulmonary problems arise late in the disease process secondary to ankylosis of the costovertebral and costochondral joints. This leads to restriction defects especially if there is kyphosis of the spine. Interestingly, the "bucket handle" motion of the ribs is held open leading to an increase in functional residual capacity.[3] Apical pulmonary fibrosis is another rare complication of AS but is usually clinically insignificant. Renal insufficiency is usually due to nonsteroidal anti-inflammatory drug (NSAID) abuse nephropathy but may be secondary to IgA nephropathy. Assess baseline renal function with blood urea nitrogen (BUN) and creatinine. Proteinuria may be evident on urinalysis. Current medications used in the treatment of AS include, but are not limited to, NSAIDs, sulfasalazine, and tumor necrosis factor alpha antagonists. Information for patients can be found at the spondylitis association of America; www.spondylitis.org.

B. Regional anesthesia can be a reasonable alternative to general anesthesia. Airway equipment for emergent intubation must always be present. Spinal, epidural, and caudal neuraxial have all been used in patients with AS. Calcified ligaments may make neuraxial anesthesia difficult or impossible. Interosseous injection has been a reported complication. Local anesthesia has been used for awake cervical osteotomy. However, if the patient appears to have a difficult airway, the anesthesiologist should consider preprocedure intubation (with appropriate airway blockade), despite doing the surgery awake. Inability to manage the patient's airway in an emergency situation during awake cervical osteotomy may be fatal for the patient.

C. General endotracheal anesthesia is most safely performed for patients with cervical ankylosis by awake fiberoptic intubation.[2] More recently the laryngeal mask airway (LMA) and intubating laryngeal mask airway (ILMA) have been used successfully.[7] Other means employed include blind nasal intubation with hooked wire stylette, retrograde wire via cricothyroid, and awake tracheostomy. Small endotracheal tubes (ETTs) may be necessary if there is cricoarytenoid dysfunction.

REFERENCES

1. Khan MA: HLA- B27 and its subtypes in world populations, *Curr Opin Rheumatol* 7:263–269, 1995.
2. Sinclair JR, Mason RA: Ankylosing spondylitis: The case for awake intubation, *Anaesthesia* 39:3–11, 1984.
3. Fleisher LA: *Anesthesia and uncommon diseases*, ed 5, Philadelphia, 2005, W.B. Saunders.
4. Ovassapian A, Land P, Schafer MF, et al.: Anesthetic management for surgical corrections of the severe flexion deformity of the cervical spine, *Anesthesiology* 58:370–372, 1983.
5. Lin BC, Chen IH: Anesthesia for ankylosing spondylitis patients undergoing transpedicle vertebrectomy, *Acta Anaesthesiol Sin* 37:73–78, 1999.
6. Schelew BL, Vaghadia H: Ankylosing spondylitis and neuraxial anesthesia- a 10 year review, *Can J Anaesth* 43:65–68, 1996.
7. Lu PP, Brimacombe J, Ho AC, et al.: The intubating laryngeal mask airway in severe ankylosing spondylitis, *Can J Anaesth* 48:1015–1019, 2001.

Patient with ANKYLOSING SPONDYLITIS

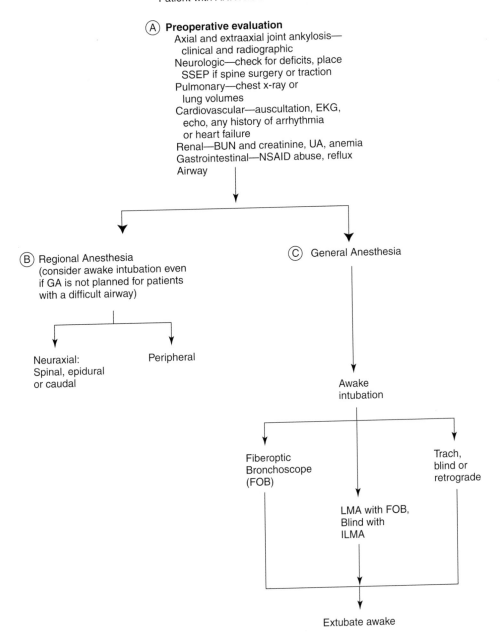

Ⓐ **Preoperative evaluation**
  Axial and extraaxial joint ankylosis—
    clinical and radiographic
  Neurologic—check for deficits, place
    SSEP if spine surgery or traction
  Pulmonary—chest x-ray or
    lung volumes
  Cardiovascular—auscultation, EKG,
    echo, any history of arrhythmia
    or heart failure
  Renal—BUN and creatinine, UA, anemia
  Gastrointestinal—NSAID abuse, reflux
  Airway

Ⓑ Regional Anesthesia
  (consider awake intubation even
  if GA is not planned for patients
  with a difficult airway)

Neuraxial: Peripheral
Spinal, epidural
or caudal

Ⓒ General Anesthesia

Awake
intubation

Fiberoptic   Trach,
Bronchoscope   blind or
(FOB)   retrograde

            LMA with FOB,
            Blind with
            ILMA

Extubate awake

Cancer Patient

ANGELA KENDRICK, M.D.

Cancer is the second leading cause of death in the United States, with more than half of all deaths occurring in patients over age 65.[1] Metastatic spread causes most deaths. In men, the most common cancers are prostate, lung, and colorectal; in women, most common are breast, lung, and colorectal cancer. In childhood, leukemia, lymphoma, and CNS tumors are most common.[2] Surgery, chemotherapy, and radiation therapy are the mainstays of cancer treatment and offer substantially increased survival rates in selected cancers. Less toxic, biologically targeted therapies are in Phase III use.[3]

A. Perform a complete and thorough review of systems and physical examination. Elderly patients may have comorbidities. Expect cardiovascular disease (e.g., hypertension, atrial arrhythmias, conduction system disease, and poor tolerance of hypovolemia or over-transfusion), pulmonary disease (e.g., chronic obstructive pulmonary disease, pneumonia, sleep apnea, postoperative ventilatory dysfunction after thoracic and upper abdominal surgery), and renal insufficiency (i.e., decreased creatinine clearance). Other abnormalities commonly seen in cancer patients include hematological alterations (e.g., anemia, thrombocytopenia, or decreased clotting factors) and neurological dysfunction (e.g., increased ICP, dementia, or peripheral weakness). Preoperative studies should be age and disease appropriate. Treat nutritional deficiencies, anemia, coagulopathy, and electrolyte abnormalities. Transfuse platelets if < 50,000.[4] Preoperative pain and anxiety can be significant in these patients. Pain may arise from nerve infiltration or metastatic spread to bones. Use an empathetic approach and aggressive multimodal management of pain, nausea, and vomiting in cancer patients.

B. Look for cancer syndromes and metabolic complications. Tumor lysis syndrome occurs after chemotherapy in tumors with a high growth rate (e.g., acute lymphocytic leukemia [ALL], Burkitt's) and may cause hyperuricemia, hyperkalemia, and hyperphosphatemia, resulting in acute renal failure. Hypercalcemia develops in a variety of tumors (e.g., lung, renal cell, multiple myeloma) and may require hydration, diuretics, steroids, and diphosphonates. Paraneoplastic syndromes are systemic manifestations including ectopic Cushing's disease; syndrome of inappropriate antidiuretic hormone (hyponatremia and hypoosmolality); and Eaton-Lambert syndrome, a myasthenia-like condition sometimes seen in patients with small cell carcinoma of the lung (patients develop skeletal weakness that does not respond to anticholinesterases).[5]

C. Chemotherapy may cause significant immunosuppression, bone marrow suppression, and cumulative toxic effects (Table 1). Doxorubicin and bleomycin therapy can cause significant morbidity. Obtain an echocardiogram (echo) to assess ventricular function if congestive heart failure has developed.

TABLE 1
Toxicities of Chemotherapeutic Agents

Chemotherapeutic agent	Toxicity	Toxic dose
Anthracycline antibiotics Doxorubicin (Adriamycin) Bleomycin	All cause pulmonary infiltrates/cardiomyopathy CHF 1–2% get severe fibrosis; avoid high FiO$_2$	>550 mg/m^2 >500 mg
Alkylating agents Cyclophosphamide (Cytoxan) Nitrosoureas (BCNU,CCNU)	All cause bone marrow depression, pulmonary toxicity, or liver/vascular disease Decreased plasma cholinesterase, hepatic disease Hepatic and renal toxicity	— — —
Antimetabolites Methotrexate Azathioprine Cis-platinum	All cause pulmonary toxicity Hypersensitivity, encephalopathy, cirrhosis Cholestasis, liver necrosis Peripheral neuropathy, ototoxicity, ATN Peripheral neuropathy, SIADH	— — — —
Vinca alkaloids Vincristine	—	— —

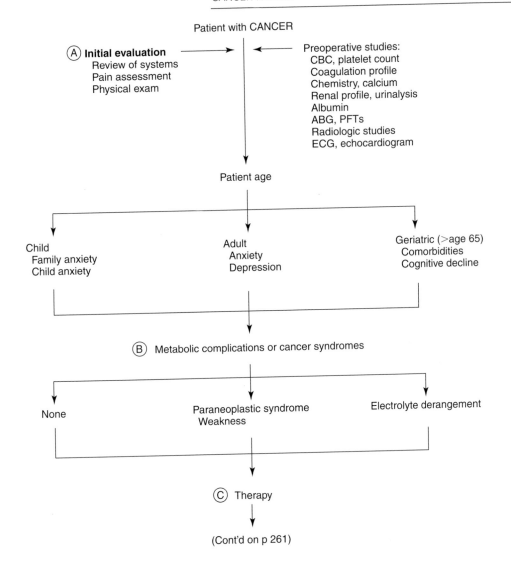

Patient with CANCER

(A) **Initial evaluation** ⟶   ⟵ Preoperative studies:
    Review of systems   CBC, platelet count
    Pain assessment   Coagulation profile
    Physical exam   Chemistry, calcium
                                           Renal profile, urinalysis
                                           Albumin
                                           ABG, PFTs
                                           Radiologic studies
                                           ECG, echocardiogram

Patient age

Child   Adult   Geriatric (>age 65)
Family anxiety   Anxiety   Comorbidities
Child anxiety   Depression   Cognitive decline

(B) Metabolic complications or cancer syndromes

None   Paraneoplastic syndrome   Electrolyte derangement
              Weakness

(C) Therapy

(Cont'd on p 261)

D. Radiation therapy damage increases with large doses and may result in synergistic toxicity with chemotherapy. Evaluate the airway for fibrosis and scarring after head and neck irradiation.

E. Steroid therapy is often used in conjunction with chemotherapy. Therefore, assess need for perioperative steroid replacement.

F. Anesthetics may be required for various indications such as biopsies, radiologic procedures, extensive operations (e.g., tumor resection and reconstructive surgery), indwelling infusion ports, or excision of recurrences. Palliative care may include spinal cord stimulators, intrathecal pumps, epidural infusions, or hospice care. Leukemia patients may require frequent lumbar punctures and bone marrow examinations. Pediatric patients usually require deep sedation or general anesthesia for such procedures. Follow strict infection control practices. Cancer patients may have significant opioid tolerance; anticipate postoperative analgesia requirements. Clarify each patient's wishes for resuscitation prior to providing an anesthetic.[6] Automatic rescinding of do-not-resuscitate (DNR) orders does not meet Joint Commission on Accreditation of Healthcare Organizations (JCAHO) standards.

G. Determine appropriate anesthetic monitoring, perioperative fluid and blood requirements, and options for postoperative pain management for the anticipated procedure. All modalities (local, MAC, regional or general anesthesia) can be used in cancer patients.

REFERENCES

1. Yancik R, Ries LA: Aging and cancer in America. Demographic and epidemiologic perspectives, *Hematol Oncol Clin North Am* 14:17, 2000.
2. National Cancer Institute: Surveillance, epidemiology, and end results database 2003, available at: www.nci.nih.gov.
3. Carney DN: Lung cancer—time to move on from chemotherapy, *N Engl J Med* 346:126, 2002.
4. Schiffer CA, Anderson KC, Bennett CL, et al.: Platelet transfusion for patients with cancer: clinical practice guidelines of the American Society of Clinical Oncology, *J Clin Oncol* 19:1519, 2001.
5. Fitch JC, Rinder CS: Cancer therapy and its anesthetic implications. In Barash PG, Cullen BF, Stoelting RK, editors: *Clinical anesthesia*, Philadelphia, 1996, Lippincott.
6. ASA Standards and Guidelines: Ethical guidelines for the anesthesia care of patients with do-not-resuscitate orders or other directives that limit treatment, Adopted 1993, amended 2001.

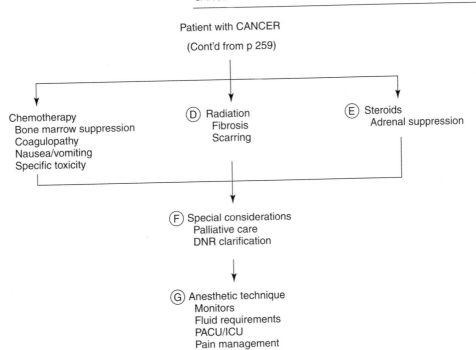

Patient with CANCER

(Cont'd from p 259)

Chemotherapy
  Bone marrow suppression
  Coagulopathy
  Nausea/vomiting
  Specific toxicity

(D) Radiation
    Fibrosis
    Scarring

(E) Steroids
    Adrenal suppression

(F) Special considerations
    Palliative care
    DNR clarification

(G) Anesthetic technique
    Monitors
    Fluid requirements
    PACU/ICU
    Pain management

Eating Disorders

ANTHONY S. POON, M.D., D.D.S., PH.D.

W. CORBETT HOLMGREEN, M.D., D.D.S.

The two most commonly encountered eating disorders are anorexia nervosa and bulimia nervosa. Both disorders occur more frequently in young females with an incidence ranging from 5 to 10% for anorexia and 3 to 30% for bulimia. While anorexia and bulimia are distinct psychopathological entities, they share common characteristics and have special implications for anesthesia.

A. Perform a careful history and physical examination. Obtain appropriate laboratory studies and preoperative tests (e.g., electrolytes, ECG). Patients suffering from anorexia nervosa refuse to maintain body weight at or above a minimally normal weight for age and height. Weight loss is mainly achieved through severe dietary restriction, with or without binging and purging, the latter being more common among bulimic patients. In severe starvation, there is a reduction in cardiac muscle mass, resulting in decreased cardiac output (hypotension, and arrhythmia. Starvation and abuse of diuretics and laxatives can all cause potentially life-threatening electrolyte imbalances. Hypokalemia predisposes the patient to cardiac dysrhythmias. Common ECG findings include T-wave flattening or inversion, ST depression, and prolonged QT interval.[1] Sinus bradycardia, atrioventricular (AV) block, Torsades, and ventricular fibrillation can also be seen. Hypomagnesemia can also cause disturbances in cardiac rhythm, as can drugs (e.g., lithium, tricyclic antidepressants) used in the treatment of anorexia. Emetine, the active ingredient in ipecac (used for emesis induction), has been found to cause dysrhythmias and a fatal form of myocarditis.[2] Repeated induced vomiting results in hypochloremic metabolic alkalosis, whereas diarrhea from laxative abuse causes a nonanion gap metabolic acidosis. Thus, prior to elective surgery, correct fluid, electrolyte, and acid-base imbalances.

B. Anorexic patients are often hypothermic and may have an impaired shivering response. Closely monitor core body temperature during the operation. Maintain a warm ambient temperature and use a warming blanket or fluid warmer. Because of the emaciated body habitus, skin fragility, and increased risk for osteoporosis, pay special note to positioning the patient and providing adequate padding and support for the extremities to reduce the risk of damage to bones, nerves, and soft tissue. Repeated cycles of starvation, binging, and purging, which is a common practice in bulimic patients, present special challenges in airway management. There is an increased risk of aspiration due to delayed gastric emptying and acute gastric dilation after binging. Administer preoperative sodium citrate, metoclopramide, or a histamine H_2-receptor blocking agent. Consider an RSI or awake intubation. Edema and inflammation of the laryngeal mucosa caused by repeated exposure to acidic gastric content can impair visualization of anatomical landmarks during direct laryngoscopy. Demineralization and erosion of dental enamel and dentin increases the risk of fracture of the anterior teeth. Frequent binging and vomiting is associated with esophageal reflux, esophagitis, Mallory-Weiss tear, esophageal stricture, and esophageal or gastric rupture.[3] Thus, insert nasogastric or orogastric tubes with great caution.

C. Pharmacokinetic changes occur in anorexic patients. This is especially true of agents that are highly lipid soluble; the abnormally low body fat content in anorexic patients reduces the volume of distribution for these drugs. Also, low serum albumin reduces plasma binding, thereby increasing the amount of free drug in circulation. Drug clearance is also expected to decrease due to a reduction in glomerular filtration secondary to dehydration and decreased drug metabolism caused by hepatic dysfunction. Administer drugs, such as sedatives and narcotics, in lower than average doses and titrate to effect in small increments. While no longer widely used, avoid halothane due to its proarrhythmic effects. Avoid hyperventilation, especially in alkalotic patients whose respiratory drive is maintained by compensatory carbon dioxide retention. Hypokalemia and hypocalcemia cause a potentiation of nondepolarizing neuromuscular blockers (NDMBs); carefully titrate doses and monitor the degree of muscular relaxation.

REFERENCES

1. Seller CA, Ravalia A: Anaesthetic implications of anorexia nervosa, *Anaesthesia* 58:437–443, 2003.
2. Sugie H, Russin R, Verity MA: Emetine myopathy: two case reports with pathobiochemical analysis, *Muscle Nerve* 7:54–59, 1984.
3. Cerami R: Anesthetic considerations with anorexia nervosa, *AANA J* 61:165–169, 1993.

Emaciated patient with suspected EATING DISORDER

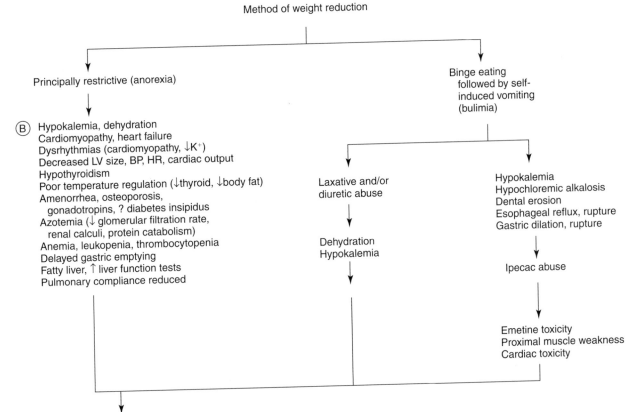

Ⓐ **Clinical evaluation** ────────────→   ←────── Electrolytes
    Young Caucasian female   CBG
    Recent history of weight loss   ECG
    Diuretic and/or laxative abuse   Chest film
    History of constipation   Thyroid function
    Body image disturbance   Pulmonary function tests
    Medications   Liver function tests
        Tricylclics
        Monoamine oxidase inhibitors

Method of weight reduction

Principally restrictive (anorexia)

Binge eating
followed by self-
induced vomiting
(bulimia)

Ⓑ Hypokalemia, dehydration
Cardiomyopathy, heart failure
Dysrhythmias (cardiomyopathy, ↓K⁺)
Decreased LV size, BP, HR, cardiac output
Hypothyroidism
Poor temperature regulation (↓thyroid, ↓body fat)
Amenorrhea, osteoporosis,
    gonadotropins, ? diabetes insipidus
Azotemia (↓ glomerular filtration rate,
    renal calculi, protein catabolism)
Anemia, leukopenia, thrombocytopenia
Delayed gastric emptying
Fatty liver, ↑ liver function tests
Pulmonary compliance reduced

Laxative and/or
diuretic abuse

Hypokalemia
Hypochloremic alkalosis
Dental erosion
Esophageal reflux, rupture
Gastric dilation, rupture

Dehydration
Hypokalemia

Ipecac abuse

Emetine toxicity
Proximal muscle weakness
Cardiac toxicity

Ⓒ Anesthetic management

    ─ If anemia severe → Transfuse

    ─ If dehydrated → Hydrate

    ─ Hypokalemia → Give potassium

    ─ Inability to maintain body temperature → Use warming blanket

    ─ Severely eroded teeth → Care during laryngoscopy

    ─ Slowed gastric emptying → Awake intubation or RSI

    ─ Decreased pulmonary compliance → Carefully adjust ventilator settings

    ─ Increased myocardial sensitivity to catecholamines → Avoid halothane use

    ─ Weakened myocardium → Caution upon rapid renourishment + intraoperative rehydration

    ─ Aspiration common→ Be alert for aspiration pneumonitis or pneumonia

    ─ Change in pharmacokinetics → Adjust medication doses

Munchausen's Syndrome

MALCOLM D. ORR, M.D., PH.D.

The patient with Munchausen's syndrome has simulated or feigned illness, which can confuse health care workers, initiate unnecessary surgery and therapy, and consume health care resources.[1-5] The syndrome is a type of factitious illness that meets the DSM-III criteria for chronic factitious illness with physical symptoms. The actions of Munchausen's patients are voluntary, deliberate, purposeful, and intentional, but they cannot control them.

A. The classic patient (usually male) has embraced disease simulation as the center of his life. He may demonstrate borderline personality disorder, is rarely schizophrenic, has a history of infrequent, discontinuous, short-term employment, and (not infrequently) is a prisoner. The clinical presentation (symptoms and signs) suggests a known disease, often life-threatening. The working, or nonprototypical, Munchausen's patient is more likely to be female; many are nurses or other health care professionals. These patients have a borderline personality disorder, and pseudologia (lying) is frequent. As in the classic form, symptoms and signs simulate life-threatening conditions. A common component of this syndrome is a transference reaction; thus romantic attachments to the health care provider (real or imagined) may be present. Diagnosis may require an elevated index of suspicion. Features commonly seen include pathological lying; wandering from hospital to hospital; and recurrent, feigned, or simulated illness. Supporting features include borderline or antisocial personality; unusual or dramatic presentation; disorders that may have been self-inflicted; acceptance of diagnostic procedures, treatments, and operations with equanimity; history of multiple hospitalizations and operations with multiple scars; and sophisticated medical knowledge. Virtually all organ systems have been involved. The most common presentations are abdominal (e.g., pain suggesting appendicitis, renal stones), hemorrhagic (hemoptysis, hematuria, hematochezia, or vaginal bleeding), and neurologic. Behavior may be bizarre, demanding, evasive, or unruly. Leaving the hospital against medical advice is common.

B. Some patients use symptoms and signs in other patients (often children) to seek the attention of the health care provider and the health care system. Presenting symptoms and signs span all of medicine and may be so convincing that the deception can be perpetuated for months or years. The perpetrator is frequently a child's parent but in some cases has been a health care worker. Such individuals go to extraordinary lengths to produce symptoms and signs, and some have been convicted in criminal prosecutions.[5]

C. Select monitoring and anesthetic technique(s) appropriate for the planned surgical or obstetric procedure. If possible, review previous anesthesia records to gain information about adverse reaction to anesthetic agents.[6] Use good judgment in advising the patient about proposed anesthetic management, disclose risks and benefits completely, and document these discussions well (see paragraph D).

D. Several Munchausen's syndrome patients have sued for malpractice on the grounds that because their symptoms and signs were feigned, the surgery was unnecessary. In one published case and two others known to the author, lawsuits were initiated by the Munchausen's syndrome patient. In the two cases scheduled for trial, both were settled out of court because the experience of such a patient with deception makes it extremely difficult to predict a jury response in favor of the defense. As lawsuits for gain would provide a definite material goal, the condition of such a patient may extend into the area of malingering: a conscious attempt to use feigned illness for substantial gain in the courts.

REFERENCES

1. Larcher V: Non-accidental injury, *Hosp Med* 65 (6):365–368, 2004.
2. Nadelson T: The Munchausen spectrum: borderline character features, *Gen Hosp Psychiatry* 1:11–17, 1979.
3. Galvin HK, Newton AW, Vandeven AM: Update on Munchausen syndrome by proxy, *Curr Opin Pediatr* 17 (2):252–257, 2005.
4. Rabinerson D, Kaplan B, Orvieto R., et al.: Munchausen syndrome in obstetrics and gynecology, *J Psychosom Obstet Gynaecol* 23 (4):215–218, 2002.
5. Mehta NJ, Khan IA: Cardiac Munchausen syndrome, *Chest* 122 (5):1649–1653, 2002.
6. Lad SP, Jobe KW, Polley J, et al.: Munchausen's syndrome in neurosurgery: report of two cases and review of the literature, *Neurosurgery* 55 (6):1436, 2004.

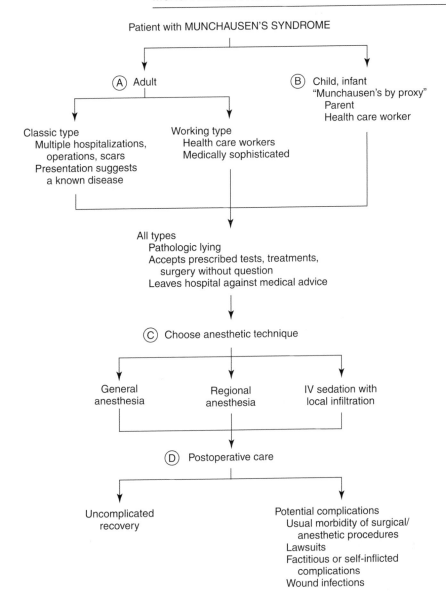

Patient with MUNCHAUSEN'S SYNDROME

A Adult

B Child, infant
"Munchausen's by proxy"
Parent
Health care worker

Classic type
Multiple hospitalizations,
operations, scars
Presentation suggests
a known disease

Working type
Health care workers
Medically sophisticated

All types
Pathologic lying
Accepts prescribed tests, treatments,
surgery without question
Leaves hospital against medical advice

C Choose anesthetic technique

General
anesthesia

Regional
anesthesia

IV sedation with
local infiltration

D Postoperative care

Uncomplicated
recovery

Potential complications
Usual morbidity of surgical/
anesthetic procedures
Lawsuits
Factitious or self-inflicted
complications
Wound infections

Thermal Injury

GARY WELCH, M.D.

The skin is the largest organ of the body, enabling thermoregulation, maintenance of the internal milieu, and barrier protection from pathogens. Skin loss (from thermal, electrical, chemical, or bacterial injury) was formerly classified as first, second, or third degree based on the depth of injury. Current classification is *superficial partial-thickness, deep partial-thickness,* and *full-thickness injury.* Partial-thickness burns are capable of healing; full-thickness burns require skin replacement. Care can be divided into three phases: (1) resuscitation, (2) convalescence, and (3) reconstruction. The patient may return to the first phase during convalescence if an infection or another medical or surgical condition arises. Each phase presents unique management challenges.[1–6]

A. During the immediate postinjury period, determine the mechanism of injury—flame, chemical, heated fluids, infection, drug reaction, or electrical. Evaluate for concomitant trauma, occurrence in a confined space/facial burns (indicating the possibility of airway injury and edema), and for preexisting comorbidities. Place a large-bore IV catheter and administer oxygen (O_2).

B. Evaluate airway patency. Early indicators of inhalation injury include singed nasal vibrissae and carbonaceous sputum. Patients with significant facial burns may develop airway edema during resuscitation, which can lead to airway occlusion. Therefore, consider early intubation to protect the airway. In some cases a surgical airway may be necessary.

C. Measure carboxyhemoglobin. Levels > 20 suggest smoke inhalation sufficient to produce cyanide toxicity.

D. Assess the depth of injury to estimate healing. Calculate the extent of the burn size based on the "rule of nines" (each of the following represents 9% of body surface area in an adult: one arm, anterior thorax, upper thigh, head). The genitalia are 1%.

E. The extent of an electrical injury can be deceiving. Usually there is an entry point (point of contact with the electrical source) and an exit point (ground); significant tissue damage often occurs between these two points resulting in underlying muscular injury. Look for myoglobinuria, hyperkalemia, renal failure, and cardiac arrhythmias.

F. Chemical injuries (strong acid or alkali) require irrigation with water; neutralization is not indicated (heat generated may cause additional injury). Do not irrigate with water in the case of exposure to agricultural lime because the mixture of lime and water produces an exothermic reaction creating heat injury. Instead, brush off as much lime as much as possible prior to irrigation with water.

G. Resuscitation formulas, based on the percent of skin damaged, are based on the Parkland formula: 3 to 4 ml of crystalloid/kg/% of burn area. Give half of the calculated fluid in the first 8 hours after injury and the rest over the next 16 hours. (This is an estimate; some patients require more and some less, depending on the response of heart rate, BP, and urine production).

H. Evaluate and intubate the airway. Consider awake intubation with a flexible bronchoscope or a video laryngoscope. Assure adequate IV access—internal jugular or subclavian catheter if necessary. In larger burns, consider CVP or pulmonary artery catheter (or noninvasive cardiac output monitor) and arterial line. Consider transesophageal echocardiography to assess regional and global wall motion. Warm all IV fluids and warm the operating room to 85° to 90°F. Blood loss during burn wound excisions can be as much as 300 ml per percent burn wound excised and grafted—plan accordingly. Induce general anesthesia with ketamine, 1 to 2 mg/kg, in patients with cardiovascular compromise. Avoid succinylcholine because it may cause hyperkalemia in burn patients; use a rapid-acting nondepolarizing agent. Maintain the anesthetic with an inhalation, balanced, or total IV anesthetic (TIVA—consider 20 ml propofol mixed with 100 mg ketamine and 5 mg of midazolam; administer as a 5 to 8 ml bolus followed by an infusion at 5 to 8 ml/hr). TIVA is useful in patients with ventilatory problems who require specialized ventilators that cannot deliver anesthetic gases. During the convalescent phase, patients require daily wound care and require frequent anesthetics. Place padding to protect fragile skin and use caution when placing the face mask if there has been facial injury. Consider use of a laryngeal mask airway (LMA) or regional anesthesia.

I. Individualize pain management—patients often require repeated operative procedures (dressing changes or debridement), and tolerance to opioids is common. IM ketamine 3 to 5 mgs/kg provides 20 minutes of intense analgesia for dressing changes and brief debridement.

REFERENCES

1. Atiyeh BS, Gunn SW, Hayek SN: State of the art in burn treatment, *World J Surg* 29 (2):131–148, 2005.
2. Hemington-Gorse SJ: Colloid or crystalloid for resuscitation of major burns, *J Wound Care* 14 (6):256–258, 2005.
3. Cartotto R, Musgrave MA, Beveridge M, et al.: Minimizing blood loss in burn surgery, *J Trauma* 49:1034–1039, 2000.
4. MacLennan N, Heimbach DM, Cullen BF: Anesthesia for major thermal injury, *Anesthesiology* 89 (3):749–770, 1998.
5. Garner JP, Jenner J, Parkhouse DA: Prediction of upper airway closure in inhalational injury, *Mil Med* 170 (8):677–82, 2005.
6. Han T, Kim H, Bae J, et al.: Neuromuscular pharmacodynamics of rocuronium in patients with major burns, *Anesth Analg* 99 (2): 386–392, 2004.

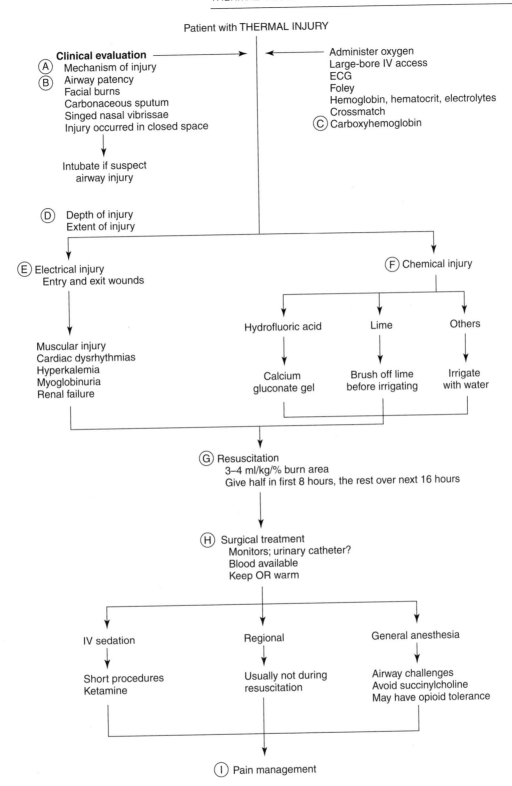

Patient with THERMAL INJURY

Clinical evaluation
(A) Mechanism of injury
(B) Airway patency
    Facial burns
    Carbonaceous sputum
    Singed nasal vibrissae
    Injury occurred in closed space

Administer oxygen
Large-bore IV access
ECG
Foley
Hemoglobin, hematocrit, electrolytes
Crossmatch
(C) Carboxyhemoglobin

Intubate if suspect
    airway injury

(D) Depth of injury
    Extent of injury

(E) Electrical injury
    Entry and exit wounds

(F) Chemical injury

Hydrofluoric acid   Lime   Others

Muscular injury
Cardiac dysrhythmias
Hyperkalemia
Myoglobinuria
Renal failure

Calcium   Brush off lime   Irrigate
gluconate gel   before irrigating   with water

(G) Resuscitation
    3–4 ml/kg/% burn area
    Give half in first 8 hours, the rest over next 16 hours

(H) Surgical treatment
    Monitors; urinary catheter?
    Blood available
    Keep OR warm

IV sedation   Regional   General anesthesia

Short procedures   Usually not during   Airway challenges
Ketamine   resuscitation   Avoid succinylcholine
                                               May have opioid tolerance

(I) Pain management

Jehovah's Witness Patient

MALCOLM D. ORR, M.D., PH.D.

"Jehovah's Witnesses" is the popular name for the Watchtower Bible and Tract Society. Their interpretation of the Bible is literal, and their faith holds that it is contrary to the teachings of their church to receive blood or blood products.[1] Although they accept other forms of medical and surgical care, most Witnesses refuse to receive blood or to authorize its administration. They believe that acceptance of blood may interfere with the pursuit of eternal life. This prohibition may extend to autologous blood as well; once completely separated from the body, it cannot be reinfused. The concept of bloodless surgery is actively promoted. Some changes in definitions, obligations, and state's rights have emerged since 1986. Because Jehovah's Witness patients have no aversion to nonblood products, bleeding problems in such patients may benefit from the use of DDAVP (desmopressin) or recombinant erythropoietin.[2] They actively request that all methods be used to reduce the need for blood.

A. Determine preoperatively whether the patient will accept RBCs or other blood products, and document the discussion in the medical record. If he or she will accept blood, proceed as usual. Before elective surgery, be sure that hemoglobin (Hb) and coagulation parameters are normal. Use erythropoietin to bring Hb to normal levels.

B. When minors must undergo emergency surgery or when blood transfusion is medically indicated for minors, it may be possible to obtain a court order permitting administration of blood products. Adult patients have the right to refuse blood. If there are no dependents, the wish to accept no blood must be honored. Added to the adult patient category is the "emancipated minor," a person less than 18 years old who is married or serving in the armed forces, financially independent, or living away from home. For adults with dependents, management is potentially more complex. The state has become interested in the care of dependents if a decision is made to withhold life-supporting treatment. If the patient then dies and the state becomes liable for all or part of the support of the dependents, the state may rule that the treatment be given to the adult patient to protect the state. If questions arise in the care of adults with dependents, pregnant women in the third trimester, or minors, the wise course in elective surgery is to take counsel with the patient and even with another impartial health care provider. If blood is refused in a life-threatening situation, recourse to a court opinion is advised. Other special situations include pregnant patients and patients of questionable competence. Consultation with the hospital's ethics committee may be helpful.

C. Employ adjunctive techniques to minimize blood loss. Position the patient so that CVP is not elevated. Use tourniquets if feasible. Consider using controlled hypotensive techniques to lower the BP and reduce arterial bleeding. There may be less blood loss if regional anesthesia techniques are used. Good surgical technique, including meticulous dissection, frequent use of the electrocautery, and careful hemostasis, is essential. Many Witnesses accept extracorporeal oxygenation, hemodialysis, or autologous transfusion (intraoperative blood salvage).[3,4] The essential feature for acceptance of these techniques is that the blood is in continuous contact with the circulation at all times. Any materials that serve as plasma expanders but do not contain active clotting factors have the potential to cause a dilutional coagulopathy. Use hetastarch, pentastarch, and other dextrans with caution.[5] Although these are acceptable to the Jehovah's Witness patient, they can reduce the ability of the blood to clot in the recipient. Such situations have developed in patients transfused with more than the usually recommended volume.

D. With experience, some centers have developed expertise in managing even extensive surgical procedures without transfusion, and their techniques may offer guidance to those who care for such patients occasionally.[6,7] After extensive unreplaced blood loss, postoperative treatment includes fluids, nutrition, and iron. With normal bone marrow function, blood cells are regenerated, although complete recovery from surgery may take longer than usual. Lawsuits for assault may be filed against the anesthesiologist who administers blood against the patient's wishes without a court order. Courts are less likely to grant permission for a lifesaving transfusion in the face of patient refusal.

REFERENCES

1. Kulvatunyou N, Heard SO: Care of the injured Jehovah's Witness patient: case report and review of the literature, *J Clin Anesth* 16 (7):548–553, 2004.
2. Price S, Pepper JR, Jaggar SI: Recombinant human erythropoietin use in a critically ill Jehovah's Witness after cardiac surgery, *Anesth Analg* 101 (2):325–327, 2005.
3. Jagannathan N, Tetzlaff JE. Epidural blood patch in a Jehovah's Witness patient with post-dural puncture cephalgia, *Can J Anaesth* 52 (1):113, 2005.
4. Holt RL, Martin TD, Hess PJ, et al.: Jehovah's Witnesses requiring complex urgent cardiothoracic surgery, *Ann Thorac Surg* 78 (2): 695–697, 2004.
5. Lockwood DN, Bullen C, Machin SJ: A severe coagulopathy following volume replacement and hydroxyethyl starch in a Jehovah's Witness, *Anaesthesia* 43:391–3, 1988.
6. Jabbour N, Gagandeep S, Mateo R, et al.: Live donor liver transplantation without blood products: strategies developed for Jehovah's Witnesses offer broad application, *Ann Surg* 240 (2): 350–357, 2004.
7. Panousis K, Rana B, Hunter J, et al.: Rapid sequence quadruple joint replacement in a rheumatoid Jehovah's Witness, *Arch Orthop Trauma Surg* 123 (2–3):128–131, 2003.

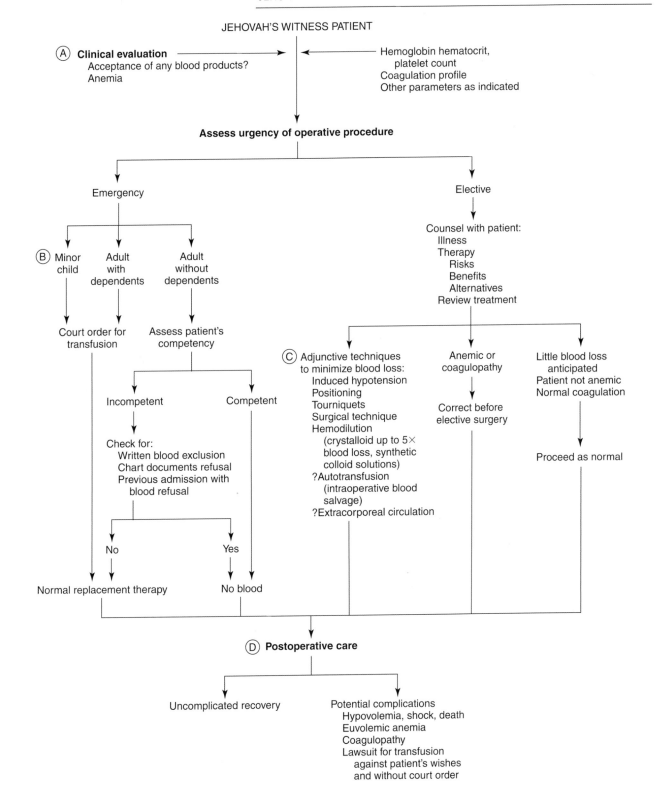

Allergic Reactions

GEORGE A. DUMITRASCU, M.D.

Significant reactions under anesthesia occur with an incidence estimated at 1:5,000 to 1:20,000 cases. Several surveys across the world show a mortality rate between 3 and 9%. Analyzing the etiology of these reactions, one must take onto account antigen-antibody interactions (immune-mediated hypersensitivity, anaphylaxis), massive release of vasoactive mediators from basophils and mast cells in response to administration of certain drugs (anaphylactoid reactions), as well as possible activation of the complement pathway. In the same patient, more than one mechanism may be involved in the production of an allergic reaction.[1-5] See Table 1.

A. Large studies have documented that regardless of the etiology, intraoperatively, hypotension may be the first and only manifestation of an allergic reaction. The diagnosis should thus be suggested by the dramatic nature of the clinical manifestations in close temporal relationship to exposure to an antigen. A review of the literature reveals that the most common agents responsible for intraoperative anaphylaxis are muscle relaxants (70% of cases), followed by latex (15% of cases), antibiotics, thiobarbiturates, and opioids; colloids and radiocontrast material account for the rest of the reported incidents.

B. Therapy should be prompt and targeted to three immediate goals: prevent hypoxemia, maintain intravascular volume, and inhibit further cellular degranulation. Rapidly expand intravascular volume with 1 to 4 L of crystalloid and colloid and assess hemodynamic status. Persistent hypotension mandates early intervention with IV epinephrine in doses of 10 to 100 μg. The dose of epinephrine should be doubled and repeated every 1 to 3 minutes until BP stabilizes. The beta agonist effects of epinephrine also serve to relax bronchial smooth muscle.

C. There is recent interest in using vasopressin intravenously in incremental doses of 5 units in the treatment of anaphylactoid reactions[6]; however, the lack of prospective, randomized studies warrants caution when comparing efficacy and safety profile to epinephrine. There is no evidence that administration of an antihistamine is effective in treating anaphylaxis once mediators have been released. Corticosteroids may be uniquely beneficial for the allergic reactions secondary to activation of the complement cascade.

REFERENCES

1. Mertes PM, Laxenaire MC: Adverse reactions to neuromuscular blocking agents, *Curr Allergy Asthma Rep* 4 (1):7–16, 2004.
2. Mertes PM, Laxenaire MC, Alla F: Anaphylactic and anaphylactoid reactions occurring during anesthesia in France in 1999–2000 *Anesthesiology* 99 (3):536–545, 2003.
3. Lieberman P: Anaphylactic reactions during surgical and medical procedures, *J Allergy Clin Immunol* 110 (2):S64–S69, 2002.
4. Fasting S, Gisvold SE: Serious intraoperative problems—a 5 year review of 83,844 anesthetics, *Can J Anaesth* 49 (6):545–553, 2002.
5. Stoelting RK, Dierdorf SF: *Anesthesia and co-existing disease*, ed 4, New York, 2002, Churchill Livingstone.
6. Williams SR, Denault AY, Pellerin M, et al.: Vasopressin for treatment of shock following aprotinin administration, *Can J Anaesth* 51 (2):169–172, 2004.

TABLE 1
Mechanisms of Allergic Reactions

Anaphylaxis
Life-threatening manifestation of an antigen-antibody interaction. Sensitization of the host occurs whenever exposure to an antigen (e.g., drug, food, or latex) incites the production of antigen-specific IgE antibodies. Subsequent exposure to a chemically similar antigen will initiate rapidly (within 10 minutes) degranulation of mast cells and basophils on a large scale. The result is a marked increase in capillary permeability, allowing the extravasation of up to 50% of the intravascular volume into the extracellular space.

Anaphylactoid reaction
Does not require prior exposure to antigens. Certain drugs possess the inherent ability to induce massive release of histamine from basophils generating a clinical picture indistinguishable from anaphylaxis.

Activation of the complement system
By immunological (IgG-antigen or heparin-protamine complexes) or nonimmunological (endotoxin) factors that results in the production of anaphylatoxins C3a, C4a, and C5a, which themselves are capable of causing mast cell and basophil mediator release.

Patient with ALLERGIC REACTIONS

Preoperative Considerations

Assess risk of an allergic reaction

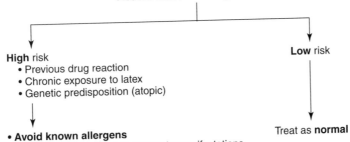

High risk
- Previous drug reaction
- Chronic exposure to latex
- Genetic predisposition (atopic)

Low risk

- **Avoid known allergens**
- **Consider pretreating** to attenuate manifestations
  - Prehydrate
  - H$_1$ and H$_2$ blockers (start 24 hrs. preop)
  - Corticosteroids
- Consider **invasive monitoring**

Treat as **normal**

Intraoperative Considerations

(A) **Suspect allergic reaction**
- **Temporal relationship to antigen exposure**
- Hypotension and tachycardia: may be the only presenting signs under GA
- Bronchospasm, airway edema: 12% of reactions involve airway edema
- Cutaneous signs: with low cardiac output there may be no cutaneous manifestations

(B) **Begin treatment**
  Stop suspected allergen
  Increase **FiO$_2$** to **100%**
  Consider **intubation** of the trachea
  Assess **hemodynamic** state

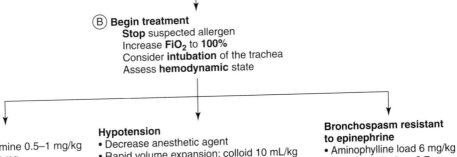

Stable
- Diphenhydramine 0.5–1 mg/kg
- Ranitidine 50 mg
- Corticosteroids

Hypotension
- Decrease anesthetic agent
- Rapid volume expansion: colloid 10 mL/kg
- Epinephrine 10 mcg IV; repeat prn

Bronchospasm resistant to epinephrine
- Aminophylline load 6 mg/kg IV over 20 min then 0.7 mg/kg/hr × 12 hr

(C) **Hypotension resistant to epinephrine**
- Epinephrine infusion
- Vasopressin 5 U IV, repeat

Postoperative Considerations

- Serum sample at **1 hr** post-reaction for **tryptase** concentration
- **ICU admission** for monitoring: ABGs, lactic acid, coagulation studies, electrolytes, urea
  ! *10% of deaths secondary to pulmonary edema*
- **Skin testing** 1 month postevent

Latex Allergy

KEVIN M. BRADY, M.D.

DOLORES B. NJOKU, M.D.

Natural rubber latex (NRL) is derived from the bark of the *Hevea brasiliensis* tree. NRL can be found in several products including gloves, Foley catheters, syringes, IV fluid containers, and tubing. Allergy to NRL was first described in 1927, when a health care provider with previous exposure to NRL developed a rash after exposure to gloves containing this product. The first anaphylactic reaction to NRL was reported in 1979; however, the first anaphylactic reaction to latex surgical gloves was reported in 1984. The first fatal latex anaphylactic reaction was reported in 1991.[1]

Latex reactions can be one of two types. Type I hypersensitivity, or immediate hypersensitivity, reactions are thought to be a response to proteins contained in latex. These reactions are immunoglobulin E-mediated (IgE-mediated) and may cause the release of vasomotor activators, such as histamine, leukotrienes, and prostaglandins. Type IV hypersensitivity, or delayed hypersensitivity, reactions are thought to be a response to antioxidants and preservatives from the manufacturing process. These reactions are T-cell mediated and may cause a contact dermatitis.

There are certain factors associated with an increased risk for latex allergy. Persons at high risk include patients with spina bifida, myelomeningocele, genitourinary malformations, health care workers, and rubber industry workers. Children with multiple surgical procedures or surgical procedures prior to one year of age have an increased incidence of latex allergy.[3] Additionally, specific epitopes of proteins from avocado, banana, chestnut, kiwi, peach, tomato, potato, and bell pepper have been reported to cross react with NRL proteins. This cross-reactivity has been termed the latex-fruit syndrome.[4]

Latex allergy appears to be increasing among specific patient populations and health care workers. However, the actual incidence of latex allergy among health care workers is unknown. Even so, multiple studies, some lacking controls and standardization, report an incidence which varies from 0 to 30%.[2] Because the most serious reaction to NRL is anaphylaxis, latex allergy should always be considered in any patient who develops anaphylaxis.

A. Identify all patients at high risk for latex allergy by performing a thorough history and physical examination. Inquire about exposure to rubber gloves, balloons, other latex products, and allergies to fruits and vegetables.

B. Create a latex-free environment for patients with known latex allergy and those who are at high risk for latex allergy. It is hoped that reducing latex exposure in high risk patients will reduce the incidence of latex allergy in the years to come. Attempt to schedule procedures as the first case in the operating room for the day.

C. Consider premedication in patients with a history of life-threatening reactions from latex exposure. If previous latex reactions were not life-threatening, premedication is not necessary; avoid latex exposure in these patients.

D. If a patient develops anaphylaxis, administer oxygen, IV fluids, epinephrine, corticosteroids, and H_1 and H_2 antagonists. Epinephrine is the antidote for anaphylaxis. Early administration of epinephrine will stop the release of vasomotor activators. In severe reactions, consider early intubation of the trachea. Patients with partial sympathectomy due to epidural and spinal anesthesia may have refractory hypotension requiring large amounts of fluid and epinephrine.

E. Differentiate between anaphylaxis and anaphylactoid reactions by obtaining serum C3, C4, and tryptase levels. These levels are elevated following anaphylaxis secondary to NRL. Obtaining diagnostic tests is extremely controversial; there is little evidence to guide decision making.

F. The following diagnostic tests are available. Radioallergosorbent (RAST) is an in vitro test for IgE anti-latex antibody. Latex IgE is specific but not sensitive (65 to 85%). While there are multiple latex IgE commercial kits available, ALA-STAT is the only test with FDA approval.[5] A patch test is available to test for contact dermatitis or type IV hypersensitivity reactions. Skin prick tests can be dangerous. There are five reported cases of anaphylaxis from skin-prick testing. Currently there is no Food and Drug Administration (FDA) approved reagent for skin-prick testing. Until such time that the FDA approves a standardized skin-prick testing reagent, skin-prick testing is not recommended.

REFERENCES

1. Ownby DR: A history of latex allergy, *J Allergy Clin Immunol* 110 (2 Suppl):S27–3S2, 2002.
2. Garabrant DH, Schweitzer S: Epidemiology of latex sensitization and allergies in health care workers, *J Allergy and Clin Immunol* 110 (2 Suppl):S82–S95, 2002.
3. Kwittken PL, Sweinberg SK, Campbell DE, et al.: Latex hypersensitivity in children: clinical presentation and detection of latex-specific immunoglobulin E, *Pediatrics* 95 (5):693–699, 1995.
4. Wagner S, Breiteneder H: The latex-fruit syndrome, *Biochem Soc Trans* 30 (Pt 6):935–940, 2002.
5. Liccardi G, Dente B, Triggiani M, et al.: A multicenter evaluation of the CARLA system for the measurement of specific IgE antibodies vs. other different methods and skin prick tests, *J Investig Allergol Clin Immunol* 12 (4):235–241, 2002.

Patient with LATEX ALLERGY

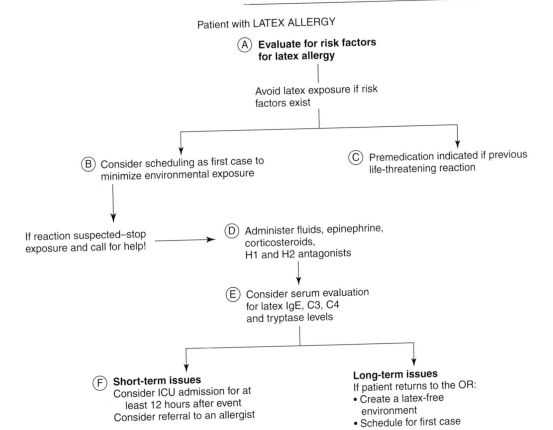

Ⓐ **Evaluate for risk factors
for latex allergy**

Avoid latex exposure if risk
factors exist

Ⓑ Consider scheduling as first case to
minimize environmental exposure

Ⓒ Premedication indicated if previous
life-threatening reaction

If reaction suspected–stop
exposure and call for help!

Ⓓ Administer fluids, epinephrine,
corticosteroids,
H1 and H2 antagonists

Ⓔ Consider serum evaluation
for latex IgE, C3, C4
and tryptase levels

Ⓕ **Short-term issues**
Consider ICU admission for at
least 12 hours after event
Consider referral to an allergist

Long-term issues
If patient returns to the OR:
• Create a latex-free
environment
• Schedule for first case
of day

Systemic Lupus Erythematosus (SLE)

MARY BLANCHETTE, M.D.

Systemic lupus erythematosus (SLE) is a disorder of immunological regulation of unknown cause that is manifested as a multisystemic inflammatory disease. The clinical manifestations, mode of presentation, and clinical course vary greatly, and therapeutic interventions are primarily designed to attenuate the symptoms of the disease. When surgery is planned for the patient with SLE, tailor the anesthetic management to the severity of the disease, the clinical manifestations present, the probability of future organ involvement, the current drug therapy, and the awareness that pregnancy and surgical stress can aggravate the disease process.[1]

A. An insightful evaluation depends on a thorough history and careful examination of the patient with focused attention on the many organ systems that can be involved. Severity of systemic involvement varies greatly. The patient may have few complaints or may manifest generalized systemic toxicity (e.g., fever, dehydration, severe infections, or septicemia). Consequently, perioperative laboratory evaluation and intraoperative management are influenced by the severity of systemic involvement. The most common drugs used include aspirin, nonsteroidal anti-inflammatory drugs (NSAIDs), antimalarial drugs (chloroquine or hydroxychloroquine), corticosteroids, and cytotoxic drugs. Aspirin and NSAIDs impair coagulation; antimalarials used on a long-term basis produce skeletal muscle myopathy, cardiomyopathy, and peripheral neuropathy; and exogenous corticosteroids cause protean systemic disorders and suppress production of steroids by the adrenal gland. Perioperative steroid "coverage" is standard for those currently or recently treated with corticosteroids. The clinical manifestations of SLE range from limited to many and complex. Nondeforming, polyarticular arthritis most commonly involves the hands, wrists, elbows, knees, and ankles. The cervical spine and the cartilages of the larynx usually are not involved. Skin lesions occur frequently. Ulcerations of the mouth and lips can occur. Alopecia is common; therefore, the scalp should be protected from prolonged pressure during operations. Renal involvement is common in SLE. Renal function varies from normal to dialysis dependent. Nervous system involvement in SLE manifests as neuropsychiatric disorders, memory impairment, disorientation, pyramidal tract signs, or cranial nerve defects. It would not be unusual for symptoms to worsen with surgery. Pericarditis is the most common finding of cardiac involvement in SLE. Pericardial tamponade is unusual. Endocarditis with noninfectious vegetations near the rings of the heart valves can occur. Coronary heart disease is frequent, as is hyperlipidemia and hypertension. Pulmonary disease is variable. Pleuritic chest pain is a common pulmonary manifestation of SLE. Chronic interstitial lung disease and pulmonary hypertension (HTN) occur. Anorexia, nausea, vomiting, and abdominal pain are common. Mesenteric vasculitis can lead to intestinal perforations and the need for emergency surgery. A hypercoagulable state may occur—the antiphospholipid syndrome manifests with in vitro prolongation of activated partial thromboplastin time (aPTT) and a strong predilection for in vivo thrombosis.[2,3] Thrombosis in both venous and arterial beds may occur. This problem often is recurrent. Myopathy, liver enlargement, and Sjögren's syndrome have been noted to occur with SLE. Anesthetic management needs to address these aspects of the disease.

B. Perioperative laboratory evaluation is dictated by the clinical assessment of the patient.

C. In general, the anesthetic management of the patient is planned to minimize surgical stress, which may exacerbate the disease manifestations. When urgency of the planned procedure is such that little time is available for complete evaluation and stabilization of disorders induced by SLE, management is rendered more challenging.

D. Select monitors as appropriate for the planned procedure and the patient's disorders. In patients with known hypercoagulable state, use invasive lines only when the benefits far outweigh the risks.

E. Regional anesthesia should be considered because of its ability to control perioperative stress. However, because of the possible presence of neurological disease, infection, and coagulopathies, a careful risk-benefit analysis needs to be made. Intraoperative and postoperative thromboses have been reported to occur in patients with antiphospholipid antibody syndrome, and vigilance should be high for these complications.[4]

REFERENCES

1. Madan R, Khoursheed M, Kukla R, et al.: The anaesthetist and the antiphospholipid syndrome, *Anaesthesia* 52 (1):72–76, 1997.
2. Kone A: Antiphospholipid antibody and anesthesia, *Acta Anaesthesiol Belg* 54 (2):169–171, 2003.
3. Wetzl RG: Anaesthesiological aspects of pregnancy in patients with rheumatic diseases, *Lupus* 13 (9):699–702, 2004.
4. Ozaki M, Minami K, Shigematsu A: Myocardial ischemia during emergency anesthesia in a patient with systemic lupus erythematosus resulting from undiagnosed antiphospholipid syndrome, *Anesth Analg* 95 (1):255, 2002.

Patient with SYSTEMIC LUPUS ERYTHEMATOSUS

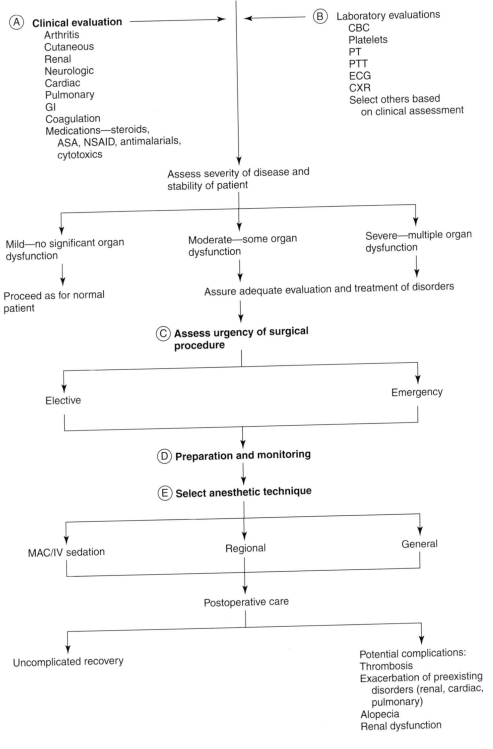

(A) **Clinical evaluation**
Arthritis
Cutaneous
Renal
Neurologic
Cardiac
Pulmonary
GI
Coagulation
Medications—steroids,
ASA, NSAID, antimalarials,
cytotoxics

(B) Laboratory evaluations
CBC
Platelets
PT
PTT
ECG
CXR
Select others based
on clinical assessment

Assess severity of disease and
stability of patient

Mild—no significant organ
dysfunction

Moderate—some organ
dysfunction

Severe—multiple organ
dysfunction

Proceed as for normal
patient

Assure adequate evaluation and treatment of disorders

(C) **Assess urgency of surgical
procedure**

Elective

Emergency

(D) **Preparation and monitoring**

(E) **Select anesthetic technique**

MAC/IV sedation

Regional

General

Postoperative care

Uncomplicated recovery

Potential complications:
Thrombosis
Exacerbation of preexisting
disorders (renal, cardiac,
pulmonary)
Alopecia
Renal dysfunction

SPECIALTY ANESTHESIA AND CARDIOTHORACIC AND VASCULAR ANESTHESIA

INVASIVE HEMODYNAMIC MONITORING

CARDIOPULMONARY BYPASS (CPB)

CORONARY ARTERY BYPASS GRAFTING (CABG)

OFF-PUMP CORONARY ARTERY BYPASS (OPCAB)

ACUTE HEART FAILURE (AHF) IN CARDIAC SURGERY

MITRAL VALVE REPLACEMENT

REPAIR OF CONGENTIAL HEART DISEASE (CHD): BYPASS

REPAIR OF CHD: NONBYPASS

ONE-LUNG ANESTHESIA

THORACOSCOPY AND VIDEO-ASSISTED THORACIC SURGERY (VATS)

MEDIASTINOSCOPY

TRACHEAL STENOSIS (TS): INJURY AND RESECTION

INTRAOPERATIVE LOSS OF PACEMAKER CAPTURE

ENDOVASCULAR PROCEDURES

AORTIC ARCH ANEURYSMS

DESCENDING AND THORACOABDOMINAL AORTIC ANEURYSMS

ABDOMINAL AORTIC ANEURYSMS

LOWER EXTREMITY BYPASS PROCEDURES

ESOPHAGOGASTRECTOMY (EG)

TRANSJUGULAR INTRAHEPATIC PORTOSYSTEMIC SHUNT (TIPS)

Invasive Hemodynamic Monitoring

SALLY COMBEST, M.D.

CHRISTOPHER A. BRACKEN, M.D., PH.D.

MARY ANN GURKOWSKI, M.D.

Invasive hemodynamic monitoring is desirable for patients with serious medical disorders or who are undergoing complex surgical procedures (e.g., cardiac, thoracic, or major vascular). Prompt recognition and accurate assessment of significant circulatory changes permit appropriate management.[1] Pediatric cases have special considerations.[2]

A. Monitor arterial pressure by direct cannulation of a peripheral artery, which provides a beat-to-beat display of the arterial pressure, and the waveform may indicate the presence of hypovolemia (a significant "dip" in BP occurs simultaneously with a delivered positive-pressure breath) as well as information about stroke volume ([SV] broad, wide curves indicate normal SV; narrowed curves indicate decreased SV). Myocardial contractility may be assessed by evaluation of the rate of rise (dp/dt) of the BP tracing. Direct cannulation of a peripheral artery also allows blood sampling for laboratory studies.

B. Central venous monitoring is useful in patients who undergo operations expected to result in extensive fluid shifts and who have no underlying cardiovascular or pulmonary disease. In healthy patients, right-sided and left-sided filling pressures can be assumed to be proportional, thus allowing CVP measurement to be a sufficient determinant of volume status and preload. Analysis of the CVP waveform may be useful in diagnosing pathological cardiac conditions. Insertion of a central venous line allows long-term IV access for hyperalimentation or antibiotic therapy. Approaches to central venous cannulation include external jugular (EJ), internal jugular (IJ), subclavian (SC), long arm (LA) basilic vein, and femoral cannulation. EJ cannulations may be difficult to thread, especially with a large catheter or a short neck but have few potential complications. SC cannulation is the most comfortable for the patient in the long term but is more difficult for the anesthesiologist to manipulate or replace intraoperatively and runs a higher risk of pneumothorax or uncontrolled hemorrhage on insertion. LA requires good arm veins and some luck in manipulating the catheter past the shoulder. Femoral cannulation is rarely used in the long term and has some potential for infection but should be considered if necessary. IJ cannulation is generally the choice for central venous cannulation by most anesthesiologists, because it allows direct access to the right atrium via the superior vena cava (SVC) and is easiest to manipulate or change. Caution is required in patients with carotid disease, and this approach is contraindicated with neck tumors or SVC obstruction.

C. The pulmonary artery (PA) catheter can be used in the differential diagnosis of low cardiac output (CO) secondary to hypovolemia, left or right ventricular failure, pulmonary embolism, chronic pulmonary hypertension (HTN), or cardiac tamponade. PA catheter placement is an invasive procedure, and potential gains must be weighed against the risk of balloon rupture, pulmonary infarction, catheter knotting, rhythm disturbances, and infection.[3] The tip of the catheter should be in the middle third of the lung field (in supine patients, determine the position by lateral chest x-rays [CXRs]).[4]

D. CO is determined by the thermodilution technique, and derived indices are calculated. Derived indices provide a working knowledge on which to base therapeutic interventions. Estimation of hemodynamic subset is straightforward and may help in choosing an appropriate therapeutic intervention. Mixed venous blood is obtained for calculation of intrapulmonary shunting. Newer PA catheters incorporate technology to assess mixed venous oxygen (O_2) saturation, right ventricular ejection fraction (EF), and CO on a continuous basis. Oximetry catheters are useful in unstable or septic shock patients in whom O_2 delivery to, and utilization by, the tissues is uncertain. Transesophageal echocardiography (TEE) is used in the OR to monitor global myocardial performance, including end-diastolic volume, EF, valvular function, and wall motion abnormalities (first indication of developing ischemia) on a real-time basis. This technology has become widely available and is useful in assessment of perioperative cardiovascular pathophysiology and hemodynamics, as well as detection of myocardial ischemia and assessment of surgical results (valvular surgery, coronary artery bypass grafting [CABG], congenital heart surgery).[5]

REFERENCES

1. Vender JS: Pulmonary artery catheter utilization: the use, misuse, or abuse, J Cardiothorac Vasc Anesth 20 (3):295–299, 2006.
2. Millar CL, Burrows FA: Invasive monitoring in the pediatric patient [review], Int Anesth Clin 30:91, 1992.
3. Bossert T, Gummert JF, Bittner HB, et al.: Swan-Ganz catheter-induced severe complications in cardiac surgery: right ventricular perforation, knotting, and rupture of a pulmonary artery, J Card Surg 21 (3):292–295, 2006.
4. Kronberg GM, Quan SF, Schlobohm RM, et al.: Anatomic locations of the tips of pulmonary-artery catheters in supine patients, Anesthesiology 51:467, 1979.
5. Kneeshaw JD: Transoesophageal echocardiography (TOE) in the operating room, Br J Anaesth 97 (1):77–84, 2006.

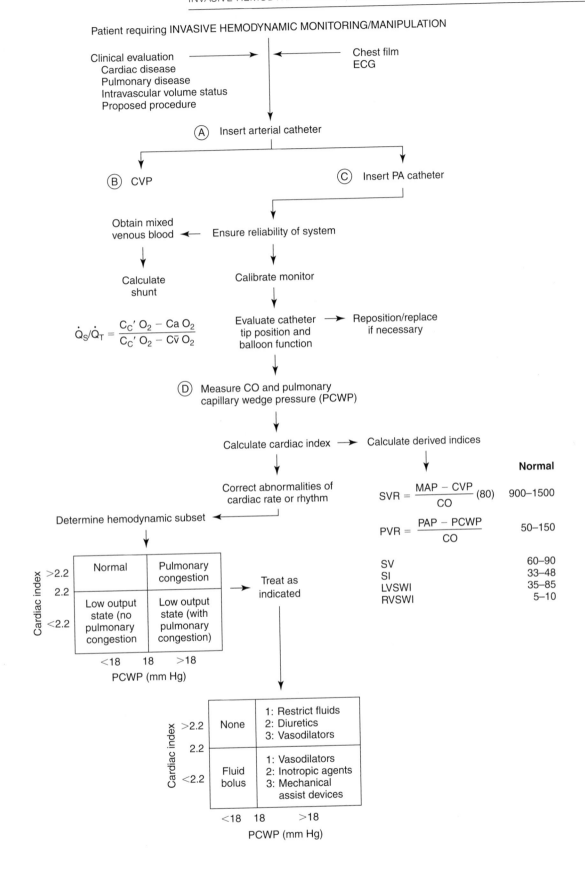

Patient requiring INVASIVE HEMODYNAMIC MONITORING/MANIPULATION

Clinical evaluation
    Cardiac disease
    Pulmonary disease
    Intravascular volume status
    Proposed procedure

Chest film
ECG

(A) Insert arterial catheter

(B) CVP

(C) Insert PA catheter

Obtain mixed venous blood

Ensure reliability of system

Calculate shunt

Calibrate monitor

$$\dot{Q}_S/\dot{Q}_T = \frac{C_{C'}O_2 - C_aO_2}{C_{C'}O_2 - C\bar{v}O_2}$$

Evaluate catheter tip position and balloon function → Reposition/replace if necessary

(D) Measure CO and pulmonary capillary wedge pressure (PCWP)

Calculate cardiac index → Calculate derived indices

Correct abnormalities of cardiac rate or rhythm

		Normal
$SVR = \dfrac{MAP - CVP}{CO}$ (80)		900–1500
$PVR = \dfrac{PAP - PCWP}{CO}$		50–150
SV		60–90
SI		33–48
LVSWI		35–85
RVSWI		5–10

Determine hemodynamic subset

Cardiac index	PCWP (mm Hg)	
	<18 18	>18
>2.2	Normal	Pulmonary congestion
<2.2	Low output state (no pulmonary congestion)	Low output state (with pulmonary congestion)

Treat as indicated

Cardiac index	PCWP (mm Hg)	
	<18 18	>18
>2.2	None	1: Restrict fluids 2: Diuretics 3: Vasodilators
<2.2	Fluid bolus	1: Vasodilators 2: Inotropic agents 3: Mechanical assist devices

Cardiopulmonary Bypass (CPB)

SALLY COMBEST, M.D.

CHRISTOPHER A. BRACKEN, M.D., PH.D.

MARY ANN GURKOWSKI, M.D.

Cardiopulmonary bypass (CPB) oxygenates blood, provides an adequate cardiac index, and facilitates surgery on the nonbeating heart. On total bypass the entire cardiac output (CO) is supplied by the pump, because the heart is excluded by aortic cross-clamping, and venous return is diverted to the pump's venous reservoir (Figure 1). During partial bypass the heart provides part of the CO.

A. Monitor arterial BP with a radial artery catheter. During normothermia, maintain mean arterial pressure (MAP) at 50 to 100 mm Hg (cerebral autoregulation permits normal cerebral blood flow at this level). During hypothermia, lower pressures are permitted because cerebral oxygen (O_2) demands are reduced. If hypotension occurs on initiation of CPB, consider hypovolemia (venous return started before arterial infusion), aortic dissection as a result of arterial cannula displacement, or equipment malfunction. Hypertension (HTN) may be caused by arterial flow in excess of venous flow, aortic cannula positioned into the innominate or subclavian artery, or generalized hypothermia, or it may be secondary to catecholamine or renin release.

B. The pulmonary artery (PA) catheter allows measurement of cardiac filling pressure and CO. Obtain mixed venous blood for calculation of pulmonary shunt, and derive hemodynamic variables. On CPB, significant rises in PA pressure may reflect overdistention of the left ventricle; pull the PA cath back 3 to 4 cm on initiation of CPB.

C. Administer heparin (fixed dose of 300 mg/kg or determined by heparin dose response) through a functioning CVP catheter, not a peripheral IV, or have the surgeon give it directly into the right atrium. Monitor anticoagulation with activated clotting time (ACT) or heparin assays (HEPCON). An ACT > 400 seconds is desirable before CPB (normal ACT < 150 seconds). Direct thrombin inhibitors are being investigated for use in patients with heparin-induced thrombocytopenia (HIT).[1-3]

D. Monitor two ECG leads (V_5 for the detection of myocardial ischemia and II for dysrhythmia diagnosis). Monitor esophageal, rectal, blood, and myocardial temperatures during CPB. Nasopharyngeal temperature is used to monitor brain temperature. Rectal or urinary bladder temperatures are considered the standard in determining the adequacy of rewarming. Determine sodium and potassium levels during CPB. Potassium levels may rise because of the high potassium (K^{++}) concentrations used in the cardioplegic solution. A urinary output of 1 ml/kg/hr during CPB is adequate. If other cardiovascular indices are normal and urinary output is low, renal hypoperfusion is the likely cause. Mannitol, furosemide, or return of pulsatile flow may be necessary to restore adequate urinary output.

E. Wean from CPB once the patient is warm; has normal acid-base status, hematocrit (Hct), and electrolyte levels; and is hemodynamically stable with adequate cardiac filling pressures. Transesophageal echocardiography (TEE) is helpful in assessing volume status and myocardial contractility. Reverse heparin with protamine.[4]

F. Longer bypass runs carry a higher incidence of complications. Embolic phenomena are major hazards (air, plaques, blood element aggregates, fat, or debris).[5] Pulmonary complications include hypoxia, fluid overload, and O_2 toxicity. Prophylactic steroid therapy is controversial. Coagulopathies may be secondary to excessive protamine, thrombocytopenia, DIC, and blood trauma[6] (especially after long pump runs).

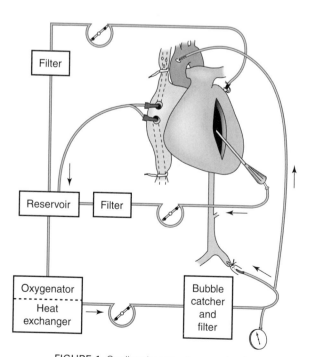

FIGURE 1 Cardiopulmonary bypass circuit.

REFERENCES

1. Vincentelli A, Jude B, Belisle S: Antithrombotic therapy in cardiac surgery, *Can J Anaesth* 53 (6 suppl):S89–S102, 2006.

Patient for CARDIOPULMONARY BYPASS

Clinical evaluation ———————→   ←——— Coagulation (PT, PTT, platelet count)
Cardiac lesion(s)   CBC, electrolytes, urinalysis, SMA-12
Pulmonary status   Blood cross-matched
Renal disease

Anesthetic management

Ⓐ Arterial blood pressure   Ⓑ Swan-Ganz   TEE   ABGs   Ⓒ Anticoagulation   Ⓓ ECG
   (50–100 mm   catheter   Volume status   Hemoglobin V_5, II
   Hg-normothermia)   PA pressures   Myocardial   saturation
   ↓ BP   CVP   function—wall
      "Bled out"   Cardiac output   motion   Heparin via   Monitor
      Dissection   (thermodilution)   abnormalities   Mixed   CVP catheter   Temperature
      Equipment failure   Systemic vascular   Valvular function venous   Fixed dose   Electrolytes
      Hemodilution   resistance   Hemodynamic   saturation   (300 µg/kg)   (Na^+, K^+)
      Nonpulsatile flow   calculations   Dose response   Urinary output
   ↑ BP   ACT (>400   (1 mL/kg/hr)
      Displaced cannula tip   Base deficit   prebypass)   HCT
      Catecholamine release
      Renin release
      Hypothermia

Ⓔ Discontinuation of CPB

Potential problems   Recovery
   Increased potassium
   ↳ **Glucose + insulin**
   Hypothermia   Uncomplicated   Ⓕ Potential complications
   ↳ **Adequate rewarming**   recovery   Emboli
   Coronary artery air   Pulmonary disorders
   ↳ **Removal of air**   Coagulopathies
   LV dysfunction   Extubate 6–24 hr   Polyuria
   ↳ **Inotropic support**   postoperatively   Hyperglycemia
   Coronary spasm/ischemia   Neurologic damage
   ↳ **IV nitroglycerin, verapamil**   Intraoperative awareness
   Myocardial infarct   Renal dysfunction
   ↳ **Prevent extension**   Reduced immunologic function
   Heart block   Protamine reactions
   ↳ **Correct dysrhythmia/AV pace**   Heparin-induced
   Hypovolemia   thrombocytopenia
   ↳ **Judicious volume expansion**
   Reverse heparin
   ↳ **Protamine**

2. Shore-Lesserson L: Hematologic aspects of cardiac surgery, *ASA Refresher Courses in Anesthesiology* 33 (1):213–223, 2005.
3. Wasowicz M, Vegas A, et al.: Bivalirudin anticoagulation for cardiopulmonary bypass in a patient with heparin-induced thrombocytopenia, *Can J Anesth* 52 (10):1093–1098, 2005.
4. Welsby IJ, Newman MF, Phillips-Bute B, et al.: Hemodynamic changes after protamine administration: association with mortality after coronary artery bypass surgery, *Anesthesiology* 102 (2):308–314, 2005.
5. Prasongsukarn K, Borger MA: Reducing cerebral emboli during cardiopulmonary bypass, *Semin Cardiothorac Vasc Anesth* 9 (2):153–158, 2005.
6. Anderson MN, Kuchiba K: Blood trauma produced by pump oxygenators: a comparative study of five different units, *J Thorac Cardiovasc Surg* 57:238, 1969.

Coronary Artery Bypass Grafting (CABG)

SALLY COMBEST, M.D.

CHARLES B. HANTLER, M.D.

Coronary artery bypass grafting (CABG) is the most frequently performed major surgical procedure in the United States. Advances and newer approaches include less invasive surgical approaches, use of intraoperative transesophageal echocardiography (TEE), and the incorporation of regional anesthesia for this procedure.[1,2] In patients with stable angina, the indications for CABG are controversial but include left main coronary artery disease (CAD) and three-vessel CAD with decreased left ventricular (LV) function. Most patients who undergo CABG show improvement of symptoms; prognosis is clearly improved only in patients with left main CAD, patients with three-vessel CAD and decreased LV function, and possibly others with diabetes mellitus (DM). Patients with unstable angina refractory to medical therapy are candidates for operation or other invasive procedures.

A. Evaluate the severity of CAD and ventricular dysfunction (history, physical examination, exercise stress test, echocardiography [echo], thallium scan, and angiography). Many patients will have a history of hypertension (HTN), DM, smoking, and treatment with aspirin or platelet-inhibiting medications. Obtain baseline coagulation studies (platelet count, prothrombin time (PT), partial thromboplastin time (PTT), international normalized ratio [INR]). Patients with carotid bruits may be at increased risk for postoperative neurological complications and probably should undergo noninvasive Doppler studies of the carotid arteries.

B. Continue cardiac medications until surgery (some discontinue digoxin the evening before surgery, because they are fearful of dysrhythmias). Withdrawal of beta-blockers may provoke myocardial ischemia. Sedate the patient to avoid myocardial ischemia, but use caution in patients with depressed LV function or severe pulmonary disease. Antibiotic prophylaxis reduces infection.

C. Arterial and central lines may be placed before induction of anesthesia without inducing myocardial ischemia. Pulmonary artery (PA) catheters should be selectively used.[3] Transesophageal echocardiography (TEE) provides the most sensitive monitor of myocardial ischemia available to the anesthesiologist.[4]

D. Tailor the anesthetic technique to the patient's LV function and extent of CAD. The classic cardiac induction consists of a slow, high-dose narcotic induction, but different induction techniques have been used to obtain the goals of hemodynamic stability and early extubation (fast track).

E. Any volatile anesthetic can be safely used as tolerated. Establish adequate anticoagulation before initiation of cardiopulmonary bypass (CPB). Administer heparin, 3 to 4 mg/kg, to achieve an activated clotting time (ACT) > 400 seconds. Resistance to heparin may be encountered in patients treated with heparin preoperatively. An adult CPB circuit needs to be primed with 1500 to 2500 ml of volume. Mean arterial pressure (MAP) commonly falls during initiation of CPB because of reduced viscosity and perhaps, circulating vasoactive substances. Cerebral autoregulation appears to be maintained during hypothermic CPB when MAP > 30 mm Hg. Catecholamine levels rise significantly as CPB proceeds and may cause increased MAP. Maintain MAP between 50 and 100 mm Hg during CPB by adjusting the flow rate of the CPB pump and using anesthetics, vasodilators, or vasopressors as necessary. Bypass flow of 2.25 L/min/m^2 is required during normothermia and can be reduced to 1.6 L/min/m^2 during hypothermia (25° and 28°C). Hypothermia may provide myocardial protection (delaying myocardial rewarming) and cerebral protection. Adverse CNS outcomes are more common than previously thought. The most likely cause is emboli from CPB or more likely, dislodgement of emboli during aortic manipulation.

F. Before termination of CPB, check hemoglobin (Hb), electrolytes, glucose, arterial acid-base status, bilateral lung inflation and deflation, core body temperature, HR, and rhythm. Decide whether to institute inotropic support, depending on the quality of anastomoses, preoperative ventricular function, adequacy of myocardial protection during aortic cross-clamping, and duration of aortic cross-clamping. If CPB cannot be terminated with maximal inotropic support,[5] an intraaortic balloon pump (IABP) or ventricular assist device should be inserted.

Patient scheduled for
CORONARY ARTERY BYPASS GRAFTING

(A) Clinical evaluation ────────────────▶   ◀──────── CBC, SMA-6 and -12, coagulation profile
      History   Urinalysis, 12-lead ECG, chest film,
      Physical examination   ABGs, type and crossmatch blood

Review catheterization data:
      Left main or severe 3-vessel disease
      Refractory unstable angina
      Postinfarction angina
      LV ejection fraction > 20%
      Bypassable vessels (no diffuse distal disease)
      Absence of debilitating concomitant disease

Maximize medical management of: ────▶   Assess for other systemic diseases:
      Angina → ? need for IABP   Carotid, renal, pulmonary, hematologic
      Congestive heart failure
      Hypertension
      Dysrhythmias

(C) Monitoring ◀──────────────── (B) Premedication
      ECG (V$_5$ or modified V$_5$, II)   Narcotic: morphine, 0.1–0.15 mg/kg IM
      Stethoscope   Sedative: diazepam (10 mg PO)
      Radial arterial line   Reduce doses if poor myocardial function
      CVP   Nitroglycerin ointment
      PA catheter (if poor LV function)   Continue beta-blockers, nitrates, calcium
      TEE   channel blockers

(D) Anesthetic technique

High dose narcotic   "Fast track"

                          Monitor ischemia
                              ECG, TEE,
                pulmonary capillary wedge pressure

Depress LV function as needed (may avoid negative
inotrope if LV function depressed preoperatively)

(E) CPB

(F) Wean from CPB

Temperature
Rhythm
Laboratory values (electrolytes, ABG)
± inotropes, vasodilators

(Cont'd on p 285)

G. When the patient is hemodynamically stable after termination of CPB, administer protamine, determining the dose according to ACT or heparin levels. Excess protamine can increase bleeding and hypotension, PA vasoconstriction, and right ventricular (RV) failure. A "wet" surgical field may result from platelet dysfunction, fibrinolysis, or inadequate heparin reversal. Administer plasma or platelets only if specifically indicated. Early extubation (<6 hours) and early discharge home (3 to 5 days) can be accomplished using fast-track techniques.[6] This is cost effective compared with the high-dose narcotic technique. Some centers are extubating patients in the recovery room and discharging them to non-ICU-monitored beds.

REFERENCES

1. Katsnelson Y, Raman J, Katsnelson F, et al.: Current state of intraoperative echocardiography, *Echocardiography* 20 (8):771, 2003.
2. Priestley MC, Cope L, Halliwell R, et al.: Thoracic epidural anesthesia for cardiac surgery: the effects on tracheal intubation time and length of hospital stay, *Anesth Analg* 94:275–282, 2002.
3. Dalen JE: The pulmonary artery catheter—friend, foe, or accomplice? *JAMA* 286:348–350, 2001.
4. Wappler F: Cardiac and thoracic vascular surgery, *Best Pract Res Clin Anaesthesiol* 17 (2):219–233, 2003.
5. McKinlay KH, Schinderle DB, Swaminathan M, et al.: Predictors of inotrope use during separation from cardiopulmonary bypass, *J Cardiothorac Vasc Anesth* 18 (4):404–408, 2004.
6. Thomas R, Smith D, Strike P: Prospective randomized double-blind comparative study of rocuronium and pancuronium in adult patients scheduled for elective "fast track" cardiac surgery involving hypothermic cardiopulmonary bypass, *Anaesthesia* 58 (3):265–271, 2003.

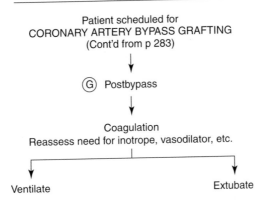

Patient scheduled for
CORONARY ARTERY BYPASS GRAFTING
(Cont'd from p 283)

Ⓖ Postbypass

Coagulation
Reassess need for inotrope, vasodilator, etc.

Ventilate   Extubate

Off-Pump Coronary Artery Bypass (OPCAB)

D.M. ANDERSON, M.D.

Coronary artery bypass grafting (CABG) performed without cardiopulmonary bypass (CPB) is called off-pump coronary artery bypass (OPCAB) and is a preferred technique of some cardiovascular surgeons. At some medical centers, nearly all CABGs are performed off pump; at others, almost none of the CABGs are done off pump; others select OPCAB on a case by case basis. CPB is associated with substantial morbidity. However, the benefits of OPCAB are still unclear.[1,2] Some evidence suggests improved early and midterm survival.[3,4] Patients having OPCABs generally are extubated sooner, spend less time in the ICU, and are discharged from the hospital more quickly.

A. Consider the following issues when planning an anesthetic for OPCAB.[5] Determine the status of the patient's cardiac function and other medical problems. Read the catheterization report to locate and assess the severity of the coronary lesions. During OPCAB, distal diseased arteries and severely stenosed coronary arteries can be occluded without significant hemodynamic effect, because distal arteries supply smaller areas of the heart and severely stenosed arteries are likely to have collateral flow. In contrast, occlusion of vessels that are proximally diseased (i.e., larger regions of the heart at risk) or less severely stenosed (i.e., less extensive collaterals) can result in severe myocardial ischemia with adverse hemodynamic consequences. Also note the presence or absence of concomitant valvular disease.

B. Monitoring is an important issue. American Society of Anesthesiologists (ASA) monitors are standard. Always place an arterial line and central venous catheter. The pulmonary artery (PA) catheter is not mandatory. Consider using transesophageal echocardiography (TEE). Not only is TEE useful in assessing cardiac function and detecting new wall motion abnormalities and their resolution, but it also helps to identify patients with severe atheromatous disease of the aorta, in whom it is prudent for the surgeon to avoid aortic manipulation. Keep the OR warm and continuously monitor patient temperature during OPCAB; it is more difficult to maintain adequate body temperature during this procedure, because the patient is not rewarmed with CPB.

C. Patients undergoing OPCAB are often selected for fast-track anesthetic techniques, which may include immediate postoperative extubation in the OR at some facilities. A variety of anesthetic techniques have been reported to be effective for this purpose. Be sure to consider postoperative pain management when planning the anesthetic. Consider placement of a thoracic epidural, intrathecal narcotics, or thoracic paravertebral blocks for postoperative analgesia.

D. Hemodynamic instability can occur during OPCAB. The patient's preoperative cardiac function and the amount of surgical manipulation of the heart are the primary determinants of hemodynamic stability. Administer appropriate volumes of fluid early during the procedure to minimize hypotension. Add vasoactive medications, such as dopamine, epinephrine, or norepinephrine, to maintain stability when necessary.

E. Anticoagulation protocols differ among medical centers. Some administer much less heparin for OPCAB than for CABG using CPB. Others administer full anticoagulation and carefully reverse with protamine at the end of the procedure. Some groups employ antiplatelet regimens after OPCAB to avoid postoperative graft occlusion.

REFERENCES

1. Reston JT, Tregear SJ, Turkelson CM: Meta-analysis of short-term and mid-term outcomes following off-pump coronary artery bypass grafting, *Ann Thorac Surg* 76 (5):1510–1515, 2003.
2. Lancey RA: Off-pump coronary artery bypass surgery, *Curr Probl Surg* 40 (11):693–802, 2003.
3. Sharony R, Bizekis CS, Kanchuger M, et al.: Off-pump coronary artery bypass grafting reduces mortality and stroke in patients with atheromatous aortas: a case control study, *Circulation* 108 (Suppl 1):II15–II20, 2003.
4. Ascione R, Narayan P, Rogers CA, et al.: Early and midterm clinical outcome in patients with severe left ventricular dysfunction undergoing coronary artery surgery, *Ann Thorac Surg* 76 (3): 793–799, 2003.
5. Shanewise JS, Ramsay JG: Off-pump coronary surgery: how do the anesthetic considerations differ? *Anesthesiol Clin North Am* 21 (3):613–623, 2003.

OFF-PUMP CABG (OPCAB)

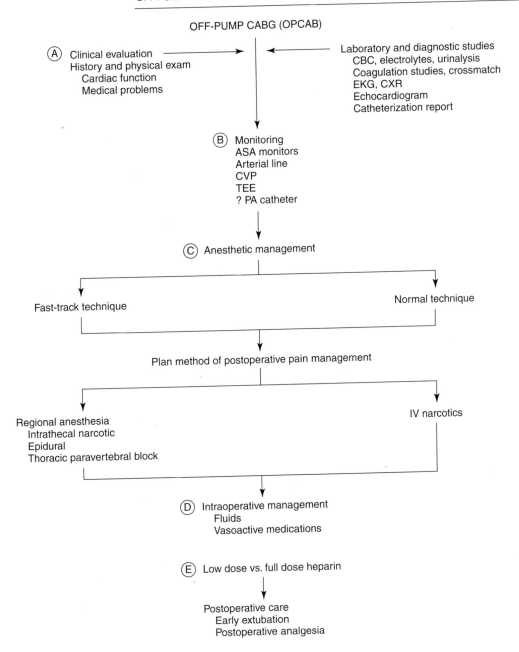

Ⓐ Clinical evaluation
  History and physical exam
    Cardiac function
    Medical problems

Laboratory and diagnostic studies
  CBC, electrolytes, urinalysis
  Coagulation studies, crossmatch
  EKG, CXR
  Echocardiogram
  Catheterization report

Ⓑ Monitoring
  ASA monitors
  Arterial line
  CVP
  TEE
  ? PA catheter

Ⓒ Anesthetic management

Fast-track technique

Normal technique

Plan method of postoperative pain management

Regional anesthesia
  Intrathecal narcotic
  Epidural
  Thoracic paravertebral block

IV narcotics

Ⓓ Intraoperative management
  Fluids
  Vasoactive medications

Ⓔ Low dose vs. full dose heparin

Postoperative care
  Early extubation
  Postoperative analgesia

Acute Heart Failure (AHF) in Cardiac Surgery

JAYDEEP S. SHAH, M.D.

MARCOS A. ZUAZU, M.D.

JOSEPH J. NAPLES, M.D.

In acute heart failure (AHF), the clinical picture is that of shock in which the BP and cardiac output (CO) are inadequate for metabolic needs. The compensatory mechanisms of the failing heart (tachycardia, vasoconstriction, and fluid retention) eventually worsen cardiac performance. Restoration of adequate perfusion pressure must be accomplished without exacerbating pulmonary congestion. Thus, the goals of pharmacological therapy for AHF in the OR setting are to optimize cardiac function at minimal expense to cardiac workload (HR, contractility, preload, and afterload). When pharmacological regimens fail, mechanical support becomes the ultimate option.

A. Determine the cause of AHF. AHF during cardiac procedures can be due to either direct or indirect myocardial insults. Direct insults include preoperatively depressed ventricular function with or without pulmonary hypertension (HTN), myocardium injury at the time of operation (e.g., ischemia, poor myocardial protection techniques, hypothermia, and iatrogenic surgical injury), increased duration of cardiopulmonary bypass (CPB), and reperfusion injury. Secondary insults include acid-base imbalance, hypoventilation, hypoxia, anemia, moderate hypocalcemia and hypomagnesemia, and cardiac dysrhythmias, all of which should be treated aggressively. Although it is not in the scope of this chapter, health care providers should be familiar with current advanced cardiac life support (ACLS) protocols. If a sinus rhythm cannot be restored, pacing wires may be applied directly to the heart for atrioventricular (AV) pacing (usually a temporary measure, as normal cardiac rhythm often follows an interval of temporary cardiac pacing).

B. The goals of inotropic therapy are to improve myocardial contractility, reduce ventricular dimension, normalize CO, optimize BP and tissue perfusion, and relieve pulmonary congestion. In the initial attempt to separate from CPB, select therapy based on information derived from arterial, venous, and pulmonary artery pressures, and CO and systemic vascular resistance (SVR). In AHF, transesophageal echocardiography (TEE) is essential for assessing ventricular function, volume status, and effect(s) of pharmacological intervention. Although calcium has been used routinely by some as a first-line agent for low CO and BP, its principal action is that of vasoconstriction with a resultant increase in mean arterial pressure. Multiple studies have been unable to demonstrate a reliable effect of calcium on CO.[1] Additionally, in certain circumstances, calcium administration may result in reducing the response to beta-adrenergic receptor (β-AR) agonists. An exception to this may be a clinical situation of hyperkalemia with a decreased serum ionized calcium level. It is routine to begin an infusion of a β-AR agonist (dopamine at 3 to 5 μg/kg/min or epinephrine at 0.03 to 0.05 μg/kg/min) in combination with nitroglycerin (NTG) at 0.5 mcg/kg/min as a starting regimen following adequate reperfusion time in the initial attempt to separate from CBP.

C. The use of phosphodiesterase inhibitors (PDEIs) results in both positive inotropic effects and systemic and pulmonary vasodilation. PDEIs may increase oxygen delivery with minimal thermogenic and metabolic effects. In addition, these agents may enhance the responsiveness to catecholamines in the situation where down-regulation of β-AR has occurred (e.g., preoperative heart failure treated with catecholamines). If the initial regimen of β-AR agonist(s) is ineffective, add milrinone with a loading dose (50 μg/kg given while the patient is on CBP) followed thereafter by continuous infusion (0.3 to 0.5 μg/kg/min). Alternatively, omit the loading dose of milrinone and begin infusion at 0.5 μg/kg/min, in addition to the existing β-AR agonist regimen. On initiation of PDEI treatment, discontinue the use of other vasodilatory drugs. The continued administration of β-AR agonists in increasing dosage may result in excessive and persistent tachycardia. The resulting tachycardia may exacerbate a low CO or low perfusion state. Consider the addition of esmolol for heart rate control and enhanced catecholamine effectiveness.

Patient with LOW BP AND LOW OUTPUT STATE INTRAOPERATIVELY

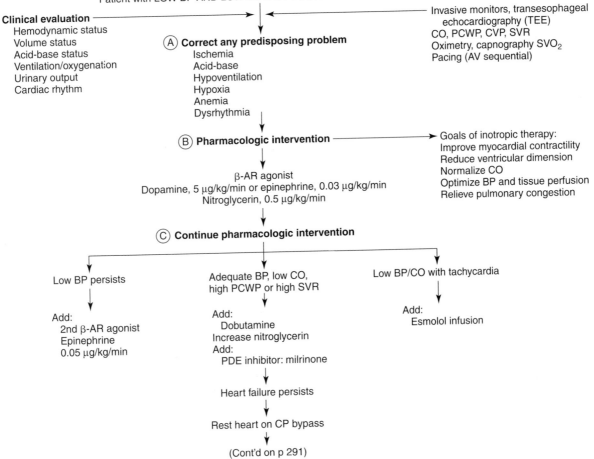

Clinical evaluation
Hemodynamic status
Volume status
Acid-base status
Ventilation/oxygenation
Urinary output
Cardiac rhythm

Invasive monitors, transesophageal
echocardiography (TEE)
CO, PCWP, CVP, SVR
Oximetry, capnography SVO_2
Pacing (AV sequential)

(A) **Correct any predisposing problem**
Ischemia
Acid-base
Hypoventilation
Hypoxia
Anemia
Dysrhythmia

(B) **Pharmacologic intervention**

Goals of inotropic therapy:
Improve myocardial contractility
Reduce ventricular dimension
Normalize CO
Optimize BP and tissue perfusion
Relieve pulmonary congestion

β-AR agonist
Dopamine, 5 µg/kg/min or epinephrine, 0.03 µg/kg/min
Nitroglycerin, 0.5 µg/kg/min

(C) **Continue pharmacologic intervention**

Low BP persists

Add:
2nd β-AR agonist
Epinephrine
0.05 µg/kg/min

Adequate BP, low CO,
high PCWP or high SVR

Add:
Dobutamine
Increase nitroglycerin
Add:
PDE inhibitor: milrinone

Heart failure persists

Rest heart on CP bypass

(Cont'd on p 291)

Low BP/CO with tachycardia

Add:
Esmolol infusion

D. If the initial pharmacological interventions are not successful, reinstitute CPB. In situations where ventricular function and CO are adequate but BP is excessively low, especially diastolic pressure, begin an infusion of norepinephrine, phenylephrine, or vasopressin.[2] AHF may be exacerbated by persistently high SVR or pulmonary vascular resistance (PVR). In these situations NTG has been useful to reduce preload, improve pulmonary congestion, and enhance subendocardial perfusion by reducing left ventricular (LV) end-diastolic volume. Nesiritide, a beta-type natriuretic peptide, although unproven for its usefulness during cardiac surgery, has been shown to compare quite favorably[3] versus NTG in recent clinical trials in patients with AHF. Impairment of LV performance resulting in low BP and CO may be secondary to right-sided heart failure (RHF), which has a negative impact on LV preload. RHF may be detected by direct observation of the heart with the TEE. Decreased right ventricular (RV) apex wall motion and increased tricuspid regurgitation are indicators of RV dysfunction. Optimize preload and decrease PVR with inodilators (e.g., dobutamine, milrinone), or inhaled nitric oxide 20 to 80 ppm.

E. Persistent failure to wean from CPB suggests need for restoration of CPB (to rest the heart for a time before a subsequent attempt to wean), insertion of an intraaortic balloon pump (IABP) for counterpulsation or a cardiac assist device. This is a surgical decision, but experience dictates that an early balloon may be lifesaving. When several potent inotrope/vasodilator combinations have been tried and failed, IABP should be instituted while the patient's heart is being rested on CPB. This technique may also "save" heart muscle that could be damaged beyond recovery. When IABP cannot be achieved or is ineffective, a temporary cardiac assist device (e.g., left-sided heart bypass, right-sided heart bypass, or biventricular assist) may be considered by the surgical team. For a temporary left-sided heart bypass, a continuous circuit is established, diverting blood from the left atrium to the aorta using a centrifugal pump without heparinization. Overall outcome with cardiac assist devices has been less than optimal.

REFERENCES

1. Royster RL, Butterworth JF IV, Prielipp RC, et al.: A randomized, blinded, placebo-controlled evaluation of calcium chloride and epinephrine for inotropic support after emergence from cardiopulmonary bypass, *Anesth Analg* 74:3–13, 1992.
2. Booth JV, Schinderle D, Welsby IJ: Pro: vasopressin is the vasoconstrictor of choice after cardiopulmonary bypass, *J Cardiothorac Vasc Anesth* 16 (6):773–775, 2002.
3. Publication Committee of the VMAC Investigators: Intravenous nesiritide vs. nitroglycerin for treatment of decompensated congestive heart failure: a randomized controlled trial, *JAMA* 287:1531–1540, 2002.
4. Rubin LJ: Primary pulmonary hypertension, *N Engl J Med* 336:111–117, 1997.

Patient with LOW BP AND LOW OUTPUT STATE INTRAOPERATIVELY
(Cont'd from p 289)

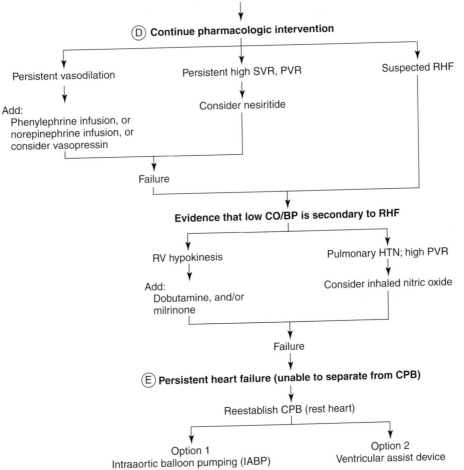

Ⓓ **Continue pharmacologic intervention**

Persistent vasodilation

Add:
  Phenylephrine infusion, or
  norepinephrine infusion, or
  consider vasopressin

Persistent high SVR, PVR

Consider nesiritide

Suspected RHF

Failure

Evidence that low CO/BP is secondary to RHF

RV hypokinesis

Add:
  Dobutamine, and/or
  milrinone

Pulmonary HTN; high PVR

Consider inhaled nitric oxide

Failure

Ⓔ **Persistent heart failure (unable to separate from CPB)**

Reestablish CPB (rest heart)

Option 1
Intraaortic balloon pumping (IABP)

Option 2
Ventricular assist device

Mitral Valve Replacement

IRENA VAITKEVICIUTE, M.D.

JOSEPH P. MATHEW, M.D.

PAUL G. BARASH, M.D.

Surgical correction of mitral valve disease (regurgitation or stenosis) may involve either repair or replacement. Myxomatous degeneration is currently the most common cause of pure mitral regurgitation (MR) in Western countries, and the vast majority of these patients are amenable to repair.[1,2] Trauma, ruptured chordae secondary to endocarditis, and papillary muscle rupture following myocardial infarction (MI) result in acute MR. Transesophageal echocardiography (TEE) quantification of MR is by the ratio of jet area to left atrial areas: mild MR, ratio <20%; moderate MR, ratio 20 to 40%; severe MR, ratio >40%. It can also be estimated using the vena contracta width: mild <0.3 cm; moderate 0.3 to 0.69 cm; severe >0.7 cm. The principal physiological change in chronic MR is a volume-overloaded left ventricle.[3] Acute MR is complicated by the addition of a pressure overload in the left atrium that can result in pulmonary edema. Mitral stenosis is almost exclusively secondary to rheumatic disease and can be treated by valvotomy or valve replacement.[1] Of patients with mitral stenosis, 40% present with coexistent MR. Mitral valve area (MVA) is commonly evaluated by TEE using the formula: 220 divided by pressure half-time. Classification of mitral stenosis is by MVA: normal 4 to 6 cm^2; mild, 1.5 to 2 cm^2; moderate, 1 to 1.5 cm^2; severe, <1 cm^2. The principal pathophysiological change in mitral stenosis is left atrial pressure (LAP) overload.[3] Chronic increases in LAP are transmitted to the pulmonary veins, but right ventricular (RV) function is normal as long as pulmonary vascular resistance (PVR) is not elevated.

A. Preoperative evaluation defines the extent of disease. Look for signs of RV failure including distended neck veins, hepatomegaly, peripheral edema, and ascites. Review the ECG, which may reveal left atrial enlargement (LAE), atrial fibrillation (AF), or RV hypertrophy (RVH). Two-dimensional TEE may demonstrate restricted motion and doming of the leaflets, prolapse of anterior or posterior cusps (mitral valve prolapse [MVP]), and ruptured chordae or papillary muscle. Doppler-TEE measures quantify the transvalvular gradients and the severity of regurgitation. Ejection fraction (EF) by radioisotope angiography is usually overestimated in patients with MR.

B. Continue antiarrhythmics if administered for control of ventricular rate. Evaluate for diuretic-induced hypokalemia. Discontinue the last four doses of warfarin to bring the international normalized ratio (INR) to 1.5 before surgery. If the INR was maintained at 3 or higher, the warfarin may need to be discontinued sooner. Start IV heparin if the risk of embolization is high.[4,5] Tailor sedative administration to the degree of ventricular dysfunction. Choose prophylactic antibiotics per guidelines of the American Heart Association.[6]

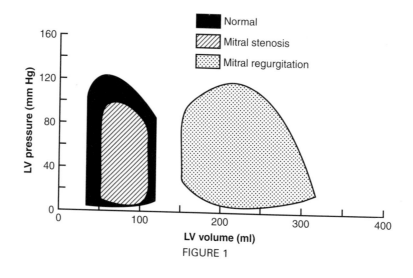

FIGURE 1

Patient for MITRAL VALVE REPLACEMENT

Ⓐ **Preoperative evaluation**
   Valvular or coronary artery disease
   Murmur
   Right heart function (↑ PVR)
   Drugs (antiarrhythmic, diuretic, anticoagulant)

Chest x-ray (cardiomegaly, pulmonary edema)
ECG (LAE, AF, RVH)
Angiography (valve area, gradient, regurgitation)
Echocardiography (valve anatomy, area, gradient, regurgitation)
CBC, coagulation profile, electrolytes, ABG

Ⓑ **Premedication**
   Antibiotics (SBE prophylaxis)
   Oxygen supplementation during transport to OR
   Continue antiarrhythmics for control of ventricular rate
   ? Potassium replacement if treated with digoxin
   Prevent sympathetic stimulation/anxiety (MS, MVP)
   ↑ Susceptibility to ventilatory depressant drugs

(Cont'd on p 295)

C. Place arterial and pulmonary artery (PA) catheters in most patients. In patients with pulmonary hypertension (HTN), weigh the benefits of PA catheterization against an increased risk of PA perforation.[7] In mitral stenosis, the pulmonary capillary wedge pressure (PCWP) overestimates the left ventricular end-diastolic pressure (LVEDP); tachycardia increases the difference between LVEDP and PCWP (Figure 1). V-wave amplitude does not correlate well with the severity of MR.[8] Place intraoperative TEE for mitral valve repair. Always assess regurgitation following mitral valve repair or replacement under normal ventricular loading conditions.

D. *Stenosis:* During induction and maintenance of anesthesia, allow minimal changes in HR (maintain sinus rhythm), systemic vascular resistance (SVR), and contractility. The Trendelenburg position is poorly tolerated.

    Regurgitation: An elevated HR (approximately 80 to 90 beats/min) is ideal, except when the MR is caused by mitral valve prolapse (MVP). Vasodilation decreases end-diastolic volume and resistance to forward flow.

E. *Stenosis:* Tachycardia other than sinus resulting in decreased BP may be treated with direct current (DC) cardioversion. Ephedrine increases contractility and cardiac output (CO) but at the expense of increased HR. Increases in ventricular afterload from phenylephrine may precipitate failure.

    Regurgitation: Decreases in BP may require inotropes. HTN can be treated with volatile agents that decrease SVR or with arterial vasodilators.

F. Postoperatively, continue antibiotics and restart anticoagulation.[5] Patients with chronic MR have decreased pulmonary compliance and increased work of breathing. Increased afterload from a newly competent valve may unmask previous contraction abnormalities.[9]

REFERENCES

1. Yacoub MH, Cohn LH: Novel approaches to cardiac valve repair: from structure to function: Part I, *Circulation* 109:942–950, 2004.
2. Yacoub MH, Cohn LH: Novel approaches to cardiac valve repair: from structure to function: Part II, *Circulation* 109:1064–1072, 2004.
3. Carabello AB, Crawford AF: Valvular heart disease, *New Engl J Med* 337:32–41, 1997.
4. Bonow RO, Carabello B, De Leon AC Jr, et al.: Guidelines for the management of patients with valvular heart disease. A report of the American College of Cardiology/American Heart Association task force on practice guidelines, *J Am Coll Cardiol* 32:1486–1588, 1998.
5. Kearon C, Hirsh J: Management of anticoagulation before and after elective surgery, *N Engl J Med* 336:1506–1511, 1997.
6. Dajani SA, Taubert KA, Wilson W, et al.: Prevention of bacterial endocarditis. Recommendations by the American Heart Association, *Circulation* 96:358–366, 1997.
7. Barash PG, Nardi D, Hammond G, et al.: Catheter-induced pulmonary artery perforation. Mechanisms, management, and modifications, *J Thorac Cardiovasc Surg* 82:5–12, 1981.
8. Pichard AD, Diaz R, Marchant E, et al.: Large V waves in the capillary wedge pressure tracing without mitral regurgitation: the influence of the pressure/volume relationship on the V wave size, *Clin Cardiol* 6:534–541, 1983.
9. Ghobashy AM, Barash PG: Valvular heart disease. In: Trojanos CA, editor: *Anesthesia for the cardiac patient*, St. Louis, 2002, Mosby.

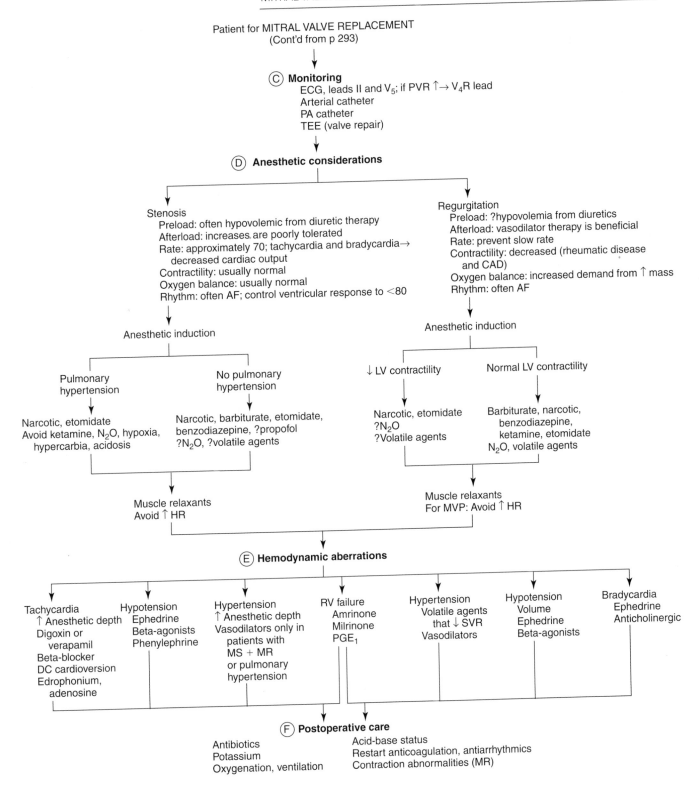

Patient for MITRAL VALVE REPLACEMENT
(Cont'd from p 293)

Ⓒ **Monitoring**
ECG, leads II and V$_5$; if PVR ↑→ V$_4$R lead
Arterial catheter
PA catheter
TEE (valve repair)

Ⓓ **Anesthetic considerations**

Stenosis
Preload: often hypovolemic from diuretic therapy
Afterload: increases are poorly tolerated
Rate: approximately 70; tachycardia and bradycardia→
decreased cardiac output
Contractility: usually normal
Oxygen balance: usually normal
Rhythm: often AF; control ventricular response to <80

Regurgitation
Preload: ?hypovolemia from diuretics
Afterload: vasodilator therapy is beneficial
Rate: prevent slow rate
Contractility: decreased (rheumatic disease
and CAD)
Oxygen balance: increased demand from ↑ mass
Rhythm: often AF

Anesthetic induction

Pulmonary
hypertension

No pulmonary
hypertension

Narcotic, etomidate
Avoid ketamine, N$_2$O, hypoxia,
hypercarbia, acidosis

Narcotic, barbiturate, etomidate,
benzodiazepine, ?propofol
?N$_2$O, ?volatile agents

Anesthetic induction

↓ LV contractility

Normal LV contractility

Narcotic, etomidate
?N$_2$O
?Volatile agents

Barbiturate, narcotic,
benzodiazepine,
ketamine, etomidate
N$_2$O, volatile agents

Muscle relaxants
Avoid ↑ HR

Muscle relaxants
For MVP: Avoid ↑ HR

Ⓔ **Hemodynamic aberrations**

Tachycardia
↑ Anesthetic depth
Digoxin or
verapamil
Beta-blocker
DC cardioversion
Edrophonium,
adenosine

Hypotension
Ephedrine
Beta-agonists
Phenylephrine

Hypertension
↑ Anesthetic depth
Vasodilators only in
patients with
MS + MR
or pulmonary
hypertension

RV failure
Amrinone
Milrinone
PGE$_1$

Hypertension
Volatile agents
that ↓ SVR
Vasodilators

Hypotension
Volume
Ephedrine
Beta-agonists

Bradycardia
Ephedrine
Anticholinergic

Ⓕ **Postoperative care**

Antibiotics
Potassium
Oxygenation, ventilation

Acid-base status
Restart anticoagulation, antiarrhythmics
Contraction abnormalities (MR)

Repair of Congenital Heart Disease (CHD): Bypass

JAYDEEP S. SHAH, M.D.

Approximately 800,000 patients in the United Stated have congenital heart disease (CHD), often with severe ventricular failure, pulmonary hypertension (HTN), dysrhythmias, and cyanosis. Once cardiovascular collapse occurs, resuscitation may be difficult in these patients; thus careful attention to detail and anticipation of potential problems is vital.[1–6]

A. The anesthesiologist must know the patient's cardiac anatomy and pathophysiology and any systemic diseases and coexisting anomalies. Even a mild upper respiratory tract infection can result in significant morbidity in children with CHD and prompts postponement of elective surgery. Document preoperative vital signs and room air SpO_2. Order laboratory tests if indicated.

B. Monitor standard American Society of Anesthesiologists (ASA) monitors, CVP, and arterial pressure monitoring. Transesophageal echocardiography (TEE) is used to assess ventricular and valvular function, volume status, regional wall motion abnormalities, and prerepair and postrepair anatomy and has become an essential tool for intraoperative management of CHD patients. More recently, neurophysiological monitoring during CHD surgeries—cerebral oxygen saturation (near-infrared spectroscopy), cerebral blood flow (transcranial Doppler ultrasound), and the depth of anesthesia (bispectral index)—has become commercially available. Evidence that neurological monitoring during complex CHD surgery improves outcomes is accumulating.

C. Tailor premedication and induction techniques to the patient's pathophysiology. Use of antifibrinolytics (Aprotinin), especially in complex CHD repairs, is highly recommended.

D. Maintain mean arterial pressure (MAP) between 20 and 50 mm Hg and normal PaO_2, $PaCO_2$, and pH. The prime volume necessary to fill the cardiopulmonary bypass (CPB) circuit and ensure that no air is pumped results in hemodilution on initiation of bypass. The prime itself is usually hyponatremic, hypocalcemic, hypomagnesemic, hypocapnic, acidotic, and hypoosmolar. Thus, the result is a state of anemia, thrombocytopenia, hypocoagulability, and hypoproteinemia. This dilutional state prompts administration of blood and blood products and additional doses of drugs. Prior to initiating bypass, achieve adequate anticoagulation with 3 to 4 mg/kg heparin intravenously. An activating clotting time (ACT) of 300 to 400 seconds is acceptable to initiate CPB; however, a value of 400 seconds or greater is necessary to ensure no microscopic evidence of aggregates. Check the ACT every 30 minutes while on CPB. Hypothermia is induced to protect both the heart and brain (maintaining myocardial ATP stores, decreasing the cerebral metabolic rate and total body oxygen consumption, and decreasing anesthetic requirements). However, hypothermia can lead to arrhythmias and decreased myocardial contractility, increased blood glucose levels, and poor rheology due to increased blood viscosity. The use of hemofiltration or ultrafiltration during or immediately after CPB has been shown to decrease the need of inotropic and ventilatory support by removing inflammatory mediators.

E. Deep hypothermic circulatory arrest (DHCA) is used for complex intracardiac and aortic repairs. Core cooling to 15°–18°C is accomplished with CPB prior to initiating DHCA. During the DHCA, administration of mannitol (0.5 g/kg), furosemide (0.25 to 1 mg/kg), H_1 and H_2 blockers, steroids, and use of alpha-blockers have been recommended. DHCA can be utilized for approximately 45 minutes, after which neuropsychological dysfunction, both transient and permanent, has been reported in up to 45% of infants.

F. Before discontinuing CPB, rewarm (usually 37°C) with no significant difference between core and peripheral temperatures. Ensure adequate cardiac rhythm (paced or normal sinus rhythm), hematocrit (Hct) level, ABG, and electrolyte balance. Ventilate with 100% oxygen. Pulmonary toilet with suctioning of endotracheal secretions and administration of inhaled albuterol will improve pulmonary compliance and reduce pulmonary vascular resistance (PVR). Both inotropic and vasodilator drugs should be available for bolus or infusion. Difficulties in discontinuation of CPB are usually multifactorial and may be due to a lengthy bypass period, electrolyte imbalance, inadequacy of the repair, or preexisting myocardial damage. Subsequent reversal of heparin is accomplished with protamine: 1 mg for every milligram of heparin. Administration of protamine should be slow (over 20 to 30 minutes) as it can cause severe hypotension, pulmonary HTN, anaphylaxis, and anaphylactoid reactions.

G. Individualize the postoperative care based on the type of repair and its physiological effects. CHD patients are (1) prone to arrhythmias in the postoperative period; (2) particularly susceptible to the deleterious effects of hypoventilation and decreases in oxyhemoglobin saturation; and (3) dependent on vasoactive and inotropic pharmacological support, which should not be discontinued abruptly. It is important that these patients be followed closely in the postoperative period by an anesthesiologist, pediatric intensivist, or cardiologist familiar with their specific cardiac disease.

Patient with
CONGENITAL CARDIAC DISEASE FOR BYPASS PROCEDURE

(A) Clinical and diagnostic evaluation ⟶
    See congential heart disease—nonbypass
    Rule out URI, especially RSV
    Evaluate for cardiac stability

(B) Monitoring
    ASA monitors
    Temperature
    Arterial line
    Central venous line
    TEE
    Neurophysiologic monitoring

(C) Premedication and induction techniques ⟶
    See congenital heart disease—nonbypass
    Aprotinin

Manipulation of SVR, PVR, myocardial function with anesthetic agents, ventilation, oxygenation:

- PPV increases PVR and decreases pulmonary flow
- Low FiO_2 will also limit pulmonary blood flow
- Hypercarbia increases PVR Hyperventilation decreases PVR
- Inhalational agents reduce SVR and improve systemic flow
- N_2O can be used to limit the amount of FiO_2
- NO decreases PVR
- High-dose narcotic (fentanyl) techniques have the least effect on failing myocardial performance while helping block the stress response
- Morphine theoretically decreases both SVR and PVR
- Ketamine increases PVR and SVR, which results in increased left-to-right shunting
- Beta-blockade (esmolol) can be used to relax dynamic outflow obstruction

(D) Cardiopulmonary bypass
    Heparin 3–4 mg/kg IV
    ACT >400 sec—
        check every 30 min
    MAP 20–50 mm Hg
    Blood and products available
    pH stat management
    Avoid hypoglycemia
    Use hemofiltration
        or ultrafiltration
    Monitor urine output

(E) Deep hypothermic circulatory arrest
    Complex congenital heart repairs
    Cooling to 15°–18°C
    Give furosemide, mannitol, H1 and H2
        blockers, steroids, alpha-blockers
    Avoid duration longer than 45 min

(F) Discontinuation of CPB
    Adequate rewarming (37°)
    Adequate ventilation (FiO_2 1.0)
    Adequate cardiac rhythm (pacing?)
    Normal ABG, electrolytes, adequate Hct
    Pulmonary toilet
    Available inotropes/pressor infusions
    Protamine once stable

(G) Postoperative care
    Avoid arrhythmias
    Avoid hypoventilation, desaturation
    Avoid sudden changes in
        pharmacological support
    Dedicated intensivist

REFERENCES

1. Warner MA, Lunn RJ, O'Leary PW, et al.: Outcomes of noncardiac surgical procedures in children and adults with congenital heart disease. Mayo Perioperative Outcomes Group, *Mayo Clin Proc,* 73 (8):728–734, 1998.
2. Bettex DA, Pretre R, Jenni R, et al.: Cost-effectiveness of routine intraoperative transesophageal echocardiography in pediatric cardiac surgery: a 10-year experience, *Anesth Analg* 100 (5):1271–1275.
3. Austin EH 3rd, Edmonds HL Jr, Auden SM, et al.: Benefit of neurophysiologic monitoring for pediatric cardiac surgery, *J Thorac Cardiovasc Surg* 114:707–717, 1997.
4. Miller BE, Tosone SR, Tam VKH, et al.: Hematologic and economic impact of Aprotinin in reoperative pediatric cardiac operations, *Ann Thorac Surg* 66:535–541, 1998.
5. Journois D, Israel-Biet D, et al.: High-volume, zero-balanced hemofiltration to reduce delayed inflammatory response to cardiopulmonary bypass in children, *Anesthesiology* 85:965–976, 1996.
6. Limperopoulos C, Majnemer A, Shevell MI, et al.: Predictors of developmental disabilities after open heart surgery in young children with congenital heart defects, *J Pediatr* 141 (1):51–58, 2002.

Repair of CHD: Nonbypass

JAYDEEP S. SHAH, M.D.

The incidence of congenital heart disease (CHD) is 6 to 8 per 1,000 births. Premature infants have a two- to threefold higher incidence of CHD. In recent years, enormous technological advances allow intervention for many congenital heart defects in the pediatric cardiac catheterization laboratory; valvuloplasty, angioplasty, stent implantation, coil embolization, and device occlusion require anesthesia support for extended periods of time in which there can be significant hemodynamic instability. It is important to understand the pathophysiology of a given defect—increased pulmonary blood flow (left-to-right shunts), decreased pulmonary blood flow (right-to-left shunts), a mixing of pulmonary and systemic circulation (complex shunt), or an obstruction to flow.

A. Most patients are on antiarrhythmics, diuretics, or anticoagulants; coordinate management with the cardiologist and consider endocarditis prophylaxis. CHD patients need not be admitted to the hospital preoperatively if in good health. Schedule preanesthetic evaluation before the day of surgery to evaluate concurrent congenital defects,[1] medication changes, review labs and studies. Perform a careful airway exam—the incidence of perioperative morbidity due to an underlying airway anomaly may be as high as 50% in CHD patients.[2] Respiratory function may be compromised (prolonged ventilator support, recurrent pleural effusions, possibly hypoplastic lungs).

B. Premedicate with great care. Sedation may diminish children's crying during separation from the parents, decreasing O_2 consumption and avoiding increases in pulmonary vascular resistance (PVR). However, even minimal respiratory depression may result in significant desaturation in children with cyanotic CHD. Oral midazolam (0.75 mg/kg) appears to be safe and efficacious in this group of patients.[3]

C. For therapeutic procedures performed in the cardiac catheterization lab, consider a deep sedation technique or a lighter level of general anesthesia that allows maintenance of the spontaneous respiration. However, this does not ensure greater hemodynamic stability. Increases in end-tidal CO_2 due to respiratory depression can lead to acute exacerbation of pulmonary artery (PA) pressures and PVR.[4] Change in myocardial contractility or systemic vascular resistance (SVR) can result in mismatching pulmonary-to-systemic blood flow ratios. More complex defects and planned therapeutic interventions usually require controlled ventilation. No evidence supports superiority of any particular anesthetic technique. Both total IV and mixed inhalation/IV techniques have been successfully employed.

D. Traditional operative repair of CHD not requiring cardiopulmonary bypass (CPB) includes repair of aortic coarctation, ligation of patent ductus arteriosus (PDA), PA artery banding, and various systemic-to-pulmonary shunt procedures for anomalies with insufficient pulmonary blood flow. The surgical approach to these defects can be either through a sternotomy or thoracotomy. The lateral decubitus position warrants careful evaluation of breath sounds after positioning. In general, the invasive nature of these procedures necessitates a deeper level of anesthesia, which will also attenuate increases in PVR and SVR. This can be accomplished with the use of larger doses of narcotics or supplemental regional anesthesia.

E. Place standard American Society of Anesthesiologists (ASA) monitors. In addition, insert CVP and arterial blood pressure monitors. Additional monitoring is case specific (e.g., the placement of a radial arterial line on the right side for coarctation surgery or contralateral to thoracotomy site for shunting procedures). Consider intraoperative transesophageal echocardiography (TEE).

F. When appropriate, perform a sevoflurane inhalation induction. Inhalation induction will theoretically be slowed in the presence of right-to-left shunting. An adequately sedated patient allows a smoother induction. If an IV induction is preferred, give titrated doses of propofol in combination with ketamine, midazolam, or narcotics.[5] In instances when preservation of SVR is crucial, consider the use of etomidate; propofol has been shown to cause a decrease in SVR in CHD patients.

G. Maintain anesthesia with narcotics in combination with an inhalation agent. Pancuronium is a useful muscle relaxation—vagolytic effects offset narcotic-induced bradycardia. Supplementary medications are procedure specific (e.g., use of a vasodilating agent for aortic cross-clamp during coarctation repair; use of atropine to block the vagal response that may occur with PDA manipulation; use of inotropic agent for the presence of cardiomyopathy during a pulmonary shunt procedure). Keep the patient warm to avoid dysrhythmias, myocardial depression, and leftward shift of the oxyhemoglobin dissociation curve.

H. At emergence, prevent airway stimulation (coughing, broncho-laryngospasm, aspiration) and ensure adequate oxygenation and ventilation. During postoperative transport, monitor pulse oximetry, ABG, and ECG. Keep resuscitation medications, airway instruments, volume expanders, cardiac pacing capability, and supplemental oxygen readily available. Address issues regarding pain control and postoperative nausea and vomiting prior to discharge.

Patient with CONGENITAL HEART DISEASE FOR NONBYPASS PROCEDURE

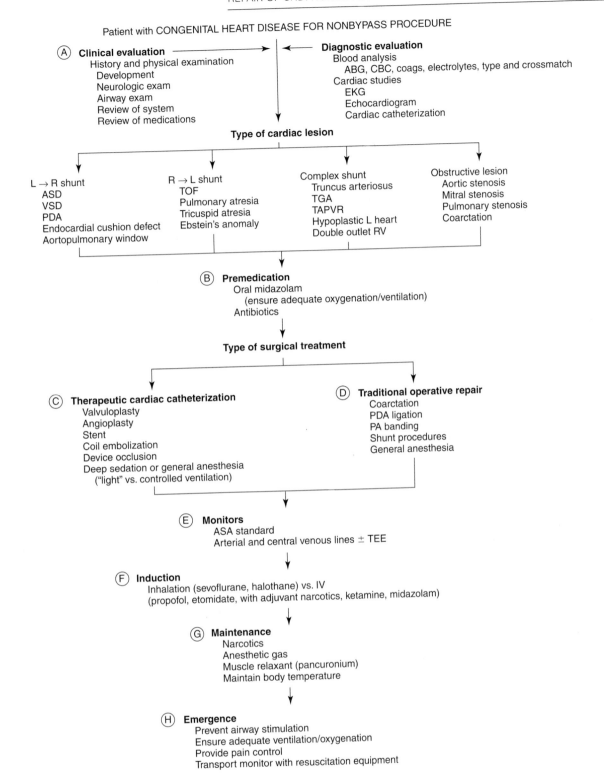

(A) **Clinical evaluation**
History and physical examination
Development
Neurologic exam
Airway exam
Review of system
Review of medications

Diagnostic evaluation
Blood analysis
ABG, CBC, coags, electrolytes, type and crossmatch
Cardiac studies
EKG
Echocardiogram
Cardiac catheterization

Type of cardiac lesion

L → R shunt
ASD
VSD
PDA
Endocardial cushion defect
Aortopulmonary window

R → L shunt
TOF
Pulmonary atresia
Tricuspid atresia
Ebstein's anomaly

Complex shunt
Truncus arteriosus
TGA
TAPVR
Hypoplastic L heart
Double outlet RV

Obstructive lesion
Aortic stenosis
Mitral stenosis
Pulmonary stenosis
Coarctation

(B) **Premedication**
Oral midazolam
(ensure adequate oxygenation/ventilation)
Antibiotics

Type of surgical treatment

(C) **Therapeutic cardiac catheterization**
Valvuloplasty
Angioplasty
Stent
Coil embolization
Device occlusion
Deep sedation or general anesthesia
("light" vs. controlled ventilation)

(D) **Traditional operative repair**
Coarctation
PDA ligation
PA banding
Shunt procedures
General anesthesia

(E) **Monitors**
ASA standard
Arterial and central venous lines ± TEE

(F) **Induction**
Inhalation (sevoflurane, halothane) vs. IV
(propofol, etomidate, with adjuvant narcotics, ketamine, midazolam)

(G) **Maintenance**
Narcotics
Anesthetic gas
Muscle relaxant (pancuronium)
Maintain body temperature

(H) **Emergence**
Prevent airway stimulation
Ensure adequate ventilation/oxygenation
Provide pain control
Transport monitor with resuscitation equipment

REFERENCES

1. Griffin KJ, Elkin TD, Smith CJ: Academic outcomes in children with congenital heart disease, *Clin Pediatr* 42 (5):401–409, 2003.
2. Kazim R, Berdon WE, Montaya CH, et al.: Tracheobronchial anomalies in children with congenital cardiac disease, *J Cardiothorac Vasc Anesth* 12:553–555, 1998.
3. Levine MF, Hartley EJ, Macpherson BA, et al.: Oral midazolam premedication for children with congenital cyanotic heart disease undergoing cardiac surgery: a comparative study, *Can J Anaesth* 40:934–938, 1993.
4. Alswang M, Friesen RH, Bangert P: Effect of preanesthetic medication on carbon dioxide tension in children with congenital heart disease, *J Cardiothorac Vasc Anesth* 8 (4):415–419, 1994.
5. Friesen RH, Alswang M: Changes in carbon dioxide tension and oxygen saturation during deep sedation for paediatric cardiac catheterization, *Paediatr Anaesth* 6 (1):15–20, 1996.

One-Lung Anesthesia

KATHERINE R. McGUIRE, M.D.

CHRISTOPHER A. BRACKEN, M.D., PH.D.

MARY ANN GURKOWSKI, M.D.

Absolute indications for lung separation include prevention of cross-contamination from a diseased to a healthy lung, bronchopulmonary lavage, and redistribution of ventilation (as in bronchopleural or bronchocutaneous fistula, major bronchial disruption, or large cysts or bullae). High-priority relative indications include surgical exposure for thoracic aortic aneurysm repair, upper lobectomy, and pneumonectomy. Lower-priority relative indications include exposure for esophageal resection, lower or middle lobectomy, and thoracoscopy.[1] A variety of airway management options for achieving lung separation and one-lung ventilation (OLV) are available.

A. Assess pulmonary function, evaluate for lung infection and comorbid cardiac disease, and determine the planned extent of pulmonary resection. Evaluate for myasthenic syndrome and syndrome of inappropriate antidiuretic hormone (SIADH) secretion in cancer patients.

B. Pulse oximetry and capnography are essential. Place an arterial catheter for BP monitoring and ABG analysis. Central access may be indicated for pressure monitoring and vasoactive drug infusion. If a pulmonary artery (PA) catheter is placed in a pneumonectomy patient, withdraw it prior to PA ligation.

C. For most thoracic procedures, use GETA with controlled ventilation.

D. For lung separation, the Robertshaw-design double-lumen endobronchial tube (DLT) is most widely used. Place the DLT through the vocal cords with the distal concavity facing anterior. Once the tip has passed the cords, remove the stylet and rotate the tube 90 degrees to the left (in the case of a left-sided DLT) and advance until resistance is met. Verify proper placement both clinically and with flexible fiberoptic bronchoscopy. (The carina should be visible through the tracheal lumen without herniation of the bronchial cuff. The upper surface of the blue bronchial cuff should be visible just below the carina.) For clinical verification of a left-sided DLT, inflate the tracheal cuff with up to 20 ml of air and verify equal ventilation of both lungs. Next, inflate the bronchial cuff with up to 3 ml of air, clamp the tracheal lumen, and ascertain that only the left lung is being ventilated. Finally, unclamp the tracheal lumen and clamp the bronchial lumen, verifying that only the right side is now being ventilated. Because the right mainstem bronchus is shorter than the left, placing a right-sided DLT is often more difficult. If a right-sided DLT is required, confirm proper position clinically and by bronchoscopic visualization of the right upper lobe bronchus orifice through the ventilating slot of the bronchial cuff. After placing the patient in the lateral decubitus position, again confirm proper tube position. Advantages of the DLT include its fixed curvature to facilitate positioning, low resistance to gas flow, and relative ease of suctioning. Disadvantages include the potential for malposition and tracheobronchial injury. Other options for lung separation include bronchoscopy-assisted placement of either a Univent tube with its incorporated bronchial blocker or an independent blocker (such as the Arndt endobronchial blocker or an arterial embolectomy catheter) passed through a standard single-lumen endotracheal tube (ETT).[2,3] With bronchial blockers, a tube change at the conclusion of surgery is unnecessary. Disadvantages include potential difficulty with placement and suctioning as well as ease of dislodgement with loss of lung separation.

Patient for ONE-LUNG ANESTHESIA

(A) Clinical evaluation ⟶ ⟵ Chest film
      Tumor—paraneoplastic syndromes   Pulmonary function tests, ABGs,
      Asthma, chronic obstructive pulmonary   split lung function, or V/Q scan
        disease, smoking history   ECG
      Infections, hemoptysis,   Electrolytes
        congestive heart failure   CBC
      Medications: bronchodilators

(B) Preparation and monitoring ⟶ Arterial line
                                ± CVP
                                Pulse oximeter
                                Capnograph

(C) Anesthetic induction

(D) Intubation with DLT. Univent, bronchial blocker

                   Confirmation of placement

Positioning, thoracotomy

(Cont'd on p 303)

E. Pulmonary circulation to the collapsed lung, while decreased due to hypoxic pulmonary vasoconstriction, still produces a large shunt. Therefore, once OLV begins, use a high FiO_2 (up to 1) to protect against hypoxemia.[4] To decrease airway pressures, consider using pressure-control ventilation and set the tidal volume lower than the traditionally recommended 10 to 12 ml/kg.[5] Adjust respiratory rate to keep the $PaCO_2$ at about 35 mm Hg. If hypoxemia worsens, verify proper DLT position and consider applying continuous positive airway pressure (CPAP) to the nondependent lung. Applying PEEP to the dependent lung improves ventilation-perfusion matching but may worsen shunt and is probably most beneficial in the hypoxemic patient with a diseased dependent lung. Intermittent two-lung ventilation also increases PaO_2. Ligation of the PA or cardiopulmonary bypass (CPB) may be necessary in extreme cases.

F. Prior to chest closure, it is customary to hold positive pressure at 35 to 40 cm H_2O to test the suture lines for leaks. If postoperative ventilatory support is needed, either change the DLT to a standard single-lumen ETT under direct vision using a tube exchanger or leave the DLT in place. Beware of acquired airway difficulty due to secretions, facial or laryngeal edema, or laryngeal trauma.

REFERENCES

1. Cohen E, Neustein SM, Eisenkraft JB: Anesthesia for thoracic surgery. In: Barash PG, Cullen BF, Stoelting RK, editors: *Clinical anesthesia*, ed 5, Philadelphia, 2006, Lippincott Williams & Wilkins.
2. Thielmeier KA, Anwar M: Complications of the Univent tube, *Anesthesiology* 84:491, 1996.
3. Arndt GA, Kranner PW, Lorenz D: Co-axial placement of endobronchial blocker, *Can J Anaesth* 41:1126, 1994.
4. Cohen E, Neustein SM, Eisenkraft JB: Anesthesia for thoracic surgery. In: Barash PG, Cullen BF, Stoelting RK, editors: *Clinical anesthesia*, ed 5, Philadelphia, 2006, Lippincott Williams & Wilkins.
5. Tugrul M, Camici E, Karadeniz H, et al.: Comparison of volume control with pressure control ventilation during one-lung anaesthesia, *Br J Anaesth* 79:306, 1997.

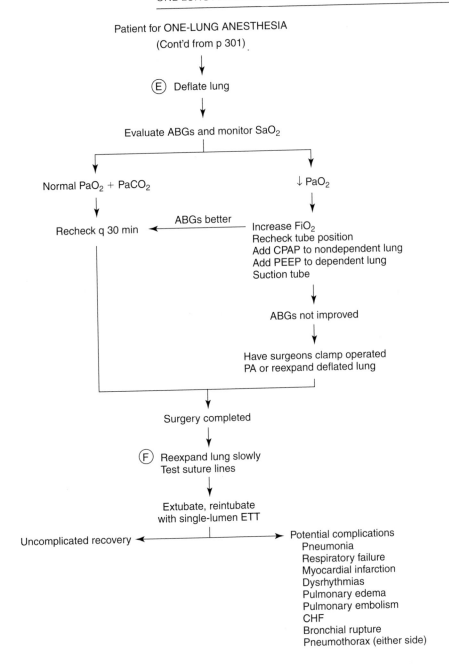

Patient for ONE-LUNG ANESTHESIA

(Cont'd from p 301)

(E) Deflate lung

Evaluate ABGs and monitor SaO$_2$

Normal PaO$_2$ + PaCO$_2$ ↓ PaO$_2$

Recheck q 30 min ←— ABGs better — Increase FiO$_2$
Recheck tube position
Add CPAP to nondependent lung
Add PEEP to dependent lung
Suction tube

ABGs not improved

Have surgeons clamp operated
PA or reexpand deflated lung

Surgery completed

(F) Reexpand lung slowly
Test suture lines

Extubate, reintubate
with single-lumen ETT

Uncomplicated recovery ←   → Potential complications
Pneumonia
Respiratory failure
Myocardial infarction
Dysrhythmias
Pulmonary edema
Pulmonary embolism
CHF
Bronchial rupture
Pneumothorax (either side)

Thoracoscopy and Video-Assisted Thoracic Surgery (VATS)

WILLIAM T. MERRITT, M.D., M.B.A.

Thoracoscopy and video-assisted thoracic surgery (VATS) are increasingly utilized for a variety of diagnostic and therapeutic procedures, including the parenchymal lung disease, pleural disease, spontaneous pneumothorax, sympathectomy, esophageal disease, and in the assessment of various mediastinal lesions.[1,2] Thoracoscopic intervention can lead to severe lung injury and is contraindicated when a patient is known or suspected to have dense pleural adhesions or postpleural space obliteration (pleural symphysis)—these prevent lung separation and collapse needed for insertion of instruments, lung visualization, and manipulation. Caution is warranted with the use of VATS in the setting of previous VATS or thoracotomy, deep parenchymal lesions, prior irradiation of the hilum, hilar lymphadenopathy, fused lung fissures, and tumor involvement of the chest wall. Large tumors, evidence of metastatic disease, and established mediastinal malignancy usually are not amenable to thoracoscopic approaches. When there is a suspected or known need for a sleeve resection for tracheal or bronchial involvement, VATS is likely to limit the needed exposure.

A. Anesthesia issues for VATS procedures relate to the condition of the patient, the needs of the surgery, surgical positioning, and the inherent potential for conversion to an open thoracotomy. Preoperative evaluation for VATS should be similar to that for bronchoscopy or open thoracotomy. A comprehensive history and physical, appropriate laboratory tests, pulmonary and cardiovascular evaluation fitting to symptoms, or the planned procedure are in order.

B. Local anesthesia or moderate sedation may be successful for minor procedures of brief duration. Regional anesthesia can be employed, and options include intercostal nerve blocks two to three spaces above and below the incision combined with an ipsilateral stellate ganglion block, thoracic paravertebral blocks, thoracic epidural anesthesia, and even field blocks. Pleural pain may require installation of local intrapleural anesthesia. Such techniques depend on a cooperative patient who will be able to breathe spontaneously throughout the procedure. Unsatisfactory surgical conditions, respiratory insufficiency, mediastinal-shift hemodynamics, or bleeding may force urgent conversion to general anesthesia and possibly an open thoracotomy.

C. General anesthesia with one-lung ventilation (OLV) is most commonly performed for thoracoscopic procedures. While a double-lumen endotracheal tube (DLT) is usually the best method for lung isolation, bronchial blockade and mainstem intubation are alternatives; institutional preference and provider experience are important. Direct arterial pressure measurement is especially useful in the setting of hypoxia, conversion to an open procedure, or in the unlikely event of major blood loss. Ensure adequate IV access. Lateral positioning requires additional attention to bony prominences, the legs, the arms, shoulders, and the neck. Sufficient padding, including a chest/"axillary" roll, is important, as is securing the torso so that shifting of position does not occur under the drapes as the table is moved to accommodate surgical needs. Fiberoptic bronchoscopy (FOB), with suction capability, adds the ability to confirm clinical judgment in DLT or bronchial blocker placement. FOB is especially useful in fine tuning correct position, redirection when initial placement is not correct, and when problems arise intraoperatively. Because VATS is less invasive, neuraxial anesthesia may not be as useful as in open thoracotomy, but certainly can be employed postoperatively if needed. Pleurodesis is commonly used for recurrent pleural effusions and pneumothoraces. Either mechanical or chemical techniques are utilized. Self-limited pleuritic pain does result and may warrant more aggressive pain therapy.[1,2] For general anesthesia use high FiO_2 and short-acting inhalational or IV agents and muscle relaxants. Goals include a quick emergence, minimal to absent pain, and the ability to effectively cough. Operative lung continuous positive airway pressure (CPAP) during VATS may not be acceptable from a surgical perspective. If hypoxia does not respond to ventilated lung PEEP, conversion to an open thoracotomy may be necessary. Attempts to improve oxygenation via administration of both nitric oxide and almitrine (an enhancer of hypoxic pulmonary vasoconstriction) have been reported to be successful in maintaining PaO_2, and such maneuvers may eventually become widely used. If CO_2 is instilled into the operative chest, limiting the pressure to <10 mm Hg and the flow to 1 to 2 L/min should prevent mediastinal-shift and associated hemodynamic changes.

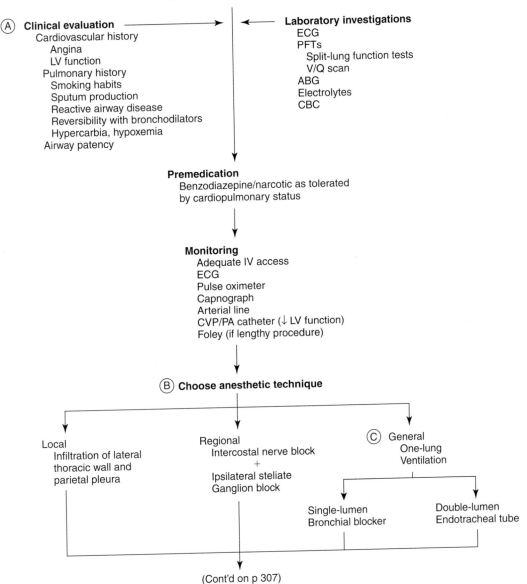

Patient for THORACOSCOPY

Ⓐ **Clinical evaluation**
    Cardiovascular history
      Angina
      LV function
    Pulmonary history
      Smoking habits
      Sputum production
      Reactive airway disease
      Reversibility with bronchodilators
      Hypercarbia, hypoxemia
    Airway patency

Laboratory investigations
    ECG
    PFTs
      Split-lung function tests
      V/Q scan
    ABG
    Electrolytes
    CBC

Premedication
Benzodiazepine/narcotic as tolerated
by cardiopulmonary status

Monitoring
    Adequate IV access
    ECG
    Pulse oximeter
    Capnograph
    Arterial line
    CVP/PA catheter (↓ LV function)
    Foley (if lengthy procedure)

Ⓑ **Choose anesthetic technique**

Local
    Infiltration of lateral
    thoracic wall and
    parietal pleura

Regional
Intercostal nerve block
    +
Ipsilateral steliate
Ganglion block

Ⓒ General
    One-lung
    Ventilation

Single-lumen
Bronchial blocker

Double-lumen
Endotracheal tube

(Cont'd on p 307)

D. Complications during or after thoracoscopy are similar to those of open thoracotomy. Intraoperative hypoxia, hypercarbia, bleeding, or findings that make thoracoscopy inadequate may require urgent or emergent conversion to open thoracotomy. Potential complications include injury to intrathoracic structures; bronchopleural fistula; tumor spillage; and inadequate procedure for the disease. If carbon dioxide insufflation is used, CO_2 embolism, subcutaneous emphysema, or mediastinal shift may occur. The latter may be moderated by adjusting tidal volume to 5 to 7 ml/kg. Postoperatively, persistent air leak or pneumothorax may occur. While often said to be less painful than open thoracotomy, inadequate IV pain control may warrant insertion of a postoperative thoracic epidural.

REFERENCES

1. Roviaro GC, Varoli F, Vergani C, et al.: State of the art in thoracoscopic surgery: a personal experience in 2000 videothoracoscopic procedures and an overview of the literature, *Surg Endosc* 16:881–892, 2002.
2. Video-assisted thoracic surgery. In: Yang SC, Cameron DE, *Current therapy in thoracic and cardiovascular surgery*, Philadelphia, 2004, Mosby.
3. Conacher ID: Anaesthesia for thoracoscopic surgery, *Best Pract & Res Clin Anaesthesiol* 16:53–62, 2002.
4. Sullivan EA, Bussieres JS, Tschernko EM. Anesthesia for specific thoracic procedures. In: Kaplan JA, Slinger PD, editors: *Thoracic anesthesia*, ed 3, Philadelphia, 2003, Churchill Livingstone.

Patient for THORACOSCOPY
(Cont'd from p 305)

↓

Ⓓ **Potential intraoperative complications**
    Hemorrhage ——————————————→ Open thoracotomy
    Perforation of diaphragm and other organs
    Gas emboli
    Tension pneumothorax
    Reduced cardiac output with high insufflation pressures
    Hypercarbia, hypoxia

Mediastinoscopy

WILLIAM T. MERRITT, M.D., M.B.A.

MARCELO QUEZADO, M.D.

Lymph drains from the hilar area to the subcarinal, paratracheal, and supraclavicular nodal regions. Because of this drainage pattern, a number of pathological conditions can be reached with the mediastinoscope—lymphoma and malignant lung tumors of the lung can be identified, as well as vascular tissue, connective tissue, and bone tumors. Secondary tumors of the mediastinum or lung may be found. Benign tumors, including thymic, thyroid, and tracheal, may be diagnosed. Other uncommon pathology includes thymoma, lipoma, myxoma, and pheochromocytoma. Even hiatal hernia and thoracic aneurysms may be present in the mediastinum. With experience, the only firm contraindication is a permanent tracheostomy, post-laryngectomy. Issues of considerable concern include ascending aortic aneurysms, goiter, innominate artery aneurysm, inoperative tumors, tracheostomy, anterior mediastinal masses, recurrent laryngeal nerve injury, previous mediastinoscopy, superior vena cava (SVC) syndrome, and thoracic inlet tumors (e.g., Pancoast-like mass; and substernal thyroid). Of the several potential approaches for mediastinoscopy, a midline suprasternal entry allows for bilateral assessment of nodal tissue.[1-4]

A. Preoperative assessment for mediastinoscopy, or any procedure in a patient with known or suspected mediastinal involvement, must be attentive to evidence of tracheobronchial compression (e.g., wheezing, dyspnea, or orthopnea), esophageal involvement (e.g., dysphagia), and changes related to exercise or position. Before anesthesia and surgery, radiation therapy may be useful for large radiosensitive masses. Chest x-rays (CXRs), CT/magnetic resonance imaging (MRI) examinations of chest and neck, echocardiography (echo), pulmonary function tests (PFTs), and flow-volume loops (supine and upright) help define the relative functional location and dynamic nature of the obstructing mass and the extent of the airway or vascular compromise. Mediastinal masses may lead to the SVC syndrome with an increased risk of major venous bleeding.

B. Place pulse oximeter and arterial catheter on the side of the mediastinoscopy and an indirect BP monitor on the contralateral arm to evaluate for innominate or subclavian artery compression by the mediastinoscope. Insert a large-bore IV line before biopsies are taken and check that blood is immediately available. Patients who are debilitated may benefit from a mediastinoscopy under local anesthesia. However, general anesthesia is preferred by most. Evidence of airway compromise requires special consideration. Those with intrathoracic tracheobronchial obstruction may benefit from intubation while spontaneously breathing. Every effort should be made to determine if the cell type is known to be radiotherapy or chemotherapy sensitive; such treatment may shrink the tumor and decrease or ablate the obstructive symptoms. Muscle paralysis, which improves surgical conditions and lessens the likelihood of sudden movement, may lead to airway collapse and inability to ventilate the patient. Availability and institution of cardiopulmonary bypass (CPB) is potentially lifesaving in such settings. Those with extrathoracic obstruction may benefit from awake intubation, assessment of the obstruction, and placement of a small diameter endotracheal tube through the narrowed area, under direct vision. Parasternal mediastinotomy (Chamberlain procedure) allows diagnosis and staging of left upper lobe lesions and the presence of mediastinal invasion. A small incision is made at the left second or third intercostal cartilage. This procedure can be done with local anesthesia, sedation, or general anesthesia with laryngeal mask airway (LMA) or endotracheal tube (ETT). Invasive monitoring should not be needed. Complications include rare bleeding, which might require a more extensive thoracotomy or sternotomy, with appropriate anesthesia interventions.

C. While mediastinoscopy by experienced surgeons and anesthesiologists is a safe procedure, with reported mortality of less than 0.1% and morbidity of about 1.5%, reported risks include hemorrhage, pneumothorax, hemo-mediastinum with cardiovascular collapse, mechanical pressure on the innominate (brachiocephalic) artery, hemiparesis, phrenic or recurrent laryngeal nerve injury, esophageal injury, tumor spread, air embolism, chylothorax, infection, and tracheal collapse after the procedure. If the mediastinoscopy is to immediately precede thoracotomy, drug selection should anticipate a shortened procedure necessitated by the findings of the mediastinoscopy. For urgent conversion to an open thoracotomy, sternotomy or lateral thoracotomy are possibilities, depending on patient stability. Lung separation will be beneficial (double-lumen endotracheal tube [DLT], or bronchial blocker).

REFERENCES

1. Ponn RB: Mediastinoscopy and mediastinotomy. In: Yang SC, Cameron DE, editors: Current therapy in thoracic and cardiovascular surgery, St. Louis, 2004. Mosby.
2. Dosios T, Theakos N, Chatziantoniou C: Cervical mediastinoscopy and anterior mediastinotomy in superior vena cava obstruction, Chest 128 (3):1551–1556, 2005.
3. Ehrenwerth J, Brull SJ: Anesthesia for thoracic diagnostic procedures, In: Kaplan JA, Slinger PD, editors: Thoracic anesthesia, ed 3, Philadelphia, 2003, Churchill Livingstone.
4. Datta D, Lahiri B: Preoperative evaluation of patients undergoing lung resection surgery, Chest 123:2096–2103, 2003.

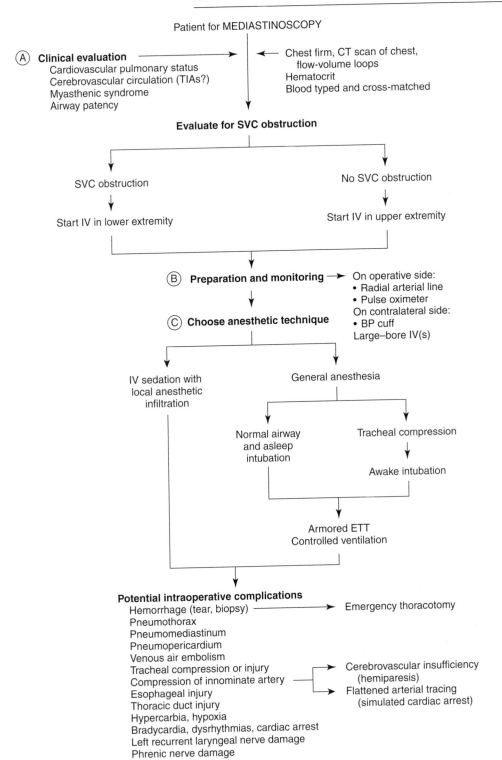

Patient for MEDIASTINOSCOPY

Ⓐ **Clinical evaluation** → ← Chest firm, CT scan of chest,
　　Cardiovascular pulmonary status 　　　flow-volume loops
　　Cerebrovascular circulation (TIAs?) 　Hematocrit
　　Myasthenic syndrome 　　　　　　　Blood typed and cross-matched
　　Airway patency

Evaluate for SVC obstruction

SVC obstruction　　　　　　　　　　No SVC obstruction

Start IV in lower extremity　　　　　　Start IV in upper extremity

Ⓑ **Preparation and monitoring** → On operative side:
　　　　　　　　　　　　　　　　　• Radial arterial line
　　　　　　　　　　　　　　　　　• Pulse oximeter
Ⓒ **Choose anesthetic technique**　On contralateral side:
　　　　　　　　　　　　　　　　　• BP cuff
　　　　　　　　　　　　　　　　　Large–bore IV(s)

IV sedation with　　　　　General anesthesia
local anesthetic
infiltration

　　　　　　Normal airway　　　Tracheal compression
　　　　　　and asleep
　　　　　　intubation　　　　　Awake intubation

　　　　　　　　Armored ETT
　　　　　　　　Controlled ventilation

Potential intraoperative complications
　　Hemorrhage (tear, biopsy) ——→ Emergency thoracotomy
　　Pneumothorax
　　Pneumomediastinum
　　Pneumopericardium
　　Venous air embolism
　　Tracheal compression or injury　　　→ Cerebrovascular insufficiency
　　Compression of innominate artery ——　　(hemiparesis)
　　Esophageal injury　　　　　　　　　→ Flattened arterial tracing
　　Thoracic duct injury　　　　　　　　　　(simulated cardiac arrest)
　　Hypercarbia, hypoxia
　　Bradycardia, dysrhythmias, cardiac arrest
　　Left recurrent laryngeal nerve damage
　　Phrenic nerve damage

Tracheal Stenosis (TS): Injury and Resection

KATHERINE R. McGUIRE, M.D.

CHRISTOPHER A. BRACKEN, M.D., PH.D.

Tracheal stenosis (TS) refers to narrowing of the tracheal lumen at any point from the glottis to the carina. Congenital causes of TS include aberrant tracheal morphology, webs, vascular rings, and laryngotracheal malacia. Acquired TS may occur with neoplasms, tracheal injury or infection, prolonged or traumatic intubation, and tracheostomy.[1] Extrinsic lesions, such as anterior mediastinal masses, may also compress the trachea.

A. Preoperative evaluation includes review of pulmonary function tests (PFTs), flow-volume loop studies, and ABG values. Estimate the size of the tracheal lumen with radiographic studies. Assess the airway, determine exercise tolerance, and evaluate for evidence of pulmonary infection and respiratory distress. Question the patient about position-dependent airway obstruction to determine the proper induction position. Decisions about premedication must balance airway risk against anxiety level. Tracheal lumen under 6 mm generally makes preoperative sedation too risky. Traumatic tracheobronchial injury, whether blunt or penetrating, may be difficult to detect but is suggested by subcutaneous emphysema, pneumomediastinum, or pneumoperitoneum.[2] In these patients, airway manipulation must be carefully considered and attempted only after appropriate diagnostic studies, such as CT scanning and bronchoscopy, have defined the location and extent of injury.

B. During an unrelated surgical procedure, if an unexpected inability to pass the endotracheal tube (ETT) beyond the vocal cords suggests TS, restore spontaneous ventilation and awaken the patient. In patients with known TS in whom intubation is deemed feasible, a routine induction and intubation sequence may be followed, but have emergency airway management equipment immediately available, including a fiberoptic bronchoscope (FOB) and multiple ETT sizes. When in doubt about airway patency, maintain spontaneous ventilation. Awake intubation or tracheostomy under local anesthesia with minimal IV sedation may be necessary to secure the airway. PTJV and translaryngeal catheter oxygen (O_2) insufflation are other options.

C. During tracheal resection and reconstruction procedures, airway management and maintenance of adequate oxygenation and ventilation can be challenging. Severe lung disease is a relative contraindication to these procedures, which most commonly entail segmental tracheal resection with primary anastomosis.[3]

Consider steroids to help minimize edema. Invasive arterial BP monitoring is indicated. During surgery, use a high FiO_2 to help protect against hypoxemia. Keep the patient in Trendelenburg position to minimize aspiration of blood and debris. With high tracheal lesions, resection can often be performed around a small ETT passed through and distal to the stenosis. More complex high tracheal lesions may necessitate ventilation through a second, sterile ETT (connected to a sterile circuit) placed distal to the lesion by the surgeon after opening the trachea. After resection, this sterile ETT is removed and the original tube (which was passed in the standard fashion either above the lesion or distal to it) is advanced across the anastomosis. Low tracheal, carinal, and bronchial lesions may require more complex airway manipulation, including unilateral or bilateral endobronchial intubation and one-lung ventilation (OLV). After resection, the distal tubes are removed and the original tube passed across the anastomotic site.[4] Other options for tracheal resection and reconstruction procedures include high-frequency positive-pressure ventilation and high-frequency jet ventilation through a small catheter placed across either the lesion or transected airway. These high-frequency ventilation modes may improve surgical access but carry the disadvantages of impaired egress of gas during exhalation and potential catheter occlusion or displacement. In some cases, cardiopulmonary bypass (CPB) may be necessary for gas exchange. Throughout surgery, close communication with the surgical team is of paramount importance. Postoperatively, extubate as early as possible. Keep the patient's neck in a flexed position to reduce tension on the tracheal anastomotic suture lines.[5]

REFERENCES

1. Cohen E, Neustein SM, Eisenkraft JB: Anesthesia for thoracic surgery. In: Barash PG, Cullen BF, Stoelting RK, editors: *Clinical anesthesia*, ed 5, Philadelphia, 2006, Lippincott Williams & Wilkins.
2. Dutton RP, McCunn M: Anesthesia for trauma. In: Miller RD, editor: *Miller's anesthesia*, ed 6, Philadelphia, 2005, Elsevier.
3. Wilson WC, Benumof JL: Anesthesia for thoracic surgery. In Miller RD, editor: *Miller's anesthesia*, ed 6, Philadelphia, 2005, Elsevier.
4. Geffin B, Bland J, Grillo HC: Anesthetic management of tracheal resection and reconstruction, *Anesth Analg* 48:884, 1969.
5. Beyer PY, Wilson RS: Anesthetic management of tracheal resection and reconstruction, *J Cardiol Anesth* 2:821, 1988.

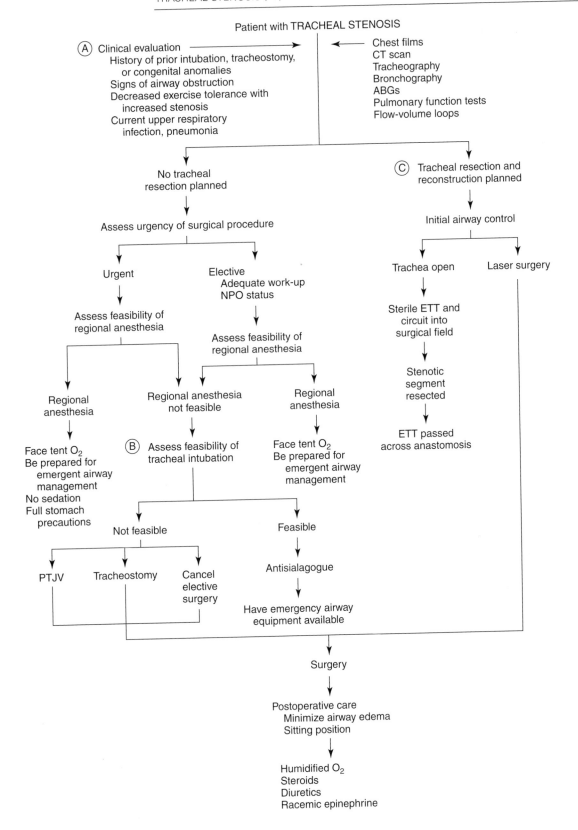

Patient with TRACHEAL STENOSIS

(A) Clinical evaluation
    History of prior intubation, tracheostomy,
      or congenital anomalies
    Signs of airway obstruction
    Decreased exercise tolerance with
      increased stenosis
    Current upper respiratory
      infection, pneumonia

Chest films
CT scan
Tracheography
Bronchography
ABGs
Pulmonary function tests
Flow-volume loops

No tracheal resection planned

Assess urgency of surgical procedure

Urgent

Elective
    Adequate work-up
    NPO status

Assess feasibility of regional anesthesia

Assess feasibility of regional anesthesia

Regional anesthesia

Regional anesthesia not feasible

Regional anesthesia

Face tent O_2
Be prepared for emergent airway management
No sedation
Full stomach precautions

(B) Assess feasibility of tracheal intubation

Face tent O_2
Be prepared for emergent airway management

Not feasible

Feasible

PTJV   Tracheostomy   Cancel elective surgery

Antisialagogue

Have emergency airway equipment available

(C) Tracheal resection and reconstruction planned

Initial airway control

Trachea open

Laser surgery

Sterile ETT and circuit into surgical field

Stenotic segment resected

ETT passed across anastomosis

Surgery

Postoperative care
    Minimize airway edema
    Sitting position

Humidified O_2
Steroids
Diuretics
Racemic epinephrine

Intraoperative Loss of Pacemaker Capture

JAMES R. ZAIDAN, M.D., M.B.A.

While pacemakers were initially inserted as simply a way to pace the ventricle to avoid severe bradycardia or asystole, with advances in technology, pacemakers have become sophisticated devices that function in a variety of ways. Standard pacemaker nomenclature is listed in Table 1. It is critical before caring for any patient with a pacemaker to know several things: (1) the underlying rhythm or indication for pacer placement, (2) what the setting of the pacemaker is, (3) what the response to magnet placement is, and (4) when the last interrogation was, especially if placement was more than 5 years ago as battery life may become an issue with older pacemakers. This knowledge will help the provider effectively treat and manage the patient in the event of pacemaker failure.

A. When the pacemaker fails to pace the ventricle, the anesthesiologist must observe the patient's escape rate and cardiac rhythm. Commonly, the rate increases after several seconds to a more physiological rate. If the rate increases but is slower than desired, consider atropine or an isoproterenol infusion (1 to 2 μg/min). Treat a patient who has no escape rhythm with CPR and as guided by the advanced cardiac life support (ACLS) protocol[1] until a temporary pacemaker (either transcutaneous or transvenous) arrives or until the infusions become effective.

B. The cause for pacemaker failure should be investigated. The main causes of failure are loss of delivered impulse and increase in pacing threshold of the myocardium. If the patient has external pacing wires, all connections with the generator and generator power should be ensured. Myocardial ischemia may cause an increase in the pacing threshold, leading to loss of capture. If this is suspected, optimize myocardial oxygen delivery with treatment of hypertension (HTN), anemia, or hypoxia. Beta-blockers will increase the pacing threshold and should be avoided in this situation. Hyperpolarization of the myocardial cell membrane can occur with alkalosis or hypocarbia leading to an increase in the pacing threshold, as will hypokalemia, which may result from hyperventilation. Hyperglycemia will also raise the threshold, as will hypothermia, and may cause failure of the pacemaker to capture.

C. Electromagnetic interference (EMI), in particular the electrocautery, can create special situations. EMI dispersal pads should be placed at a location remote from the generator on the patient. If feasible, bipolar cautery should be used as it is less likely to cause interference with the pacemaker function. Generators can reprogram even if they are programmed to asynchronous activity. However, as long as they remain in the DOO or VOO mode of activity, they, at least, will not be inhibited by the electrocautery. Placing a magnet on the generator can increase the likelihood of reprogramming; however, this change will not manifest itself until the magnet is removed. One option is to reprogram the pacemaker to the asynchronous mode preoperatively and have the magnet immediately available. If reprogramming occurs as manifested by a change in paced rate or a loss of capture, place the magnet over the pacemaker, proceed with surgery, and reprogram the pacemaker in the postoperative period. In an emergency, proceed without reprogramming, keep the magnet immediately available and apply it over the pacemaker if noticeable reprogramming occurs. Once surgery is over, interrogate the pacemaker to assure that parameters are correct for the patient, and reprogram to VVI/DDD.

REFERENCES

1. American Heart Association: 2005 guidelines for cardiopulmonary resuscitation and emergency cardiovascular care. Part 7.3: Management of symptomatic bradycardia and tachycardia, *Circulation* 112 (24 Supplt): IV-67–77, 2005.
2. Salukhe TV, Dob D, Sutton R: Pacemakers and defibrillators: anaesthetic implications, *Br J Anaesth* 93:95–104, 2004.
3. Anand NK, Maguire DP. Anesthetic implications for patients with rate-responsive pacemakers, *Semin Cardiothorac Vasc Anesth* 9 (3):251–259, 2005.

TABLE 1
The North American Pacing and Electrophysiology Group Pacemaker Codes

Position	Action	Letter designation
I	Chamber paced	A (atrial), V (ventricular), D (dual)
II	Chamber sensed	A (atrial), V (ventricular), O (asynchronous)
III	Mode of action	I (inhibited), T (triggered), D (dual), O (asynchronous)
IV	Rate modulation	O (no rate modulation), R (rate adaptable)
V	Anti-tachycardia	O (none), P (pace), S (shock), D (pace and shock)

INTRAOPERATIVE LOSS OF PACEMAKER CAPTURE

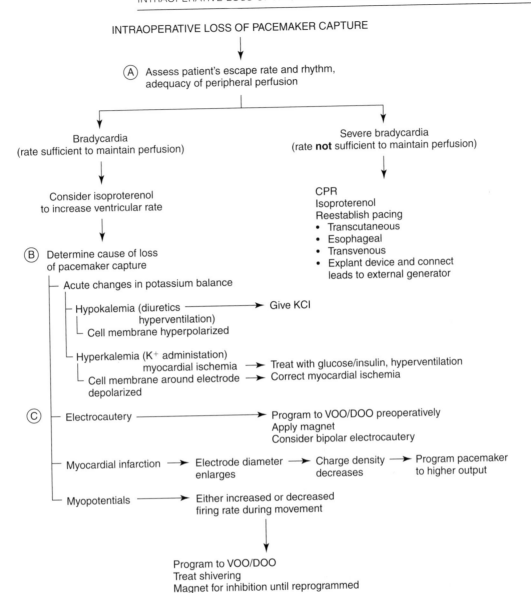

Endovascular Procedures

MARCOS A. ZUAZU, M.D.

JOSEPH J. NAPLES, M.D.

Among the many challenges and innovations facing the practicing anesthesiologist on a daily basis, few are as complex as that of minimally invasive vascular surgery, more properly termed "endovascular surgery". This rapidly growing new field involves management of high-risk patients using low–impact closed procedures, which are often performed outside the OR by a wide variety of different medical specialists (e.g., vascular surgeons, cardiologists, interventional radiologists, neurosurgeons, and cardiac surgeons.) Medical staff turf battles in this environment are not unheard of.

In 1991, Parodi and Palmaz first reported a series of patients with abdominal aortic aneurysms (AAA) treated with endoluminal stenting performed by deploying a vascular graft with self-expanding hooked fixation devices at each end through a catheter inserted via femoral cutdown.[1] Since their pioneering work, an explosive growth of high-technology applications has expanded to carotid stenting and almost every other arterial repair procedure. Despite shorter hospital stays and recovery periods, the costs of these technologies are quite high. Endovascular stenting for aortic aneurysm repair can cost considerably more than open surgery. Recent data for patient outcomes following AAA repair utilizing endovascular surgery are encouraging, and reports from carotid and vertebral stenting are similar, with success rates of >95% in midterm followup studies.[2,3] Thoracic aortic stenting is more controversial, although results are encouraging and spinal cord ischemic complications are not different from those of open procedures. Earlier problems seen in repair of severe aorto-iliac occlusive disease are being resolved by technological advances, such as modular ("kissing") stents to address aortic bifurcation anatomy. Known complications, such as restenosis and endovascular leaks, are being addressed by implant modifications, the design of extension cuffs, and other device improvements. Filters built into carotid stents have reduced embolization of cerebral debris during manipulation to rates similar to those of carotid shunt insertions. Recent data suggest that the cost of surveillance after endovascular surgery to assess durability, as well as increased mortality due to these procedures, are of lessening concern and sicker patients are now being included in these procedures.

A. The usual paradigms for the evaluation of high-risk vascular patients apply here. Patients selected for endovascular intervention tend to be sicker and have more comorbidities than those for open repair. Rigorous cardiac evaluation is basic for proper risk management. Coronary artery disease (CAD) is prevalent in these patients; diagnosis and therapeutic optimization is mandatory. Complications are usually related to cardiovascular events. Target organ dysfunction is frequent; therefore evaluate for renal and hepatic disease. Because endovascular surgery is basically an angiographic procedure, large doses of contrast dye are used (100 to 200 ml) and contrast nephropathy can result. Interventions with fenoldopam infusions have been associated with reduced mortality and dialysis requirements. A type and screen is sufficient for some procedures. In aorto-iliac stenting, blood loss is reportedly high, averaging 800 to 1,000 ml; therefore obtain a type and cross-match in these patients so that blood products are available on short notice.

B. Select monitors that are used for open vascular surgical procedures. Despite a low rate of conversion to open repair, aggressive hemodynamic management with strict BP, HR, and ST segment control is required; invasive monitoring is standard. Place large-bore peripheral IV lines. Employ heat conservation strategies; a large body surface is exposed during some procedures (often nipple to toes) for long periods of time.

C. A wide range of anesthetic management techniques have been used successfully.[4,5] Regional anesthesia is a common choice; both spinal and epidural anesthesia are well suited for these procedures. Prior to placing an epidural, determine if the patient will be started on a postoperative anticoagulation protocol. Because groin incisions are standard and are amenable to infiltration with long-duration local anesthetics, MAC anesthesia has been used with good results. In the specific area of carotid stenting, neurological status must be evaluated during occlusion and opening of the device; therefore, provide only light sedation. Tailor sedation to allow patient arousal and cooperation in following of commands. With sedation techniques, there is always a risk of hypoxia during lengthy procedures. The cumulative effect of sedatives and analgesics in elderly patients with chronic obstructive pulmonary disease (COPD), obesity, and sleep apnea is of concern; therefore, in some cases, a general anesthetic is a better choice, as it allows airway control. Also consider procedure duration when choosing a regional anesthetic technique. If spinal anesthesia is chosen for a long procedure, choose longer acting agents (e.g., isobaric mixtures or opiates) and techniques (e.g., continuous spinal). General anesthesia is commonly administered for aorto-iliac stenting; no differences in the occurrence of major cardiovascular events have been in series comparing patients with similar risk profiles.

Patient for ENDOVASCULAR SURGICAL PROCEDURES

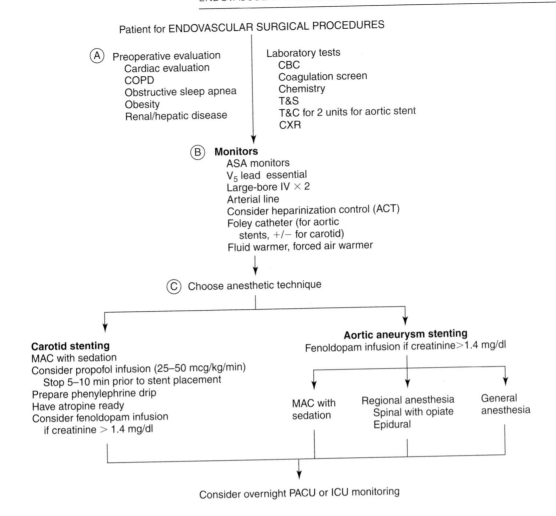

Ⓐ Preoperative evaluation
    Cardiac evaluation
    COPD
    Obstructive sleep apnea
    Obesity
    Renal/hepatic disease

Laboratory tests
    CBC
    Coagulation screen
    Chemistry
    T&S
    T&C for 2 units for aortic stent
    CXR

Ⓑ **Monitors**
    ASA monitors
    V_5 lead essential
    Large-bore IV × 2
    Arterial line
    Consider heparinization control (ACT)
    Foley catheter (for aortic
        stents, +/− for carotid)
    Fluid warmer, forced air warmer

Ⓒ Choose anesthetic technique

Carotid stenting
MAC with sedation
Consider propofol infusion (25–50 mcg/kg/min)
    Stop 5–10 min prior to stent placement
Prepare phenylephrine drip
Have atropine ready
Consider fenoldopam infusion
    if creatinine > 1.4 mg/dl

Aortic aneurysm stenting
Fenoldopam infusion if creatinine>1.4 mg/dl

MAC with sedation

Regional anesthesia
Spinal with opiate
Epidural

General anesthesia

Consider overnight PACU or ICU monitoring

REFERENCES

1. Parodi JC, Palmaz JC, Barone HD: Transfemoral intraluminal graft implantation for abdominal aortic aneurysms, *Ann Vasc Surg* 5 (6): 491, 1991.
2. Carpenter JP, Anderson WN, Brester DC et al.: Multicenter pivotal trial results of the Lifepath System for endovascular aortic aneurysm repair, *J Vasc Surg* 39 (1):34, 2004.
3. Wholey M, Wholey MH, Jarmolowski CR, et al.: Endovascular stents for carotid artery occlusive disease, *J Endovasc Surg* 4 (4): 326, 1997.
4. De Virgilio C, Romero L, Donayre C, et al.: Endovascular abdominal aortic aneurysm repair with general versus local anesthesia: a comparison of cardiopulmonary morbidity and mortality rates, *J Vasc Surg* 36 (5):988, 2002.
5. Riddell JM, Black JH, Brewster DC, et al.: Endovascular abdominal aortic aneurysm repair, *Int Anesthesiol Clin* 43 (1):79–91, 2005.

Aortic Arch Aneurysms

MARCOS A. ZUAZU, M.D.

JOSEPH J. NAPLES, M.D.

Common causes of aneurysm formation include myxomatous degeneration, Marfan syndrome, atherosclerotic degeneration, and aortic dissection. The DeBakey classification of aortic dissection divides this disease into three types depending on location. The arch is involved in types I and II.[1] Anesthetic management of arch repair is the same for aneurysm or dissection; the terms will be used interchangeably. The surgical repair of an aortic arch aneurysm requires interruption of cerebral blood flow; replacement of the aortic valve is sometimes combined. Endovascular repairs are performed in some centers.[2]

A. Assess comorbidities—evaluate severity of atherosclerotic disease and aortic valve function. Patients with acute dissection are often unstable; urgency of care may preclude complete evaluation. Review CT studies to determine the extent of dissection or aneurysmal disease. Because dissection may cause visceral ischemia, evaluate territories at risk. Anticipate hypertension and renal dysfunction (may be worsened by angiographic contrast dye). Consider mannitol and fenoldopam in such cases.

B. Plan for major blood loss and severe coagulopathies, as profound hypothermia will be an integral part of the operation. Ensure availability of blood products (PRBCs, FFP, platelet concentrates, and cryoprecipitate). Arrange for RBC recovery and autotransfusion equipment to decrease banked blood usage.

C. Prepare the patient for surgery in an area with good monitoring capabilities. Insert two large-bore peripheral IV catheters (14-gauge or rapid infusion catheters [7 to 8 French] if available). Place a 20-gauge arterial line in the left or right radial artery depending on the extension of the dissection, if present. Insert an additional femoral arterial line after induction to assist in the accuracy of BP recordings during CPB and hypothermia. Place an oximetry-capable pulmonary artery (PA) catheter in the right internal jugular vein if possible, using a large-bore introducer containing a pair of additional channels (12 French) to assist in large-volume rapid replacement. Although transesophageal echocardiography (TEE) is useful during major aortic surgery, the PA catheter will be valuable in assessing volume status and in the management of postoperative hemodynamic alterations that may lead to low cardiac output (CO). Apply EEG leads. Monitor at least two temperatures, usually nasopharyngeal (reflecting brain temperature) and rectal. (The temperature thermistors in PA catheters are not accurate at the low temperatures of profound hypothermic arrest.)

D. Induction and maintenance of anesthesia is similar to that used for other complex cardiac operations, with goals of adequate anesthesia and hemodynamic stability. Choose a gentle induction technique including moderate doses of an opiate and maintenance with benzodiazepine and inhalation agent. This will allow neurological evaluation in the postoperative period. Obtain a baseline ABG and activated clotting time prior to cardiopulmonary bypass (CPB) and monitor every 30 minutes. Aprotinin use during deep hypothermic cooling is controversial; adjust heparin doses as required if aprotinin is used.[3]

E. Aortic arch repair generally requires deep hypothermic circulatory arrest to reduce neurological injury and allow a bloodless field. Attempt a slow, gradual cooling with CPB to prevent prolonged cardiac fibrillatory activity. The EEG will show initial slowing followed by burst suppression near 24°C. A silent (isoelectric) EEG and suppression of SSEPs requires nasopharyngeal temperatures below 17°C in 40% of patients.[4] Temperatures of 12° to 15°C are sometimes necessary for brain protection, because there is considerable variability among patients.[5] For additional cerebral protection, cold blood is pumped in a retrograde fashion through a superior vena cava (SVC) cannula at a rate of up to 400 to 600 ml/min while CPB is not operational; do not exceed retrograde pressures of 25 mm Hg. It is currently thought that barbiturates add little to cerebral protection and may interfere with electrophysiological monitoring.

F. Temperature—correct ABG values to achieve normocarbia and normal pH during cooling and consider using corticosteroids to minimize cerebral edema.

G. After completion of arch repair, restart CPB after deairing maneuvers by the surgeon. Begin rewarming with rates of about 1°C every 3 minutes. When normothermia is achieved, attempt to separate from CPB. After weaning from CPB, assure hemostasis. Assess coagulation parameters frequently; use the thromboelastogram or Sonoclot tests to guide therapy. Maintain adequate CO in the post-CPB and early ICU periods with inotropic and vasodilator infusions.

Patient with an AORTIC ARCH ANEURYSM

(A) **Clinical evaluation** ⟶
    Cardiology evaluation
    Aortic valve status (replacement ?)
    Aneurysm vs. dissection
    Acute vs. chronic
    Medical history, systems assessment
    Medication history

⟵ Preoperative testing
    EKG, echocardiogram, catheterization
    CT scan, CXR
    ABG, acid-base status
    Blood counts, coagulation studies
    BUN, creatinine, electrolytes, urinalysis

(B) **Alert blood bank**
    Type and crossmatch: RBCs, FFPs, Platelets 20 units each, cryoprecipitate
    Request cell-saver equipment

(C) **Preparation and monitoring** (pre- and postinduction)

ASA monitors
EKG including V_5 lead
Arterial catheters: radial (right vs. left
    depending on site of dissection)
    and femoral (postinduction)
TEE (postinduction)

Large-bore peripheral IV lines
Oxymetric PA catheter, R IJV, with introducer
    double lumen, VIP for drug infusion
EEG: unprocessed or processed
Consider cerebral oximetry
Temperature (rectal *and* naso-pharyngeal)

(D) **Anesthetic induction and maintenance**
    Cardiac induction, moderate opioid dose (fentanyl 25–50 μg/kg)
    Midazolam, up to 0.1 mg/kg (neurological evaluation affected by large dose)
    Nondepolarizer for intubation; if indicated, consider infusion and continue in ICU
    Baseline ABG, ACT (to be repeated every 30 min)

(E) **Hypothermia and circulatory arrest**
    Rectal temperature < 17°
    EEG isoelectric
    Retrograde venous cerebral perfusion (pressure < 25 mmHg), flows 400–600 ml/min

(F) **Acid-base strategies**
    pH-stat management

(G) **Rewarming and air extraction maneuvers**
    TEE
    Separate from CPB
    Assess hemostasis (coagulation studies, TEG, sonoclot)
    Treat coagulopathies aggressively (TEA or aminocaroic acid for fibrinolysis)
    Inotropic and/or vasodilator infusions to maintain adequate cardiac output

ICU

REFERENCES

1. Debakey ME, Henly WS, Cooley DA, et al.: Surgical management of dissecting aneurysms of the aorta, *J Thoracic Cardiovasc Surg* 49:130–149, 1965.
2. Malina M, Sonesson B, Ivancev K: Endografting of thoracic aortic aneurysms and dissections, *J Cardiovasc Surg (Torino)* 46 (4): 333–348, 2005.
3. Ehrlich M, Grabenwoger M, Cartes-Zumelzu F, et al.: Operations of the thoracic aorta and hypothermic circulatory arrest: is aprotinin safe? *J Thorac Cardiovasc Surg* 115:220–225, 1998.
4. Stecker MM, Cheung AT, Pochettino A, et al.: Deep hypothermic circulatory arrest: I. Effects of cooling on electroencephalogram and evoked potentials, *Ann Thorac Surg* 71 (1):14–21, 2001.
5. Coselli JS, Crawford ES, Beall AC Jr, et al.: Determination of brain temperatures for safe circulatory arrest during cardiovascular operation, *Ann Thorac Surg* 45:638–642, 1988.

Descending and Thoracoabdominal Aortic Aneurysms

MARCOS A. ZUAZU, M.D.

JOSEPH J. NAPLES, M.D.

The complexity of repair of an aortic lesion is dependent on the type and extent of the lesion. The Crawford classification system is the most comprehensive system used to discriminate among these pathologies and divides them into four types (extents) depending on the aortic segment involved.[1] Extent I is confined to the descending thoracic aorta (with or without involvement of the distal aortic arch); Extent II involves the entire thoracic and abdominal aorta; Extent III involves the distal thoracic and the abdominal aorta; Extent IV involves only the abdominal aorta below the diaphragm. Although the lesion type is a major determinant of surgical risk,[2] anesthetic management is essentially the same because management problems are similar.

A. Perform a complete history and physical examination. Evaluation should be as extensive as possible. In acute situations, such as unstable dissection with visceral ischemia or a leaking aneurysm, this may not be possible. In stable situations, obtain a thorough cardiology workup to define the severity of valvular and coronary artery disease (CAD). Assess renal, pulmonary, hepatic, and hematological abnormalities; optimize any problems and make preparations for interventions to benefit organ systems at risk. Manage hypertension (HTN) and rule out the presence of cerebrovascular disease. Review aortography, magnetic resonance imaging (MRI), and CT scans to determine the extent of the patient's lesion and its surgical repair. Additional problems may be revealed, such as false and true aortic channels in dissections or left mainstem bronchus narrowing by a large aneurysm. Angiographic determination of the location of the "critical intercostal vessel" (the one feeding the artery of Adamkiewicz) has been recommended; reimplantation of this vessel into the graph may decrease the risk of spinal cord ischemia and resulting postoperative paraplegia. The blood loss can be considerable for these repairs; notify the blood bank preoperatively. Cross-match for 15 to 20 units of RBCs and other blood products (i.e., FFP, platelet concentrates, and possibly cryoprecipitate); coagulopathy is the norm after major blood loss. Have autotransfusion equipment available and ready, as its use can significantly reduce the need for blood components.

B. Prepare the patient for anesthesia. Insert 14-gauge IV catheters or preferably, 7- or 8-gauge French rapid infusion catheters for volume replacement. Place an arterial catheter in the left radial artery. If possible, sedate the patient and place a lumbar CSF drainage catheter at L3–L4. With the patient in the lateral decubitus position, connect the catheter to a drainage system and calibrate it to drain at 10 mm Hg. This will serve to protect the spinal cord from injury.[3] Insert an Arrow-type MAC catheter with pulmonary artery (PA) insertion port in the internal jugular vein. Connect the 10-gauge lumens to the appropriate tubing of a high volume replacement device and to the cell recovery unit. Insert an oxymetric-type PA catheter. This is especially useful for postoperative ICU care. Consider placing a femoral arterial catheter for pressure monitoring during left-sided heart bypass and distal aortic perfusion.

C. Induce anesthesia using a cardiac anesthetic technique; maintain tight hemodynamic control. After adequate muscle relaxation, insert a left-sided endobronchial double-lumen tube (DLT); guide its placement with fiberoptic bronchoscopy (FOB). An endobronchial blocker or a Univent tube is a useful alternative. Insert a transesophageal echocardiography (TEE) probe. Maintain anesthesia by titrating narcotics and muscle relaxants throughout the procedure, aided by moderate levels of inhalation anesthetics. After the patient is positioned for surgery in the right lateral decubitus position, recalibrate the CSF drainage catheter at 10 mm Hg and ensure free flow. Place monitoring electrodes for somato-sensory or somato-motor evoked potentials. Electrophysiological monitoring can require changes in anesthetic technique and depth.[4]

Patient with DESCENDING THORACIC AND THORACOABDOMINAL AORTIC ANEURYSM OR DISSECTION

Ⓐ **Clinical evaluation** ⟶   ⟵ EKG, chest film
　　Cardiology evaluation   CT, aortography, MR angiography
　　Renal, pulmonary, hepatic, heme   　Define extent
　　Diabetic history   　Dissection or aneurysm
　　Medications   　Acute vs. chronic
          　Traumatic transection
          Echocardiography, EF
          CBC, electrolytes, glucose, BUN, creatinine
          Coagulation profile
          Urinalysis
          Notify blood bank: ensure blood product availability
          Notify autotransfusion service
          Notify electrophysiology personnel

Ⓑ Preparation of patient and selection of monitors

ASA monitors   Right radial and femoral line (for distal perfusion)
2 large-bore IVs   Lumbar CSF drainage catheter
Fluid warmers   　Connect to drainage system (Becker-type)
IV midazolam for sedation   　Calibrate to drain at 5–10 mm Hg
R IJ arrow MAC type catheter   　(Recalibrate after right lateral decubitus positioning)
　and SVO$_2$ type PA catheter
12 Fr lumen for rapid infusion

Ⓒ Induction and maintenance

          Electrophysiology monitor
          　(SSEPs, SMEPs)
Preoxygenate   TEE
Fentanyl 25 µg/kg or sufentanil 3–4 µg/kg
Hypnotic of choice
NMB for intubation (succinylcholine if necessary)
Intubate with left DLT (vs. univent or bronchial blocker)
Maintenance with opiate, midazolam, volatile agent, NMB

(Cont'd on p 321)

D. In most cases, left-sided heart bypass and distal aortic perfusion are required to prevent organ damage due to the ischemia from the aortic cross-clamp. Bypass with CSF drainage is reported to prevent paraplegia, which is a catastrophic complication.[5] Prepare infusion pumps for administration of inotropic agents, beta-blockers, and vasodilators. Connect high-flow fluid warmers to all transfusion lines. Provide pharmacological protection against renal dysfunction; fenoldopam, mannitol, and bicarbonate infusions have been used.[6] Pay strict attention to hemodynamic parameters and treat unstable situations promptly. Rapid volume replacement is especially important if simple cross-clamping is used without shunts. Regional hypothermic techniques, such as epidural cooling, have been used by some as an adjunct to prevent spinal cord ischemia during complex repairs.[7] Monitor for coagulation abnormalities; treat with appropriate blood component administration. At the end of the procedure, change the DLT to a single-lumen endotracheal tube. Transport the patient to the ICU for overnight ventilation with appropriate sedative and analgesic coverage to minimize discomfort. Postoperative epidural analgesia is not recommended for use in the immediate postoperative period in these patients, because it may obscure neurological examination. Continue spinal fluid drainage for at least 48 hours postoperatively; resumption of CSF drainage in the ICU may reverse delayed onset paraplegia.[8]

REFERENCES

1. Crawford ES, Crawford JL, Safi HJ, et al.: Thoracoabdominal aortic aneurysms: preoperative and intraoperative factors determining immediate and long-term results of operations in 605 patients, *J Vasc Surg* 3:389–404, 1986.
2. LeMaire SA, Miller CC, Conklin LD, et al.: Estimating group mortality and paraplegia rates after thoracoabdominal aortic aneurysm repair, *Ann Thorac Surg* 75 (2):508–513, 2003.
3. Coselli JS, LeMaire SA, Koksoy C, et al.: Cerebrospinal fluid drainage reduces paraplegia after thoracoabdominal aortic aneurysm repair: results of a randomized clinical trial, *J Vasc Surg* 35 (4):631–639, 2002.
4. Dong CC, MacDonald DB, Janusz MT: Intraoperative spinal cord monitoring during descending thoracic and thoracoabdominal aneurysm surgery, *Ann Thorac Surg* 74 (5):S1873–S1876; discussion S1892–S1898, 2002.
5. Estrera AL, Rubenstein FS, Miller CC, et al.: Descending thoracic aortic aneurysm: surgical approach and treatment using the adjuncts cerebrospinal fluid drainage and distal aortic perfusion, *Ann Thorac Surg* 72:481–486, 2001.
6. Merten GJ, Burgess WP, Gray LV, et al.: Prevention of contrast-induced nephropathy with sodium bicarbonate: a randomized controlled trial, *JAMA* 291:2328–2334, 2004.
7. Black JH, Davison JK, Cambria RP: Regional hypothermia with epidural cooling for prevention of spinal cord ischemic complications after thoracoabdominal aneurysm surgery, *Semin Thorac Cardiovasc Surg* 15 (4):345–352, 2003.
8. Fleck TM, Koinig H, Hutschala D, et al.: Cerebrospinal fluid drainage duration after thoracoabdominal aortic aneurysm repair, *Anesthesiology* 99:1019–1020, 2003.

Patient with DESCENDING THORACIC AND THORACOABDOMINAL AORTIC ANEURYSM OR DISSECTION
(Cont'd from p 319)

   ↓

(D) Intraoperative management
    Assess ventilation and oxygenation (ABGs), perfusion (SVO_2), perfusion pressure
    Maintain cardiac output (inotropes, vasodilators, vasoconstrictors)
    Maintain heart rate and myocardial O2 consumption (beta-blocker)
    Maintain anticoagulation, follow ACT
    Blood transfusion as necessary for HCT > 25
    Frequent coagulation checks
      Administer blood components to optimize clotting (FFP, platelets, cryo)
    Maintain CSF drainage < 10 mm Hg
    Consider epidural cooling
    Renal protection protocol:
      Mannitol 0.5 gm/kg prior to aortic cross-clamp
      Fenoldopam infusion
    Acid-base management

               ↓

        Postoperative care
          Overnight ventilation
          CSF drainage for 72 hours

Abdominal Aortic Aneurysms

MELBA W.G. SWAFFORD, M.D.

Abdominal aortic aneurysms, the 13th leading cause of death in the United States, are most commonly due to degeneration from arteriosclerosis. They comprise 65% of all aortic aneurysms; 90% occur below the renal arteries. Symptoms range from none to pain in the abdomen, back, flank, shoulder, or groin. Progression may ultimately lead to life-threatening rupture. Prior to 1999, treatment was limited to open surgical repair. However, endovascular stent placement is an increasingly popular therapy. Several studies show that complications, mortality, and hospital stays have been less than those encountered with open surgical procedures.[1–4] With the use of endovascular stent correction of aneurysms, all avenues of anesthetic management, including local anesthesia, are available.

A. Perform a thorough preoperative evaluation. Myocardial infarction (MI) is a major cause of perioperative morbidity and mortality. Although cardiac risk is reduced with endovascular repair, no data suggest that cardiology evaluations should be minimized.[5] Review diagnostic studies to optimize cardiac, pulmonary, and renal performance during the perioperative period. This information will help intraoperative planning if a suprarenal aortic cross-clamp is required.

B. At a minimum, monitor SpO_2, end-tidal carbon dioxide (CO_2), ECG, temperature, urinary output, intraarterial BP, and CVP. Consider other monitors, e.g., pulmonary artery (PA) catheter, transesophageal echocardiography (TEE), in patients with compromised myocardial function or who require a suprarenal aortic cross-clamp.

C. The patient with an abdominal aortic aneurysm is at an increased risk for hemodynamic instability because of the potential for rupture. Have all necessary apparatus and pharmacological agents ready and working when the patient arrives in the OR. For volume replacement, this includes functional large-bore peripheral or central IV catheters, a blood warmer device, cell-saver unit, blood, and coagulation factors. Pharmacological agents that should be available include vasodilators, inotropic agents (if indicated by cardiac status), and minidose heparin. For suprarenal aortic cross-clamp, consider osmotic diuretics (e.g., mannitol) to support renal function.

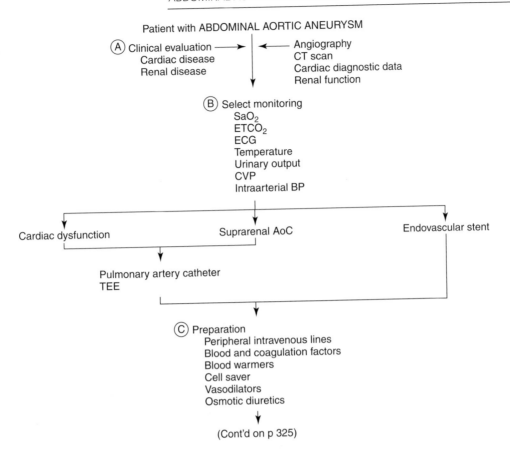

Patient with ABDOMINAL AORTIC ANEURYSM

Ⓐ Clinical evaluation ⟶   ⟵ Angiography
      Cardiac disease   CT scan
      Renal disease   Cardiac diagnostic data
                                   Renal function

Ⓑ Select monitoring
      SaO$_2$
      ETCO$_2$
      ECG
      Temperature
      Urinary output
      CVP
      Intraarterial BP

Cardiac dysfunction   Suprarenal AoC   Endovascular stent

Pulmonary artery catheter
TEE

Ⓒ Preparation
      Peripheral intravenous lines
      Blood and coagulation factors
      Blood warmers
      Cell saver
      Vasodilators
      Osmotic diuretics

(Cont'd on p 325)

D. Plan intraoperative management taking into account both procedure and patient co-existing diseases. For open procedures, consider either epidural anesthesia with sedation or general anesthetic techniques. Tailor induction of anesthesia and intubation to the patient's cardiac status. For maintenance, use a combination of narcotics and inhalation anesthetics in most cases. Connect volume replacement devices before incision. During surgical exposure, prepare for aortic cross-clamp. Consistent responses to cross-clamping of the aorta include increases in MAP and systemic vascular resistance (SVR). Therefore, initiate vasodilator therapy during surgical exposure rather than at the moment of cross-clamping to minimize these responses. Infrarenal aortic cross-clamp is usually associated with a less marked increase in SVR and MAP than is suprarenal aortic cross-clamp. Aortic cross-clamp effects that are not as consistent involve changes in cardiac output (CO) and filling pressures; these have been reported to increase, decrease, or have no change.[6] Placement of aortic cross-clamp is critical in patients with coronary artery disease (CAD) who may experience brief left ventricular (LV) failure in response to the aortic cross-clamp. In such patients, consider adding inotropic support to vasodilator therapy to improve tolerance of aortic occlusion. Blood volume redistribution is a critical element that lends support to the practice of volume loading during aortic cross-clamp. All cell-saver blood should be reinfused immediately, and additional RBCs and plasma should be infused as needed to increase filling pressures.

E. Administer a volume load in preparation for aortic cross-clamp release, because it results in a consistent decrease in MAP and SVR. Because vasodilating metabolites accumulate distal to the aortic cross-clamp, initiate sodium bicarbonate therapy and hyperventilation to minimize the vasodilating effect after aortic cross-clamp release. A gradual release of the aortic cross-clamp is preferred as this will minimize decreases in MAP and SVR. In patients who have undergone suprarenal aortic cross-clamp, administer indigo carmine after aortic cross-clamp release to determine the adequacy of renal blood flow and its effect on urine production. The appearance of blue urine indicates the return of kidney function after this ischemic period. Insure adequate hemostasis prior to transporting the patient to the ICU.

F. For endovascular stent placement, choose from a variety of anesthetic techniques including local anesthesia with sedation, neuraxial anesthesia (e.g., epidural), and general anesthesia.[7] After the graft is deployed, digital subtraction angiography is utilized to verify graft position and evaluate for leaks. Multistage grafts may be inserted requiring angiography after each deployment. A motionless field enhances the quality of such angiographic images; motion caused by breathing must be eliminated. Therefore, if sedation is used, titrate to insure that patients can cooperate during this phase.

REFERENCES

1. Arko FR, Hill BB, Olcott C, et al.: Endovascular repair reduces early and late morbidity compared to open surgery for abdominal aortic aneurysm, *J Endovasc Ther* 9 (6):711–718, 2002.
2. Towne JB: Endovascular treatment of abdominal aortic aneurysms, *Am J Surg* 189:140–149, 2005.
3. Faries PL, Bernheim J, Kilaru S, et al.: Selecting stent grafts for the endovascular treatment of abdominal aortic aneurysms, *J Cardiovasc Surg (Torino)* 44 (4):511–518, 2003.
4. Marin ML, Hollier LH, Ellozy SH, et al.: Endovascular stent graft repair of abdominal and thoracic aortic aneurysms: a ten-year experience with 817 patients, *Ann Surg* 238 (4):586–593, 2003.
5. Cuypers PWM, Buth J: Does endovascular aortic aneurysm repair justify a reduced cardiology work-up? *J Cardiovasc Surg (Torino)* 44 (3):437–442, 2003.
6. Gelman S: The pathophysiology of aortic cross-clamping and unclamping, *Anesthesiology* 82:1026–1060, 1995.
7. Mordecai MM, Crawford CC: Intraoperative management: endovascular stents, *Anesthesiol Clin North Am* 22:319–332, vii, 2004.

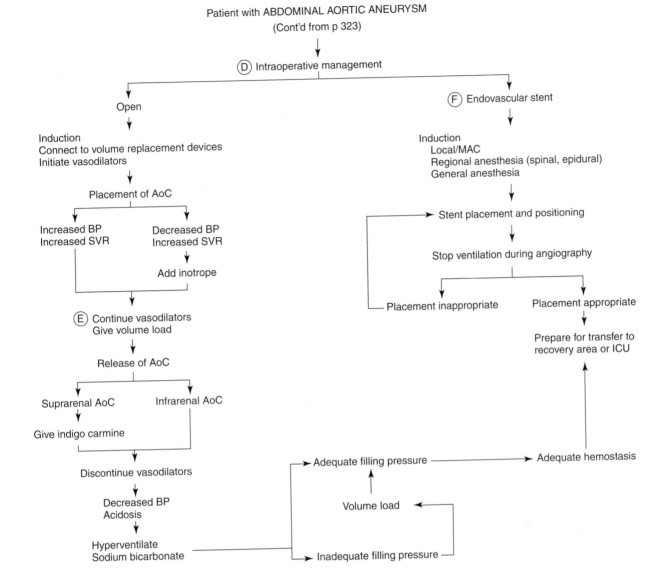

Patient with ABDOMINAL AORTIC ANEURYSM
(Cont'd from p 323)

Ⓓ Intraoperative management

Open

Induction
Connect to volume replacement devices
Initiate vasodilators

Placement of AoC

Increased BP   Decreased BP
Increased SVR   Increased SVR

Add inotrope

Ⓔ Continue vasodilators
Give volume load

Release of AoC

Suprarenal AoC   Infrarenal AoC

Give indigo carmine

Discontinue vasodilators

Decreased BP
Acidosis

Hyperventilate
Sodium bicarbonate

Ⓕ Endovascular stent

Induction
Local/MAC
Regional anesthesia (spinal, epidural)
General anesthesia

Stent placement and positioning

Stop ventilation during angiography

Placement inappropriate   Placement appropriate

Prepare for transfer to
recovery area or ICU

Adequate filling pressure ——————→ Adequate hemostasis

Volume load

Inadequate filling pressure

Lower Extremity Bypass Procedures

WENDY B. KANG, M.D., J.D.

The stereotypical patient for lower extremity bypass surgery is a high-risk candidate for anesthesia. The patient is often a hypertensive, geriatric patient with coronary artery disease (CAD), chronic obstructive pulmonary disease (COPD), renal insufficiency or failure requiring dialysis, and the multiorgan deteriorations of diabetes.[1-5]

A. Perform a history and physical examination. Order appropriate laboratory studies. Ischemia to the lower limb can be acute or chronic. Acute formation of thrombus creates the mnemonic situation of pain, pallor, pulselessness, paresthesia, or paralysis. This limb-threatening ischemia mandates rapid preparations despite inadequate patient conditions (e.g., full stomach). In contrast, electively scheduled patients demonstrate chronic poor blood flow to the legs resulting in intermittent claudication. A vicious cycle is established whereby such patients cannot sustain physical reconditioning due to leg pains, and leg pains are aggravated by lack of muscle tone and chronic venous stasis.

B. Discuss the planned surgical procedure with the surgeon. Open vascular procedures remain the standard. However, more surgeons are using endovascular stents. Experienced surgeons place stents under fluoroscopic guidance within the time frame of local anesthesia with monitored anesthesia care or subarachnoid block. Be aware that although the surgeon may initially expose the infrainguinal region, the incision may be extended for aorto-iliac or aorto-femoral jumps.

C. Practice diligence in anesthetic preparations to minimize complications. Preoperatively, optimize the cardiac, pulmonary, and renal systems. Coronary ischemia remains the major cause of perioperative and postoperative mortality in patients with peripheral vascular disease. Administer beta-blockers and antihypertensive medications orally or intravenously before surgery. Encourage cessation of smoking. For patients who do smoke, provide preanesthetic nebulizer, supplement with oxygen, and plan for rapid postoperative return to the patient's pulmonary homeostasis (i.e., extubation). Provide thoughtful volume replacement, ensuring adequate hemoglobin (Hb) and hematocrit (Hct) to augment the cardiopulmonary and renal systems. Dialyze patients with severe renal failure preoperatively; avoid hypotension in a coronary patient who has been aggressively dialyzed to a "dry weight." In diabetic patients, decide whether to tightly or loosely regulate blood sugars intraoperatively. Normal blood sugar levels tend to be associated with improved wound healing and lower infection rates.

D. Select anesthetic monitors carefully. Even with a limited incision below the infrainguinal region, extensive blood loss remains a possibility. Place a large-bore IV cannula (preferably distal to the wrist in the patient who may require future atrioventricular [AV] fistula sites). If the surgeon decides that both legs must be prepped for vein grafts, consider central venous access. Place standard American Society of Anesthesiologists (ASA) monitors. Monitor ECG leads II and V to detect possible myocardial ischemia. Follow patient temperature, keeping the patient warm with thermal blankets and warmed IV fluids to prevent shivering. Do not place a blood pressure cuff on the same upper extremity as an arterio-venous fistula, which must be kept warm and flowing during surgery. The unfortunate result is a BP cuff on the same arm as the IV site. Maintain adequate BP for tissue perfusion. Consider placing an arterial line. Remember that placing an arterial line can sometimes involve more frustration and blood loss than the surgery itself. If available, enhance patient monitoring with noninvasive nasal oximetry probes and LiDCO.

E. Choose anesthetic technique. The scientific literature does not cite any statistically significant differences in patient outcomes with a particular anesthetic technique.

F. Surgery for the lower extremity is quite conducive to regional anesthesia. However, anticoagulation (e.g., heparin, low molecular weight heparin, Dextran) is often routinely administered as part of the surgery, and each anesthesiologist must decide on a comfort zone in performing major conduction anesthesia in such cases. Central conduction catheter techniques provide the most coverage if the surgeon extends the incision. Epidural anesthesia has been associated with a tendency toward better patient outcomes and better graft patency. Review preoperative laboratory studies including prothrombin time (PT) or international normalized ratio (INR), partial thromboplastin time (PTT), and platelet count. Verify that the patient is not taking herbal supplements that can affect coagulation. (I have encountered a patient who stopped taking warfarin due to insurance problems and began ingesting garlic, ginseng, and gingko pills. His INR was 4.2.)

G. Continuous peripheral nerve blocks only minimally disturb patient physiology. Consider posterior lumbar plexus blocks, which cover the lumbar dermatomes involved in femoral arterial and venous bypasses. The anterior lumbar 3-in-1 plexus block is feasible but may become an unintentional part of the surgical field. Perform a sciatic nerve block—single or continuous—to maintain total patient comfort when the surgeon contacts the posterior aspect of the leg. Avoid injury to blood vessels; if a blood vessel is penetrated, apply pressure to minimize hematoma formation.

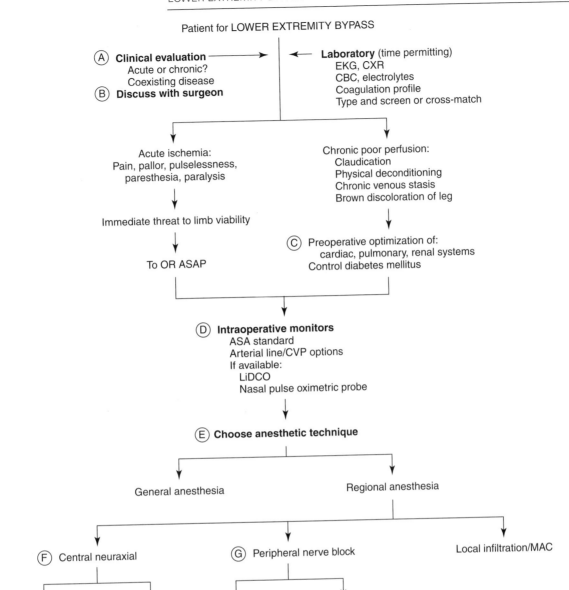

Patient for LOWER EXTREMITY BYPASS

Ⓐ **Clinical evaluation**
  Acute or chronic?
  Coexisting disease
Ⓑ **Discuss with surgeon**

Laboratory (time permitting)
  EKG, CXR
  CBC, electrolytes
  Coagulation profile
  Type and screen or cross-match

Acute ischemia:
Pain, pallor, pulselessness,
paresthesia, paralysis

Chronic poor perfusion:
  Claudication
  Physical deconditioning
  Chronic venous stasis
  Brown discoloration of leg

Immediate threat to limb viability

Ⓒ Preoperative optimization of:
  cardiac, pulmonary, renal systems
  Control diabetes mellitus

To OR ASAP

Ⓓ **Intraoperative monitors**
  ASA standard
  Arterial line/CVP options
  If available:
    LiDCO
    Nasal pulse oximetric probe

Ⓔ **Choose anesthetic technique**

General anesthesia

Regional anesthesia

Ⓕ Central neuraxial

Ⓖ Peripheral nerve block

Local infiltration/MAC

Single injection
Spinal
Epidural

Continuous
Spinal
CSE
Epidural

Single injection

Continuous
catheter techniques

REFERENCES

1. Block BM, Liu SS, Rowlingson AJ, et al.: Efficacy of postoperative epidural analgesia: a meta-analysis, *JAMA* 290:2455–2463, 2003.
2. Christopherson R, Beattie C, Frank SM, et al.: Perioperative morbidity in patients randomized to epidural or general anesthesia for lower extremity vascular surgery. Perioperative Ischemia Randomized Anesthesia Trial Study Group, *Anesthesiology* 79 (3):422–434, 1993.
3. Duggan J, Isaacson IJ: Peripheral vascular surgery. In: Youngberg JA, Lake CL, Roizen MF, et al., editors: *Cardiac, vascular and thoracic anesthesia.* New York, 2000, Churchill Livingstone.
4. Neal J: Perioperative outcome: does regional anesthesia make a difference? *ASA Annual Refresher Courses,* #431, 2003.
5. Rock P: Regional versus general anesthesia for vascular surgery patients, *ASA Annual Refresher Courses,* #114, 2003.

Esophagogastrectomy (EG)

STACEY ALLEN, M.D.

Esophagogastrectomy (EG) is a potentially curative surgical procedure to treat cancer of the esophagus, Barrett's esophagus (which is premalignant), or dilation-resistant esophageal stricture. Esophageal squamous cell carcinoma is usually associated with alcohol and tobacco abuse as well as hot beverage and caustic ingestion injury. It is usually located in the upper two thirds of the esophagus. Squamous cell carcinoma is more common than adenocarcinoma. Adenocarcinoma, which is associated with Barrett's esophagus and is usually located in the distal one third of the esophagus, is increasing in frequency. Five-year survival rates approach only 20 to 40%; when EG is combined with preoperative chemotherapy and radiotherapy, 5-year cure rates as high as 70% can be achieved when there is a complete response. Unfortunately, this occurs in only 20 to 30% of treated patients. Metastatic disease is often present at diagnosis, possibly because of the lack of an esophageal serosa and the presence of a rich lymphatic system. EG is usually not performed as a palliative procedure for metastatic disease, because the cumulative convalescence time approaches the expected survival time. Instead, limited palliative procedures (stent placement, photodynamic therapy, and laser therapy) are done.[1-3]

A. Perform a history and physical examination. Evaluate and optimize the patient's medical condition. Dehydration is common and can cause hemodynamic instability; malnutrition can impair immunity, wound healing, and muscle strength. Chronic aspiration and tobacco abuse may cause significant pulmonary disease. Chemotherapeutic agents may result in renal impairment, pulmonary fibrosis, or cardiomyopathy. Patients often have anemia, thrombocytopenia, and leukopenia. Consider the possibility of mediastinal lymphadenopathy leading to tracheal compression.

B. The common surgical approaches are transhiatal esophagectomy, right thoracotomy approach, and left thoracotomy approach. Each has advantages and disadvantages. The tumor location and prognosis will dictate the best procedure. The thoracotomy approaches will necessitate one-lung ventilation (OLV). In such cases, a double-lumen endotracheal tube (DLT) allows better pulmonary suctioning and continuous positive airway pressure (CPAP) capability in patients likely to have lung disease; it is usually exchanged for a single lumen endotracheal tube (ETT) in patients who will remain ventilated. In such cases, or in cases of difficult airway, consider using a bronchial blocker.

C. Insert large-bore IV access, because a large-volume blood loss is possible. Consider an arterial catheter when the surgical approach includes OLV; it will also allow detection of hypotension during transhiatal dissection, which can cause cardiac compression. Consider a CVP catheter to help optimize volume status and for postoperative parenteral nutrition. If the surgical approach includes a cervical anastomosis, do not place the CVP in the left neck. Consider a pulmonary artery (PA) catheter in patients with significant left ventricular dysfunction; transesophageal echocardiography (TEE) will not be an option. Avoid hypothermia (fluid warmers, appropriate room temperature, and forced air warmers); a large area of the body will be prepped and exposed to evaporative heat loss, often in a thin, malnourished patient. Hypotension, arrhythmias, and the potential for a posterior membranous tracheal tear may occur during the transhiatal dissection. Should a tear occur, OLV may be accomplished simply by right mainstem placement of the ETT if a DLT is not already in place. Avoid use of nitrous oxide. Recurrent laryngeal nerve injury may occur during cervical anastomosis; severity is variable (i.e., temporary hoarseness or permanent vocal cord paralysis). Treat hypoxia during OLV in the usual manner: adequate tidal volumes, high FiO_2, CPAP to the nonventilated lung, and judicious PEEP to the ventilated lung.

D. Consider placing an epidural for pain control, particularly for a thoracotomy approach; the dermatomal area is large in the transhiatal approach (laparotomy and cervical incision) and may be difficult to cover. However, a thoracic epidural may reduce anastomotic failure by increasing blood flow to the area, as well as reduce the risk for pneumonia and reintubation.[4,5] Intercostal or paravertebral nerve blocks may be employed if epidural is not chosen. Evaluate each patient individually for extubation. Postoperative ventilation may be preferred in a patient with poor pulmonary function secondary to preexisting lung disease, intraoperative atelectasis, large-volume resuscitation, or postoperative splinting, especially with thoracotomy. The cervical anastomosis can be damaged if immediate reintubation is required. Assure adequate pain control, temperature, volume status, pulmonary function, and ability to protect the airway from aspiration for a successful extubation. As always, communicate with the surgeon preoperatively, intraoperatively, and postoperatively to optimize patient outcome.

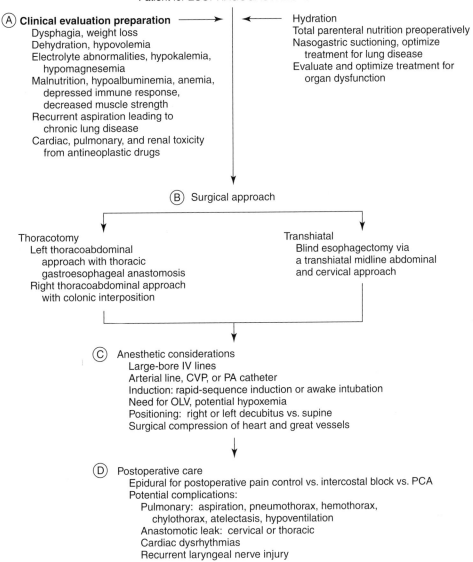

Patient for ESOPHAGOGASTRECTOMY

(A) **Clinical evaluation preparation** ⟶   ⟵   Hydration
      Dysphagia, weight loss   Total parenteral nutrition preoperatively
      Dehydration, hypovolemia   Nasogastric suctioning, optimize
      Electrolyte abnormalities, hypokalemia,   treatment for lung disease
        hypomagnesemia   Evaluate and optimize treatment for
      Malnutrition, hypoalbuminemia, anemia,   organ dysfunction
        depressed immune response,
        decreased muscle strength
      Recurrent aspiration leading to
        chronic lung disease
      Cardiac, pulmonary, and renal toxicity
        from antineoplastic drugs

(B) Surgical approach

Thoracotomy   Transhiatal
   Left thoracoabdominal   Blind esophagectomy via
     approach with thoracic   a transhiatal midline abdominal
     gastroesophageal anastomosis   and cervical approach
   Right thoracoabdominal approach
     with colonic interposition

(C) Anesthetic considerations
      Large-bore IV lines
      Arterial line, CVP, or PA catheter
      Induction: rapid-sequence induction or awake intubation
      Need for OLV, potential hypoxemia
      Positioning: right or left decubitus vs. supine
      Surgical compression of heart and great vessels

(D) Postoperative care
      Epidural for postoperative pain control vs. intercostal block vs. PCA
      Potential complications:
        Pulmonary: aspiration, pneumothorax, hemothorax,
          chylothorax, atelectasis, hypoventilation
        Anastomotic leak: cervical or thoracic
        Cardiac dysrhythmias
        Recurrent laryngeal nerve injury

REFERENCES

1. Shields T, Locicero J, Ponn R, et al.: *General thoracic surgery*, ed 6, Philadelphia, 2004, Lippincott Williams & Wilkins.
2. Karamanoukian H, Soltoski PR, Salerno TA: *Thoracic surgery secrets*, Philadelphia, 2001, Hanley & Belfus.
3. American Cancer Society Website, available at: www.cancer.org.
4. Michelet P, D'Journo XB, Roch A, et al.: Perioperative risk factors for anastomotic leakage after esophagectomy: influence of thoracic epidural analgesia, *Chest* 128 (5):3461–3466, 2005.
5. Cense HA, Lagarde SM, de Jong K, et al.: Association of no epidural analgesia with postoperative morbidity and mortality after transthoracic esophageal cancer resection, *J Am Coll Surg* 202 (3):395–400, 2006.

Transjugular Intrahepatic Portosystemic Shunt (TIPS)

JUDITH A. FREEMAN, M.B., C.H.B.

Transjugular intrahepatic portosystemic shunt (TIPS) is a transcutaneous shunt placed through the liver, connecting the right or left portal vein to one of the three main hepatic veins.[1] TIPS, performed under radiologic guidance, functions to decompress the portal circulation in patients with portal hypertension (HTN) and fulfills the same physiological function as a surgically performed side-to-side portocaval shunt. Usually the right internal jugular (IJ) vein is cannulated (straightest course to inferior vena cava [IVC]), but the left IJ, right external jugular, or femoral veins may be used. A catheter is advanced through right atrium into the IVC and then into the right hepatic vein. A wedged hepatic venogram localizes the portal vein. A puncture needle is placed through the liver into the portal vein. The transhepatic tract is then dilated with a balloon and an expandable stent is deployed and dilated to 8 to 12 mm. diameter.[1] TIPS offers advantages over surgical shunts: it is performed instead of laparotomy in critically ill patients and does not alter extra-hepatic vascular anatomy in transplant candidates.

Indications[2]	Contraindications
Esophageal and gastric variceal bleeding (acute and recurrent)	Right-sided heart failure
Refractory ascites	Cavernous portal vein thrombosis
Hepatic hydrothorax	Severe hepatic failure
Hypersplenism	Polycystic liver disease
Budd Chiari syndrome	Primary pulmonary HTN
Hepatorenal syndrome	Hepatic encephalopathy
Hepatopulmonary syndrome	—

A. Perform a careful history and physical examination. Physiological derangements include all features of severe liver disease, especially those listed as indications for this procedure. Compromised respiratory function manifesting as hypoxia may be due to V/Q mismatch from ascites, pleural effusion, hepatopulmonary syndrome, or acute respiratory distress syndrome (ARDS). Consider endotracheal intubation for airway protection. Coexisting cardiac disease is likely in cirrhosis due to alcoholic liver disease and hemochromatosis. Manage acute variceal bleeding with transfusion, medical therapy, endoscopic sclerotherapy, or balloon tamponade if necessary. Transfuse blood products to keep the platelet count above 50,000 and the international normalized ratio (INR) below 1.8. Paracentesis and thoracentesis may be necessary to improve respiratory mechanics and restore the normal position of the liver.

B. Because the radiology suite is often located away from the blood bank, anesthesia personnel, and equipment for prolonged resuscitation, prepare a complete anesthesia setup with appropriate monitors that can be easily visualized.[3,4] Atrial and ventricular dysrhythmias are common during passage of the wire through the right atrium. Plan for volume resuscitation and ensure availability of backup support personnel. Have ready access to the patient for placement of additional IV lines.

C. A TIPS procedure usually takes 2 to 3 hours. The patient must remain immobile. Creation of the transhepatic tract to the portal vein can be painful. In elective cases with an experienced radiologist, consider local anesthesia with light sedation. Avoid loss of consciousness and maintain airway reflexes; these patients have potential full stomachs and aspiration is a recognized complication. Use short-acting drugs (e.g., midazolam, fentanyl, or remifentanil) sparingly due to altered pharmacokinetics.

If patients are uncooperative, unstable, or local anesthesia is not practical, administer general anesthesia. This has been conducted successfully using propofol and laryngeal mask airway (LMA),[5] but RSI with endotracheal intubation ensures a secure airway. All induction and inhalation agents have been used.[3] Remember changes in pharmacokinetics (decreased protein binding, increased volume of distribution, decreased hepatic metabolism, and altered CNS sensitivity.) Have at least one large-bore IV; place additional IVs and invasive monitors for critically ill and actively bleeding patients. The radiologist usually passes a catheter through the right atrium, so avoid additional, unnecessary central lines. Monitor acid-base status, hematocrit (Hct), electrolytes, and glucose during long procedures. Monitor urine output (radiographic dye may induce or aggravate renal failure). Avoid hypothermia by using fluid warmers and forced air heaters.

Complications include hypotension due to bleeding varices or liver disruption, cardiac dysrhythmias (SVT, AF, VF, sinus bradycardia), hypoxemia due to preexisting pleural effusions or new onset tension pneumothorax, acute right atrial pressure increase following portal vein decompression, and aspiration during extubation.[3]

D. Extubate stable patients at the end of the procedure. Do not extubate unstable patients who require postoperative monitoring in an ICU. Monitor for potential postoperative complications including encephalopathy, pulmonary edema, sepsis, hemodynamic instability, and shunt malfunction or thrombosis.

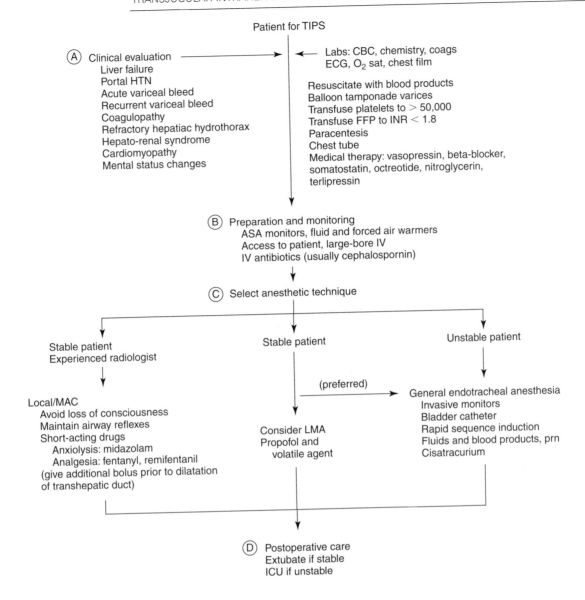

Patient for TIPS

(A) Clinical evaluation
   Liver failure
   Portal HTN
   Acute variceal bleed
   Recurrent variceal bleed
   Coagulopathy
   Refractory hepatiac hydrothorax
   Hepato-renal syndrome
   Cardiomyopathy
   Mental status changes

Labs: CBC, chemistry, coags
ECG, O₂ sat, chest film

Resuscitate with blood products
Balloon tamponade varices
Transfuse platelets to > 50,000
Transfuse FFP to INR < 1.8
Paracentesis
Chest tube
Medical therapy: vasopressin, beta-blocker,
somatostatin, octreotide, nitroglycerin,
terlipressin

(B) Preparation and monitoring
   ASA monitors, fluid and forced air warmers
   Access to patient, large-bore IV
   IV antibiotics (usually cephalospornin)

(C) Select anesthetic technique

Stable patient
Experienced radiologist

Stable patient

Unstable patient

Local/MAC
   Avoid loss of consciousness
   Maintain airway reflexes
   Short-acting drugs
      Anxiolysis: midazolam
      Analgesia: fentanyl, remifentanil
   (give additional bolus prior to dilatation
   of transhepatic duct)

(preferred)

Consider LMA
Propofol and
   volatile agent

General endotracheal anesthesia
Invasive monitors
Bladder catheter
Rapid sequence induction
Fluids and blood products, prn
Cisatracurium

(D) Postoperative care
   Extubate if stable
   ICU if unstable

REFERENCES

1. Kaufman JA, Lee MJ: *Vascular and interventional radiology: the requisites*, Philadelphia, 2004, Mosby.
2. Ong JP, Sands M, Younossi ZM: Transjugular intrahepatic portosystemic shunts (TIPS): a decade later, *J Clin Gastrenterol* 30 (1):14–28, 2000.
3. Kam PC, Tay TM: The role of the anaesthetist during the transjugular intrahepatic porto-systemic stent shunt procedure (TIPPS), *Anaesth Intensive Care* 25:385–389, 1997.
4. Kelhoffer ER, Osborn IP. The gastroenterology suite and TIPS, *Int Anesthesiol Clin* 41 (2):51–61, 2003.
5. Sampietro G, Rossi P, Di Marco P: Use of a laryngeal mask in transjugular intrahepatic portosystemic shunt procedures, *J Vasc Interv Radiol* 9:169–170, 1998.

NEUROANESTHESIA

SURGERY IN THE SITTING POSITION

CONTROLLED HYPOTENSION

INTRACRANIAL HYPERTENSION (HTN)

ACUTE SPINAL CORD INJURY (SCI)

AIRWAY MANAGEMENT IN CERVICAL FRACTURE

CONTROLLED MILD HYPOTHERMIA

CAROTID ENDARTERECTOMY (CEA)

INTRACEREBRAL ANEURYSM

ANESTHESIA DURING AWAKE CRANIOTOMY FOR EPILEPSY SURGERY

Surgery in the Sitting Position

ROSEMARY HICKEY, M.D.

Sitting position for neurosurgery provides good surgical access for posterior fossa, pineal, and cervical spinal cord procedures. Other advantages are access to midline lesions, gravity drainage of blood and CSF, reduction of ICP, and provision of an unobstructed view of the patient's face (enabling observation of motor responses to cranial nerve stimulation).[1] Potential hazards include hemodynamic instability, venous air embolism (VAE), and dysrhythmias from surgical manipulation of the brainstem and cranial nerves.

A. Evaluate for cardiovascular disease and optimize cardiac function. Limited cardiac reserve may preclude use of the sitting position. If intracranial hypertension (HTN) is present, begin measures to reduce ICP (ventricular drainage, diuretics, osmotic agents, steroids, and hyperventilation). Preoperative respiratory insufficiency may necessitate postoperative ventilation. Replace volume in dehydrated patients to attenuate changes in fluid distribution and cardiac filling pressure when the anesthetized patient is moved into the sitting position. Consider preoperative screening for a patent foramen ovale (PFO) with contrast enhanced transesophageal echocardiography (TEE) or transcranial Doppler ultrasonagraphy.[2] Recent pneumoencephalography contraindicates use of nitrous oxide (N_2O).

B. Place a Doppler precordial monitor over the right atrium (third to fifth intercostal space, right parasternal border) to detect VAE's characteristic turbulence. Insert a multiorificed-end CVP catheter (tip located near the junction of the superior vena cava [SVC] and right atrium). Monitor end-tidal carbon dioxide ([CO_2] VAE causes an increase in dead-space ventilation and a decrease in end-tidal CO_2). TEE, the most sensitive detector of VAE, allows quantification of air entrained and detection of paradoxic air embolism through a PFO or other intracardiac defect.[3] Pulmonary artery (PA) pressure increases with VAE, as air entering the pulmonary circulation causes mechanical vascular obstruction and reflex pulmonary vasoconstriction. Brainstem auditory evoked responses (BAER) are useful to monitor the auditory pathways (e.g., during acoustic neuroma surgery where the eighth cranial nerve is at risk) or as a monitor of compression or ischemia of the brainstem (e.g., monitoring the auditory tracts in the brainstem).[4] Use facial nerve monitoring (electrodes are placed in the muscles innervated by the facial nerve) in procedures involving large acoustic neuromas where facial nerve injury is common. Insert an arterial catheter for BP and ABG monitoring, and place the pressure transducer at head level to ensure adequate CPP. Wrap the legs with compression stockings to minimize venous pooling, and monitor urine output.

C. Choose an anesthetic technique that will maintain CPP (CPP = MAP − ICP), such as narcotic/muscle relaxant/low-dose inhalational technique. Avoid N_2O because it may increase the size of entrained air bubbles and exacerbate the consequences of VAE. Use nondepolarizing relaxants and control ventilation.

D. Pad all pressure points to avoid nerve compression. Make positional changes gradually; monitor BP and bilateral breath sounds as each change is made. Avoid hyperflexion of the neck, which can cause kinking of the endotracheal tube (ETT), obstruction of jugular venous drainage, and spinal cord ischemia. Examine the puncture sites if multiple attempts at pin headholder placement were made, and seal to avoid VAE from cranial diploë.

E. Cardiovascular instability is a potential complication of the sitting position. Maintain adequate preload to attenuate hypotension with positioning. Should VAE occur, notify surgeons to stop air entrainment (have them flood operative field with saline and wax the bone edges). Small volumes of air may be eliminated by the pulmonary circulation; large volumes produce an air lock in the right side of the heart impeding cardiac output (CO). Attempt to aspirate air from the multiorificed CVP catheter. If possible, lower the operative site to reduce the gradient between the operative site and the heart to lessen the amount of air entry. If surgical conditions permit, consider positioning the patient in the left lateral decubitus position to allow air to accumulate on the right side of the heart so it can be more easily aspirated from the CVP. Although PEEP and valsalva have been used to decrease the gravitational gradient between the cerebral venous system and the heart, they may be hazardous because of a reversal of the left-to-right atrial pressure gradient,[5] which can cause paradoxic air embolus through a PFO. VAE may also occur during PEEP release and during repositioning to supine.[6]

F. Surgical manipulation, brain retraction, and transmission of heat from electrocoagulation near the brainstem and cranial nerves may cause dysrhythmias and hypotension that require intervention. Damage to cranial nerves IX, X, and XII, which provide sensory and motor innervation to the larynx and pharynx, may lead to postoperative stridor, inability to handle secretions, poor swallowing, and aspiration. Intraaxial air should be considered in a patient who remains comatose after surgery. Obtain a magnetic resonance imaging (MRI) scan for diagnosis, and if intraaxial air is present, consider hyperbaric oxygenation.

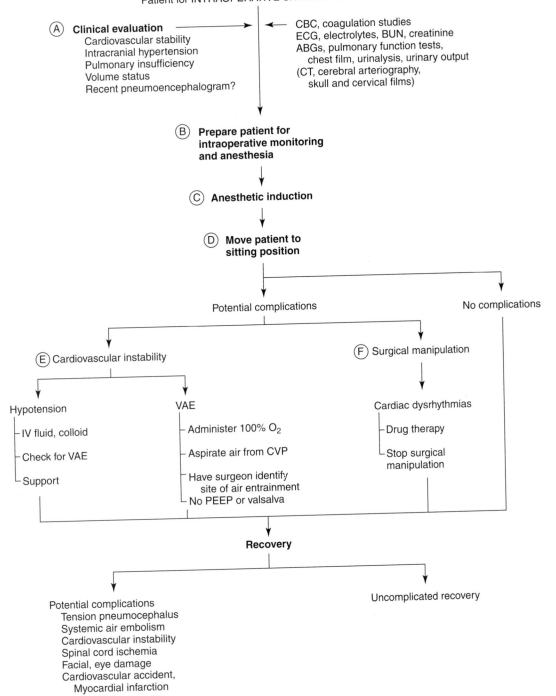

Patient for INTRAOPERATIVE SITTING POSITION

(A) **Clinical evaluation**
  Cardiovascular stability
  Intracranial hypertension
  Pulmonary insufficiency
  Volume status
  Recent pneumoencephalogram?

CBC, coagulation studies
ECG, electrolytes, BUN, creatinine
ABGs, pulmonary function tests,
  chest film, urinalysis, urinary output
(CT, cerebral arteriography,
  skull and cervical films)

(B) **Prepare patient for
intraoperative monitoring
and anesthesia**

(C) **Anesthetic induction**

(D) **Move patient to
sitting position**

Potential complications

No complications

(E) Cardiovascular instability

(F) Surgical manipulation

Hypotension
─ IV fluid, colloid
─ Check for VAE
└ Support

VAE
─ Administer 100% O_2
─ Aspirate air from CVP
─ Have surgeon identify
   site of air entrainment
└ No PEEP or valsalva

Cardiac dysrhythmias
─ Drug therapy
└ Stop surgical
   manipulation

Recovery

Potential complications
  Tension pneumocephalus
  Systemic air embolism
  Cardiovascular instability
  Spinal cord ischemia
  Facial, eye damage
  Cardiovascular accident,
    Myocardial infarction

Uncomplicated recovery

REFERENCES

1. Leonard IE, Cunningham AJ. Editorial I: The sitting position in neurosurgery—not yet obsolete! *Brit J Anaesth* 88:1–3, 2002.
2. Stendel R, Gramm HJ, Schroder K, et al.: Transcranial Doppler ultrasonography as a screening technique for detection of a patent foramen ovale before surgery in the sitting position, *Anesthesiology* 93:971–975, 2000.
3. Cucchiara RF, Seward JB, Nishimura RA, et al.: Identification of patent foramen ovale during sitting position craniotomy by transesophageal echocardiography with positive airway pressure, *Anesthesiology* 63:107–109, 1985.
4. Hickey R, Sloan TB, Albin MS: Anesthesia for posterior fossa surgery. In: Eisenkraft JB, editor: *Progress in anesthesia*, San Antonio, 1991, Dannemiller Memorial Educational Foundation.
5. Perkins NA, Bedford RF: Hemodynamic consequences of PEEP in seated neurological patients—implications for paradoxical air embolism, *Anesth Analg* 63:429–432, 1984.
6. Schmitt HJ, Hemmerling TM: Venous air emboli occur during release of positive end-expiratory pressure and repositioning after sitting position surgery, *Anesth Analg* 94:400–403, 2002.

Controlled Hypotension

ROBERT H. OVERBAUGH, M.D.

Controlled hypotensive anesthesia (CHA) is defined as the deliberate decrease of intraoperative BP to 25% to 30% below preoperative values or to a MAP of 50 to 65 mm Hg.[1] This technique has been advocated during specific operative procedures to improve surgical conditions and decrease perioperative blood loss and need for transfusion.

A. CHA is utilized in both elective procedures and emergency situations to improve operative conditions. CHA can improve operating conditions in orthopedic and facial surgery, as well as decrease blood loss in urological and neurosurgical procedures. CHA significantly decreased blood loss and improved ease of dissection during Le Fort I osteotomies.[2] CHA is superior to acute normovolemic hemodilution for decreasing the need for PRBC transfusion during radical prostatectomy procedures.[3] CHA is a commonly used technique in pediatric patients undergoing spinal fusion and scoliosis repair. CHA may be indicated in both elective and emergent intracerebral aneurysm clipping, removal of cerebral arterial-venous malformations,[4] and endoscopic sinus surgery. CHA not only decreases blood loss in patients undergoing total hip replacement, but when combined with epidural anesthesia, has been shown to decrease the incidence of venous thromboembolism (VTE).[5] CHA may be employed during radical neck dissection and repair of aortic dissections. Certain patient factors, such as religious prohibition of transfused blood products (e.g., Jehovah's Witness), may also support the use of CHA.

B. Perform a complete preoperative evaluation. Rule out any history of cardiac disease, including angina, coronary artery disease (CAD), congestive heart failure (CHF), and valvulopathies (specifically aortic or mitral stenosis). Patients with a history of cerebrovascular accident (CVA), TIA, or carotid occlusive disease are poor candidates. Other contraindications include concomitant hypovolemia, ventilatory insufficiency, hypoxemia, acidosis, and chronic anemias including sickle cell disease. Probable contraindications may include uncontrolled hypertension (HTN), hepatic or renal insufficiency, and glaucoma. Continue preoperative antihypertensive agents (including beta-blockers, calcium channel blockers, and alpha-blockers) in the perioperative period to prevent rebound HTN.

C. Place standard American Society of Anesthesiologists (ASA) monitors including a 5-lead ECG (monitoring leads II and V3) to monitor for myocardial ischemia and dysrhythmia. With few exceptions, place a continuous intraarterial catheter for BP monitoring. If large-volume shifts or changes in cardiac function are expected, consider CVP, pulmonary artery (PA) catheter, or transesophageal echocardiography (TEE). Place a urinary catheter to monitor volume status and renal perfusion. Monitor motor and sensory-evoked potentials for spinal fusion and scoliosis surgery. Consider intraoperative EEG, brainstem auditory evoked–potentials, and visual-evoked potentials for information about cerebral perfusion during CHA.

D. Determine the target MAP preoperatively, commonly 25% to 30% below preoperative values or to a MAP of 50 to 65 mm Hg. Establish the lowest acceptable level and duration of hypotension. Profound hypotension, as may be necessary to control hemorrhage in procedures such as cerebral aneurysm clipping, is tolerated for short durations. Patients with chronic HTN may not tolerate the same reduction in BP as normotensive patients; cerebral and renal autoregulatory function undergoes a rightward shift in these patients.

Patient with CONTROLLED HYPERTENSION

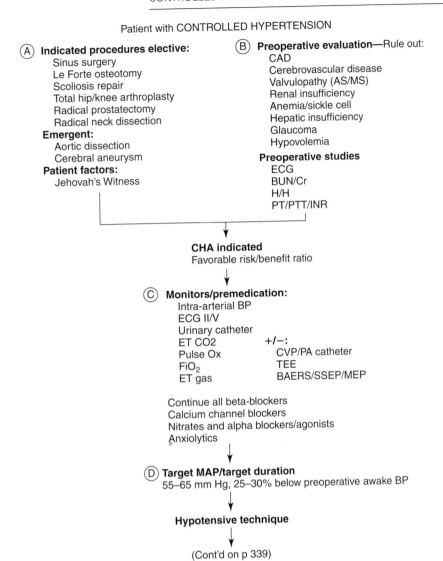

Ⓐ **Indicated procedures elective:**
    Sinus surgery
    Le Forte osteotomy
    Scoliosis repair
    Total hip/knee arthroplasty
    Radical prostatectomy
    Radical neck dissection
Emergent:
    Aortic dissection
    Cerebral aneurysm
Patient factors:
    Jehovah's Witness

Ⓑ **Preoperative evaluation—Rule out:**
    CAD
    Cerebrovascular disease
    Valvulopathy (AS/MS)
    Renal insufficiency
    Anemia/sickle cell
    Hepatic insufficiency
    Glaucoma
    Hypovolemia
Preoperative studies
    ECG
    BUN/Cr
    H/H
    PT/PTT/INR

CHA indicated
Favorable risk/benefit ratio

Ⓒ **Monitors/premedication:**
    Intra-arterial BP
    ECG II/V
    Urinary catheter
    ET CO_2
    Pulse Ox
    FiO_2
    ET gas

+/−:
    CVP/PA catheter
    TEE
    BAERS/SSEP/MEP

Continue all beta-blockers
Calcium channel blockers
Nitrates and alpha blockers/agonists
Anxiolytics

Ⓓ **Target MAP/target duration**
55–65 mm Hg, 25–30% below preoperative awake BP

Hypotensive technique

(Cont'd on p 339)

E. The choice of anesthetic technique plays an integral role in CHA and should compliment the hypotensive technique. An increase in the concentration of volatile agent, such as isoflurane (causes a dose-dependent reduction in systemic vascular resistance [SVR]), can provide CHA. Use of lumbar epidural to produce hypotension in patients undergoing hip arthroplasty significantly reduces not only operative blood loss but also decreases the risk of VTE.[5] IV anesthetics, such as propofol, can also produce dose-dependent decreases in MAP, especially in older patients.[6]

F. Consider the surgical procedure, patient characteristics, and physiological goals when selecting a hypotensive technique. Ideally, the technique should be easily titratable and have minimal potential for adverse effect or toxicity. Nitroglycerin (NTG) and sodium nitroprusside (SNP) have been commonly utilized but have drawbacks. SNP, when administered for prolonged durations, is associated with rebound HTN, tachyphylaxis, and cyanide toxicity. NTG may increase ICP and may not be an appropriate choice for cerebral procedures. It also has been shown to abolish hypoxic pulmonary vasoconstriction, which may worsen intrapulmonary shunt. Nicardipine offers rapid control of BP, is easily titrated, and does not interfere with neurophysiological monitoring during spinal surgery.[7] Esmolol, a selective beta$_1$-atagonist, provides superior surgical conditions when compared to SNP for inducing CHA for endoscopic sinus surgery.[8] Other agents that can be used for CHA include prostaglandin E$_1$ (PGE$_1$), hydralazine, adenosine, and fenoldopam. Before utilizing any hypotensive agent, consider the onset, duration of action, and potential side effect profiles.

G. Observe the patient postoperatively for persistent hypotension, rebound HTN, and tachycardia in a monitored setting. Watch for ongoing blood loss and evidence of coagulopathy. Monitor for hypoxemia, ischemia, diminished urine output, and alteration in neurological or cognitive status. Ensure that end-organ compromise has not occurred as a result of the hypotensive period.

REFERENCES

1. Van Aken H, Miller E: Deliberate hypotension. In: Miller RD, editor: *Anesthesia*, ed 5, Philadelphia, 2000, Churchill Livingstone.
2. Dolman RM, Bentley KC, Head TW, et al.: Effect of hypotensive anesthesia on blood loss and operative time during Le Fort I osteotomies, *J Oral Maxillofac Surg* 58 (8):834–839, 2000.
3. Boldt J, Weber A, Mailer K, et al.: Acute normovolaemic haemodilution vs controlled hypotension for reducing the use of allogenic blood in patients undergoing radical prostatectomy, *Br J Anaesth* 82 (2):170–174, 1999.
4. Massoud TF, Hademenos GJ: Transvenous retrograde nidus sclerotherapy under controlled hypotension (TRENSH): a newly proposed treatment for brain arteriovenous malformations-concepts and rationale, *Neurosurgery* 45 (2):351–363, 1999.
5. Westrich GH, Farrell C, Bono JV, et al.: The incidence of venous thromboembolism after total hip arthroplasty: a specific hypotensive epidural anesthesia protocol, *J Arthroplasty* 14 (4):456–463, 1999.
6. Schnider TW, Minto CF, Shafer SL, et al.: The influence of age on propofol pharmacodynamics, *Anesthesiology* 90:1502–1516, 1990.
7. Tobias JD: Controlled hypotension in children: a critical review of available agents. *Paediatr Drugs* (4) 7:439–453, 2002.
8. Boezaart AP, van der Merwe J, Coetzee A: Comparison of sodium nitroprusside- and esmolol-induced hypotension for functional endoscopic sinus surgery, *Can J Anaesth* 42 (5):373–376, 1995.

Patient with CONTROLLED HYPERTENSION
(Cont'd from p 337)

(E) **Anesthetic based:**
Decrease MAP via:
Epidural/subarachnoid anesthesia
Increasing concentration of volatile agent
Peripheral vasodilation via hypnotic agent
(propofol, thiopental)

(F) **Hypotensive agents:**

Beta-blockers:
Esmolol
Labetalol,
Metoprolol

Calcium channel blockers:
Nicardipine

Direct vasodilators:
NTG
SNP
Hydralazine

Other:
Fenoldopam
Trimethaphan,
PGE-1, Adenosine

(G) **Postoperative monitoring**

PACU:
No evidence of intra/post-operative sequela
No persistent hypotension
Tachycardia
Hypoxemia
Cardiac ischemia
Decreased urine output
Hypercarbia or altered mental status

Intensive care unit:
Evidence of end-organ sequela:
Persistent hypotension
Tacchycardia
Hypoxemia
Cardiac ischemia
Decreased urine output
Alteration in neurological/cognitive status
Ongoing bleeding
Coagulopathy

Intracranial Hypertension (HTN)

ROSEMARY HICKEY, M.D.

Intracranial hypertension (HTN) is a common sequela of severe head injury and occurs in other cerebral disorders (e.g., subarachnoid hemorrhage, brain tumors, posthypoxic brain damage, and Reye's syndrome). A sustained elevation in ICP results in a decrease in CPP (CPP = MAP – ICP) and is associated with a poor outcome. Anesthetic management of the patient with elevated ICP involves measures to reduce ICP pending definitive surgical therapy.

A. Perform a history and physical examination, including a neurological assessment. Focus on level of consciousness, signs of elevated ICP, and existence of focal neurological deficits. Assess cardiovascular, pulmonary, and renal systems, as well as airway patency and anticipated difficulty of intubation. Evaluate drug therapy preoperatively. Anticonvulsants accelerate the metabolism of steroidal muscle relaxants and steroids may produce hyperglycemia. Review the results of special studies (CT, magnetic resonance imaging [MRI], arteriography). Give minimal preoperative medication to avoid obscuring the neurological examination and to prevent increases in ICP from hypoventilation.

B. Choose anesthetic medications. Prevent coughing, straining, vomiting, and hypoventilation. Avoid ketamine, which can increase ICP.

C. Select intraoperative monitors including ICP monitor (advisable), esophageal stethoscope, ECG, arterial line, temperature probe, urinary catheter, and CVP line or pulmonary artery (PA) catheter. Monitor for venous air embolism with precordial Doppler, end-tidal carbon dioxide (CO_2) monitor, and CVP catheter (tip located near the junction of the right atrium and superior vena cava [SVC][1]). For elective procedures, place monitors before induction. In an emergency situation, the need for rapid surgical decompression may preclude preoperative placement of some monitors.

D. If a difficult intubation is not suspected in the full stomach patient, perform an RSI. Succinylcholine (SCC) may increase ICP through cortical stimulation by increases in muscle afferent activity,[2] but the effect on ICP is transient. Rocuronium has the advantage of relatively rapid onset and is not associated with increases in ICP.[3] In the case of a difficult airway, perform an awake, fiberoptic intubation after topical anesthesia.

E. For the patient who has fasted, choose propofol or thiopental for induction. In the patient who is unstable or volume depleted, etomidate may be preferable. Achieve muscle relaxation with a nondepolarizing muscle relaxant ([NDMR] vecuronium, rocuronium, pancuronium, cis-atracurium). Titrate narcotics (fentanyl, sufentanil, alfentanil, or remifentanil) to provide a smooth induction; narcotics do not increase ICP in the absence of a reduction in blood pressure. Intubate after confirmation of muscle relaxation with a nerve stimulator.

F. In the patient with a head injury in whom a cervical spine fracture has not been excluded by radiographic evaluation, perform manual inline stabilization (have an assistant stabilize the patient's head by positioning his or her hands along the side of the head, with fingertips on the mastoid to hold the occiput down).

G. In the patient with a basilar skull fracture, avoid nasal intubation to decrease the risk of intracranial passage of the endotracheal tube (ETT).

H. Employ techniques for decreasing ICP including proper head positioning to maximize venous drainage (head elevated 15 to 30 degrees without excessive rotation or flexion), moderate hyperventilation ($PaCO_2$ 25 to 30 mm Hg), barbiturates, diuretics, and avoidance of hyposmolar IV solutions. The effects of hyperventilation on ICP are immediate, but the effect is not sustained because the level of bicarbonate in the CSF decreases. Hyperventilation can cause cerebral ischemia; utilize the minimum amount that is effective. Consider monitoring jugular venous oxygen saturation (fiberoptic catheter inserted into the jugular bulb) to assess the effects of hyperventilation.[4] Mannitol (0.25 to 1 mg/kg) raises the osmolality of plasma so that brain water is withdrawn into the intravascular compartment. It maximally reduces ICP within 10 minutes of administration and the reduction in ICP persists for 3 to 4 hours. Loop diuretics (furosemide) reduce ICP by brain dehydration and by reduction in CSF formation. Given along with mannitol, furosemide results in a greater and more sustained decrease in ICP than mannitol alone.[5] Avoid glucose-containing solutions because hyperglycemia can aggravate ischemic injury[6] by increasing lactic acid production and decreasing cerebral pH. Steroids reduce ICP in patients with brain tumors but are not helpful in patients with a head injury.

I. Inhalational agents cause cerebral vasodilation and may increase ICP. These effects can be attenuated or abolished by hyperventilation. Nitrous oxide causes an increase in cerebral blood flow (CBF) and has the disadvantage of augmenting air pneumocephalus. The use of inhalational agents as the primary anesthetic technique (in combination with low-to-moderate doses of narcotic) is appropriate in patients with less severe injury.

J. In patients with severe injury who are not expected to be extubated at the end of the procedure, use a primary IV technique with continuous infusions of narcotic and thiopental or propofol. These agents have the advantage of reducing CBF, cerebral blood volume, and ICP, as well as reducing cerebral metabolic oxygen consumption ($CMRO_2$).

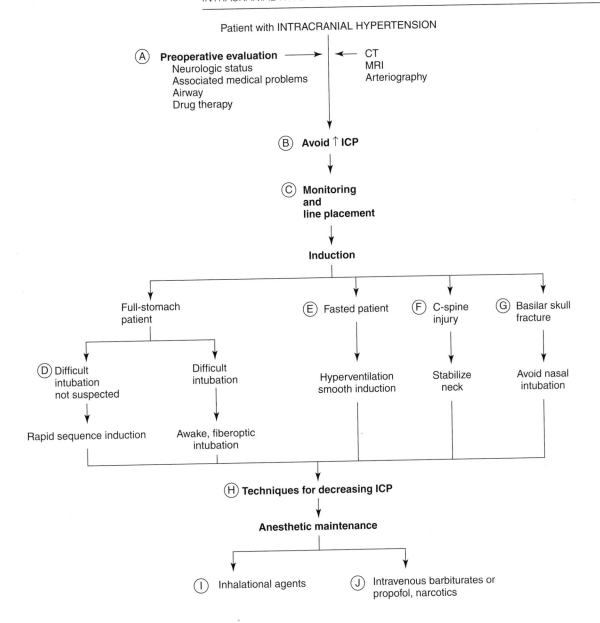

Patient with INTRACRANIAL HYPERTENSION

Ⓐ **Preoperative evaluation** ⟶   ← CT
    Neurologic status   MRI
    Associated medical problems Arteriography
    Airway
    Drug therapy

Ⓑ **Avoid ↑ ICP**

Ⓒ **Monitoring
and
line placement**

Induction

Full-stomach patient   Ⓔ Fasted patient   Ⓕ C-spine injury   Ⓖ Basilar skull fracture

Ⓓ Difficult intubation not suspected   Difficult intubation   Hyperventilation smooth induction   Stabilize neck   Avoid nasal intubation

Rapid sequence induction   Awake, fiberoptic intubation

Ⓗ **Techniques for decreasing ICP**

Anesthetic maintenance

Ⓘ Inhalational agents   Ⓙ Intravenous barbiturates or propofol, narcotics

REFERENCES

1. Bunegin L, Albin MS, Helsel PE, et al.: Positioning the right atrial catheter: a model for reappraisal, *Anesthesiology* 55:343–348, 1981.
2. Lanier WL, Milde JH, Michenfelder JD: Cerebral stimulation following succinylcholine in dogs, *Anesthesiology* 64:551–559,1986.
3. Schramm WM, Strasser K, Bartunek A, et al.: Effects of rocuronium and vecuronium on intracranial pressure, mean arterial pressure and heart rate in neurosurgical patients, *Br J Anaesth* 77:607–611, 1996.
4. Oertel M, Kelly DF, Lee JH, et al.: Efficacy of hyperventilation, blood pressure elevation, and metabolic suppression therapy in controlling intracranial pressure after head injury, *J Neurosurg* 97 (5):1045–1053, 2002.
5. Thenuwara K, Todd MM, Brian JE Jr.: Effect of mannitol and furosemide on plasma osmolality and brain water, *Anesthesiology* 96 (2):416–421, 2002.
6. Lam AM, Winn HR, Cullen BF, et al.: Hyperglycemia and neurological outcome in patients with head injury, *J Neurosurg* 75:545–551, 1991.

Acute Spinal Cord Injury (SCI)

TOD B. SLOAN, M.D., PH.D.

Suspect spinal cord injuries (SCIs) in all patients with multiple trauma, particularly those with neck complaints, neurological abnormalities, head trauma, or comatose patients with hypotension and absent reflexes.[1-3] Treat patients with suspected SCI as if they have spinal injury until it is proved otherwise. Because most cervical SCI occurs in the C4–C6 region, lateral cervical spine films visualizing through C7 usually confirm the bony injury in the common region of C4–C6; however, spine instability can be missed (up to 30% of cases), and a more extensive radiographic evaluation and cognitive participation of the patient is necessary to rule out injury.[4] SCI without radiologic abnormality (SCIWORA) can occur, especially in infants and geriatric patients, and requires magnetic resonance imaging (MRI) for diagnosis.

A. For initial management of acute SCI, control the airway, breathing, and circulation; medically manage coexisting injury; and prevent secondary SCI. Stabilize the spine (preferably with traction) in a neutral position. When possible, evaluate for comorbidities before inducing anesthesia; often, however, the first priority is securing the airway. Administer methylprednisolone to reduce the extent of neurological injury.[5]

B. Assess the need for instrumentation of the airway. If immediate intubation is needed, perform direct laryngoscopy with midline stabilization (not traction). If used, base dosages of short-acting anesthetics (to allow rapid recovery of neurological examination) such as thiopental and etomidate on cardiovascular stability. Succinylcholine (SCC) may be used until 24 hours after SCI; after that time, it may cause lethal hyperkalemia if neurological injury has occurred. If facial trauma prohibits oral intubation, consider a surgical airway (tracheostomy or cricothyrotomy) or transtracheal ventilation. In patients with head trauma, avoid the nasal route if a basilar skull fracture is possible ("battle sign," "raccoon eyes," CSF rhinorrhea).

C. After the airway is secured, ensure adequate oxygenation and ventilation. Pulmonary function studies usually reveal reduced total lung capacity, vital capacity (VC), expiratory reserve volume, FEV_1, and increased residual volume. VC appears to be an excellent measure of pulmonary compromise; patients with VC < 15 ml/kg may require intubation and ventilation support (very likely <8 ml/kg). Factors contributing to reduced ventilation include gastric distention, ileus, aspiration pneumonitis, loss of expiratory reserve and the ability to cough due to loss of abdominal (T_2–L_1) and intercostal (T_{1-11}) muscle control, fat emboli from long-bone fractures, chest trauma (rib fractures, pulmonary contusion, pneumothorax and hemothorax), loss of phrenic nerve (C3–C5) control of the diaphragm, and depressed consciousness from head injury, alcohol, or drugs. In patients with head trauma, raised ICP may need treatment. Pulmonary failure may also result from pulmonary edema secondary to myocardial injury from catecholamine surge at injury or volume overload. Hypotension is common (loss of sympathetic tone from SCI, hypovolemia, and trauma). Consider expansion of blood volume to restore adequate cardiac performance and BP (to ensure adequate organ and spinal cord perfusion). Pulmonary artery (PA) catheterization may be required, as excessive fluid infusion may lead to pulmonary edema. Use vasoconstrictor agents to treat low systemic vascular resistance (SVR) if volume is ineffective.

D. Use monitors as appropriate for the patient's overall condition and planned surgical procedure; place them before induction. Position the patient for surgery, document neurological function in the planned position (e.g., prone, lateral), and then proceed. Sudden positional changes may cause marked changes of BP. Bradycardia (including ventricular ectopy and asystole) occurs as a result of loss of cardiac accelerators (T1–T4), and is aggravated by maneuvers that increase vagal tone (airway manipulation). Treat bradycardia with atropine. Maintain normal $ETCO_2$ and BP (for optimal spinal cord blood flow) and administer vasopressors if needed (low systemic vascular resistance from SCI). If evoked potentials are used intraoperatively, choose a narcotic-based anesthetic. Electromyographic recordings with motor evoked potentials require severely restricted muscle relaxation. Monitor temperature and keep the patient warm (loss of sympathetic tone increases heat loss or gain). Monitor serum glucose because high levels may worsen ischemic injury.

E. Observe for associated injury accompanying the trauma producing the SCI. Unexplained hypotension may indicate unrecognized intraabdominal or retroperitoneal bleeding.

F. Delay extubation until adequate ventilatory function has been demonstrated; postoperative ventilation may be needed. Emergent reintubation is undesirable but if needed, use midline stabilization.

REFERENCES

1. Sloan TB, Hickey R, Albin MS: Anesthesia management of the patient with acute spinal cord injury, *Adv Anesth* 8:55, 1991.
2. Stier GR, Schell R, Cole D: Spinal Cord Injury. In: J Cottrell, DH Smith, editors: *Anesthesia and neurosurgery*, ed 4, Philadelphia, 2001, Mosby.

Patient with ACUTE SPINAL CORD INJURY

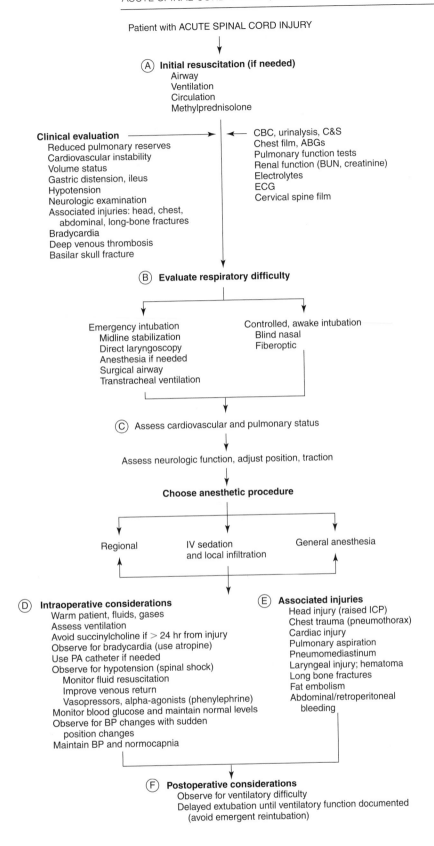

(A) **Initial resuscitation (if needed)**
Airway
Ventilation
Circulation
Methylprednisolone

Clinical evaluation
Reduced pulmonary reserves
Cardiovascular instability
Volume status
Gastric distension, ileus
Hypotension
Neurologic examination
Associated injuries: head, chest,
abdominal, long-bone fractures
Bradycardia
Deep venous thrombosis
Basilar skull fracture

CBC, urinalysis, C&S
Chest film, ABGs
Pulmonary function tests
Renal function (BUN, creatinine)
Electrolytes
ECG
Cervical spine film

(B) **Evaluate respiratory difficulty**

Emergency intubation
Midline stabilization
Direct laryngoscopy
Anesthesia if needed
Surgical airway
Transtracheal ventilation

Controlled, awake intubation
Blind nasal
Fiberoptic

(C) Assess cardiovascular and pulmonary status

Assess neurologic function, adjust position, traction

Choose anesthetic procedure

Regional

IV sedation
and local infiltration

General anesthesia

(D) **Intraoperative considerations**
Warm patient, fluids, gases
Assess ventilation
Avoid succinylcholine if > 24 hr from injury
Observe for bradycardia (use atropine)
Use PA catheter if needed
Observe for hypotension (spinal shock)
Monitor fluid resuscitation
Improve venous return
Vasopressors, alpha-agonists (phenylephrine)
Monitor blood glucose and maintain normal levels
Observe for BP changes with sudden
position changes
Maintain BP and normocapnia

(E) **Associated injuries**
Head injury (raised ICP)
Chest trauma (pneumothorax)
Cardiac injury
Pulmonary aspiration
Pneumomediastinum
Laryngeal injury; hematoma
Long bone fractures
Fat embolism
Abdominal/retroperitoneal
bleeding

(F) **Postoperative considerations**
Observe for ventilatory difficulty
Delayed extubation until ventilatory function documented
(avoid emergent reintubation)

3. Mackensie CF, Geisler FH: Management of acute cervical spinal cord injury. In: Albin MS, editor, *Textbook of neuroanesthesia with neurosurgical and neuroscience perspectives*, New York, 1996, McGraw-Hill.

4. Woodring JH, Lee C: Limitations of cervical radiography in the evaluation of acute cervical trauma, *J Trauma* 34:32–39, 1993.

5. Bracken MB, Shepard MJ, Collins WF Jr, et al.: Methylprednisolone or naloxone treatment after acute spinal cord injury: one year follow-up data. Results of the Second National Acute Spinal Cord Injury Study, *J Neurosurg* 76:23–31, 1992.

Airway Management in Cervical Fracture

LAUREN BERKOW, M.D.

Airway management in the patient with a cervical spine injury can be potentially hazardous, resulting in further neurological injury, loss of the airway, and even death.[1] Many cervical spine injuries are not immediately diagnosed, so any trauma patient should be considered to have a cervical spine injury until proven otherwise. The trauma patient should also be considered to have a full stomach; aspiration precautions should be taken and a RSI or awake intubation should be considered. The potential for difficult mask ventilation or intubation should be considered in these patients, and the availability of special airway equipment may be beneficial.

A. *Acute, unstable cervical spine injury*—Unstable cervical spine injury is most commonly a result of trauma. Certain disease processes, such as osteoarthritis and rheumatoid arthritis, may predispose the patient to injury. Injury to the upper cervical spine may lead to respiratory insufficiency and even death. These patients often need emergent airway management. Injuries to lower levels of the cervical spine usually result in weakness or neurological deficit. Associated vascular injury as well as edema may lead to rapid progression of symptoms. Other potentially life-threatening injuries may be present (head trauma or major vascular injury) and should be considered prior to administering medications. Administer oxygen and place monitors, including pulse oximetry. Stabilize the cervical spine via a collar or backboard. If the patient is obtunded, apneic, or the airway is not patent, perform emergent intubation using inline cervical stabilization, minimizing neck movement. If intubation or ventilation is not possible, place a laryngeal mask airway (LMA) to provide adequate oxygenation and ventilation.[2] If LMA placement is inadequate or not possible, consider a surgical airway, such as a cricothyroidotomy or tracheotomy.

If the patient is awake and cooperative and airway management is required, consider awake intubation after adequate airway topicalization; this allows continual assessment of neurological status. Indirect techniques, such as fiberoptic or light wand-guided intubation, do not require movement of the cervical spine and can easily be performed in cervical traction. Confirm proper placement of the endotracheal tube (ETT). Continue to assess the patient after airway management is complete.

B. *Chronic cervical spine injury*—Patients may have chronic cervical spine injury as a result of chronic disorders, such as osteoarthritis or rheumatoid arthritis, congenital abnormalities (Down's syndrome), or tumors (primary or metastatic). These patients may need airway management for surgical procedures. Perform careful intubation, with minimal neck movement and cervical stabilization. There is an increased incidence of difficult laryngoscopy and intubation in these patients, so have alternative airway devices immediately available.[3] Perform a thorough history and airway assessment to elicit a history of difficult intubation.

C. *Methods of intubation*—There is no consensus regarding the best technique for securing the airway in a patient with cervical spine injury. Direct laryngoscopy, even with inline stabilization, has been shown to cause some upper cervical spine movement and distraction.[4,5] Direct laryngoscopy may also be difficult in the presence of a cervical collar or immobilization device. Indirect techniques, such as fiberoptic intubation and light wand intubation, may result in less cervical motion and reduce the risk of further injury. It is crucial to minimize head and neck motion and maintain cervical stabilization during any type of airway intervention. Fiberoptic intubation can be performed with minimal movement of the cervical spine. When performed in the awake patient, neurological status can be assessed. Alternative airway devices such as the intubating LMA (ILMA) and the light wand stylette may also play a role in airway management of the patient with cervical spine injury.[6–8]

REFERENCES

1. Crosby E: Airway management after upper cervical spine injury: what have we learned? Can J Anaesth 49:733–744, 2002.
2. American Society of Anesthesiologist's Task Force on Management of the Difficult Airway: Practice guidelines for management of the difficult airway: an updated report by the American Society of Anesthesiologists Task Force on Management of the Difficult Airway, Anesthesiology 98:1269–1277, 2003.
3. Calder I, Calder J, Crockard HA: Difficult direct laryngoscopy in patients with cervical spine disease, Anaesthesia 50:756–763, 1995.
4. Brimacombe J, Keller C, Kunzel KH, et al.: Cervical spine motion during airway management: a cinefluoroscopic study of the posteriorly destabilized third cervical vertebrae in human cadavers, Anesth Analg 91:1274–1278, 2000.
5. Fitzgerald RD, Krafft P, Skrbensky G, et al.: Excursions of the cervical spine during tracheal intubation: blind oral intubation compared with direct laryngoscopy, Anaesthesia 49:111–115, 1994.
6. Nakazawa K, Tanaka N, Ishikawa S, et al.: Using the intubating laryngeal mask airway (LMA-Fastrach™) for blind endotracheal intubation in patients undergoing cervical spine operation, Anesth Analg 89:1319–1321, 1999.
7. Wong JK, Tongier WK, Armbruster SC, et al.: Use of the intubating laryngeal mask airway to facilitate awake orotracheal intubation in patients with cervical spine disorders, J Clin Anesth 11:346–348, 1999.
8. Inoue Y, Koga K, Shigematsu A: A comparison of two tracheal intubation techniques with Trachlight™ and Fastrach™ in patients with cervical spine disorders, Anesth Analg 94:667–671, 2002.

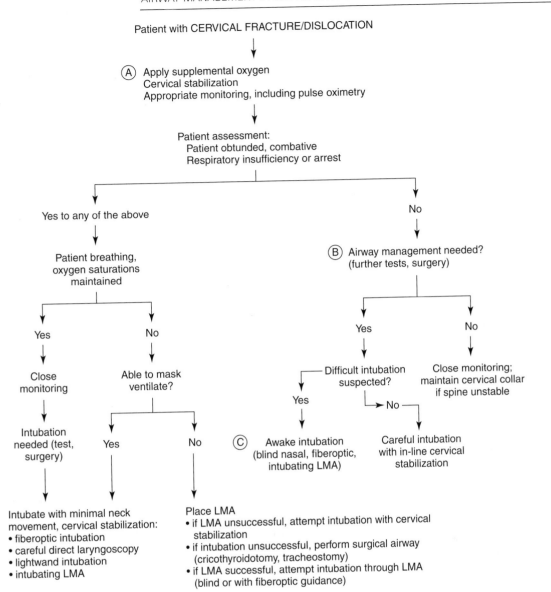

Controlled Mild Hypothermia

THOMAS FRIETSCH, M.D.

Hypothermia is commonly employed for cardiac arrest and heart surgery. Although there is no evidence-based proof of benefit when hypothermia is employed for other indications, mild or moderate hypothermia during anesthesia is practiced in many institutions. In most cases, the patient is allowed to cool passively to mild hypothermia during anesthesia.[1,2] The optimal time of onset (preischemic versus intraischemic), depth (mild, moderate or severe), duration, pH-management, and rate of cooling and rewarming are unknown. During hypothermia, oxygen is redistributed in the brain.[3] The cerebral metabolic rate, cerebral ICP, and neurotoxic sequelae of ischemia all decrease. Cerebral blood flow decreases with alpha-stat pH management of ABG but is maintained with pH-stat management (see D). The immune response decreases during hypothermia, which can result in an increased infection rate.[4] Hypothermia also results in impaired coagulation.[4] Hypothermia can lead to prolonged action of anesthetic drugs. Mild hypothermia = 34°C to 36°C, moderate hypothermia = 32°C to 34°C, and severe hypothermia = 28°C to 32°C.

A. Perform a history and physical examination and obtain appropriate preoperative labs. Determine whether the patient is a candidate for intraoperative hypothermia. Significant cardiac disease and cold autoimmune disease (CAID) are contraindications. Consider the impact of coagulopathy on the surgical outcome. Possible indications for hypothermia include: recommended following cardiac resuscitation and delayed mental recovery.[3,4] In debate: following head trauma.[5,6] Possibly effective for carotid and aneurysm surgery with expected long ischemic periods,[7] craniotomy for tumor resection, posterior fossa surgery.

B. Place standard American Society of Anesthesiologists (ASA) monitors, including a monitor of core temperature. Place an arterial line for continuous BP and ABG analysis.

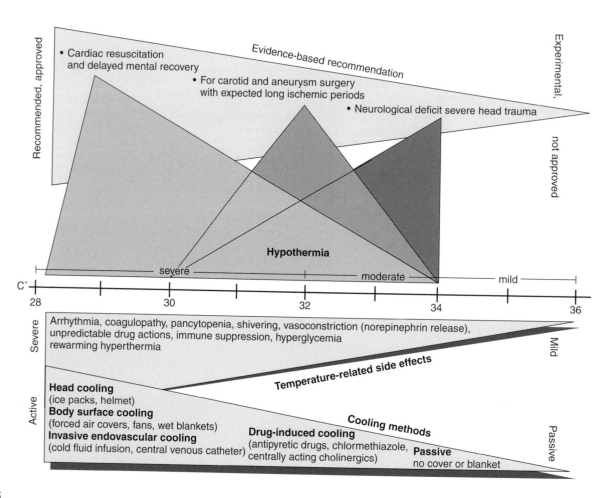

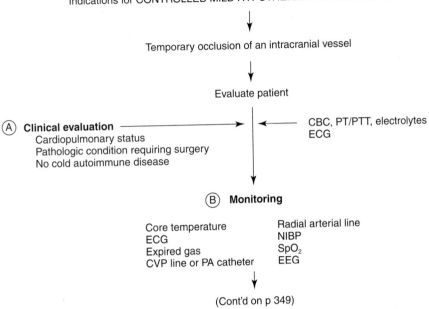

Indications for CONTROLLED MILD HYPOTHERMIA BY SURFACE COOLING

↓

Temporary occlusion of an intracranial vessel

↓

Evaluate patient

(A) **Clinical evaluation** ——————→ ←—— CBC, PT/PTT, electrolytes
    Cardiopulmonary status   ECG
    Pathologic condition requiring surgery
    No cold autoimmune disease

↓

(B) **Monitoring**

Core temperature   Radial arterial line
ECG   NIBP
Expired gas SpO_2
CVP line or PA catheter   EEG

↓

(Cont'd on p 349)

C. Cooling can be passive or active. For passive cooling, allow radiation heat loss from the uncovered, anesthetized body.[7,10] To actively cool, surface cool the body using forced air and water covers and mattresses, fans, or wet blankets,[11] cool the head with ice packs or special helmet, infuse cold fluids through a central venous catheter, or induce cooling with drugs (antipyretic drugs, clomethiazole, centrally acting cholinergics, vasodilators).

D. Monitor the patient closely. Maintain cardiac index. Watch for arrhythmias. Monitor ABGs. Cerebral blood flow is either maintained (pH-stat) or decreased (alpha-stat), depending on the adjustment of the ventilator settings to a $PaCO_2$ measured at actual body temperature (pH-stat) or at normal analysis temperature of 37°C (alpha-stat). This is due to increased gas solubility during hypothermia. Autoregulation seems to be better preserved by alpha-stat management.

E. Rewarm the patient prior to emergence and extubation. Avoid rapid rewarming (axonal damage); this can result in hyperglycemia and hyperthermia, which can lead to brain damage. Posthypothermic shivering will increase oxygen (O_2) consumption. Patients may require prolonged intubation and postoperative ICU care.

REFERENCES

1. Himmelseher S, Pfenninger E: Neuroprotection in neuroanesthesia: current practices in Germany, *Anaesthesist* 49 (5):412–419, 2000.
2. Pemberton PL, Dinsmore J: The use of hypothermia as a method of neuroprotection during neurosurgical procedures and after traumatic brain injury: a survey of clinical practice in Great Britain and Ireland, *Anaesthesia* 58 (4):370–373, 2003.
3. Sakoh M, Gjedde A: Neuroprotection in hypothermia linked to redistribution of oxygen in brain, *Am J Physiol Heart Circ Physiol* 285 (1):H17–H25, 2003.
4. Hildebrand F, Giannoudis PV, van Griensven M, et al.: Pathophysiologic changes and effects of hypothermia on outcome in elective surgery and trauma patients, *Am J Surg* 187 (3):363–371, 2004.
5. Hypothermia after Cardiac Arrest Study Group: Mild therapeutic hypothermia to improve the neurologic outcome after cardiac arrest, *N Engl J Med* 346 (8):549–556, 2002.
6. Bernard SA, Gray TW, Buist MD, et al.: Treatment of comatose survivors of out-of-hospital cardiac arrest with induced hypothermia, *N Engl J Med* 346 (8):557–563, 2002.
7. Gadkary CS, Alderson P, Signorini DF: Therapeutic hypothermia for head injury, *Cochrane Database Syst Rev* (1): CD001048, 2002.
8. Clifton GL, Miller ER, Choi SC, et al.: Lack of effect of induction of hypothermia after acute brain injury, *N Engl J Med* 344 (8):556–563, 2001.
9. Hindman BJ, Todd MM, Gelb AW, et al.: Mild hypothermia as a protective therapy during intracranial aneurysm surgery: a randomized prospective pilot trial, *Neurosurgery* 44 (1):23–32, 1999.
10. Auer RN: Non-pharmacologic (physiologic) neuroprotection in the treatment of brain ischemia, *Ann N Y Acad Sci* 939:271–282, 2001.
11. Marion DW: Therapeutic moderate hypothermia and fever, *Curr Pharm Des* 7 (15):1533–1536, 2001.

Indications for CONTROLLED MILD HYPOTHERMIA BY SURFACE COOLING
(Cont'd from p 347)

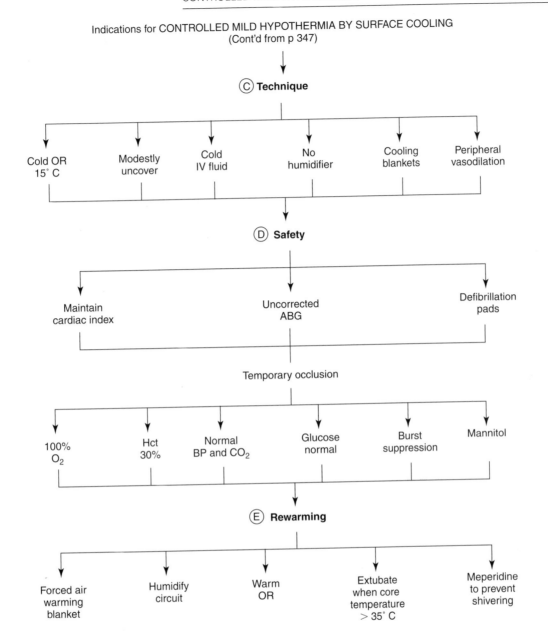

Carotid Endarterectomy (CEA)

DARIN BRANDT, D.O.

The diagnosis of carotid artery disease (CAD) is usually confirmed by carotid duplex studies. Symptomatic patients with >70% stenosis benefit from surgical over medical treatment; there is less benefit from operating on lesions with >50% stenosis. Although the ACAS study has shown benefit in CEA for asymptomatic patients with >60% stenosis, the patient's comorbid conditions need to be assessed to determine the overall risk of surgery.[1] Carotid angioplasty and stenting is just as effective as CEA in asymptomatic patients.

A. Perform a history and physical examination. Assess comorbid conditions. Approximately 50% of the complications from CEA are cardiac in origin.[2] Maintain strict perioperative glucose control in diabetic patients due to the adverse effects of hyperglycemia in the face of cerebral ischemia. Maximize antihypertensive therapy because of the associated risks of stroke and bleeding at the surgical site. Neurological risk factors that increase the likelihood of stroke include a deficit within 24 hours, stroke within 7 days, crescendo TIAs, global cerebral ischemia, and CT evidence of stroke.[1]

B. Choose intraoperative monitors and anesthetic technique. In addition to standard American Society of Anesthesiologists (ASA) monitors, place a 5-lead ECG to facilitate detection of myocardial ischemia and an arterial catheter to optimize beat-to-beat hemodynamics. Regional (superficial ± deep cervical plexus block) and general anesthesia are both acceptable anesthetic choices for CEA. Regional anesthesia allows for optimal evaluation of neurological function during carotid occlusion and is associated with greater hemodynamic stability. Its disadvantages include the risk of intravascular injection of local anesthetic and patient intolerance of being awake. A general anesthetic allows superior operating conditions and improved cerebral protection (i.e., high inspired oxygen concentration, inhaled or IV anesthetics), but monitoring of neurological function is difficult.[3] EEG is the most commonly used technique to determine the need for shunting after carotid occlusion. Other less reliable techniques include monitoring of somatosensory evoked potentials, stump pressures, Xenon perfusion scanning, and transcranial Doppler.[4]

C. Normotension is recommended during the procedure. Promptly treat hypotension; the patient will tolerate hypertension (HTN) up to 20% above baseline. Prevent tachycardia by increasing anesthetic depth or administering opiates or beta-blockers. At times, with dissection of the carotid bifurcation, bradycardia and hypotension may be seen. Prompt cessation of surgical manipulation usually reverses the situation, although atropine may be needed in some cases. Ask the surgeon to infiltrate the area of the carotid sinus with 1% lidocaine to prevent subsequent episodes. If the patient has onset of neurological dysfunction (diagnosed in the awake patient or by neurological monitoring during general anesthesia), increase the BP or institute shunting to attempt to reverse the deficit. Maintain normocarbia. Heparin usage is recommended during the procedure but routine reversal is debated.[5] Assess neurological function and avoid large BP variations and coughing on emergence.

D. During the postoperative period, hemodynamic instability involving bradycardia, hypotension, or HTN occurs frequently; only HTN appears linked to stroke, death, and cardiac complications.[6] Neck hematoma with airway compromise occurs in 1% to 3% of cases and has been associated with intraoperative hypotension, nonreversal of heparin, and carotid shunt placement.[7] Other problems include postoperative stroke and myocardial infarction (MI).

REFERENCES

1. Ailawadi G, Stanley JC, Rajagopalan S, et al.: Carotid stenosis: medical and surgical aspects, *Cardiol Clin* 20 (4):599–609, 2002.
2. Sbarigia E, Dario Vizza C, Antonini M, et al.: Locoregional versus general anesthesia in carotid surgery: is there an impact on perioperative myocardial ischemia? Results of a prospective monocentric randomized trial, *J Vasc Surg* 30 (1):131–138, 1999.
3. Mutch WA: Anaesthesia for carotid artery surgery, *Can J Anaesth* 44 (5 Pt 2):R90–R100, 1997.
4. Manninen PH, Tan TK, Sarjeant RM: Somatosensory evoked potential monitoring during carotid endarterectomy in patients with a stroke, *Anesth Analg* 93:39–44, 2001.
5. Loftus CM, Quest DO: Technical issues in carotid artery surgery, *Neurosurgery* 36 (4):629–647, 1995.
6. Wong JH, Findlay JM, Suarez-Almazor ME: Hemodynamic instability after carotid endarterectomy: risk factors and associations with operative complications, *Neurosurgery* 41 (1):35–43, 1997.
7. Self DD, Bryson GL, Sullivan PJ: Risk factors for post-carotid endarterectomy hematoma formation, *Can J Anaesth* 46 (7):635–640, 1999.

Patient presents CAROTID ENDARTERECTOMY

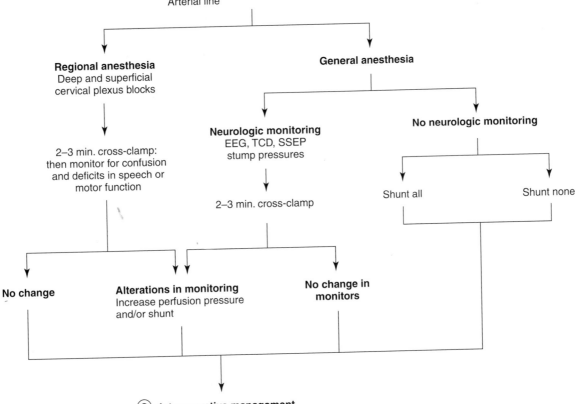

Ⓐ **Preoperative evaluation**

Medical
Maximally controlled DM and HTN
Cardiac evaluation and testing
Define preexisting neurologic deficit

Lab and tests
Hct, Gluc, K+, BUN/Cr
12 lead ECG
Note baseline BP in both arms

Ⓑ **Monitors and anesthetic choice**

Standard monitors
5-lead ECG with ST segment analysis
Arterial line

Regional anesthesia
Deep and superficial
cervical plexus blocks

General anesthesia

Neurologic monitoring
EEG, TCD, SSEP
stump pressures

No neurologic monitoring

2–3 min. cross-clamp:
then monitor for confusion
and deficits in speech or
motor function

2–3 min. cross-clamp

Shunt all

Shunt none

No change

Alterations in monitoring
Increase perfusion pressure
and/or shunt

**No change in
monitors**

Ⓒ **Intraoperative management**

Maintain normocarbia
Keep BP at baseline or 20% above
Watch for bradycardia
Heparin therapy +/− reversal
Prompt waking to allow neurologic exam
Monitor for ischemia and tachycardia

Ⓓ **Postoperative management**

Maintain stable BP and HR
Monitor for myocardial ischemia
Frequent neurologic exams
Monitor for wound hematoma and airway compromise

Intracerebral Aneurysm

RENATA RUSA, M.D.

Despite recent advances in surgical and anesthetic techniques, subarachnoid hemorrhage (SAH) associated with ruptured cerebral aneurysms still carries significant morbidity and mortality. Understanding the mechanisms of altered brain physiology and the effects of SAH on other organ systems is important for making a sound patient management plan. The primary goals of the anesthetic plan are: (1) meticulous BP control to minimize the risk of rebleeding while optimizing cerebral perfusion and minimizing the risk of cerebral ischemia, (2) optimal conditions for surgical clipping, (3) appropriate fluid therapy, and (4) timely neurological assessment on emergence.

A. Aneurysmal rupture leads to SAH and potentially, intraparenchymal or ventricular hemorrhages. This insult may result in brain edema, hydrocephalus, elevated ICP, seizures, and altered cerebral autoregulation. Determine the severity of SAH. The modified Hunt and Hess (H&H) classification system has been widely used to grade the severity of SAH. Higher H&H grades have been associated with higher mortality and morbidity, and are more likely to develop elevated ICP, impaired cerebral autoregulation, intravascular volume depletion and hyponatremia, myocardial dysfunction, and risk of delayed cerebral ischemia or vasospasm.[1,2] Look for any hemodynamically dependent changes in neurological status to aid in perioperative BP management. Review head CT or magnetic resonance imaging (MRI) to evaluate for evidence of elevated ICP, cerebral angiogram for location and number of aneurysm(s), and transcranial Doppler (TCD) for presence of vasospasm.

Catecholamine discharge during SAH can lead to severe hypertension (HTN), dysrhythmias, elevated isozymes, and left ventricular (LV) dysfunction, even in patients without cardiac disease. ECG changes include ST segment and T wave abnormalities, prolonged QTc, and U waves. Dysrhythmias can range from SVT to Vtach/Vfib. Studies suggest that ECG abnormalities are more a reflection of the severity of neurological injury and not predictive of all-cause mortality.[3] Hypokalemia and hyponatremia are common.

B. Place routine monitors and an arterial line in the awake patient, if possible. Consider CVP or pulmonary artery (PA) line in patients in need of close fluid management (e.g., high H&H grade, coexisting disease). Apply a precordial Doppler to detect air embolism. Consider EEG and evoked potentials to help assess cerebral function.

C. During induction and maintenance of anesthesia, aim for meticulous hemodynamic control and avoiding rises in ICP as primary goals. A low CPP (CPP = MAP−ICP) may compromise oxygen delivery to areas with impaired cerebral autoregulation. Increasing transmural pressure across the aneurysm may lead to rupture.

Assess the need for hyperventilation as means of achieving brain relaxation; lowering $PaCO_2$ to the low 30s can worsen ischemia. Avoid IV solutions containing glucose. Mild hypothermia (T = 33°C to 34°C) is probably beneficial in the case of SAH but not in elective aneurysm surgery.[4] Maintain a stable level of anesthesia when evoked potentials and EEG are monitored.

D. The surgeon will apply a temporary clip to an artery proximal to the aneurysm to facilitate final dissection of the aneurysm. At this time, maintain BP at high normal levels to optimize collateral flow. Avoid nitrous oxide; it worsens the neurological consequences of focal ischemia. When neuroprotection is requested prior to temporary clipping, administer incremental doses of the chosen drug (e.g., desflurane or IV boluses of thiopental[5]) until burst suppression is achieved on EEG. The use of etomidate or propofol as neuroprotective agents is controversial.

E. Endovascular coiling of aneurysms serves as an alternative to surgical clipping and is usually employed in patients with aneurysms of the posterior circulation and those who are poor surgical candidates.

F. Consider extubating patients with good H&H grades and uneventful intraoperative courses. Exceptions may be aneurysms in the vertebrobasilar system. HTN after a successful aneurysm clipping is usually desirable, but it is reasonable to treat systolic blood pressure (SBP) > 160 mm Hg with labetalol or nicardipine to decrease the chance of cerebral edema or hemorrhage. Avoid hypovolemia. All patients with SAH now receive nimodipine as prophylaxis for delayed cerebral ischemia. When vasospasm develops, the traditional approach has been induced hypertensive hypervolemic therapy.[6] CT angiography and CT perfusion scans are emerging radiologic modalities for detecting vasospasm in vessels beyond the circle of Willis demonstrated by TCD.

REFERENCES

1. Manno EM: Subarachnoid hemorrhage, *Neurol Clin* 22 (2): 347–366, 2004.
2. Mayer SA, Lin J, Homma S, et al.: Myocardial injury and left ventricular performance after subarachnoid hemorrhage, *Stroke* 30 (4):780–786, 1999.
3. Zaroff JG, Rordorf GA, Newell JB, et al.: Cardiac outcome in patients with subarachnoid hemorrhage and electrocardiographic abnormalities, *Neurosurgery* 44 (1):34–39, discussion 39–40, 1999.
4. Hindman BJ, Todd MM, Gelb AW, et al.: Mild hypothermia as a protective therapy during intracranial aneurysm surgery: a randomized prospective pilot trial, *Neurosurgery* 44 (1):23–32; discussion 32–33, 1999.
5. Hoffman WE, Charbel FT, Edelman G, et al.: Thiopental and desflurane treatment for brain protection, *Neurosurgery* 43 (5): 1050–1053, 1998.
6. McGrath BJ, Guy J, Borel CO, et al.: Perioperative management of aneurysmal subarachnoid hemorrhage: Part 2. Postoperative management, *Anesth Analg* 81 (6):1295–1302, 1995.

Patient with INTRACEREBRAL ANEURYSM

(A) **Preoperative assessment** ⟶ ⟵ **Special studies**
Neurologic status   CT, MRI, TCD, angiogram
  History of SAH   (elevated ICP, location of aneurysm(s))
  Hunt and hess grade
Cardiovascular status
Electrolyte abnormalities

Ablation of aneurysm ⟶ (E) **Endovascular therapy**
                                    May require general anesthesia
                                    and invasive monitoring

Craniotomy ⟵- - - - - Unsuccessful ⟵ ⟶ Successful
                          (consider craniotomy)

(B) **Monitoring**
                  Routine
Arterial line ⟶ Cardiovascular
CVP, PA line,   Electrophysiologic (EEG, evoked potentials)   EtCO$_2$, N$_2$
(TEE)   Assess risk of air embolism ⟵   precordial Doppler

(C) **Induction and anesthetic technique**
Meticulous BP control
Normovolemia
Mild hypothermia

Aneurysm clip application

Direct permanent clipping   (D) **Temporary clipping**
Avoid paroxysmal HTN   Optimize cerebral perfusion
                                       Burst suppression

(F) **Emergence and postoperative care**

Decreased neurologic status   Uncomplicated course

Rule out   **Delayed cerebral ischemia (vasospasm)**
Hypoxia, hypercarbia   Nimodipine
Electrolyte and metabolic abnormalities   Hypertensive hypervolemic therapy
Residual anesthetic effects   Consider angioplasty in extreme situations
Seizures
Pneumocephalus, hydrocephalus
Hemorrhage
Ischemic stroke

Anesthesia during Awake Craniotomy for Epilepsy Surgery

ETHAN GAUMOND, M.D.

JEFFREY R. KIRSCH, M.D.

Epilepsy affects 0.5% to 2% of the population; 20% are medically uncontrolled, and 13% of those with poor control may be surgical candidates (isolated seizure focus within an area of functionally silent cortex). Preoperative or awake intraoperative electrocorticography (ECoG) is used to identify epileptogenic areas. Functional mapping identifies cortex for motor and sensory function, language, and memory.

A. Evaluate patient's neurological status, antiepileptic medication schedule, and airway. Suspected difficult airway is a relative contraindication (possible intraoperative need to control airway). Additional contraindications include immaturity, communication barriers, and inability to cooperate.

B. Use standard monitors including capnometry. Invasive BP monitoring is used routinely in many centers. A urinary catheter is inserted for patient comfort. Surgical draping allows access to the face for neurological assessment during the fully awake portion of the procedure. Choices for anesthetic management during the initial portion of the procedure include sedation or transient general anesthesia maintained with short-acting agents. Propofol along with a short acting opioid provides easy titratability, antiemetic effects, anticonvulsant effects, and lack of interference with ECoG.[1] In a randomized trial of patient-controlled propofol or opioid sedation versus neuroleptanalgesia, there was a significant decrease in the occurrence of intraoperative seizures with use of propofol.[2] Remifentanil produces patient satisfaction equivalent to fentanyl and has the theoretic advantage of facilitating localization of the epileptogenic zone.[3,4] Dexmedetomidine has successfully been used for sedation during awake craniotomy.[5]

C. Several different approaches to airway management and sedation have been described for transient general anesthetic (asleep-awake-asleep) techniques. In combination with a propofol-based anesthetic, some authors describe use of positive-pressure ventilation through a nasal airway, a BiPAP machine, laryngeal mask airway (LMA), or specially designed endotracheal tubes (ETTs). The advantage of using a technique that allows for positive-pressure ventilation is the opportunity to quickly initiate hyperventilation for brain relaxation in an emergency situation. One series evaluating 332 patients with spontaneous ventilation with only a nasal trumpet found six episodes of airway/ventilation complications, three of which needed LMA or ETT placement (all were obese). Desaturation was significantly more common in obese patients as well.[6]

D. The patient's head is often placed in a stereotactic head holder after using local anesthetic at the pin sites to prevent skin and periosteal pain. After patient positioning and induction of sedation or anesthesia, a scalp block is performed. Depending on the site of incision, use a complete or unilateral scalp block. During the procedure the neurosurgeons will infiltrate the dura with local anesthetic. Painful portions of the procedure include scalp block, application of the cranial pins, craniotomy, dural manipulation, and closure. Titrate depth of anesthesia to maintain patient comfort during these periods, and track total dose of local anesthetic to avoid toxicity. Discontinue anesthetic infusions 15 to 30 minutes before ECoG. Once the patient is awake, direct ECoG recordings are performed using interictal spiking to identify the seizure focus and delineate the extent of the necessary resection. After the surgeon ensures location of the seizure focus and functional areas have been identified, cortical resection is initiated and the patient may be resedated for comfort.

E. Intraoperative complications include patient discomfort, airway obstruction, vomiting, seizures, or hypercarbia leading to inadequate brain relaxation. Manage discomfort (opioids, sedation, or adding local anesthetic to the surgical field), airway obstruction or hypoventilation (decreased anesthetic depth, nasal airway, or rarely, securing the airway). Treat nausea with ondansetron or droperidol, and prolonged seizure activity with propofol, a short-acting barbiturate, or a benzodiazepine after the ECoG is completed.

F. Postoperatively, plan frequent monitoring of antiepileptic drug levels. The onset of new neurological deficits is rare and usually limited to minor visual field and memory deficits. Postoperative persistence of seizures typical for the patient may indicate a poorer prognosis.

Patient for AWAKE CRANIOTOMY FOR EPILEPSY

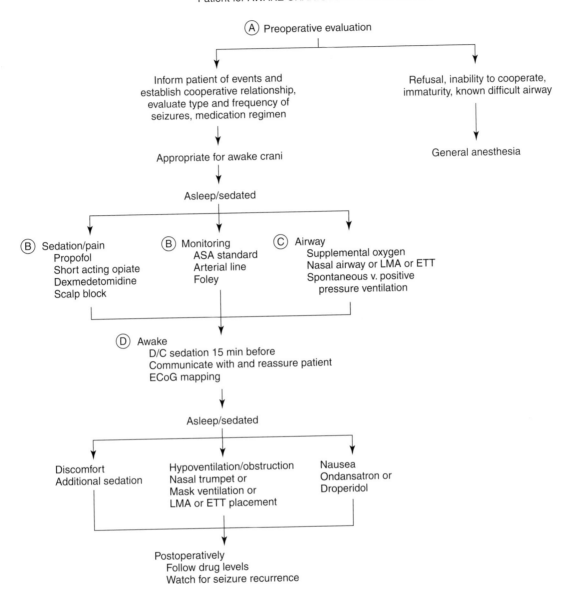

REFERENCES

1. Herrick IA, Craen RA, Gelb AW, et al.: Propofol sedation during awake craniotomy for seizures: electrocorticographic and epileptogenic effects, *Anesth Analg* 84 (6):1280–1284, 1997.
2. Herrick IA, Craen RA, Gelb AW, et al.: Propofol sedation during awake craniotomy for seizures: patient-controlled administration versus neurolept analgesia, *Anesth Analg* 84 (6):1285–1291, 1997.
3. Manninen PH, Balki M, Lukitto M, et al.: Patient satisfaction with awake craniotomy for tumor surgery: a comparison of remifentanil with fentanyl in conjunction with propofol, *Anesth Analg* 102: 237–242, 2006.

4. Wass CT, Grady RE, Fessler AJ, et al.: The effects of remifentanil on epileptiform discharges during intraoperative electrocorticography in patients undergoing epilepsy surgery, *Epilepsia* 42 (10): 1340–1344, 2001.
5. Mack PF, Perrine K, Kobylarz E, et al.: Dexmedetomidine and neurocognitive testing in awake craniotomy, *J Neurosurg Anesthesiol* 16 (1):20–25, 2004.
6. Skucas AP, Artru AA: Anesthetic complications of awake craniotomies for epilepsy surgery, *Anesth Analg* 102:882–887, 2006.

PEDIATRIC ANESTHESIA

PREMATURE INFANT

CONGENITAL DIAPHRAGMATIC HERNIA

OMPHALOCELE AND GASTROSCHISIS

TRACHEOESOPHAGEAL FISTULA (TEF)

NECROTIZING ENTEROCOLITIS (NEC)

FORMER PRETERM INFANTS UNDERGOING
MINOR SURGERY

PYLORIC STENOSIS

PEDIATRIC FLUID THERAPY IN THE
PERIOPERATIVE PERIOD

PEDIATRIC REGIONAL ANESTHESIA

Premature Infant

DEBORAH K. RASCH, M.D.

RAJAM S. RAMAMURTHY, M.D.

Premature and low-birth-weight infants (<2500 g at birth) encounter similar difficulties adapting to extrauterine life and present a distinct set of management problems for the anesthetist.[1]

A. Determine the estimated gestational age and associated disorders (hyaline membrane disease, apnea and bradycardia, hyperbilirubinemia, hypoglycemia, hypocalcemia, hemolysis from Rh or ABO incompatibility, and congenital anomalies). Hematocrit (Hct) should be >45%. Assess hydration and electrolytes. Review clinical evaluation with the neonatologist. If the infant has received supplemental oxygen (O_2), determine whether retinopathy of prematurity (ROP) has been diagnosed. Infants are not kept NPO for prolonged periods, usually 3 to 4 hours.

B. Some surgical procedures may be performed in the neonatal ICU. This practice reduces the risks of cooling and extubation associated with transport. Ensure adequate room, proper lighting, and access to patient. When a planned procedure is to be performed in the OR, accompany the infant en route to the OR, as well as on return to the ICU. Wash hands and follow all sterile precautions.

C. Use a transport isolette with stable temperature (37 to 38°C) and air/O_2 blender; monitor temperature, HR, and pulse oximetry (SpO_2); and bring resuscitation equipment. Calculate all drug dosages and fluid requirements in advance, and prepare labeled syringes. Use proper battery-operated pumps on IV and arterial lines and appropriate tubing. Use one line for drugs and another (with injection port beyond bubble filter) for fluids and blood. In general, choose 10% dextrose infusion. Call the elevator in advance. Ensure a warm environment (radiant warmer, warming mattress, forced air warmer, heat lamps). Set up a heater/humidifier in the anesthesia circuit and obtain other monitors and equipment of appropriate size. Certain procedures can be performed under regional anesthesia alone (herniorrhaphy, circumcision, or lower extremity procedures); this technique can reduce or eliminate the need for postoperative ventilation in premature infants with apnea or severe BPD.[2] Pretreatment with caffeine, 10 mg/kg, has been shown to reduce postoperative apnea and bradycardia in preterm infants undergoing general anesthesia.[3,4]

D. Except in very ill infants or those likely to have a full stomach, induce anesthesia prior to intubation to avoid hypertension (HTN), increased ICP, and the risk of intracranial hemorrhage. Possible agents include fentanyl 10 to 20 µg/kg intravenously, thiopental 4 to 6 mg/kg intravenously, and inhalational agents (sevoflurane, isoflurane) 0.3 to 0.75 MAC, with controlled ventilation. Administer muscle relaxant (pancuronium 0.1 mg/kg, vecuronium 0.1 mg/kg, or rocuronium 1 mg/kg.) Consider pretreatment with atropine, 0.1 mg, as a minimal vagolytic dose may be necessary if pancuronium is not used. Insert a 2.5- to 3.5- mm endotracheal tube (ETT). Secure the tube and periodically recheck bilateral breath sounds. Ventilate by hand initially to assess changing lung compliance and select an FiO_2 that maintains PaO_2 at 70 to 100 mm Hg. Use SaO_2 and $ETCO_2$ monitors for rapid feedback about oxygenation, ventilation, and adequacy of circulating blood volume. For improved correlation of $ETCO_2$ and $PaCO_2$, connect a surfactant adapter (Figure 1) to the ETT. Maintain PaO_2 at 70 to 100 mm Hg, $PaCO_2$ at 35 to 45 mm Hg, and pH at 7.3 to 7.45. A PaO_2 of 150 mm Hg for only 1 to 2 hours may cause ROP in infants <34 weeks gestational age. Consider blood volume to be 90 ml/kg in preterm and 85 ml/kg in term infants. Replace blood loss of >10%; treat lesser degrees of hypovolemia with plasma protein fraction, 5% albumin, or balanced salt solution, 10 ml/kg.

PREMATURE INFANT FOR SURGERY

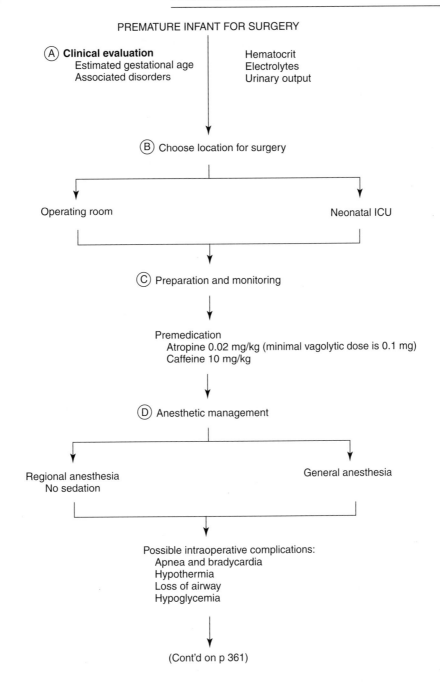

Ⓐ **Clinical evaluation**
  Estimated gestational age
  Associated disorders

Hematocrit
Electrolytes
Urinary output

Ⓑ Choose location for surgery

Operating room   Neonatal ICU

Ⓒ Preparation and monitoring

Premedication
  Atropine 0.02 mg/kg (minimal vagolytic dose is 0.1 mg)
  Caffeine 10 mg/kg

Ⓓ Anesthetic management

Regional anesthesia
No sedation   General anesthesia

Possible intraoperative complications:
  Apnea and bradycardia
  Hypothermia
  Loss of airway
  Hypoglycemia

(Cont'd on p 361)

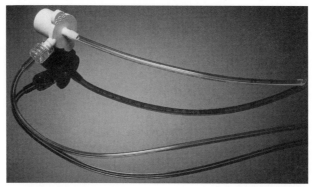

FIGURE 1 Surfactant adapter in the circuit helps measure a more accurate $ETCO_2$.

E. Airway reflexes are immature in the preterm infant and gastric emptying is delayed. Most premature infants require postoperative ventilation for several hours to days. Transport to the NICU with the tube in place. Extubation or mainstem intubation may occur easily. Request a chest x-ray (CXR) if the infant is to remain intubated to check for tube placement. The tip of the tube should be in the middle of the trachea, which is about the level of the clavicles. In the very low-birth weight infant the trachea is about 1.5 to 2 cm in length. Once the infant is stabilized and normothermia is present, reverse all muscle relaxants and observe carefully for apnea or respiratory distress if extubation is feasible. Suction the stomach before extubation to reduce gastric distention and risk of regurgitation and aspiration.

REFERENCES

1. Hillier SC, Krishna G, Brasoveanu E: Neonatal anesthesia, *Semin Pediatr Surg* 13 (3):142–151, 2004.
2. Craven PD, Badawi N, Henderson-Smart DJ, et al.: Regional (spinal, epidural, caudal) versus general anaesthesia in preterm infants undergoing inguinal herniorrhaphy in early infancy, *Cochrane Database Syst Rev* (3):CD003669, 2003.
3. Welborn LG, Greenspun JC: Anesthesia and apnea perioperative considerations in the former preterm infant, *Pediatr Clin North Am* 41 (1):181–198, 1994.
4. Henderson-Smart DJ, Steer P: Prophylactic caffeine to prevent postoperative apnea following general anesthesia in preterm infants, *Cochrane Database Syst Rev* (4):CD000048, 2001.

PREMATURE INFANT FOR SURGERY

(Cont'd from p 359)

Ⓔ Recovery

Uncomplicated recovery

Possible postoperative complications
Apnea and bradycardia
Hypothermia
Loss of airway
Barotrauma
Aspiration

Congenital Diaphragmatic Hernia

DEBORAH K. RASCH, M.D.

RAJAM S. RAMAMURTHY, M.D.

Congenital herniation of abdominal viscera through the diaphragm is associated with varying degrees of pulmonary hypoplasia, which determines the prognosis. The most common location is posterolateral on the left, but both sides may be affected. Elevated pulmonary vascular resistance (PVR) may result in persistent pulmonary hypertension of the newborn (PPHN), and perioperative mortality is high (33 to 66%).[1–3] In some centers, intrauterine surgery is performed on these patients.

A. In the past, congenital diaphragmatic hernia was considered a true surgical emergency. However, presently, infants are stabilized for at least 12 to 48 hours prior to surgical repair. Preoperative stabilization (often using extracorporeal membrane oxygenation [ECMO] and inhaled nitric oxide) has resulted in a lower mortality rate.[4–6] Prenatal diagnosis is increasingly common, but many diagnoses are postnatal, suggested by a scaphoid abdomen and bowel sounds heard in the chest. Respiratory distress may or may not be present. Chest radiography shows mediastinal shift and bowel in the chest (Figure 1). If preoperative ventilatory support is required, intubate the trachea (bag-and-mask ventilation distends the stomach, thus further compressing the ipsilateral hypoplastic lung) and insert a nasogastric (NG) tube to decompress the stomach. High airway pressure may cause pneumothorax on the unaffected side; the hypoplastic lung cannot be reinflated. Evaluate for associated anomalies (cardiovascular in 23% of patients and intestinal malrotation in 50% of patients).

B. Prepare anesthesia equipment and the OR with attention to neonatal considerations. Monitor SpO_2, ECG, temperature, BP, ABGs (right radial line for preductal samples), and $ETCO_2$. Insert a manometer in the anesthesia circuit and use a heater/humidifier for gases.

C. If the patient is not already intubated, preoxygenate and intubate awake. Anesthetize with small doses of fentanyl and paralyze with a nondepolarizing relaxant. Administer an FiO_2 of 1 and decrease gradually by 3 to 5% (a sudden drop may lead to pulmonary vasoconstriction). Check ABGs and acid-base status frequently. Avoid inhalational agents because of myocardial depression and enhancement of pulmonary shunting. Omit N_2O to avoid bowel distention. Ventilate by hand, maintaining airway pressure below 25 to 30 cm H_2O. A sudden deterioration may be a sign of pneumothorax on the normal side.

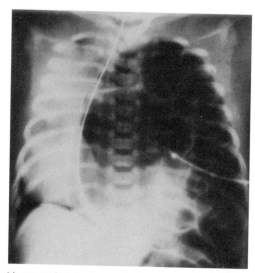

FIGURE 1 Chest x-ray (CXR) of an infant with congenital diaphragmatic hernia. Note the gas-filled bowel in the left hemithorax, with mediastinal shift.

Patient with CONGENITAL DIAPHRAGMATIC HERNIA

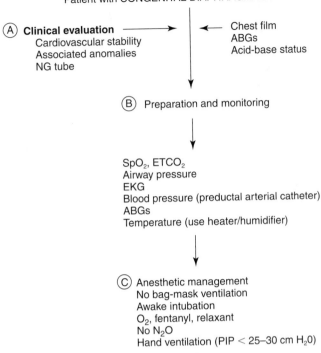

(A) **Clinical evaluation** ⟶ ⟵ Chest film
Cardiovascular stability   ABGs
Associated anomalies   Acid-base status
NG tube

(B) Preparation and monitoring

SpO_2, $ETCO_2$
Airway pressure
EKG
Blood pressure (preductal arterial catheter)
ABGs
Temperature (use heater/humidifier)

(C) Anesthetic management
No bag-mask ventilation
Awake intubation
O_2, fentanyl, relaxant
No N_2O
Hand ventilation (PIP < 25–30 cm H_2O)

(Cont'd on p 365)

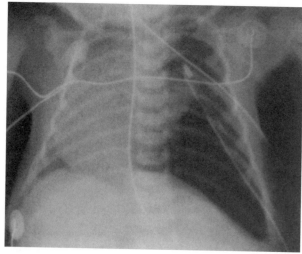

FIGURE 2 CXR taken after repair of congenital diaphragmatic hernia. Despite the presence of a functioning chest tube, the left lung is hypoplastic and thus will not expand to fill the hemithorax.

D. The abdominal cavity is underdeveloped, and primary closure may result in increased intraabdominal pressure, cephalad displacement of the diaphragm, diminished FRC, and vena caval compression. Hypotension may result from impaired venous return as well as high PVR, ventricular failure, and low cardiac output (CO). Third-space loss and blood loss are usually minimal, and dopamine support is preferable to administration of large volumes of fluid or colloid. Occasionally, primary abdominal closure is impossible. Under these circumstances a Silastic patch is used to create a ventral hernia, similar to an omphalocele repair. Closure is planned for a few days later.

E. A honeymoon period, when oxygenation is good, may follow surgery, but deterioration may be caused by increasing right-to-left shunts via fetal channels.[1] Pulmonary vasodilation with IV agents (milrinone, sodium nitroprusside, nitroglycerin) has been used with some success, but inhaled nitric oxide (NO) is the preferred pulmonary dilator in these patients. With NO, systemic vascular resistance (SVR) is preserved, resulting in less R to L shunting at the cardiac level. Prediction of survival has been based on A-aO$_2$ gradients. The hypoplastic lung may be small (Figure 2). Plan to continue ventilator, relaxant, and vasopressor support postoperatively.

REFERENCES

1. Leveque C, Hamza J, Berg AE, et al.: Successful repair of a severe left congenital diaphragmatic hernia during continuous inhalation of nitric oxide, *Anesthesiology* 80:1171–1175, 1994.
2. Rasch DK, Ramamurthy RS, Gurkowski MA: Newborn emergencies. In: Rasch DK, Webster DE, editors: *Clinical manual of pediatric anesthesia*, New York, 1993, McGraw-Hill.
3. Hall SC: Anesthesia for the neonate. In: Badgwell JM, editor: *Clinical pediatric anesthesia*, Philadelphia, 1997, Lippincott-Raven.
4. Downard CD, Jaksic T, Garza JJ, et al.: Analysis of an improved survival rate for congenital diaphragmatic hernia, *J Pediatr Surg* 38 (5):729–732, 2002.
5. Kinsella JP, Parker TA, Ivy DD, et al.: Noninvasive delivery of inhaled nitric oxide therapy for late pulmonary hypertension in newborn infants with congenital diaphragmatic hernia, *J Pediatr* 142 (4):397–401, 2003.
6. Thibeault DW, Olsen SL, Truog WE, et al.: Pre-ECMO predictors of nonsurvival in congenital diaphragmatic hernia, *J Perinatol* 22 (8):682–683, 2002.

Patient with CONGENITAL DIAPHRAGMATIC HERNIA
(Cont'd from p 363)

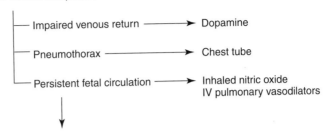

Ⓓ Potential complications

      ── Impaired venous return ────────► Dopamine

      ── Pneumothorax ────────► Chest tube

      ── Persistent fetal circulation ────────► Inhaled nitric oxide
                                            IV pulmonary vasodilators

Ⓔ Postoperative care
    Ventilator
    Muscle relaxants
    Dopamine
    Pulmonary vasodilators (inhaled NO)
    ECMO

Omphalocele and Gastroschisis

RAJAM S. RAMAMURTHY, M.D.

DEBORAH K. RASCH, M.D.

Omphalocele (a hernia through the umbilicus) and gastroschisis (eventration of abdominal contents caused by a defect of the anterior abdominal wall) are different disorders with similar anesthetic considerations. Other congenital anomalies occur commonly (76%) with omphalocele (Table 1), and a mortality rate of 30% is largely a result of cardiac anomalies and prematurity.[1-3] Gastroschisis is rarely associated with other anomalies, but more infants (58%) are premature and a similar mortality rate is caused by intestinal (malrotation and atresias) and wound complications.[1] The size of the hernia and intactness of peritoneal covering determine the urgency of surgical correction.

A. Determine gestational age and the presence of associated anomalies. In infants with gastroschisis and ruptured omphalocele, there is great loss of protein and third-space fluid, which leads to hemoconcentration, hypoperfusion, oliguria, and metabolic acidosis. Maintain normal perfusion to vital organs by monitoring BP and urinary output and by replacing volume loss (bolus 10 ml/kg plasma substitutes). Significant evaporative heat and fluid loss occurs from exposed bowel.[4,5] Cover the exposed intestine with a sterile gauze and keep moist with warm sterile saline. Place the infant in a thermoneutral environment. Decompress the stomach with a nasogastric (NG) tube, sometimes with low suction.

B. Maintain body temperature and continue fluid resuscitation. Set up warming lights, a heating blanket, and an airway heater/humidifier. Use a manometer in the breathing circuit to monitor inflation pressure. Use sterile precautions and premature infant considerations when appropriate. Monitor temperature, pulse oximetry, $ETCO_2$, arterial BP, ABGs, and electrolyte status. Aspirate the NG tube frequently.

C. The stable infant with a small hernia that is covered with peritoneum requires less aggressive surgical management and monitoring. If there is no tension on the abdominal wall with closure of the defect and if muscle relaxants (MRs) are not required to facilitate return of the contents of the abdominal cavity, significant postoperative respiratory difficulty is unlikely and extubation in the OR or after transport to the neonatal ICU is feasible. Unstable infants with large hernias or exposed abdominal contents require emergency repair.[6] Intubate the patient awake after volume replacement has been instituted, and titrate small doses of narcotics (fentanyl, 10 to 20 µg/kg) and MRs. Avoid N_2O to prevent bowel distention. Work closely with the surgeon to determine whether primary closure can be accomplished. Closure with maximal relaxation may result in excessive intraabdominal pressure, obstruction of the inferior vena cava, lowered cardiac output (CO), hypotension, and elevation of the diaphragm with respiratory embarrassment. Monitor airway pressure to detect impaired compliance. The alternative to primary closure is construction of a Silastic silo that encloses the viscera. The size of the silo is gradually reduced as the abdominal cavity enlarges.

D. Postoperatively, gradually withdraw MRs and ventilatory support. This may take a few days.

TABLE 1
Congenital Anomalies Associated with Omphalocele

Congenital heart disease
Wilms' tumor
Beckwith-Wiedemann syndrome
Intestinal malrotation
Intestinal atresia

REFERENCES

1. Rasch DK, Ramamurthy RS, Gurkowski MA: Newborn emergencies. In: Rasch DK, Webster DE, editors: *Clinical manual of pediatric anesthesia*, New York, 1993, McGraw-Hill.
2. Gibbin C, Touch S, Broth RE, et al.: Abdominal wall defects and congenital heart disease, *Ultrasound Obstet Gynecol* 21 (4): 334–337, 2003.
3. Salihu HM, Boos R, Schmidt W: Omphalocele and gastroschisis, *J Obstet Gynaecol* 22 (5):489–492, 2002.
4. Philippart AI, Canty TG, Filler RM: Acute fluid volume requirements in infants with anterior abdominal wall defects, *J Pediatr Surg* 7:553–558, 1972.
5. Amata AO: Anaesthetic considerations in exomphalos repair: a report of two cases, *Afr J Med Med Sci* 24 (4):403–406, 1995.
6. Towne BH, Peters G, Chang JH: The problem of "giant" omphalocele, *J Pediatr Surg* 15:543–548, 1980.

Neonate with OMPHALOCELE OR GATROSCHISIS

(A) **Clinical evaluation** ———→   ←— CBC, platelet count
　　Associated anomalies   Serum albumin, colloid oncotic pressure
　　Gestational age   Blood glucose

(B) Preparation and monitoring
　　Administer fluid, colloid

(C) Assess stability of infant
　　and size of hernia

Stable infant,   Unstable infant,
small hernia   large hernia

Awake intubation   Awake intubation
or RSI   Narcotics/relaxants

Neonatal precautions   Fluids, colloid

Abdomen closed   Abdomen closed
                                                or silo created

No tension   Tension

Extubate

**Transport to neonatal ICU
intubated and paralyzed**

(D) Postoperative management

　── Wean from relaxants and
　　ventilator over 24–48 hr

　── Daily cinching or silo
　　(no anesthesia)

Uncomplicated   Potential complications
recovery   Sepsis/wound complications
                              Complications of prematurity
                              Barotrauma
                              Death (30%)

Tracheoesophageal Fistula (TEF)

DEBORAH K. RASCH, M.D.

RAJAM S. RAMAMURTHY, M.D.

Tracheoesophageal fistula (TEF) is a congenital malformation of the distal trachea and esophagus that occurs in 1 per 3,000 live births. Approximately 22% of these infants have a major cardiovascular anomaly, and 30 to 40% are premature. The most common defect is a blind upper esophageal pouch and a fistulous tract between the lower esophagus and trachea (Figure 1). At birth the infant has copious frothy secretions in the mouth. Bag-and-mask ventilation will distend the stomach. Diagnosis is suggested by failure of catheter passage to the stomach, the presence of coughing, and cyanosis during feeding and is confirmed by x-ray (radiopaque catheter is in a blind pouch approximately 10 cm from the gum line). Aspiration causes pulmonary compromise.[1-5]

A. Determine gestational age and presence of other congenital anomalies, such as vertebral defects, imperforate anus, TEF, and radial and renal dysplasia (VATER association). If there is a question of cyanotic congenital heart disease (CHD), cardiac catheterization or echocardiography (echo) precedes surgical repair. Evaluate x-rays for abdominal air (confirms a fistula between trachea and lower esophagus) and pulmonary infiltrates.

B. Rarely, emergency gastrostomy may be performed under local anesthesia in the neonatal ICU to relieve gastric distention and respiratory compromise and allow cardiopulmonary stabilization before definitive repair at 48 to 72 hours. The blind upper pouch is suctioned continuously. Prepare for management of the premature infant, and monitor arterial BP, pulse oximetry, and urinary output. Auscultate heart and breath sounds with a precordial stethoscope (not esophageal) positioned in the left axilla.

C. For type I TEF (no communication between esophagus and trachea) induce anesthesia with routine neonatal technique; all other types of TEF require awake intubation after atropine and preoxygenation. The fistula is usually in the posterior wall of the trachea, close to the carina. Achieve satisfactory endotracheal tube (ETT) position (avoid right endobronchial intubation and excessive distention of the stomach). The right lung will be compressed during right thoracotomy for TEF repair. If right endobronchial intubation occurs, hypoxemia develops rapidly.

D. Try to prevent gastric distention intraoperatively to avoid gastric rupture, ventilatory impedance, and cardiac arrest. Gastrostomy may be needed if distention is unavoidable. Have the patient breathe spontaneously or assist ventilation by hand to assess changing compliance. Do not give muscle relaxants until the chest is opened, and if possible, until the fistula is ligated. Watch for obstruction of the ETT (secretions, surgical manipulation).

E. Plan postoperative ventilation for sick infants. Bloody tracheal secretions continue to be a problem during the postoperative period. Avoid esophageal suction and extension of the neck to protect the surgical repair. Tracheomalacia, tracheal compression, or recurrent laryngeal nerve injury may cause upper airway obstruction immediately after extubation.

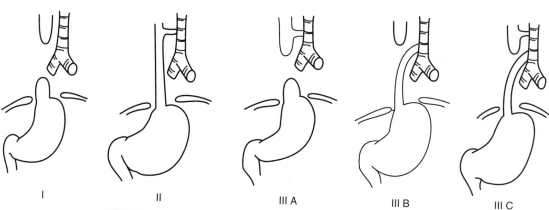

FIGURE 1 Types of tracheoesophageal fistula. Type IIIB is most common.

| I | II | III A | III B | III C |

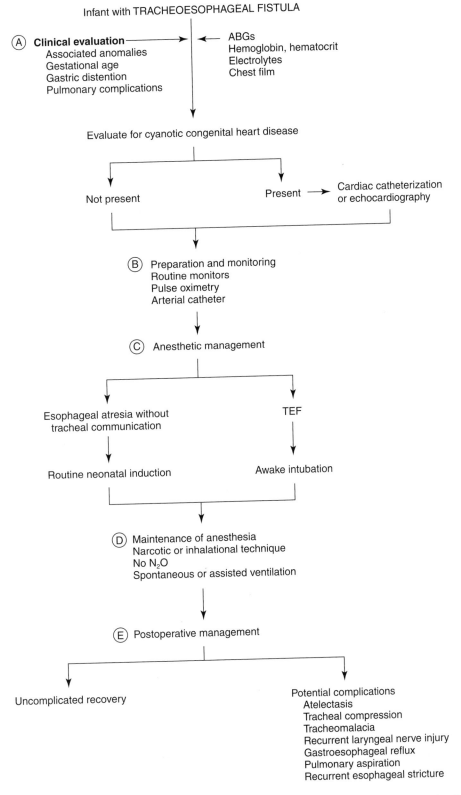

Infant with TRACHEOESOPHAGEAL FISTULA

Ⓐ **Clinical evaluation**
Associated anomalies
Gestational age
Gastric distention
Pulmonary complications

ABGs
Hemoglobin, hematocrit
Electrolytes
Chest film

Evaluate for cyanotic congenital heart disease

Not present

Present → Cardiac catheterization or echocardiography

Ⓑ Preparation and monitoring
Routine monitors
Pulse oximetry
Arterial catheter

Ⓒ Anesthetic management

Esophageal atresia without tracheal communication

TEF

Routine neonatal induction

Awake intubation

Ⓓ Maintenance of anesthesia
Narcotic or inhalational technique
No N_2O
Spontaneous or assisted ventilation

Ⓔ Postoperative management

Uncomplicated recovery

Potential complications
Atelectasis
Tracheal compression
Tracheomalacia
Recurrent laryngeal nerve injury
Gastroesophageal reflux
Pulmonary aspiration
Recurrent esophageal stricture

REFERENCES

1. Diaz LK, Akpek EA, Dinavahi R, et al.: Tracheoesophageal fistula and associated congenital heart disease: implications for anesthetic management and survival, *Paediatr Anaesth* 15:862–869, 2005.
2. Hillier SC, Krishna G, Brasoveanu E: Neonatal anesthesia, *Semin Pediatr Surg* 13 (3):142–151, 2004.
3. Orford J, Cass DT, Glasson MJ: Advances in the treatment of oesophageal atresia over three decades: the 1970s and the 1990s, *Pediatr Surg Int* 20:402–407, 2004.
4. Tercan E, Sungun MB, Boyaci A, et al.: One-lung ventilation of a preterm newborn during esophageal atresia and tracheoesophageal fistula repair, *Acta Anaesthesiol Scand* 46:332–333, 2002.
5. Spoon JM: VATER Association, *Neonatal Netw* 22 (3):71–75, 2003.

Necrotizing Enterocolitis (NEC)

DEBORAH K. RASCH, M.D.

RAJAM S. RAMAMURTHY, M.D.

Necrotizing enterocolitis (NEC) is thought to be the pathological response of the immature intestine to hypoxic, ischemic injury, probably caused by asphyxia of the fetus or newborn baby. Bacterial invasion through damaged mucosa and generalized sepsis occurs in 50% of infants with NEC.[1] Patients at greatest risk are premature infants ≤32 weeks' gestation and weighing <1500 g.[1,2] Other risk factors are hyaline membrane disease, hypotension, patent ductus arteriosus (PDA), hypothermia, umbilical-vessel catheterization, exchange transfusion, and polycythemia.[1,3] Early signs are increased gastric residuals, abdominal distention, vomiting of feedings, ileus, and bloody stools, progressing to intestinal perforation, peritonitis, and septic shock. Pneumatosis intestinalis and intrahepatic venous gas on x-ray examination confirm NEC. Presence of gastric pneumatosis, although rare, signifies fulminant NEC.[4]

A. Evaluate as for the premature infant and assess hydration (peripheral perfusion, urinary output, vital signs, acid-base status). Give volume expanders (fluid, colloid, or blood) to correct hypovolemia caused by endotoxic shock and intraabdominal third-space fluid losses. Weight is not a reliable measure of volume status. Correct metabolic acidosis to pH > 7.20. Consider vasopressor support with dopamine. Evaluate coagulation studies, and give platelet concentrate preoperatively to thrombocytopenic, bleeding infants. Apnea may be caused by hypoxia, shock, or abdominal distention[1] and may necessitate preoperative intubation. Review chest films, ABGs or capillary blood gases (CBGs), and chest x-ray (CXR) results. Medical management includes nasogastric (NG) suction, IV fluids, and antibiotics. Surgery is reserved for infants with bowel perforation or progressive acidosis;[2] these patients may be gravely ill.

B. In addition to usual preparation for a neonate, calculate resuscitation drug doses (including dextrose 25%, calcium chloride, or sodium bicarbonate) preoperatively. Have a dopamine infusion available. Monitor direct BP, glucose, and ABGs. Umbilical arterial lines are usually removed in infants suspected to have NEC; thus consider inserting a peripheral arterial catheter. Set up blood warmers and a heater or humidifier, and have blood available in the OR. Have a suction trap inserted in the surgical suction equipment and arrange for sponges to be weighed.

C. Intubate the patient awake because of debilitated status, borderline hemodynamics, and the potential for regurgitation and aspiration. Rarely, RSI may be indicated. Rapid fluid resuscitation is often necessary as the abdomen is opened, so prepare at least two functioning IV lines before the skin is incised.

D. Induction and maintenance of GETA is with ketamine (1 to 2 mg/kg intravenously) in the hypovolemic infant or fentanyl (10 to 20 μg/kg) if the infant is stable. Oxygen and air are mixed to produce PaO_2 of 80 to 100 mm Hg. Avoid N_2O because it may increase the size of gas bubbles in the bowel wall and hepatic portal system. Use vecuronium or pancuronium, 0.1 to 0.2 mg/kg, for surgical relaxation. Control ventilation by hand to assess changing compliance. If pressor support is needed, give dopamine (start at 5 μg/kg/min and titrate to effect). For each one third of blood volume replaced, consider giving calcium chloride, 20 mg/kg intravenously, to prevent hypotension and dysrhythmias associated with citrate (chelation of calcium) and to improve myocardial contractility. Intraoperative consultation with the neonatologist may be helpful for management of fluids, electrolytes, and acid-base status.

E. Keep patients intubated and maintain mechanical ventilation. Postoperative abdominal distention, massive fluid resuscitation, and persistent acidosis may cause respiratory compromise for several days.

REFERENCES

1. Kliegman RM, Fanaroff AA: Necrotizing enterocolitis, N Engl J Med 310:1093–1103, 1984.
2. Rasch DK, Ramamurthy RS, Gurkowski MA: Newborn emergencies. In: Rasch DK, Webster DE, editors: Clinical manual of pediatric anesthesia, New York, 1993 McGraw-Hill.
3. Noerr B: Current controversies in the understanding of necrotizing enterocolitis. Part 1, Adv Neonatal Care 3 (3):107–120, 2003.
4. Travadi JN, Patole SK, Simmer K: Gastric pneumatosis in neonates: revisited, J Paediatr Child Health 39 (7):560–562, 2003.

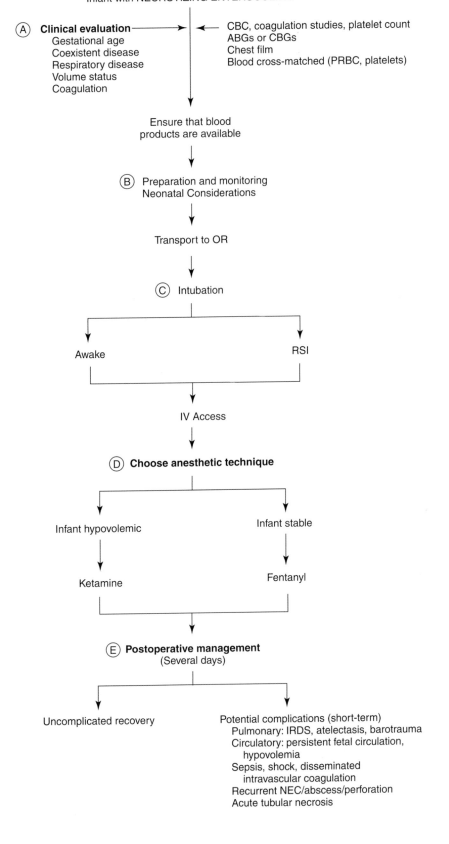

Infant with NECROTIZING ENTEROCOLITIS

Ⓐ **Clinical evaluation** ────────→   ←──── CBC, coagulation studies, platelet count
    Gestational age   ABGs or CBGs
    Coexistent disease   Chest film
    Respiratory disease   Blood cross-matched (PRBC, platelets)
    Volume status
    Coagulation

Ensure that blood
products are available

Ⓑ Preparation and monitoring
    Neonatal Considerations

Transport to OR

Ⓒ Intubation

Awake   RSI

IV Access

Ⓓ **Choose anesthetic technique**

Infant hypovolemic   Infant stable

Ketamine   Fentanyl

Ⓔ **Postoperative management**
    (Several days)

Uncomplicated recovery   Potential complications (short-term)
    Pulmonary: IRDS, atelectasis, barotrauma
    Circulatory: persistent fetal circulation,
      hypovolemia
    Sepsis, shock, disseminated
      intravascular coagulation
    Recurrent NEC/abscess/perforation
    Acute tubular necrosis

Former Preterm Infants Undergoing Minor Surgery

LEILA G. WELBORN, M.D.

Premature infants represent a significant operative risk because they have many immature organ systems. The incidence of apneic episodes is inversely related to postconceptual age and is influenced by patient, surgical, and anesthetic factors. Although some continue to be extremely ill and require multiple emergency operations to survive, most are relatively well and require minor surgical procedures (e.g., herniorrhaphy) than can be scheduled electively. Former preterm infants are prone to develop apnea or bradycardia after general anesthesia.

A. In evaluating infants with a history of prematurity, beware that preterm infants of <44 to 46 weeks are at high risk for developing postoperative ventilatory dysfunction.[1] Apnea may be related to many causes; if it occurs after an operative procedure, however, it is most likely related to metabolic derangements, pharmacological effects, or CNS immaturity. Metabolic causes of apnea such as hypothermia, hypoglycemia, hypocalcemia, acidosis, and hypoxemia can be avoided by meticulous attention to details of the anesthetic management of neonates. If possible, delay nonessential surgery until the infant is beyond 44 to 46 weeks' postconceptual age and not anemic. Review records for oxygen (O_2) therapy, intubation, residual lung damage, neurological damage (intraventricular hemorrhage), cardiac or metabolic derangements, and growth and development.

B. In the OR, monitor HR, heart sounds, BP, ECG, temperature, O_2 saturation, and end-tidal carbon dioxide (CO_2).

C. Choose an anesthetic technique. Supplement GETA with neuromuscular blockade and controlled ventilation. Consider spinal or caudal anesthesia without sedation, which may decrease the incidence of postoperative apnea compared with general inhalational anesthesia. Avoid using opioids and barbiturates. Most anesthetic drugs affect the respiratory system, directly or indirectly. Most inhalational agents, narcotics, and sedatives probably produce respiratory depression in neonates who have an immature respiratory center. Although the cause of apnea after anesthesia is unknown, studies have speculated that the respiratory center in preterm infants is easily inhibited by trace concentrations of anesthetics, endorphins, or hypoxemia; central respiratory stimulants, such as methylxanthines, may prevent apnea when given postoperatively. The perioperative use of IV caffeine (10 mg/kg) as a respiratory stimulant has proved effective in the management of neonatal apnea and postoperative ventilatory dysfunction in otherwise healthy former preterm infants.[2] Spinal anesthesia without ketamine sedation in former premature infants was not associated with postoperative apnea, whereas infants receiving either general anesthesia or spinal anesthesia with ketamine sedation experienced a significant incidence of postoperative apnea.[3] Other studies have not shown a clear relationship between anesthetic approach and postoperative apnea.[4] Anemia in former preterm infants can be associated with an increased incidence of postoperative apnea. Anemic infants have a high percentage of fetal hemoglobin and low 2,3 diphosphoglycerate (2,3-DPG) levels; the O_2 dissociation curve shifts to the left and thereby decreases O_2 availability to the tissues.[5] If surgery cannot be deferred long enough to allow for correction of anemia, make plans for postoperative overnight hospital admission to allow close observation and monitoring.

D. Postoperatively, plan for at least 12 hours of monitoring (for apnea and bradycardia) for all infants with risk of postoperative apnea following all anesthetics. Infants with greater degrees of preoperative dysfunction need correspondingly longer periods of postoperative observation.

REFERENCES

1. Welborn LG, Ramirez N, Oh TH, et al.: Postanesthetic apnea and periodic breathing in infants, *Anesthesiology* 65:658–661, 1986.
2. McNamara DG, Nixon GM, Anderson BJ: Methylxanthines for the treatment of apnea associated with bronchiolitis and anesthesia, *Paediatr Anaesth* 14 (7):541–550, 2004.
3. Welborn LG, Rice LJ, Hannallah RS, et al.: Postoperative apnea in former preterm infants: prospective comparison of spinal and general anesthesia, *Anesthesiology* 72:838–842, 1990.
4. Craven PD, Badawi N, Henderson-Smart DJ, et al.: Regional (spinal, epidural, caudal) versus general anaesthesia in preterm infants undergoing inguinal herniorrhaphy in early infancy, *Cochrane Database Syst Rev* (3):CD003669, 2003.
5. Cote CJ, Zaslavsky A, Downes JJ, et al.: Postoperative apnea in former preterm infants after inguinal herniorrhaphy. A combined analysis, *Anesthesiology* 82 (4):809–822, 1995.

FORMER PRETERM INFANT FOR MINOR SURGERY

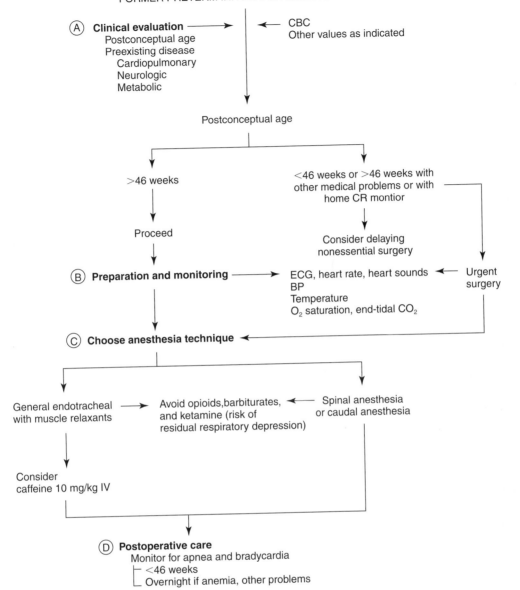

(A) **Clinical evaluation** → ← CBC
    Postconceptual age   Other values as indicated
    Preexisting disease
      Cardiopulmonary
      Neurologic
      Metabolic

Postconceptual age

>46 weeks   <46 weeks or >46 weeks with
                   other medical problems or with
                     home CR montior

Proceed   Consider delaying
                    nonessential surgery

(B) **Preparation and monitoring** → ECG, heart rate, heart sounds ← Urgent
                     BP   surgery
                     Temperature
                     O_2 saturation, end-tidal CO_2

(C) **Choose anesthesia technique** ←

General endotracheal → Avoid opioids,barbiturates, ← Spinal anesthesia
with muscle relaxants   and ketamine (risk of   or caudal anesthesia
                  residual respiratory depression)

Consider
caffeine 10 mg/kg IV

(D) **Postoperative care**
    Monitor for apnea and bradycardia
      ⊢ <46 weeks
      ∟ Overnight if anemia, other problems

Pyloric Stenosis

DEBORAH K. RASCH, M.D.

Congenital hypertrophic pyloric stenosis (CHPS) is a common GI malformation that classically occurs in the first male offspring of a family. Recently, postnatal administration of macrolide antibiotic (i.e., erythromycin derivatives to breastfeeding mothers) has been shown to increase the risk of CHPS.[1] Infants present at 4 to 6 weeks of age with projectile, nonbile-stained vomiting, visible gastric peristalsis after a feeding, and often a palpable, olive-shaped abdominal mass that corresponds to hypertrophied pyloric muscle. Diagnosis depends on the presence of an abdominal mass and characteristic history. In patients in whom the "olive" cannot be palpated, diagnosis is confirmed by gastric dilation on x-ray, abdominal ultrasound demonstrating an enlarged pylorus, or barium contrast studies that show a narrow, elongated pyloric sphincter. Severe dehydration and electrolyte imbalance must be corrected before surgery is performed.[3] CHPS is a medical, not surgical, emergency.[1–3]

A. Assess hydration by physical examination (e.g., skin turgor, orbits, mucous membrane moisture, warmth of extremities, pulses); laboratory values (blood urea nitrogen [BUN] ≤ 10, creatinine [Cr] ≤ 0.8); and vital signs, including weight (the infant should show weight gain after admission to the hospital as an indication of rehydration) and urinary output (at least 1 ml/kg/hr).

B. Correct hypokalemic, hypochloremic metabolic alkalosis which is common in CHPS. Administer IV 0.45% sodium chloride (NaCl) or 0.9% NaCl with potassium chloride (KCl) added. (Metabolic alkalosis will be corrected by the kidneys after adequate chloride (Cl^-) and potassium (K) supplementation.) Serum HCO_3 should be ≤30 prior to surgery.

C. Unlike normal infants of the same age who have rapid gastric emptying, these infants retain feedings for 24 hours or more. Barium contrast poses an additional risk if perioperative aspiration of gastric contents occurs. Treat the infant with continuous gastric suction before anesthesia while other parameters are being corrected.

D. Preparation for pyloromyotomy typically takes a minimum of 4 to 8 hours of IV hydration. Severely dehydrated, malnourished infants may require 3 to 4 days to safely restore electrolytes, fluids, proteins, and blood.

E. Warm the OR, humidify all gases, ensure the availability of pediatric airway and suction equipment, and have a functioning IV line. Place the infant in the left lateral decubitus position and aspirate the stomach with a soft catheter, even if the infant received previous gastric suction. Preoxygenate with 100% oxygen (O_2) by face mask with the infant in the supine position.

F. Depending on the skill of the anesthetist and the physical condition of the infant, perform either awake intubation or RSI using cricoid pressure with thiopental 5 TO 6 mg/kg, or etomidate 0.3 mg/kg; atropine 0.02 mg/kg; and succinylcholine (SCC) 2 mg/kg IV.[4] Etomidate may be preferred over thiopental due to its shorter half-life; debilitated infants do not metabolize barbiturates normally and sedative effects may last 30 to 60 minutes after a single induction dose. Avoid hyperventilation; maintain end-tidal carbon dioxide (CO_2) in the 40 to 50 mm Hg range to prevent worsening of CNS alkalosis and postoperative respiratory depression.

G. Maintain the anesthetic with an inhalational agent. Muscle relaxant may facilitate surgical access. Coughing or straining by the infant may result in surgical perforation of the mucosa. Regional anesthesia has been suggested as an alternative to general anesthesia, but this is reserved for infants with other congenital or acquired conditions that increase the risk of general anesthesia.[5] Intraoperative transfusion of blood products is rarely indicated because blood loss is usually insignificant.

REFERENCES

1. Sorensen HT, Skriver MV, Pederson L, et al.: Risk of infantile hypertrophic pyloric stenosis after maternal postnatal use of macrolides, *Scand J Infect Dis* 35 (2):104–106, 2003.
2. Bissonnette B, Sullivan PJ: Pyloric stenosis, *Can J Anaesth* 38:668–676, 1991.
3. Cook-Sather SD, Tulloch HV, Liacouras CA, et al.: Gastric fluid volume in infants for pyloromyotomy, *Can J Anaesth* 44:278–283, 1997.
4. Cook-Sather SD, Tulloch HV, Cnaan A, et al.: A comparison of awake versus paralyzed tracheal intubation for infants with pyloric stenosis, *Anesth Analg* 86:945–951, 1998.
5. Somri M, Gaitini LA, Vaida SJ, et al.: The effectiveness and safety of spinal anaesthesia in the pyloromyotomy procedure, *Paediatr Anaesth* 13 (1):32–37, 2003.

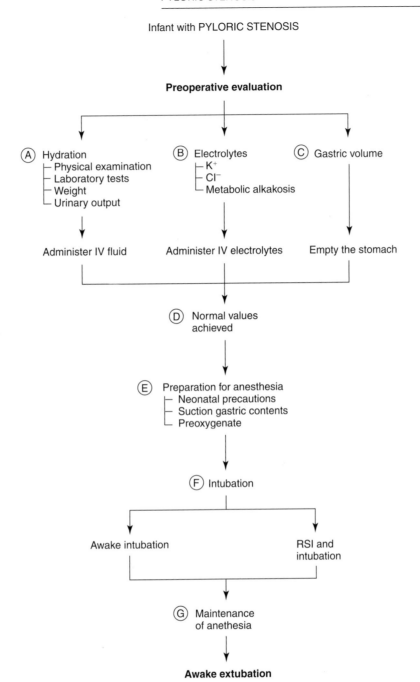

Infant with PYLORIC STENOSIS

Preoperative evaluation

(A) Hydration
— Physical examination
— Laboratory tests
— Weight
— Urinary output

(B) Electrolytes
— K⁺
— Cl⁻
— Metabolic alkakosis

(C) Gastric volume

Administer IV fluid

Administer IV electrolytes

Empty the stomach

(D) Normal values achieved

(E) Preparation for anesthesia
— Neonatal precautions
— Suction gastric contents
— Preoxygenate

(F) Intubation

Awake intubation

RSI and intubation

(G) Maintenance of anethesia

Awake extubation

Pediatric Fluid Therapy in the Perioperative Period

LEILA G. WELBORN, M.D.

A thorough knowledge of fluid and electrolyte therapy is necessary for adequate perioperative care of children. The exact fluid regimen depends on the patient's age, preoperative state of health, hydration, fluid electrolyte balance, and surgical procedure. Infants and small children are particularly at risk from alterations in fluid balance secondary to deprivation of fluid intake. Neonates have certain unique physiological features; many organ systems undergo maturation after birth. Renal function, although immature at birth, matures rapidly. Full function is reached by 1 year of age. A major goal of fluid therapy is to provide the kidney with a volume of fluid sufficient to allow excretion of the solute load at a urine concentration that will not tax the kidney's diluting or concentrating ability. The glomerular filtration rate (GFR) of newborns is only 25% that of older children and many of the tubular transport systems are not fully functional. Neonates' kidneys are less able to concentrate urine and have limited ability to conserve or excrete sodium. However, recent evidence indicates that the young kidney is able to increase its clearance of free water when faced with an acute fluid load. Compared with adults, infants have a large body surface area relative to body weight. Therefore, even without abnormal losses, they have a higher rate of water exchange relative to total body water. Dehydration is likely if fluid intake is curtailed or if excessive losses occur.

A. Perform a preoperative evaluation. Pay special attention to cardiovascular and renal status and state of hydration. Tachycardia or hypotension may signify hypovolemia, whereas pulmonary edema in a normal healthy child may indicate fluid overload. Decreased urinary output may be caused by renal failure or cardiovascular dysfunction, but in a normal child generally indicates abnormalities of fluid balance.

B. Correct anemia if possible before administering anesthesia. Neonates requiring surgery usually have life-threatening disorders and are likely to have abnormal fluid and electrolyte imbalances. Correct these abnormalities whenever possible before the patient is brought to the OR. A trend toward shorter and more reasonable periods of fasting has developed in recent years.[1,2] Current recommendations are an NPO period prior to induction of 8 hours for solids and 3 to 4 hours for clear liquids.

C. Intraoperative fluid therapy may involve initiation of fluid management or may be a continuation of ongoing fluid therapy. It can be as simple as replacing the deficits from the preoperative NPO status and providing maintenance fluids or as complex as correcting preoperative abnormal deficits, intraoperative translocated fluids, and variable blood loss in addition to providing maintenance fluids. Assuming that a healthy child is in water and electrolyte balance at the time oral feedings are discontinued, estimate the fluid deficit at the time of induction by multiplying the child's hourly maintenance fluid requirement by the number of hours since the last feeding. Replace this deficit by giving half of the calculated volume during the first hour of anesthesia and the other half over the next 1 to 2 hours, in addition to intraoperative maintenance fluids. Determine the hourly maintenance rate (ml/hr) of fluids to be infused during surgery on the basis of body weight:

$$\leq 10 \text{ kg} = \text{weight} \times 4;$$
$$11\text{--}20 \text{ kg} = 20 + \text{weight} \times 2;$$
$$> 20 \text{ kg} = \text{weight} + 40$$

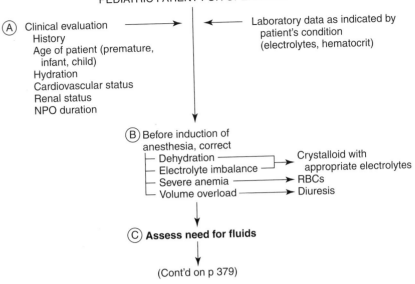

PEDIATRIC PATIENT FOR OPERATION

(A) Clinical evaluation
   History
   Age of patient (premature,
      infant, child)
   Hydration
   Cardiovascular status
   Renal status
   NPO duration

Laboratory data as indicated by
   patient's condition
   (electrolytes, hematocrit)

(B) Before induction of
   anesthesia, correct
   — Dehydration ⎫
   — Electrolyte imbalance ⎭ → Crystalloid with
                                 appropriate electrolytes
   — Severe anemia ——→ RBCs
   — Volume overload ——→ Diuresis

(C) **Assess need for fluids**

(Cont'd on p 379)

D. When planning intraoperative glucose administration, consider newborns and premature infants as separate groups. Assume that all such patients are hypoglycemic until proven otherwise. Replacement fluid should approximate the composition of the fluid lost, requiring administration of either normal saline or a balanced salt solution (e.g., lactated Ringers [LR]). The literature gives conflicting data about the intraoperative use of glucose. Clinical signs of hypoglycemia in the perioperative period may not be observed (masked by preanesthetic medication or general anesthesia) or may be misinterpreted (sympathetic nervous system hyperactivity erroneously ascribed to anxiety). Most authors recommend the routine use of solutions containing glucose during surgery. To decide what concentration of glucose, if any, to use for routine intraoperative IV administration in pediatric patients, weigh the risks of hypoglycemia (blood glucose [BG] <50 mg/dl^{-1}) versus hyperglycemia (BG >200 mg/dl^{-1}) at the infusion rates selected. There are two known adverse effects of intraoperative hyperglycemia: an osmotic diuresis and the potential for an adverse neurological outcome should cerebral ischemia occur.[3] Neurological damage is known to occur with hypoglycemia in children, and many of the signs of hypoglycemia are masked by general anesthesia. Asymptomatic hypoglycemia is a rare but ever-present possibility in healthy children with prolonged fasting before anesthesia. Contrary to accepted opinion, a stress-induced intraoperative BG increase does not occur in all patients. If a solution with no glucose is used for intraoperative infusion, monitor intraoperative BG. Administration of solutions containing 5% dextrose can result in intraoperative hyperglycemia.[4] Therefore, use a less concentrated glucose solution (e.g., 2.5% dextrose in LR) at recommended infusion rates to provide adequate glucose for healthy children (300 mg/kg/hr) and adequate volume replacement, while avoiding hyperglycemia and hypoglycemia.[5] Because 2.5% dextrose in LR is not commercially available, it must be prepared by the individual practitioner using 50% dextrose solution. Neither giving nor avoiding solutions containing glucose produces a predictable BG level as a result of the interplay between homeostatic mechanisms due to the hormonal responses to surgical stress and the availability of substrate for gluconeogenesis. When tight control of glucose is required, perform serial BG measurements and adjust the amount of dextrose given accordingly.

Risk factors for preoperative fasting hypoglycemia include prematurity (infants), discontinuation or reduction of preoperative dextrose infusion, myopathies, glycogen storage diseases, hyperinsulinemic conditions (infants of diabetic mothers, insulinomas), malnourishment (including small-for-gestational age neonates), and abnormalities of lipolysis or amino acid metabolism. Risk factors for intraoperative hypoglycemia when fluids that do not contain dextrose are given include long surgical procedures, pediatric patients, discontinuation or reduction of glucose-based parenteral hyperalimentation, drugs (e.g., propranolol, alcohol), and certain disease states (pancreatic islet cell adenoma or carcinoma, hepatoma, fibroma, or adrenal insufficiency). Risk factors for intraoperative hyperglycemia include exogenous dextrose administration, alteration of hormone levels affecting glucose homeostasis, and decreased peripheral glucose utilization.

REFERENCES

1. Crawford M, Lerman J, Christensen S, et al.: Effects of duration of fasting on gastric fluid pH and volume in healthy children, *Anesth Analg* 71:400–403, 1990.
2. Cote CJ: NPO after midnight for children: a reappraisal, *Anesthesiology* 72:589–592, 1990.
3. Sieber FE, Smith DS, Traystman RJ, et al.: Glucose: a reevaluation of its intraoperative use, *Anesthesiology* 67:72–81, 1987.
4. Welborn LG, McGill WA, Hannallah RS, et al.: Perioperative blood glucose concentrations in pediatric outpatients, *Anesthesiology* 65:543–547, 1986.
5. Welborn LG, Hannallah RS, McGill WA, et al.: Glucose concentrations for routine intravenous infusion in pediatric outpatient surgery, *Anesthesiology* 67:427–430, 1987.

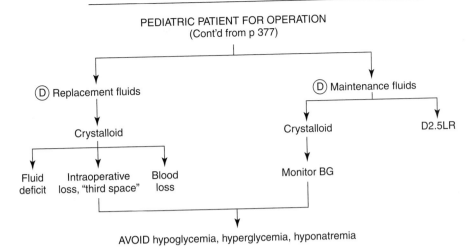

PEDIATRIC PATIENT FOR OPERATION
(Cont'd from p 377)

Ⓓ Replacement fluids

Crystalloid

Fluid deficit

Intraoperative loss, "third space"

Blood loss

Ⓓ Maintenance fluids

Crystalloid

D2.5LR

Monitor BG

AVOID hypoglycemia, hyperglycemia, hyponatremia

Pediatric Regional Anesthesia

DEBORAH K. RASCH, M.D.

LYNDA T. WELLS, M.D.

Regional anesthesia for pediatric patients is safe and effective.[1] Regional anesthesia has received renewed interest because of the recent focus on perioperative analgesia as a health care quality issue and because increasing numbers of premature nursery graduates with residual lung disease are presenting for operation. The latter may be at greater risk than age-matched healthy infants for development of apnea and respiratory compromise when general anesthesia is employed,[2,3] although this has been questioned in recent studies.[4,5] The differences in pediatric and adult anatomy should be appreciated, as should the recommended doses of local anesthetic[6] and adjunctive drugs at various stages of development. Peripheral nerve blocks are safer than neuraxis blocks.[1]

A. Consider operative site, patient age, other medical problems, and parental preference before administering regional anesthesia. Advantages of regional anesthesia include provision of excellent analgesia, profound muscle relaxation below the level of the block obviating or reducing the need for other muscle relaxants, reduction of the depth of general anesthesia required, and decreased variability in vital signs caused by changes in surgical stimulus. Spinal (Table 1) and caudal (Table 2) anesthesia also eliminate the bradycardic response to manipulation of the mesentery or spermatic cord during operations of the lower abdomen or genitourinary tract. Other advantages include immobility of the extremity after tendon or nerve repair in young children who are unable to follow postoperative instructions not to use the involved extremity.

B. Perform plexus and peripheral nerve blocks using a nerve stimulator with insulated, blunt bevel needles of appropriate length. Thread a catheter if a continuous technique is desired or to allow a block of prolonged duration. Calculate the total dose of local anesthesia recommended per hour and give in an appropriate volume to achieve the desired effect. Consider the addition of clonidine (1 μcg/kg) to prolong the duration of the block.[7] There are limitations to providing regional anesthesia in children: (1) lack of expertise among anesthesiologists in placing regional blocks, and (2) the need for two people experienced in managing pediatric patients when blocks are placed under general anesthesia (one ensures the safe administration of general anesthesia while the other places the regional block).

C. Determine if the patient will require sedation or anesthesia for the administration of regional anesthesia. Neonates often tolerate regional anesthesia with only a pacifier to calm them. However, it is not realistic to expect most children to lie still for the insertion of a regional block without first inducing general anesthesia or administering significant sedation.

D. Select appropriate medications for patients who will be sedated during placement of regional anesthesia. In infants up to about 6 months of age, ketamine 4 to 5 mg/kg intramuscularly with 0.01 mg/kg atropine mixed in the same syringe works nicely to induce the calm needed for performance of a block. Note, however, that ketamine increases the risk of apnea in premature infants. In older children, place an IV catheter preoperatively for administration of sedation. A variety of agents can be used. In our experience, midazolam given in incremental doses of up to 0.1mg/kg combined with fentanyl (1 to 2 μg/kg) affords excellent sedation for insertion of blocks. Consider topical local anesthetic (EMLA, 4% lidocaine) to minimize the discomfort of venous cannulation and block needle insertion.

E. For outpatient procedures, consider induction of general anesthesia prior to placement of the block; ketamine and other sedatives may cause prolonged sedation in children, which might delay discharge.

TABLE 1
Recommended Dosages for Subarachnoid Block in Children

Author	Anesthetic solution	Dosage	Volume D₁₀W
Gouveia[8]	Lidocaine 5%	1 to 2 mg/kg	Equal part
Berkowitz[9]	Tetracaine 1%	0.2 mg/kg	Equal part
Melman, et al.[10]	Hyperbaric lidocaine 5%	1.5 to 2.5 mg/kg*	None

*Infants up to 10 kg.

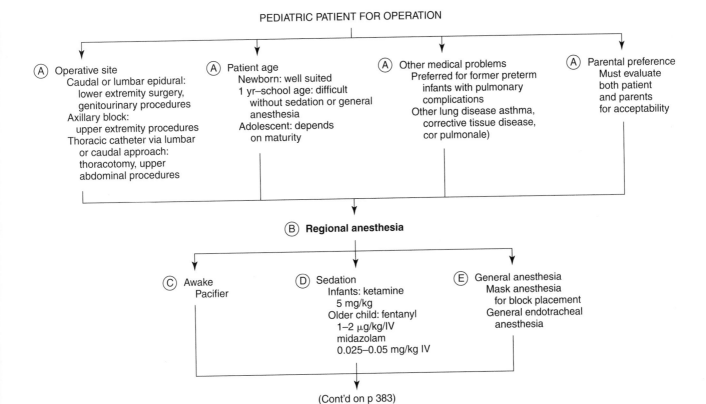

PEDIATRIC PATIENT FOR OPERATION

(A) Operative site
  Caudal or lumbar epidural:
    lower extremity surgery,
    genitourinary procedures
  Axillary block:
    upper extremity procedures
  Thoracic catheter via lumbar
    or caudal approach:
    thoracotomy, upper
    abdominal procedures

(A) Patient age
  Newborn: well suited
  1 yr–school age: difficult
    without sedation or general
    anesthesia
  Adolescent: depends
    on maturity

(A) Other medical problems
  Preferred for former preterm
    infants with pulmonary
    complications
  Other lung disease asthma,
    corrective tissue disease,
    cor pulmonale)

(A) Parental preference
  Must evaluate
    both patient
    and parents
    for acceptability

(B) **Regional anesthesia**

(C) Awake
  Pacifier

(D) Sedation
  Infants: ketamine
    5 mg/kg
  Older child: fentanyl
    1–2 μg/kg/IV
    midazolam
    0.025–0.05 mg/kg IV

(E) General anesthesia
  Mask anesthesia
    for block placement
  General endotracheal
    anesthesia

(Cont'd on p 383)

TABLE 2
Dosage Example for Caudal Anesthesia

For infants <15 kg, volume of LA = (0.1 ml LA solution) × (kg wt) × (no. spinal segments blocked)

For example, in a 3-kg infant presenting for herniorrhaphy, a T_{10} level is required.

Volume needed = (0.1 ml LA) × (3 kg wt) × (12* segments) = 3.6 ml of LA solution.

*12 segments = 5 sacral + 5 lumbar + 2 thoracic.

F. Choose a method of providing postoperative analgesia. Epidural administration of preservative-free morphine sulfate, 0.05 mg/kg/dose, results in excellent analgesia for 12 to 36 hours. Epidural fentanyl by continuous infusion may offer some advantages because of greater lipid solubility. In neonates, start the infusion at 0.25 μcg/kg/h and titrate to effect. For outpatients, local anesthesia (e.g., bupivacaine, ropivacaine) is safest as a single injection at the end of the procedure to allow 6 to 8 hours of postoperative pain relief. Observe children who have received epidural narcotics in a monitored setting postoperatively to watch for apnea. Be sure that patients with diminished sensory or motor function are carefully supervised to prevent accidental damage to skin and joints and to prevent falls.

REFERENCES

1. Giaufre E, Dalens B, Gombert A: Epidemiology and morbidity of regional anesthesia in children: a one-year prospective survey of the French-Language Society of Pediatric Anesthesiologists, *Anesth Analg* 83 (5):904–912, 1996.
2. Somri M, Gaitini L, Vaida S, et al.: Postoperative outcome in high-risk infants undergoing herniorrhaphy: comparison between spinal and general anaesthesia, *Anaesthesia* 53 (8):762–766, 1998.
3. Frumiento C, Abajian JC, Vane DW: Spinal anesthesia for preterm infants undergoing inguinal hernia repair, *Arch Surg* 135 (4): 445–451, 2000.
4. Craven PD, Badawi N, Henderson-Smart DJ, et al.: Regional (spinal, epidural, caudal) versus general anaesthesia in preterm infants undergoing inguinal herniorrhaphy in early infancy, *Cochrane Database Syst Rev* (3):CD003669, 2003.
5. Kunst G, Linderkamp O, Holle R, et al.: The proportion of high risk preterm infants with postoperative apnea and bradycardia is the same after general and spinal anesthesia, *Can J Anaesth* 46 (1): 94–95, 1999.
6. Berde C. Local anesthetics in infants and children: an update, *Paediatr Anaesth* 14 (5):387–393, 2004.
7. Rochette A, Raux O, Troncin R, et al.: Clonidine prolongs spinal anesthesia in newborns: a prospective dose-ranging study, *Anesth Analg* 98 (1):56–59, 2004.
8. Gouveia MA: Raquinaesthesia para pacientes pediatricos, *Rev Bras Anestesiol* 4:503, 1970.
9. Berkowitz S, Greene BA: Spinal anesthesia in children: report based on 350 patients under 13 years of age, *Anesthesiology* 12:376–387, 1951.
10. Melman E, Penuelas JA, Marrufo J: Regional anesthesia in children, *Anesth Analg* 54:387–390, 1975.

PEDIATRIC PATIENT FOR OPERATION
(Cont'd from p 381)

(F) **Postoperative analgesia**

Preservative-free morphine,
0.05 mg/kg/dose

Fentanyl,
1 μg/kg/load
0.25–1 μg/kg/hr

Local anesthetics
Best as single shot
for outpatients

OBSTETRIC AND GYNECOLOGIC ANESTHESIA

Analgesia for Labor and Delivery

Anesthesia Management of Preterm Labor (PTL)

Difficult Airway in Pregnancy

Obstetric Hemorrhage

Preeclampsia and Eclampsia

Cesarean Delivery

Pregnant Diabetic Patient

Pregnant Cardiac Patient

Nonobstetric Surgery in Pregnancy

Maternal Infections and Anesthesia

Labor and Delivery in the Patient Susceptible to Malignant Hyperthermia (MH)

Amniotic Fluid Embolism (AFE)

Morbidly Obese Parturient

Anesthesia for the Patient with Multiple Gestation

Fetal Monitoring

Postpartum Tubal Ligation (PPTL)

Fetal Surgery

Neonatal Resuscitation

Analgesia for Labor and Delivery

SUSAN H. NOORILY, M.D.

Labor is usually a painful experience but this varies from patient to patient. Of parturients, 80% describe labor pain as "very severe or intolerable," and 50% note that their pain management is inadequate.[1] An ideal anesthetic would provide rapid pain relief lasting throughout the labor and delivery period and have no adverse effect on the mother, fetus, or progress of labor.

A. Labor pain has two components. During the first stage, a visceral pain results from cervical dilatation and distension of the lower uterine segment with contractions. Pain is referred to dermatomes T10–L1, the same spinal cord segments that receive input from the uterus and cervix. During the late first and second stage, pain results from vaginal and perineal distension during fetal descent. This somatic pain is transmitted via the pudendal nerve through S2–S4.

B. Perform a thorough preanesthetic evaluation on any patient requesting analgesia for labor and delivery. Assess obstetric diagnoses, fetal status, and progress of labor. Obtain pertinent laboratory information (e.g., coagulation studies in preeclamptic patients).

C. Discuss the analgesic options with the patient. Counsel the patient regarding the risks and benefits of each. Education decreases anxiety and allows the parturient to give informed consent.

D. Nonpharmacological methods of pain control in labor have several different mechanisms of action, including competitive sensory stimulation, alteration of the biological response to pain, and amelioration of negative psychological issues. Nonpharmacological methods include psychosocial support, psychoprophylaxis (e.g., Lamaze), hypnosis, biofeedback, massage, acupuncture, hydrotherapy (e.g., warm water baths), intradermal sterile water blocks for back pain, transcutaneous electrical nerve stimulation (TENS), and movement and positioning.[3]

E. Systemic medications, including opioids, sedatives, and amnestic drugs are available for use during labor.[4] Of these, opioids are the most commonly used but have limited analgesic efficacy for labor pain and poor patient satisfaction. In addition, high doses of opioids result in unwanted side effects in the mother (i.e., nausea and vomiting, sedation, respiratory depression, disorientation, delayed gastric emptying) and baby (i.e., respiratory depression and low neurobehavioral scores). Narcotics should be avoided in the last 2 to 4 hours of labor. Meperidine is the most widely used labor narcotic and is often given in conjunction with an antiemetic to prevent nausea and vomiting. Fentanyl is a highly lipid-soluble, rapid acting narcotic that is useful for labor analgesia. Patient-controlled analgesia (PCA) is available in some institutions; remifentanil is currently being studied for this use.[5]

F. Paracervical block provides excellent analgesia for a period of up to 2 hours during the first stage of labor. This block has the potential for severe complications (i.e., fetal bradycardia, distress, and death) and is not commonly used for this purpose.[4] Lumbar sympathetic block can provide analgesia for the first stage of labor. Pudendal nerve block is useful during the second stage of labor and to augment an epidural that does not provide good sacral analgesia.

G. Neuraxial analgesia is the most effective method of labor analgesia.[2] In addition to excellent pain relief, neuraxial analgesia helps decrease circulating catecholamine concentrations, maintain adequate maternal and fetal oxygenation with a decrease in maternal hyperventilation, and decrease the incidence of maternal and fetal acidosis. If neuraxial is chosen, obtain informed consent and prepare the patient. Place the appropriate monitors on the patient and administer IV fluids for preload.

ANALGESIA FOR LABOR AND DELIVERY

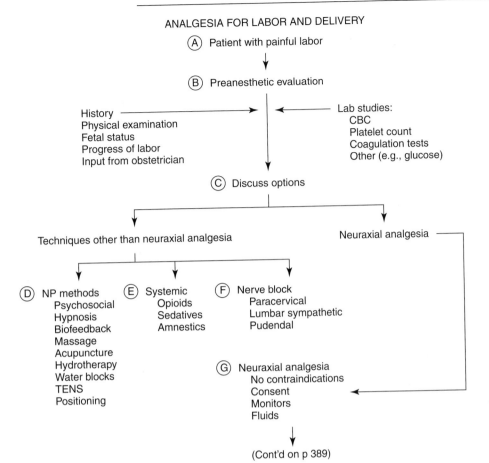

(A) Patient with painful labor

(B) Preanesthetic evaluation

History
Physical examination
Fetal status
Progress of labor
Input from obstetrician

Lab studies:
CBC
Platelet count
Coagulation tests
Other (e.g., glucose)

(C) Discuss options

Techniques other than neuraxial analgesia

Neuraxial analgesia

(D) NP methods
Psychosocial
Hypnosis
Biofeedback
Massage
Acupuncture
Hydrotherapy
Water blocks
TENS
Positioning

(E) Systemic
Opioids
Sedatives
Amnestics

(F) Nerve block
Paracervical
Lumbar sympathetic
Pudendal

(G) Neuraxial analgesia
No contraindications
Consent
Monitors
Fluids

(Cont'd on p 389)

H. Lumbar epidural analgesia (LEA) provides excellent pain relief throughout the course of labor and can be extended to provide anesthesia for instrumented delivery or cesarean section. A continuous infusion of dilute local anesthetic with the addition of lipid-soluble opioid to reduce local anesthetic requirement produces reliable analgesia with minimal motor blockade as well as minimal effect on uterine activity and fetal well-being. Potential complications include accidental dural puncture causing postdural puncture headache (PDPH), postpartum low back pain, nerve injury, infection, maternal fever, hematoma, hypotension, nausea and vomiting, urinary retention, respiratory depression, pruritus, inadequate pain relief, and possibly an increased risk of prolonged labor and instrumented delivery (controversial).[6] The risks of inadvertent subarachnoid and intravascular injection are prevented by performing a test dose and incremental drug injection. Patient-controlled epidural analgesia is a safe and effective approach, best achieved with low-concentration local anesthetic and opioid combinations.[4]

I. Intrathecal opioids (IT) provide effective, rapid analgesia during early labor without motor blockade. Maternal hypotension, when it occurs, is due to analgesia and decreased circulating catecholamines and opioid-induced preganglionic sympathetic block.[4] Several early case reports described sudden fetal bradycardia after administration of IT, but the changes were usually transient and resolved spontaneously. Other complications include pruritus, nausea and vomiting, urinary retention, respiratory depression, risk of PDPH (1 to 2% with pencil-point spinal needle), nerve injury, and infection. A combination of IT with a small dose of local anesthesia increases the duration of analgesia and provides perineal anesthesia. IT clonidine is also safe and effective but can have hemodynamic effects.[4] Consider using continuous spinal analgesia after accidental dural puncture with an epidural needle, in patients who are to receive only IT opioids during labor, and in cases where the epidural failure rate is expected to be high (e.g., morbid obesity).[4]

J. Combined spinal-epidural (CSE) analgesia for labor offers the advantages of both IT (i.e., rapid onset) and LEA (i.e., placement of catheter for prolonged use). With CSE, the IT injection takes place prior to threading the epidural catheter. The catheter can be used immediately or at a later time. Administer a test dose prior to activating the LEA catheter.

K. Carefully monitor patients who have received labor analgesia. Follow the progress of labor and fetal status in all patients. Anesthetic requirements may change throughout labor. Some patients will require assistance with pain management after delivery.

REFERENCES

1. Ranta P, Spalding M, Kangas-Saarela T, et al.: Maternal expectations and experiences of labour pain-opinions of 1091 Finnish parturients, *Acta Anaesthesiol Scand* 39 (1):60–66, 1995.
2. Halpern SH, Leighton BL: Misconceptions about neuraxial analgesia, *Anesthesiol Clin North Am* 21 (1):59–70, 2003.
3. Simkin PP, O'hara M: Nonpharmacologic relief of pain during labor: systematic reviews of five methods, *Am J Obstet Gynecol* 186:S131–S159, 2002.
4. Paech M: Newer techniques of labor analgesia, *Anesthesiol Clin North Am* 21 (1):1–17, 2003.
5. Evron S, Glezerman M, Sadan O, et al.: Remifentanil: a novel systemic analgesic for labor pain, *Anesth Analg* 100 (1):233–238, 2005.
6. Leighton BL: The impact of neuraxial analgesia on the progress and outcome of labor, *Tech Reg Anesth Pain Manage* 7 (4):197–203, 2003.

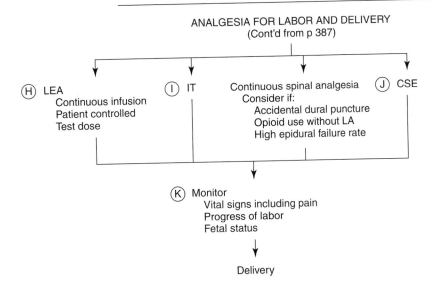

ANALGESIA FOR LABOR AND DELIVERY
(Cont'd from p 387)

(H) LEA
    Continuous infusion
    Patient controlled
    Test dose

(I) IT
    Continuous spinal analgesia
    Consider if:
        Accidental dural puncture
        Opioid use without LA
        High epidural failure rate

(J) CSE

(K) Monitor
    Vital signs including pain
    Progress of labor
    Fetal status

Delivery

Anesthesia Management of Preterm Labor (PTL)

JINNY KIM HARTMAN, M.D.

Preterm labor (PTL) has severe implications for both mother and fetus and is the most common cause of antenatal hospitalization. PTL is commonly defined as contractions occurring between 20 and 36 weeks' gestation at a rate of four in 20 minutes or eight in 1 hour, associated with at least one of the following: cervical change over time or dilation greater than or equal to 2 cm.[1] Preterm delivery (PTD) is defined as birth occurring before 37 full weeks of gestation.[2] Preterm deliveries account for up to 11% (or 440,000) of all births in the United States.[1] Between 69 and 83% of all neonatal deaths occur in preterm infants; if infants survive, 50% of long-term neurological impairment is due to PTD.[1] Thus, effective management of PTL and prevention of PTD is crucial. Pharmacological therapy of PTL and delivery of a premature infant have significant anesthetic implications. A discussion of tocolytic therapies is included. The risks of therapy may outweigh the benefits in many patients, especially after 32 to 36 weeks' gestation. The primary goal of anesthetic management is maternal and fetal safety. Maternal safety can be greatly influenced by the anesthesiologist. In contrast, fetal morbidity and mortality are largely dependent on gestational age rather than anesthetic technique.

A. Management of PTL is difficult and largely ineffective. The majority of preterm laboring patients deliver. Identification of patients at risk for PTL is nonspecific and nonsensitive. When identified, not all patients are candidates for tocolysis. Up to 33% of women in PTL will have premature rupture of membranes, a relative contraindication to tocolysis. Another 25% of patients in PTL require immediate delivery.[2-4] A recent retrospective study showed that only 9% of PTD patients were candidates for tocolysis.[5] For the majority of patients in PTL, prepare for inevitable delivery of a premature infant, either vaginally or by cesarean section. Anesthetic concerns for the parturient include difficult airway, propensity to hypoxia and hypotension, full stomach, hypoglycemia, hypocarbia, and decreased MAC. Concerns for the premature infant include asphyxia and drug depression; a premature fetus is more susceptible to drug effects. The anesthesiologist must be skilled in neonatal resuscitation. Regional anesthesia is preferred due to the unpredictability of the maternal airway. If general anesthesia is required, employ left uterine displacement, provide reflux prophylaxis, preoxygenation, and RSI with cricoid pressure.

B. Commonly used tocolytics include magnesium sulfate, beta-adrenergic agents, and prostaglandin synthetase inhibitors.[6,7] Other agents include calcium channel blockers (nifedipine), and oxytocin receptor antagonists. Magnesium sulfate ($MgSO_4$) is often first-line tocolytic therapy. It acts via the CNS to decrease seizures and block neuromuscular transmission. $MgSO_4$ can cause respiratory depression and profound muscular weakness.[1,6,8] It can significantly potentiate the effects of muscle relaxants; therefore, carefully monitor neuromuscular blockade. Diligently assess alertness and strength prior to maternal extubation. $MgSO_4$ can also cause hypotension, but in sheep studies it does not decrease uterine blood flow.[8] Lastly, $MgSO_4$ can cause pulmonary edema. Treatment $MgSO_4$ overdose with calcium gluconate. Beta-adrenergic agonists (e.g., terbutaline) act by stimulation of $beta_2$-adrenergic receptors in the myometrium causing uterine relaxation. These agonists are not specific for myometrial $beta_2$ receptors. They can affect $beta_1$ and $beta_2$ receptors at multiple organ sites causing hypotension, tachycardia, cardiac arrhythmias (SVT), hypoglycemia, and pulmonary edema.[6,9] Beta-adrenergic side effects, especially hypotension, are of concern when regional anesthesia is used; studies to date do not show an increase in adverse outcome with this combination, and hypotension can be treated with ephedrine.[9] Prostaglandin synthetase inhibitors (e.g., indomethacin) inhibit cyclooxygenase, decreasing the formation of prostaglandins and preventing the rise in intracellular calcium levels.[7] These drugs have been implicated in hepatitis, renal failure, and GI bleeding. They may also increase bleeding time, but in the absence of a significant bleeding history, regional anesthesia is not contraindicated.

REFERENCES

1. AHRQ: Management of preterm labor. Summary, evidence report/technology assessment, Number 18. AHRQ Publication No. 01-E020, October 2000.
2. Resnik R: Issues in the management of preterm labor, *J Obstet Gynaecol Res* 31:354–358, 2005.
3. Lockwood CJ: The diagnosis of preterm labor and the prediction of preterm delivery, *Clin Obstet Gynecol* 38:675–687, 1995.
4. Dewan DM: Anesthesia for preterm delivery, breech presentation, and multiple gestation, *Clin Obstet Gynecol* 30:566–578, 1987.
5. Thangaratinam S, Coomarasamy A: Progestational agents to prevent preterm birth: a meta-analysis of randomized controlled trials, *Obstet Gynecol* 105:1483–1484, 2005.
6. Berkman ND, Thorp JM Jr, Lohr KN, et al.: Tocolytic treatment for the management of preterm labor: a review of the evidence, *Am J Obstet Gynecol* 188:1648–1659, 2003.
7. Ingemarsson I, Lamont RF: An update on the controversies of tocolytic therapy for the prevention of preterm birth, *Acta Obstet Gynecol Scand* 82:1–9, 2003.
8. Vincent RD Jr, Chestnut DH, Sipes SL, et al.: Magnesium sulfate decreases maternal blood pressure but not uterine blood flow during epidural anesthesia in gravid ewes, *Anesthesiology* 74:77–82, 1991.
9. McGrath JM, Chestnut DH, Vincent RD, et al.: Ephedrine remains the vasopressor of choice for treatment of hypotension during ritodrine infusion and epidural anesthesia, *Anesthesiology* 80:1073–1081, 1994.

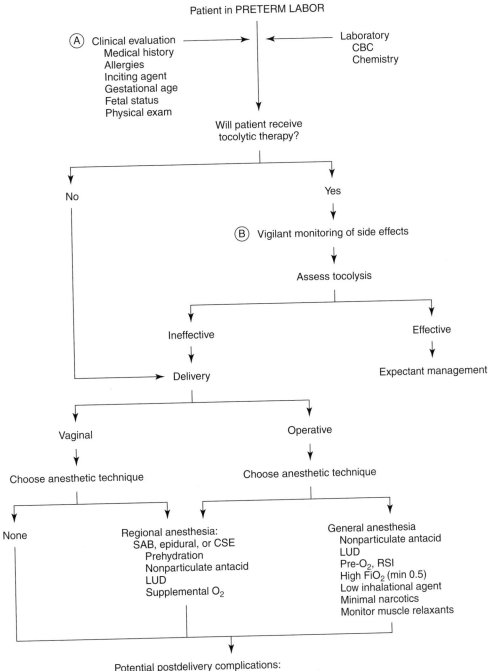

Patient in PRETERM LABOR

Ⓐ Clinical evaluation
   Medical history
   Allergies
   Inciting agent
   Gestational age
   Fetal status
   Physical exam

Laboratory
CBC
Chemistry

Will patient receive
tocolytic therapy?

No

Yes

Ⓑ Vigilant monitoring of side effects

Assess tocolysis

Ineffective

Effective

Delivery

Expectant management

Vaginal

Operative

Choose anesthetic technique

Choose anesthetic technique

None

Regional anesthesia:
   SAB, epidural, or CSE
   Prehydration
   Nonparticulate antacid
   LUD
   Supplemental O_2

General anesthesia
   Nonparticulate antacid
   LUD
   Pre-O_2, RSI
   High FiO_2 (min 0.5)
   Low inhalational agent
   Minimal narcotics
   Monitor muscle relaxants

Potential postdelivery complications:
   Maternal hypoxia, hypotension
   Fetal asphyxia, fetal drug depression, fetal death

Difficult Airway in Pregnancy

BONNY CARTER, M.D.

Pregnant patients are at risk for difficult airway management from upper airway edema, increased soft tissue, and enlarged breasts. Oxygen (O_2) reserves decrease (increased metabolism and decreased FRC). Delayed gastric emptying and incompetent lower esophageal sphincter tone predispose to aspiration. Systemic and epidural opioid analgesics further delay gastric emptying.[1-3]

A. Evaluate the airway carefully. The incidence of a severe grade III or IV laryngoscopic view ranges from 0.05 to 0.35% in the general population, and expect a higher incidence in obstetrics. Failed intubation and mask ventilation ranges from 0.0001 to 0.02%. Administer an oral nonparticulate antacid. Consider an H_2 antagonist and metoclopramide for patients who are to receive GETA. Place the patient in "sniffing" position—a shoulder roll can optimize this position. Preoxygenate the patient (100% O_2 via face mask) for 3 minutes or have her take four vital capacity breaths.

B. Encourage early epidural analgesia for patients at high risk for cesarean delivery (i.e., preeclampsia, gestational diabetes, obesity, previous cesarean delivery, or signs of fetal or maternal compromise). Emergency GETA can often be avoided when a functioning epidural catheter is in place. Encourage patients presenting for elective cesarean delivery to choose regional anesthesia. Regional anesthesia does not completely avoid airway risk.

C. If awake intubation is required, give adequate topical local anesthesia. Options include direct laryngoscopy, retrograde wire, blind nasal, and fiberoptic laryngoscopy. Direct laryngoscopy is stimulating and often poorly tolerated. The nasal mucosa of the parturient is swollen and friable and prone to bleeding; topical ephedrine (5%) has been used as a vasoconstrictor.

D. After induction of GETA, restrict attempts at laryngoscopy to two to three; the pharyngeal mucosa is friable, and numerous attempts may compromise subsequent efforts to mask ventilate the patient. With each attempt, change patient position, the laryngoscope blade, or the laryngoscopist. If intubation is unsuccessful, maintain oxygenation by mask with cricoid pressure and call for help (e.g., anesthesia personnel, an otolaryngologist who can perform a tracheotomy).

E. If cesarean delivery is not urgent, maintain oxygenation by mask ventilation with cricoid pressure until the patient awakens. Then consider regional anesthesia or an awake intubation.

F. If delivery of the fetus is emergently necessary and mask ventilation with cricoid pressure is adequate, proceed with cesarean delivery under mask general anesthesia. Weigh ease of mask ventilation against the clinical urgency of the situation. Discuss the relative risks with the obstetrician. Maintain cricoid pressure throughout the procedure.

G. If both intubation and mask ventilation have failed, oxygenating the patient is an urgent priority. Accomplish oxygenation first and, if possible, protect the airway from aspiration of gastric contents.

H. The laryngeal mask airway (LMA) is now recognized as part of the ASA Difficult Airway Algorithm. The LMA has been found to be a lifesaving device in parturients undergoing emergency cesarean section who could not be ventilated or intubated by conventional methods. The limits to the classical LMA are that it does not protect against aspiration and may be difficult to use with positive-pressure ventilation (PPV). The ProSeal laryngeal mask airway (PLMA) is a new device with a modified cuff and drainage tube designed to allow drainage of the digestive tract and thereby lessen the risk of aspiration. The PLMA allows PPV more reliably than the classic LMA.

I. The esophageal Combitube is a double-lumen tube (DLT) with one lumen ending at the distal tip and the other lumen exiting through perforations 4 to 8 cm from the distal tip. The distal tip enters the esophagus the majority of the time; if both cuffs are inflated, the trachea is ventilated via the perforations positioned in the oropharynx. If the distal tip enters the trachea, it can be used as a conventional endotracheal tube (ETT). In both positions, the Combitube protects against aspiration.

J. Cricothyrotomy and transtracheal jet ventilation (TTJV) allow rapid oxygenation in an emergency situation. Ventilation may be inadequate. Risks include barotrauma, subcutaneous emphysema, and bleeding (trauma to the thyroid artery). Maintain cricoid pressure, ensure that the upper airway is patent to allow exhalation, and hold the catheter firmly at all times to prevent dislodgment and soft tissue injury.

K. Retrograde wire intubation is performed by threading a long guidewire through a transtracheal needle, retrieving the end through the nose or mouth, and passing an ETT over the wire. The tube may meet resistance at the glottis. Threading the wire through the suction port of a fiberoptic bronchoscopy (FOB) allows visualization of the glottis during intubation.

L. At times, a surgical airway is the only option.

M. When delivery is not emergent and oxygenation is achieved without aspiration protection (e.g., LMA, TTJV), awaken the patient and proceed with regional anesthesia or an awake intubation. If the fetus is distressed, compare the potential risk to the parturient to that of the fetus if cesarean delivery proceeds. In some cases (i.e., placental abruption, maternal hemorrhage, or cardiac arrest), delivery may be lifesaving to both the mother and the baby.

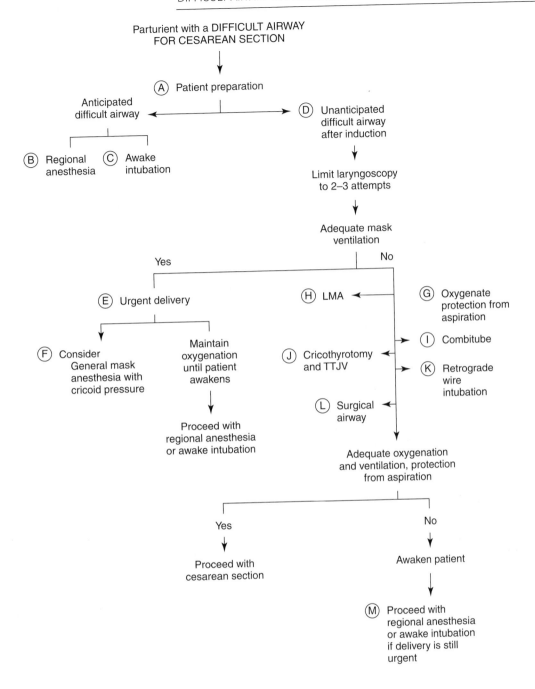

REFERENCES

1. Kuczkowski K: The difficult airway. In: Chestnut DH, editor: *Obstetric anesthesia: principles and practice,* ed 3, St. Louis, 2004, Mosby Year Book.
2. Rasmussen GE, Malinow AM: Toward reducing maternal mortality: the problem airway in obstetrics, *Int Anesthesiol Clin* 32:83, 1994.
3. Cook TM, Nolan JP, Verghese C, et al.: Randomized crossover comparison of proseal with the classic laryngeal mask airway in unparalysed anaesthetized patients, *Br J Anaesth* 88:527–533, 2000.

Obstetric Hemorrhage

MOHAMED TIOURIRINE, M.D.

Despite advances in management, obstetric hemorrhage remains a leading cause of maternal morbidity and mortality.[1] In a normal pregnancy, the expected blood loss is 500 ml during vaginal delivery and up to 1,000 ml during cesarean delivery. Due to the physiological changes of pregnancy, parturients tolerate up to 1,000 ml of blood loss without major change in hematocrit (Hct), BP, or cardiac output (CO). Vital signs may remain normal until greater than 30% of the blood volume is lost.[2] Obstetric hemorrhage is an acute, usually unexpected blood loss that occurs before, during, or after delivery. Major causes are placental abnormalities, coagulopathy, trauma, uterine atony, and retained uterine contents. Successful management of obstetric hemorrhage depends on prevention, early suspicion, and rapid intervention. Maternal hemorrhage is classified as antepartum or postpartum by the time of occurrence. Causes of antepartum hemorrhage include placenta previa, placental abruption, and uterine rupture. Postpartum hemorrhage can occur early (within 24 hours) or late (up to 6 weeks); causes include uterine atony, genital laceration, placental abnormalities, uterine inversion, and coagulation disorders.

A. Always maintain good communication with the obstetric team when the diagnosis of obstetric hemorrhage is suspected. Discuss the etiology and severity of the hemorrhage. Estimate blood loss. Remember that a healthy parturient can lose large volumes of blood without significant changes in vital signs. Orthostatic changes suggest tenuous volume status. Send blood for cross-match and assessment of Hct and coagulation status. In cases of antepartum or intrapartum hemorrhage, determine fetal condition and obstetrical plan.

B. Follow the general rules of resuscitation: airway, breathing, and circulation. Call for help. Ensure adequate IV access. Start a rapid infusion device. Administer IV fluid (e.g., crystalloid/colloid) to maintain normovolemia. Consider blood transfusion when the patient exhibits signs of hypovolemia despite adequate volume replacement or in the presence of fetal distress and ongoing blood loss. Consider placement of a central venous catheter to guide volume replacement. Place an arterial line if frequent blood sampling is expected. Monitor urine output, BP, and CVP (if catheter placed). Consider use of vasopressors. Recheck the hematocrit and coagulation parameters; treat abnormalities promptly as necessary. Keep the patient warm.

C. Discuss the obstetric management of the patient with the obstetricians. Management of obstetric hemorrhage depends on a multitude of factors, including severity of the hemorrhage, gestational age and condition of the fetus, and timing (i.e., antepartum versus postpartum). Maternal or fetal deterioration mandates urgent intervention including maternal resuscitation, delivery of the fetus, and uterine hemostasis (e.g., contraction, tamponade, embolization of hypogastric or uterine arteries, surgical repair of tissue lacerations, and possibly hysterectomy.)

D. Mild antepartum bleeding in a laboring patient is often managed by vaginal delivery. Place an epidural for labor analgesia only in the absence of coagulopathy and maternal hypovolemia. Severe antepartum hemorrhage is an indication for emergent cesarean delivery. Sympathetic blockade produced by regional anesthesia may impair normal compensatory mechanisms and exacerbate hypotension. Consider general anesthesia as the preferred method of anesthesia in such cases. Choose an induction agent that supports hemodynamic stability (e.g., ketamine or etomidate). In cases of fetal distress, provide 100% oxygen to maximize delivery to the fetus. Minimize inhaled anesthetic concentrations, because these promote uterine relaxation and bleeding. If obstetric bleeding occurs in a parturient with a functioning regional anesthetic, continue to utilize this technique if normovolemia can be maintained and the patient remains comfortable. Convert to a general anesthetic to protect the patient's airway in the presence of hemodynamic instability or to improve patient comfort.

E. Postpartum hemorrhage is most frequently caused by uterine atony. Attempt pharmacological control whenever possible (e.g., oxytocin, Hemabate, or ergonovine). Only a small percentage of patients will require hysterectomy. Genital lacerations can usually be repaired with local anesthetic and IV sedation or under regional anesthesia. Detachment of a retained placenta may require uterine relaxation, or in the case of a placenta accreta, surgical treatment (i.e., hysterectomy). Accreta occurs most commonly in the setting of placenta previa and prior cesarean section. If uterine inversion occurs, the uterus must be replaced rapidly, requiring uterine relaxation. In the awake patient, attempt uterine relaxation by administering nitroglycerin (50 to 100 μg intravenously); if this is not successful and preexisting regional anesthesia does not provide adequate conditions, induce GETA and administer a volatile agent.

F. The postoperative course may be uneventful. However, be on the alert for complications including disseminated intravascular coagulation, acute renal failure, Sheehan syndrome (hypopituitarism), and infection. Admit the patient to an ICU in the event of massive transfusion.

REFERENCES

1. Esler MD, Douglas MJ: Planning for hemorrhage: Steps an anesthesiologist can take to limit and treat hemorrhage in the obstetric patient, *Anesthesiol Clin North Am* 21 (1):127–144, 2003.
2. Crochetiere C: Obstetric emergencies, *Anesthesiol Clin North Am* 21 (1):111–125, 2003.

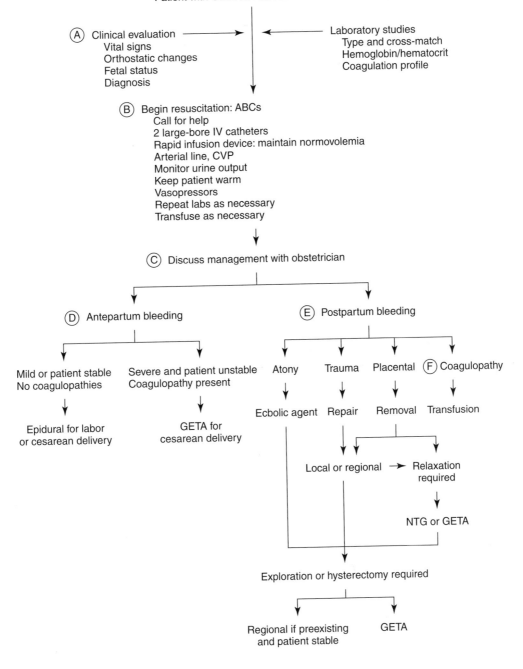

Patient with OBSTETRIC HEMORRHAGE

Ⓐ Clinical evaluation
    Vital signs
    Orthostatic changes
    Fetal status
    Diagnosis

Laboratory studies
    Type and cross-match
    Hemoglobin/hematocrit
    Coagulation profile

Ⓑ Begin resuscitation: ABCs
    Call for help
    2 large-bore IV catheters
    Rapid infusion device: maintain normovolemia
    Arterial line, CVP
    Monitor urine output
    Keep patient warm
    Vasopressors
    Repeat labs as necessary
    Transfuse as necessary

Ⓒ Discuss management with obstetrician

Ⓓ Antepartum bleeding

Ⓔ Postpartum bleeding

Mild or patient stable
No coagulopathies

Severe and patient unstable
Coagulopathy present

Atony

Trauma

Placental

Ⓕ Coagulopathy

Epidural for labor
or cesarean delivery

GETA for
cesarean delivery

Ecbolic agent

Repair

Removal

Transfusion

Local or regional → Relaxation
required

NTG or GETA

Exploration or hysterectomy required

Regional if preexisting
and patient stable

GETA

Preeclampsia and Eclampsia

SUSAN H. NOORILY, M.D.

Preeclampsia is classically defined by a triad of symptoms: hypertension (HTN) with proteinuria or edema and is a leading cause of maternal and neonatal morbidity and mortality.[1] Preeclampsia involves every major organ system. A small percentage of preeclamptic women develop eclampsia (seizures).

A. Preeclampsia is associated with an elevated systemic vascular resistance (SVR) and contracted plasma volume. Edema is present and can involve airway structures. Pulmonary edema is one of the most severe manifestations. Thrombocytopenia is common; other coagulation abnormalities can occur. HELLP (hemolysis, elevated liver enzymes, and low platelet count) syndrome is a variant of severe preeclampsia; patients present with GI complaints. Preeclamptic women may have renal and hepatocellular dysfunction. Headaches, visual disturbances, and seizures are manifestations of CNS involvement. In the United States, seizure prophylaxis with magnesium sulfate ($MgSO_4$) is standard therapy. Magnesium causes muscle weakness, potentiates muscle relaxants, causes transient decreases in blood pressure and may exaggerate the hypotensive effects of regional anesthesia, and can depress pulmonary and cardiac function; therefore deep tendon reflexes (DTRs) and blood levels are closely monitored.

B. Preeclamptic women are classified as mild or severe. The goal of treatment is stabilization and delivery. HTN is controlled with antihypertensive agents, such as hydralazine, labetalol, and nifedipine or nicardipine. Oliguria is treated with a fluid challenge; if there is no response, central pressure monitoring may be useful to guide fluid management. Pulmonary edema is more common postpartum; treatment involves supportive therapy, diuretics, and occasionally vasodilators and mechanical ventilation. Eclamptic seizures require conservative airway management, supplemental oxygen (O_2), $MgSO_4$, and small doses of anticonvulsant (e.g., thiopental 50 to 75 mg). Rarely, airway protection and intubation are necessary. Immediate cesarean section is not attempted until the parturient is stable.

C. Routine monitoring for preeclampsia includes close nursing supervision, continuous fetal heart rate (FHR) monitoring, noninvasive BP, input and output (I&O) with urinary catheter, DTR checks, and pulse oximetry if available. Place arterial lines in patients with BP refractory to treatment, when potent vasodilators are required, and for frequent blood sampling (especially ABGs or if coagulopathy is present). Invasive central monitoring is controversial and is not essential for fluid management in every severely preeclamptic patient.[1] CVP and pulmonary artery (PA) pressure may not correlate.[2] Indications for PA catheters in preeclamptic women are: severe HTN resistant to treatment, pulmonary edema, oliguria not responsive to fluids, and coexisting maternal cardiac disease. Use of the antecubital vein approach may decrease the risks of hematoma and pneumothorax. New noninvasive monitoring is available at some centers and may be useful.

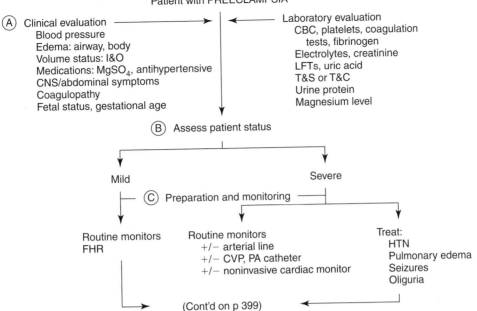

Patient with PREECLAMPSIA

Ⓐ Clinical evaluation
    Blood pressure
    Edema: airway, body
    Volume status: I&O
    Medications: $MgSO_4$, antihypertensive
    CNS/abdominal symptoms
    Coagulopathy
    Fetal status, gestational age

Laboratory evaluation
    CBC, platelets, coagulation
        tests, fibrinogen
    Electrolytes, creatinine
    LFTs, uric acid
    T&S or T&C
    Urine protein
    Magnesium level

Ⓑ Assess patient status

Mild

Severe

Ⓒ Preparation and monitoring

Routine monitors
FHR

Routine monitors
    +/− arterial line
    +/− CVP, PA catheter
    +/− noninvasive cardiac monitor

Treat:
    HTN
    Pulmonary edema
    Seizures
    Oliguria

(Cont'd on p 399)

D. Consult with the obstetrician regarding the planned mode of delivery; good communication is essential. Regional anesthesia is usually the technique of choice. Evaluate coagulation and volume status prior to proceeding. The platelet count is a useful predictor of functional clotting. Treat hypotension promptly. In nonoliguric patients, administer a cautious preload of a balanced salt solution or colloid. For labor and delivery, continuous lumbar epidural analgesia (LEA) provides excellent pain relief with improved intervillous blood flow, control of HTN, and improved cardiac output (CO). Intrathecal narcotic (ITN), alone or in combination with LEA (combined spinal-epidural [CSE]), is useful early in labor. Continuous spinal analgesia may be advantageous in morbidly obese preeclamptic women but has a risk of postdural puncture headache (PDPH). When regional anesthesia is contraindicated, use of parenteral narcotics may be necessary.

E. Preeclamptic women are at increased risk for cesarean section. The indication and urgency of cesarean section will dictate the choice of anesthetic. Regional anesthesia is preferred. "Single-shot" subarachnoid block (SAB) is safe in mild preeclampsia and is an alternative to GETA in emergent situations. Recent findings suggest that SAB is safe in severe preeclampsia as well.[4,5] LEA has been a longstanding choice in severe preeclampsia because local anesthetic can be slowly titrated. LEA blunts stress responses during cesarean section. Epinephrine (used with caution) and narcotic will improve the block. Continuous SAB is an alternative useful in morbidly obese patients. If an urgent or emergency cesarean section is required in a patient who has a functioning labor LEA or SAB catheter in place, the sensory level can usually be elevated rapidly in time for incision.

F. Plan GETA when regional anesthesia is contraindicated, for eclampsia with increased ICP and refractory seizures, and when there is not time to establish an adequate regional block. Stabilize BP prior to induction (diastolic BP < 105 mm Hg); labetalol, lidocaine, narcotic, nitroglycerin (NTG), and nitroprusside have all been used. Patients may have upper airway edema. Induce GETA by RSI or do an awake intubation. Do not defasciculate. Choose a small endotracheal tube ([ETT] 6.0 to 6.5 mm). Monitor paralysis. Use small doses of maintenance muscle relaxant. Extubate only when the patient is fully awake. Antihypertensives attenuate the hypertensive response to extubation. Observe preeclamptic patients closely for 24 hours postpartum; seizures and pulmonary edema can develop during this period.

REFERENCES

1. Ramanathan J, Bennett K: Pre-eclampsia: fluids, drugs, and anesthetic management, *Anesthesiol Clin N Am* 21:145–163, 2003.
2. Bolte AC, Dekker GA, van Eyck J, et al.: Lack of agreement between central venous pressure and pulmonary capillary wedge pressure in preeclampsia, *Hypertens Pregnancy* 19:261–271, 2000.
3. Jouppila P, Jouppila R, Hollmen A, et al.: Lumbar epidural analgesia to improve intervillous blood flow during labor in severe preeclampsia, *Obstet Gynecol* 59:158–161, 1982.
4. Aya AGM, Mangin R, Vialles N, et al.: Patients with severe preeclampsia experience less hypotension during spinal anesthesia for elective cesarean delivery than healthy parturients: a prospective cohort comparison, *Anesth Analg* 97:867–872, 2003.
5. Hood D, Curry R: Spinal versus epidural anesthesia for cesarean section in severely preeclamptic patients: a retrospective survey, *Anesthesiology* 90:1276–1282, 1999.

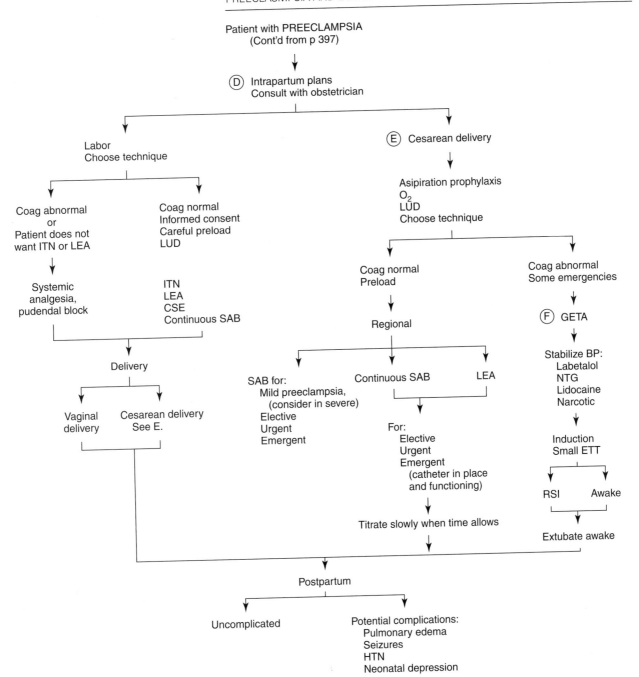

Patient with PREECLAMPSIA
(Cont'd from p 397)

Ⓓ Intrapartum plans
Consult with obstetrician

Labor
Choose technique

Coag abnormal
or
Patient does not
want ITN or LEA

Coag normal
Informed consent
Careful preload
LUD

Systemic
analgesia,
pudendal block

ITN
LEA
CSE
Continuous SAB

Delivery

Vaginal
delivery

Cesarean delivery
See E.

Ⓔ Cesarean delivery

Asipiration prophylaxis
O₂
LUD
Choose technique

Coag normal
Preload

Coag abnormal
Some emergencies

Regional

Ⓕ GETA

SAB for:
Mild preeclampsia,
(consider in severe)
Elective
Urgent
Emergent

Continuous SAB

LEA

Stabilize BP:
Labetalol
NTG
Lidocaine
Narcotic

For:
Elective
Urgent
Emergent
(catheter in place
and functioning)

Induction
Small ETT

RSI   Awake

Titrate slowly when time allows

Extubate awake

Postpartum

Uncomplicated

Potential complications:
Pulmonary edema
Seizures
HTN
Neonatal depression

Cesarean Delivery

DANIEL MARTIN BITNER, M.D., M.S.

Cesarean deliveries now exceed 24% in the United States. Physiological changes increase the possibility of failures in intubation or ventilation (difficult intubations 10 times more likely) and aspiration. Anesthetic complications account for 3 to 12% of maternal deaths. Thus, regional anesthesia is preferred. Maternal safety is paramount, even in a crisis situation.[1]

A. Determine urgency of cesarean section and assess the fetal heart rate tracing. Examine patient; a comprehensive assessment is not always possible in crisis situations, but assess the airway. Evaluate comorbidities: prior cesarean section (increased placenta accreta and previa), pregnancy-induced hypertension (HTN) or preeclampsia, and cardiac disease. In preeclamptic patients, obtain platelet and coagulation studies, if possible. Typical blood loss is 1,000 ml. Obtain informed consent.

B. Administer aspiration prophylaxis (nonparticulate oral antacid and IV H_2 antagonist [e.g., ranitidine] or proton pump inhibitor [e.g., omeprazole]), preferably 30 minutes prior to the anesthetic. Metoclopramide enhances gastric emptying, increases lower esophageal tone, and has antiemetic properties. Avoid or minimize preoperative sedation.

C. Maintain left uterine displacement (LUD) to avoid aortocaval compression. Administer supplemental oxygen (O_2). Place standard American Society of Anesthesiologists (ASA) monitors. Insert two large-bore IV catheters. Prehydrate with 15 to 20 ml/kg. Colloid solutions may be beneficial when pulmonary edema is a concern. Limit hetastarch (coagulopathy) and normal saline (hyperchloremic metabolic acidosis). Avoid boluses of solutions containing glucose; these may precipitate postdelivery neonatal hypoglycemia and jaundice.

CESAREAN DELIVERY

Urgency assessment

↓

(A) **Pre-operative evaluation**
  • Airway exam
  • Focused H&P
  • Pre-op labs/studies

↓

(B) **Aspiration prophylaxis/pre-op meds**
  • Sodium citrate with H_2 blocker or proton inhibitor
  • +/− metoclopramide
  • Difficult airway prep

↓

(C) **LUD position**
Fluid bolus
ASA monitors +/− invasive monitoring

↓

(Cont'd on p 403)

D. Choose anesthetic technique based on fetal and maternal factors.[2] GETA is indicated for profound fetal distress (prolapsed umbilical cord, placental abruption); anticipated severe maternal hemorrhage (placenta accreta/increta/percreta, uterine rupture); maternal thrombocytopenia/coagulopathy (hemolysis, elevated liver enzymes, and low platelet count [HELLP]); systemic maternal sepsis; and contraindication to, patient refusal of, or inadequate regional anesthesia. Otherwise, regional anesthesia is preferred (minimal fetal drug exposure, no intubation, mother is awake during delivery). Parturients have decreased anesthetic requirements.

E. Regional anesthesia techniques include spinal (continuous or single shot), epidural, and combined spinal epidural (CSE). Infiltration of local anesthetic can be a primary technique but is generally used to supplement inadequate regional anesthesia or when an anesthesia provider is unavailable and either mother or fetus is in extremis. Spinal anesthesia is technically simpler, rapidly produces a dense block, and minimizes risk of local anesthetic toxicity but has a finite duration (unless a catheter is placed), increased maternal hypotension (sympathectomy), and possibility of postdural puncture headache (PDPH). Local anesthetics used include lidocaine, bupivacaine, tetracaine, procaine, ropivacaine, and levobupivacaine with opioids (enhanced anesthetic quality, postoperative analgesia), and possibly epinephrine (prolonged duration). Treat hypotension with exaggerated LUD, IV fluids, and vasopressors (ephedrine or phenylephrine). Spinal anesthesia is safe in preeclamptic patients.[3,4] Labor epidurals can be dosed further for cesarean section. Local anesthesia agents include 3% 2-chloroprocaine or 2% lidocaine with 1 mEq of sodium bicarbonate per 10 ml (rapid onset), with opioids (enhanced block quality of block, postoperative analgesia). Avoid 2-chloroprocaine if epidural opioids are planned. Add epinephrine (1:400,000) to prolong the duration of lidocaine. Bupivacaine 0.5% and ropivacaine 0.5% have longer durations of action than lidocaine. Ropivacaine is thought to be less cardiotoxic than bupivacaine; do not use 0.75% bupivacaine in this setting. Disadvantages of epidural anesthesia include risks of local anesthetic toxicity (intravascular injection) and high spinal or subdural block, slower onset time, a less dense or patchy block, and a high incidence of PDPH when the dura is pierced. Administer a test dose. Think of each dose as a test dose; limit boluses to 5 ml every 2 to 5 minutes until the desired level is achieved. Aspirate prior to each bolus. Treat hypotension. If a high spinal occurs, aggressively manage the airway, provide positive-pressure ventilation with 100% oxygen (O_2), maintain exaggerated LUD, and provide IV fluids and vasopressors, including epinephrine. Exercise caution when considering spinal anesthesia after a failed epidural. Consider CSE as an alternative combining the advantages of spinal (i.e., faster onset and denser blockade) and epidural (i.e., titratable, continuous anesthesia, less profound hypotension) techniques. Evaluate the pros and cons of regional anesthesia in patients with thrombocytopenia or coagulopathy (risk of spinal or epidural hematoma). With regional anesthesia, consider supplemental sedation after delivery of the neonate, especially if the uterus is externalized.

F. For GETA, prep and drape prior to induction to minimize fetal drug exposure. Preoxygenate and perform an RSI with thiopental, propofol, ketamine, or etomidate (significance of neonatal serum cortisol suppression is controversial), and succinylcholine (SCC) or rocuronium, or perform awake, fiberoptic intubation. Use a short-handled laryngoscope and insert a smaller than normal endotracheal tube (ETT). Have difficult airway equipment immediately available. Monitor neuromuscular blockade (NMB)—may be prolonged in patients receiving $MgSO_4$ or metoclopramide. Maternal muscle relaxant rarely affects neonatal neuromuscular function. Maintain GETA with up to 50% N_2O (if fetal distress, administer 100% O_2) and <0.5 MAC volatile agents to prevent uterine atony.

G. After clamping of the umbilical cord, infuse oxytocin in crystalloid over 30 minutes to control postpartum hemorrhage; give prophylactic antibiotics if required. Administer methylergonovine or prostaglandin $F_{2\text{-alpha}}$ via IM or intramyometrial injection to treat refractory hemorrhage. Avoid IV administration of these agents (severe hypertension [HTN]). In addition, prostaglandin $F_{2\text{-alpha}}$ may produce profound bronchospasm; use with caution in patients with reactive airway disease.

REFERENCES

1. Kuczkowski KM, Reisner LS, Lin D: Anesthesia for cesarean section. In: Chestnut DH, editor: Obstetric anesthesia principles and practice, ed 3, Philadelphia, 2004, Elsevier Mosby.
2. Yaakov B: Stat cesarean delivery in the parturient with a difficult airway–regional or general anesthesia, *Curr Rev Clin Anesth* 22 (15):185–196, 2002.
3. Aya AG, Mangin R, Vialles N, et al.: Patients with severe preeclampsia experience less hypotension during spinal anesthesia for elective cesarean delivery than healthy parturients: a prospective cohort comparison, *Anesth Analg* 97:867–872, 2003.
4. Gaiser, RR: Changes in the provision of anesthesia for the parturient undergoing cesarean section, *Clin Obstet Gynecol* 46 (3): 646–656, 2003.

CESAREAN DELIVERY
(Cont'd from p 401)

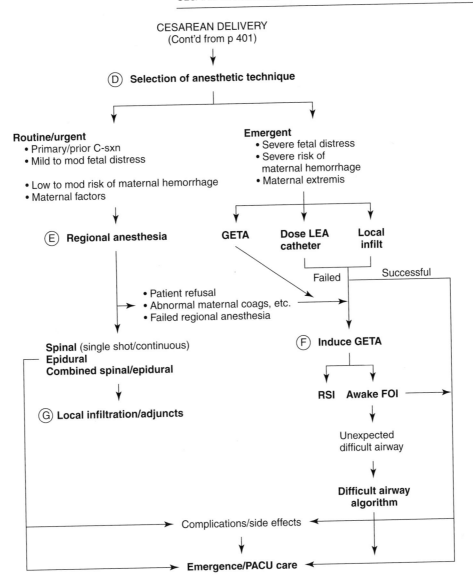

Ⓓ **Selection of anesthetic technique**

Routine/urgent
• Primary/prior C-sxn
• Mild to mod fetal distress

• Low to mod risk of maternal hemorrhage
• Maternal factors

Emergent
• Severe fetal distress
• Severe risk of
  maternal hemorrhage
• Maternal extremis

Ⓔ **Regional anesthesia**   **GETA**   **Dose LEA catheter**   **Local infilt**

Failed   Successful

• Patient refusal
• Abnormal maternal coags, etc.
• Failed regional anesthesia

Spinal (single shot/continuous)   Ⓕ **Induce GETA**
Epidural
Combined spinal/epidural

Ⓖ **Local infiltration/adjuncts**   **RSI   Awake FOI**

Unexpected
difficult airway

**Difficult airway
algorithm**

Complications/side effects

Emergence/PACU care

Pregnant Diabetic Patient

MOHAMED TIOURIRINE, M.D.

Diabetes mellitus (DM) occurring during pregnancy is divided into two categories. Parturients with pregestational DM have a diagnosis of diabetes mellitus type 1 or 2 prior to pregnancy. Parturients with gestational diabetes (GDM) have the onset of carbohydrate intolerance during pregnancy. Parturients with both GDM and pregestational DM have an increased risk of pregnancy-related complications.[1] Complications can be maternal (hypoglycemia, hyperglycemia, ketoacidosis, hyperosmolar hyperglycemic nonketotic coma [HHNC], superimposed hypertension [HTN], and nephropathy) or fetal (macrosomia, respiratory distress, preterm labor, hypoglycemia, hypocalcemia, fetal anomalies, and fetal demise). Diabetic patients who plan pregnancies should undergo preconceptual evaluation; tight glycemic control is an important part of the management of pregestational diabetes. Similarly, early diagnosis of GDM is important in improving fetal outcome. Anesthetic management of these patients can be challenging.

A. Review the patient's medical record. Determine the type (e.g., 1, 2, GDM) and classification of diabetes as an indication of the severity of the disease. Perform a history and physical examination. The most important clinical features to consider are the recognition of the "stiff joint syndrome, "autonomic dysfunction," and "gastroparesis," which is usually characteristic of long-standing DM. Another consideration is the presence of obesity; this is more typical of GDM and type 2 DM. Assess for the presence of long-term complications of DM (e.g., nephropathy, retinopathy, or vasculopathy) as well as short-term complications (e.g., adequacy of glucose control and preeclampsia). The presence of these clinical features increases the risk of aspiration, difficult intubation, and difficult epidural placement.

B. If vaginal delivery is expected, consider regional analgesia for labor. Epidural or combined spinal-epidural (CSE) are the preferred techniques. The advantages of regional techniques include patient comfort, reduction of maternal stress, and because an epidural catheter is in place, the ability to provide rapid anesthesia for an emergency procedure. There is a case report of severe maternal hypoglycemia following CSE analgesia for labor.[2] Therefore, monitor glucose levels throughout labor to detect complications such as DKA, HHNC, or hypoglycemic episodes.

C. If an elective cesarean delivery is planned, consider spinal, epidural, or CSE; all have all been used safely. Provide aspiration prophylaxis, avoid aorto-caval compression, and monitor glucose levels. In the case of an urgent or emergency cesarean delivery, avoid general anesthesia when possible because airway and aspiration risks are greater (due to stiff joint syndrome, obesity, gastroparesis, and autonomic dysfunction).

D. In the immediate postpartum period, be mindful of the risk of hypoglycemia; insulin requirements decrease dramatically after delivery. Postpartum hemorrhage can occur secondary to uterine atony. In the long term, patients with GDM must be followed; there is a risk that these patients will develop type 2 DM after delivery.

REFERENCES

1. Landon MB, Catalano PM, Gabbe SG: Diabetes mellitus. In Gabbe SG, Niebyl JR, and Simpson JL, editors: *Obstetrics: normal and problem pregnancies*, ed 4, New York, 2002, Churchill Livingstone.
2. Crites J, Ramanathan J: Acute hypoglycemia following combined spinal-epidural anesthesia (CSE) in a parturient with diabetes mellitus, *Anesthesiology* 93:591–592, 2000.

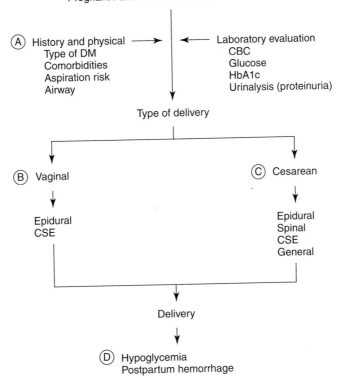

Pregnant Patient with DIABETES MELLITUS

(A) History and physical → ← Laboratory evaluation
    Type of DM   CBC
    Comorbidities   Glucose
    Aspiration risk   HbA1c
    Airway   Urinalysis (proteinuria)

Type of delivery

(B) Vaginal   (C) Cesarean

Epidural   Epidural
CSE   Spinal
                               CSE
                               General

Delivery

(D) Hypoglycemia
    Postpartum hemorrhage

Pregnant Cardiac Patient

JOY L. HAWKINS, M.D.

Cardiac disease during pregnancy is uncommon but remains the leading cause of maternal death caused by preexisting disease. With advances in neonatology, cardiology, and cardiac surgery, more women are reaching childbearing age with a congenital cardiac lesion. Fewer parturients have valvular lesions from rheumatic disease, but more have had valvular prosthetic replacements for congenital lesions.

A. Functional status before and during pregnancy is the best predictor of maternal outcome and helps determine the need for invasive monitoring at the time of delivery. The New York Heart Association (NYHA) classification is useful:

Class I: Asymptomatic
Class II: Symptoms with greater than normal activity
Class III: Symptoms with normal activity
Class IV: Symptoms at rest

In general, patients in Class I or II have a good prognosis, but functional status may deteriorate during pregnancy, especially when volume increases and cardiac output (CO) are maximal (28 to 30 weeks gestation and immediately postpartum).

B. The type of cardiac lesion also influences maternal risk.[1] Mortality may be 25 to 50% in patients with pulmonary hypertension (HTN), Eisenmenger's Syndrome, coarctation of the aorta with valvular involvement, and Marfan syndrome with aortic involvement. These women should be counseled to consider sterilization or first-trimester termination. If a pregnancy is carried to term, a 5 to 15% mortality rate may be expected in patients with severe mitral stenosis (Classes III and IV or with atrial fibrillation), severe aortic stenosis, and previous myocardial infarction (MI).

C. Physiological changes during pregnancy may significantly affect the course of cardiac disease. Increased intravascular volume leads to volume overload. Decreased systemic vascular resistance (SVR) causes more right-to-left shunting. Hypercoagulability increases the need for anticoagulation. CO and HR increase during labor. Volume shifts occur at delivery. Optimize the patient's antepartum status in consultation with her cardiologist (bed rest, aggressive medical management, and invasive monitoring if needed). Replace warfarin with dalteparin. Change to subcutaneous heparin at 36 weeks gestation (approximately 10,000 units every 8 to 12 hours) and maintain a partial thromboplastin time (PTT) at twice control.[2] If necessary, heparin may be reversed intrapartum with protamine. Cardiac surgery should not be automatically withheld during pregnancy. Maternal mortality is comparable to the nonpregnant patient, although fetal mortality may be high if preterm delivery occurs. If possible, schedule surgery during the second trimester to decrease risks of teratogenicity and preterm labor. Use high pump flows and pressures to maximize uterine blood flow, and use fetal monitoring after 24 weeks' gestation to optimize the intrauterine environment. Expect fetal bradycardia to occur at the onset of cardiopulmonary bypass. Hypothermia may be used.[3]

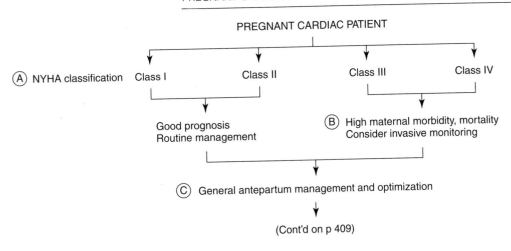

(Cont'd on p 409)

TABLE 1
Vaginal versus Cesarean Delivery

	Vaginal delivery	Elective cesarean delivery
Advantages	Less blood loss Avoids surgical stress Hemodynamic stability Early ambulation	Able to time delivery Avoids need for emergency cesarean
Disadvantages	Labor can be prolonged, unpredictable	Major surgery Major anesthetic Increased risk of hemorrhage Postoperative infection Postoperative pulmonary complications

TABLE 2
Cardiovascular Effects of Obstetric Drugs

Side Effect	Medication
↑ HR	Beta-agonist tocolytic agents, meperidine
↑ Pulmonary vascular resistance (PVR)	Carboprost tromethamine, methylergonovine, parenteral narcotics (↑PCO_2)
↑ SVR	Carboprost tromethamine, methylergonovine
↓ SVR	Regional anesthesia, morphine, prostaglandin E_2 (PGE_2), beta-agonist tocolytic agents, oxytocin (bolus), magnesium (bolus)

D. Use antepartum and intrapartum left uterine displacement and supplemental oxygen. Use regional analgesia for most lesions to minimize fluctuations in CO. Deliver in a setting in which specialized management, especially critical care nursing, is available. Plan a shortened second stage of labor with instrumented delivery if necessary. The route of delivery (vaginal versus cesarean delivery) should be based on obstetric, not cardiac considerations (Table 1). Most patients should receive bacterial endocarditis prophylaxis using ampicillin 2 g (vancomycin 1 g if allergic) and gentamicin 1.5 mg/kg. Regional anesthetic techniques such as continuous lumbar epidural (CLE) or spinal (CSA) or combined spinal-epidural (CSE) anesthetics are usually well tolerated. Support SVR as needed with phenylephrine. Parturients with severely stenotic valvular lesions or right-to-left shunts (severe mitral or aortic stenosis, pulmonary HTN, or cyanotic congenital lesions) may not tolerate decreased SVR or decreased venous return to the right ventricle. Labor analgesia for these patients may be managed with intrathecal narcotics, either single shot or through a continuous spinal catheter, or with IV patient-controlled narcotics and a pudendal block for delivery. If general anesthesia is required for cesarean delivery, a controlled cardiac induction using opioids as needed should be preceded by aspiration prophylaxis using an H_2-receptor antagonist, metoclopramide, and a non-particulate antacid.[4–7]

E. Many obstetric drugs have hemodynamic consequences, and their side effects could be harmful with specific cardiac lesions.

REFERENCES

1. Poppas A, Carson MP, Rosene-Montella K, Powrie RO: Cardiovascular disease. In: Lee RV, Rosene-Montella K, Barbour LA, Garner PR, Keely E, editors, *Medical care of the pregnant patient*. Philadelphia, 2000, American College of Physicians.
2. American College of Obstetricians and Gynecologists: *Thromboembolism in pregnancy*. ACOG Practice Bulletin #19, Washington DC, 2000.
3. Strickland RA, Oliver WC, Chantigian RC, et al.: Anesthesia, cardiopulmonary bypass, and the pregnant patient. *Mayo Clin Proc* 66:411–429, 1991.
4. Ridley DM, Smiley RM: The parturient with cardiac disease. *Anesthesiol Clin North Am*, 16:419–440, 1998.
5. Camann WR, Thornhill ML: Cardiovascular disease. In: Chestnut DH, editor: *Obstetric anesthesia*, St. Louis, 1999, Mosby.
6. Cox PB, Gogarten W, Marcus MA: Maternal cardiac disease, *Curr Opin Anaesthesiol* 18 (3):257–262, 2005.
7. Gomar C, Errando CL: Neuroaxial anaesthesia in obstetrical patients with cardiac disease, *Curr Opin Anaesthesiol* 18 (5): 507–512, 2005.

PREGNANT CARDIAC PATIENT
(Cont'd from p 407)

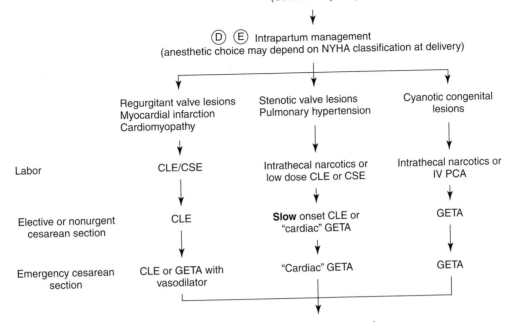

Ⓓ Ⓔ Intrapartum management
(anesthetic choice may depend on NYHA classification at delivery)

	Regurgitant valve lesions Myocardial infarction Cardiomyopathy	Stenotic valve lesions Pulmonary hypertension	Cyanotic congenital lesions
Labor	CLE/CSE	Intrathecal narcotics or low dose CLE or CSE	Intrathecal narcotics or IV PCA
Elective or nonurgent cesarean section	CLE	**Slow** onset CLE or "cardiac" GETA	GETA
Emergency cesarean section	CLE or GETA with vasodilator	"Cardiac" GETA	GETA

Postpartum management
Consider transfer to ICU for monitoring and nursing care

Nonobstetric Surgery in Pregnancy

JINNY KIM HARTMAN, M.D.

Approximately 2% of pregnant women in the United States undergo surgery and anesthesia each year for indications unrelated to gestation (i.e., appendicitis, adnexal and cervical diseases, cholelithiasis, breast tumors, or trauma).[1-3] Anesthesia during pregnancy is unique in that it requires careful consideration of two patients simultaneously—mother and fetus. Risks to the mother are due to the physiological changes of pregnancy most significant of which involve the airway, pulmonary, cardiac, CNS, and GI systems. Parturients are at increased risk for aspiration, difficult airway, hypoxemia, hypotension, anesthetic overdose, and embolic phenomena. The risks to the fetus include the potential for teratogenicity, asphyxia, and preterm delivery. Elective surgery should be delayed until about 6 weeks after delivery. Urgent surgery should be delayed until the second trimester when organogenesis (15 to 56 days) is complete. Emergency surgery cannot be delayed and should be performed under local or regional anesthesia when possible. It is important to note that to date, no correlation has been made between anesthesia and poor fetal outcome. The more critical factors are severity of underlying maternal illness and site or invasiveness of surgery.

A. A complete history and physical examination is essential. Airway examination is especially important in the pregnant patient. Pregnancy can cause increased airway vascularity and edema and thus increase the likelihood of a difficult intubation. There is an increased risk of aspiration caused by mechanical and hormonal factors and is greatest after 12 to 14 weeks' gestation. Gastric volume is increased due to delayed gastric emptying and increased secretion, and pH is lowered due to increased parietal cell activity. Parturients are at increased risk for hypoxemia, because of a decrease in FRC and RV as well as an increase in oxygen consumption (about 20% for all by the second trimester). Hypotension from aortocaval compression can occur in up to 30% of parturients. Left uterine displacement (LUD) is necessary when placing patients in the supine position. Pregnant women have increased sensitivity to inhalational, IV, and regional anesthetics. MAC is decreased (20 to 40%), presumably from the sedative effects of progesterone. Local anesthetic requirements are also decreased (30%). All anesthetic doses must be adjusted accordingly.

410

Pregnant patient for NONOBSTETRIC SURGERY

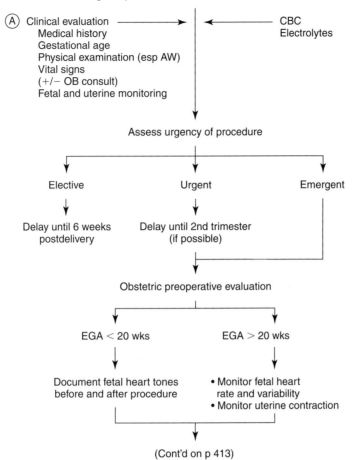

Ⓐ Clinical evaluation
   Medical history
   Gestational age
   Physical examination (esp AW)
   Vital signs
   (+/− OB consult)
   Fetal and uterine monitoring

CBC
Electrolytes

Assess urgency of procedure

Elective   Urgent   Emergent

Delay until 6 weeks   Delay until 2nd trimester
   postdelivery   (if possible)

Obstetric preoperative evaluation

EGA < 20 wks   EGA > 20 wks

Document fetal heart tones   • Monitor fetal heart
before and after procedure   rate and variability
                                    • Monitor uterine contraction

(Cont'd on p 413)

B. Main concerns for both mother and fetus are to prevent maternal hypoxemia and hypotension. This will in turn prevent fetal asphyxia and distress. Considerations for the fetus are mainly teratogenicity of anesthetic agents and premature delivery. Administer supplemental oxygen (O_2). The effects of anesthetic agents on fetal development and hemostasis have been evaluated by three main classes of studies: (1) small animal studies, (2) epidemiologic surveys of health care workers chronically exposed to inhalational anesthetics in the work environment, and (3) outcome studies in women who have undergone surgery during pregnancy. To date, no currently used anesthetic agent (excluding cocaine) has been proven to be teratogenic or abortifacient in humans.[4–7] However, some controversy remains, especially with regard to nitrous oxide. Nitrous oxide is known to oxidize vitamin B_{12}, a coenzyme needed for DNA synthesis. Nitrous also increases adrenergic tone, possibly constricting uterine vasculature and decreasing uterine blood flow. Early small animal studies showed a high incidence of organ anomalies and fetal resorption in rats exposed to 50 to 75% nitrous oxide. It should be noted however that the duration of exposure was not typical of clinical anesthetic use (24 hours). In addition, findings in rats cannot necessarily be applied to humans. Benzodiazepines were also controversial; the Centers for Disease Control and Prevention (CDC) reported an increase in cleft lip anomalies in infants born to women exposed to diazepam. Further studies have failed to support the original findings. Ultimately, it is best to choose agents with a long history of safe use in humans (e.g., thiopental, etomidate, ketamine, fentanyl, morphine, isoflurane, muscle relaxants, or local anesthetics). Let it be emphasized that to date, no correlation has been found between anesthesia and outcome of pregnancy.

C. Local or regional anesthesia is preferable to general anesthesia because they minimize drug exposure to the mother and fetus. Administer a nonparticulate antacid within 30 minutes of the procedure. Adequately preload with a balanced salt solution, maintain LUD position, and give supplemental O_2. Monitor as for general anesthesia. Avoid hypoxia, hypotension, hyperglycemia, and hypoglycemia. If a vasopressor is needed, use ephedrine first. Always be ready to induce general anesthesia should the need arise.

D. If general anesthesia is required, place the patient in LUD position to avoid hypotension and decreased uteroplacental blood flow. Again, avoid hypoxemia hypotension, hypoglycemia, and hyperglycemia. Give anxiolytics if necessary to prevent hyperventilation and alkalosis which can cause vasoconstriction and decreased oxygen transfer to the fetus. Administer a nonparticulate antacid with an H_2-receptor blocking agent or metoclopramide. Carefully evaluate the airway, monitor BP, ECG, oxygenation, ventilation and temperature. Preoxygenate, choose an RSI with cricoid pressure. If the fetus is 20 to 24 weeks estimated gestational age, apply an external Doppler monitor and a tocodynamometer as per obstetric/gynecologic consult.[8] It is common for baseline HR and beat to beat variability to decrease under anesthesia. Decelerations are not normal, however, and indicate fetal stress. Use drugs that have a safe history as previously mentioned. Administer at least 50% O_2 and decreased doses of inhalational agents. A combination of narcotic, volatile agent, and muscle relaxant is a safe and effective technique. Extubate when the patient is fully awake and reversed (because of full stomach).

REFERENCES

1. Kuczkowski KM: Nonobstetric surgery during pregnancy: what are the risks of anesthesia? *Obstet Gynecol Surv* 59 (1):52–56, 2004.
2. Cohen-Kerem R, Railton C, Oren D, et al.: Pregnancy outcome following non-obstetric surgical intervention, *Am J Surg* 190 (3): 467–473, 2005.
3. Logsdon-Poborny VK: Gynecologic surgery during pregnancy, *Clin Obstet Gynecol* 37:294–305, 1994.
4. Boivin JF: Risk of spontaneous abortion in women occupationally exposed to anesthetic gases: a meta-analysis, *Occup Environ Med* 54:541–548, 1997.
5. Fink BR, Shepard TH, Blandau RJ: Teratogenic activity of nitrous oxide, *Nature* 214:146–148, 1967.
6. Masse RI, Fujinaga M, Rice SA, et al.: Reproductive and teratogenic effects of nitrous oxide, halothane, isoflurane and enflurane in Sprague-Dawley rats, *Anesthesiology* 64:339–344, 1986.
7. Safra MJ, Oadley GP: Association between cleft lip with or without cleft palate and prenatal exposure to diazepam, *Lancet* 2:478, 1975.
8. Ong BY, Baron K, Stearns EL, et al.: Severe fetal bradycardia in a pregnant surgical patient despite normal oxygenation and blood pressure, *Can J Anaesth* 50 (9):922–935, 2003.

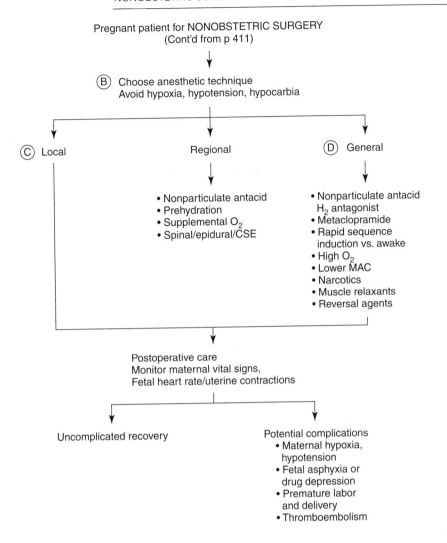

Pregnant patient for NONOBSTETRIC SURGERY
(Cont'd from p 411)

(B) Choose anesthetic technique
Avoid hypoxia, hypotension, hypocarbia

(C) Local

Regional
• Nonparticulate antacid
• Prehydration
• Supplemental O_2
• Spinal/epidural/CSE

(D) General
• Nonparticulate antacid
  H_2 antagonist
• Metaclopramide
• Rapid sequence
  induction vs. awake
• High O_2
• Lower MAC
• Narcotics
• Muscle relaxants
• Reversal agents

Postoperative care
Monitor maternal vital signs,
Fetal heart rate/uterine contractions

Uncomplicated recovery

Potential complications
• Maternal hypoxia,
  hypotension
• Fetal asphyxia or
  drug depression
• Premature labor
  and delivery
• Thromboembolism

Maternal Infections and Anesthesia

FRED J. SPIELMAN, M.D.

DAVID C. MAYER, M.D.

During pregnancy, immunoglobulin levels decrease and lymphocyte function and numbers are diminished. Invasive maternal and fetal monitoring, prolonged labor, vaginal examinations, uterine catheters, and fetal scalp electrodes may increase intrauterine infections. Pregnant women may have viral infections (e.g., herpes simplex virus [HSV] or human immunodeficiency virus [HIV]) or acute bacterial infections (e.g., chorioamnionitis). Maternal infection is associated with preterm delivery and the direct fetal effects, such as meningitis, sepsis, and pneumonia. Extreme temperature elevations may have a deleterious effect on the fetus and mother due to tachycardia and increased oxygen consumption and catecholamine production.

A. Perform a physical examination. Maternal fever is abnormal and etiology must be determined. Obtain a complete blood count (CBC) with differential, appropriate cultures, and radiography, if indicated. When fetal well-being is compromised, consider urgent delivery.

B. Intraamniotic infections (IAI) such as chorioamnionitis occur in 1% of pregnancies, especially during premature rupture of membranes due to ascending passage of Bacteroides, group B streptococci, or *Escherichia coli*. Look for fever, maternal or fetal tachycardia, malodorous amniotic fluid, and uterine tenderness. Bacteremia occurs in 10% of cases. Therefore, institute antibiotic therapy early and deliver the baby expeditiously. Uterine infections may affect uterine contractility and result in dysfunctional labor, increased hemorrhage, and cesarean delivery.[1] Perform regional anesthesia cautiously in the febrile patient, after antibiotic therapy is initiated and a stable or declining temperature is documented. Development of meningitis or epidural abscess is a rare event in patients with IAI. Two retrospective studies of regional anesthesia in women with IAI did not demonstrate an increase in meningitis or epidural abscess even when patients did not receive antibiotics prior to epidural catheter insertion.[2,3] In another study, bacteremic rats pretreated with antibiotics prior to dural puncture did not develop meningitis.[4]

C. HIV is associated with an increased incidence of premature rupture of membranes, low birth weight, and preterm birth. For the best neonatal outcome, minimize the infant's exposure to maternal blood and vaginal secretions; the use of zidovudine during pregnancy and elective cesarean delivery has dramatically reduced the vertical transmission.[5] Apply universal precautions (meticulous handling of needles, airway devices, and the patient's body secretions). Perform regional anesthesia after careful neurological examination. The virus infects the CNS early in the course of disease; therefore, even in asymptomatic patients, regional anesthesia is not contraindicated. In a study of 30 HIV-positive parturients receiving spinal, epidural, or parenteral analgesia-anesthesia, there was no acceleration or progression of neurological or infectious complications during a 6-month followup period.[6] Three patients in the study had inadvertent dural punctures with an epidural needle; epidural blood patch (EBP) was not performed. Although EBP has been used safely in HIV-positive patients, the procedure, although most likely safe, is controversial.[7] Alternatively, consider an infusion of normal saline. Avoid regional anesthesia in the presence of multiorgan involvement and unstable cardiorespiratory or neurological function.

D. Genital herpes infections are caused by herpes simplex virus-2 (HSV-2). The greatest risk during pregnancy is the development of neonatal herpes infection, which can cause CNS damage or death. Transmission occurs with fetal passage during vaginal delivery. Cesarean delivery is performed in a laboring patient with visible lesions to reduce neonatal viral exposure. Consider regional anesthesia; regional anesthesia has not been associated with neurological infections or sequelae in parturients with recurrent HSV infections.[8] Use of regional anesthesia in patients with primary HSV is controversial, because viremia may be present. Neuraxial morphine has been associated with recrudescence of oral herpetic lesions (HSV-1), possibly resulting from immunological changes that occur in the trigeminal nerve ganglia.[9] However, most anesthesiologists do not consider a history of oral herpes to be a contraindication to epidural or spinal morphine.

E. Epidural analgesia has been suggested as a cause of maternal pyrexia. The etiology is unclear, but an infectious source is unlikely and no fetal ill effects have been noted. Investigations of temperature changes during labor have found that epidural analgesia causes, at most, mild elevation in maternal temperature that should not be confused with fever secondary to IAI.[10]

REFERENCES

1. Duff P, Sanders R, Gibbs RS: The course of labor in term patients with chorioamnionitis, Am J Obstet Gynecol 147:391–395, 1983.
2. Bader AM, Gilbertson L, Kirz L, et al.: Regional anesthesia in women with chorioamnionitis, Reg Anesth 17:84–86, 1992.
3. Ramanathan J, Vaddadi A, Mercer BM, et al.: Epidural anesthesia in women with chorioamnionitis, Anesthesiol Rev 19:35, 1992.
4. Carp H, Bailey S: The association between meningitis and dural puncture in bacteremic rats, Anesthesiology 76:739–742, 1992.
5. Connor EM, Sperling RS, Gelber R, et al.: Reduction of maternal-infant transmission of human immunodeficiency virus type 1 with

MATERNAL INFECTION AT TERM

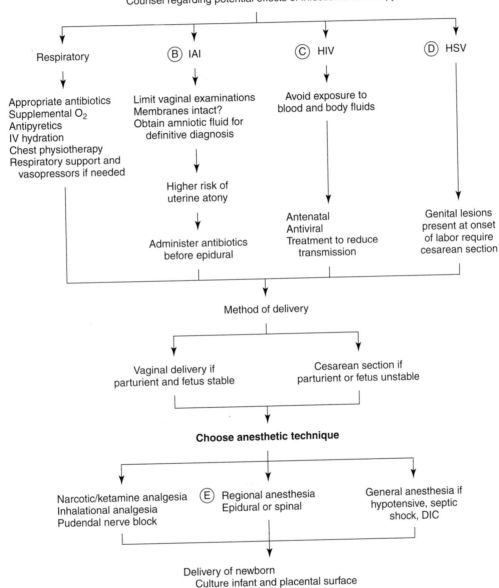

Ⓐ Clinical evaluation/risk factors ——————→   ←—— Laboratory values
   History and physical examination: CBC, differential, urinalysis
      Invasive maternal and fetal monitoring   Cultures and sensitivity
      Fetal tachycardia   Radiography
      Malodorous amniotic fluid

Predelivery assessment
   Specific infection (IAI, HIV, HSV)
   Consultations (perinatologist, neonatologist, infectious
      disease specialist)
   Planned route of delivery
   Counsel regarding potential effects of infection and therapy

Respiratory   Ⓑ IAI   Ⓒ HIV   Ⓓ HSV

Appropriate antibiotics   Limit vaginal examinations   Avoid exposure to   Genital lesions
Supplemental O₂   Membranes intact?   blood and body fluids   present at onset
Antipyretics   Obtain amniotic fluid for   of labor require
IV hydration   definitive diagnosis   cesarean section
Chest physiotherapy
Respiratory support and
   vasopressors if needed

                            Higher risk of
                            uterine atony

                            Administer antibiotics   Antenatal
                            before epidural   Antiviral
                                                           Treatment to reduce
                                                           transmission

Method of delivery

Vaginal delivery if   Cesarean section if
parturient and fetus stable   parturient or fetus unstable

Choose anesthetic technique

Narcotic/ketamine analgesia   Ⓔ Regional anesthesia   General anesthesia if
Inhalational analgesia   Epidural or spinal   hypotensive, septic
Pudendal nerve block   shock, DIC

Delivery of newborn
   Culture infant and placental surface
   Observe and monitor newborn for
      sepsis, colonization, acidemia

zidovudine treatment. Pediatric AIDS Clinical Trials Group Protocol 076 Study Group, *N Engl J Med* 331:1173–1180, 1994.

6. Hughes SC, Dailey PA, Landers D, et al.: Parturients infected with human immunodeficiency virus and regional anesthesia. Clinical and immunologic response, *Anesthesiology* 82:32–37, 1995.

7. Tom DJ, Gulevich SJ, Shapiro HM, et al.: Epidural blood patch in the HIV-positive patient: review of clinical experience. San Diego HIV Neurobehavioral Research Center, *Anesthesiology* 76:943–947, 1992.

8. Bader AM, Camann WR, Datta S: Anesthesia for cesarean delivery in patients with herpes simplex virus type-2 infections, *Reg Anesth* 15:261–263, 1990.

9. Boyle RK: A review of the anatomical and immunological links between epidural morphine and herpes simplex labialis in obstetric patients, *Anaesth Intens Care* 23:425–432, 1995.

10. Vallejo MC, Kaul B, Adler LJ, et al.: Chorioamnionitis, not epidural analgesia, is associated with maternal fever during labour, *Can J Anaesth* 48:1122–1126, 2001.

Labor and Delivery in the Patient Susceptible to Malignant Hyperthermia (MH)

M. JOANNE DOUGLAS, M.D.

Malignant hyperthermia (MH), an inherited disorder of skeletal muscle, may present as a life-threatening hypermetabolic crisis when affected patients are exposed to triggers, such as succinylcholine (SCC) or volatile anesthetics. Reported episodes of MH during labor and delivery are rare, but death has occurred. Management of MH-susceptible (MHS) parturients involves avoiding known triggers and instituting prompt intervention and treatment when a reaction is diagnosed.

A. Consider the parturient at risk for MH if she has a positive caffeine halothane contracture test (CHCT) or, in the absence of muscle biopsy, an unequivocal MH reaction or a positive family history. Deoxyribonucleic acid (DNA) linkage markers are of limited benefit to certain families because MH is a multigenic disorder.[1] Creatine kinase (CK) levels are not diagnostic of MH.

B. Previous anesthesia consultation and immediate notification of admission to the labor suite ensure that equipment and appropriate medications are immediately available. Inform the neonatologist in case dantrolene is to be used before delivery (the infant will need to be observed for sedation and hypotonia if dantrolene is administered before birth).

C. Early institution of an epidural block provides effective analgesia, which can be extended for operative delivery, if required, thus avoiding general anesthesia. Safe agents include local anesthetics, narcotics, and nitrous oxide. The use of ephedrine is controversial, although other adrenergic agents have not been shown to trigger MH.[2] The signs of an MH reaction (tachycardia, tachypnea, labile BP, or fever) are also signs of infection. Remember, not all that is hot is MH.

D. Cesarean section should be performed only for obstetric reasons. A regional technique is preferred. If contraindicated, use nontriggering anesthetic agents (thiopental, nondepolarizing muscle relaxants [NDMRs], narcotics, nitrous oxide, or oxygen). Rocuronium (0.6 to 0.9 mg/kg) is an alternative to SCC for intubation but adequate relaxation requires an induction dose of thiopental (4 to 6 mg/kg).[3] Oxytocin is safe. If the cesarean section is elective, prepare the anesthesia machine by changing the soda lime and breathing circuit. Remove the vaporizers and flush with oxygen (O$_2$) at 10 L/min for 10 to 20 min.[4] If a reaction develops unexpectedly it is unnecessary to change the machine immediately (see G).

E. Prepare or obtain MH equipment and drugs, including dantrolene, sterile water for mixing, other resuscitative drugs (sodium bicarbonate or procainamide), ABG and CVP monitoring equipment and a cooling blanket. It is essential to monitor BP, ECG, temperature with two probes (axillary and core), end-tidal carbon dioxide (CO$_2$), and pulse oximetry. Cold IV solutions and ice should be available.

F. Only one case of possible MH in a newborn has been reported.[5] Although dantrolene crosses the placenta, adverse reactions in neonates have not been reported.[6] Watch the infant for sedation and hypotonia if dantrolene is administered before birth.

G. Dantrolene prophylaxis is not recommended for the parturient because of placental transfer. Uterine atony has been reported with dantrolene[7] and is most likely related to mannitol (carrier vehicle).[8] If a reaction develops, it is no longer considered necessary to change the anesthetic tubing or soda lime. Initiate treatment as listed in chapters 58, 59, and 60.

H. Following an MH episode, monitor for 24 hours or longer; continue dantrolene for at least 24 hours (1 mg/kg). Measure CK levels at the time of the reaction and repeat 24 hours later when peak levels occur.[9] Offer genetic counseling and diagnostic muscle biopsy testing (CHCT) to family members.

REFERENCES

1. Sambuughin N, Sei Y, Gallagher KL, et al.: North American malignant hyperthermia population: screening of the ryanodine receptor gene and identification of novel mutations, Anesthesiology 95:594–599, 2001.
2. Urwyler A, Censier K, Seeberger MD, et al.: In vitro effect of ephedrine, adrenaline, noradrenaline and isoprenaline on halothane-induced contractures in skeletal muscle from patients potentially susceptible to malignant hyperthermia, Br J Anaesth 70:76–79, 1993.
3. Abouleish E, Abboud T, Lechevalier T, et al.: Rocuronium (Org 9426) for caesarean section, Br J Anaesth 73:336–341, 1994.
4. Beebe JJ, Sessler DI: Preparation of anesthesia machines for patients susceptible to malignant hyperthermia, Anesthesiology 69:395–400, 1988.
5. Sewall K, Flowerdew RM, Bromberger P: Severe muscular rigidity at birth: malignant hyperthermia syndrome? Can Anaesth Soc J 27:279–282, 1980.
6. Craft JB, Goldberg NH, Lim M, et al.: Cardiovascular effects and placental passage of dantrolene in the maternal-fetal sheep model, Anesthesiology 68:68–71, 1988.
7. Weingarten AE, Korsh JI, Neuman GG, et al.: Postpartum uterine atony after intravenous dantrolene, Anesth Analg 66:269–270, 1987.
8. Shin YK, Kim YD, Collea JV, et al.: Effect of dantrolene sodium on contractility of isolated human uterine muscle, Int J Obstet Anesth 4:197–200, 1995.
9. Antognini JF: Creatine kinase alterations after acute malignant hyperthermia episodes and common surgical procedures, Anesth Analg 81:1039–1042, 1995.

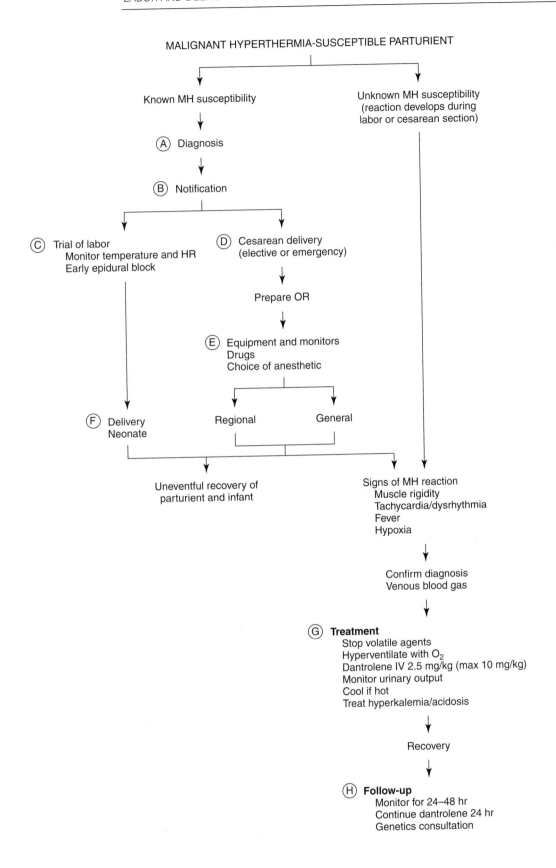

MALIGNANT HYPERTHERMIA-SUSCEPTIBLE PARTURIENT

Known MH susceptibility

Unknown MH susceptibility
(reaction develops during
labor or cesarean section)

(A) Diagnosis

(B) Notification

(C) Trial of labor
    Monitor temperature and HR
    Early epidural block

(D) Cesarean delivery
    (elective or emergency)

Prepare OR

(E) Equipment and monitors
    Drugs
    Choice of anesthetic

Regional   General

(F) Delivery
    Neonate

Uneventful recovery of
parturient and infant

Signs of MH reaction
Muscle rigidity
Tachycardia/dysrhythmia
Fever
Hypoxia

Confirm diagnosis
Venous blood gas

(G) **Treatment**
    Stop volatile agents
    Hyperventilate with O_2
    Dantrolene IV 2.5 mg/kg (max 10 mg/kg)
    Monitor urinary output
    Cool if hot
    Treat hyperkalemia/acidosis

Recovery

(H) **Follow-up**
    Monitor for 24–48 hr
    Continue dantrolene 24 hr
    Genetics consultation

Amniotic Fluid Embolism (AFE)

MOHAMED TIOURIRINE, M.D.

Amniotic fluid embolism (AFE) is an unpredictable, unpreventable, uncommon disorder of pregnancy (incidence between 1 in 8,000 and 1 in 80,000) with a high morbidity and mortality (mortality reported between 61 and 86%).[1-3] Survivors often have irreversible neurological sequelae. Early recognition and supportive treatment are necessary for improved outcomes. AFE is defined as the abrupt entry of amniotic fluid (AF) through the uteroplacental or endocervical veins into the maternal circulation. The pathophysiology is not completely understood, but it is no longer thought to be an embolic problem. Rather, the injury is thought to be a result of an inflammatory response to circulating AF.[3] It has been suggested that the process be renamed the "Anaphylactoid Syndrome of Pregnancy."[4] Three phases are described.[1] First, the acute cardiopulmonary insult (dyspnea, cyanosis, hypoxemia, hypotension, pulmonary edema, seizures, coma) occurs. Second, coagulopathy develops. Third, end-organ damage is apparent. Most patients die within the first hour after the onset of symptoms.[4]

A. Three conditions are necessary for the occurrence of AFE: rupture of membranes (spontaneous or artificial), an open uterine or endocervical vein, and a pressure gradient to force fluid into the venous system. Meconium may be an aggravating factor. Other reported predisposing factors include advanced maternal age, multiparity, use of uterine stimulants, short or tumultuous labor, uterine distension, cephalopelvic disproportion, fetal demise, cesarean delivery, amniocentesis, and uterine rupture. AFE has also been reported following amnioinfusion, cervical suture removal, and intrauterine injection of hypertonic saline to induce abortion.[1]

B. AFE usually presents suddenly and progresses rapidly to cardiopulmonary collapse. AFE may be heralded by the abrupt onset of chills, vomiting, anxiety, chest discomfort, coughing, and a sensation of exhaustion and impending doom. This is followed by respiratory distress, cardiovascular collapse, shock, seizures, coma, and death. Cardiovascular collapse is the result of left ventricular (LV) dysfunction.[2] Most patients develop noncardiogenic pulmonary edema; patients have frothy pink sputum, jugular venous distension, and rales. Patients surviving the cardiopulmonary insult often develop a consumptive coagulopathy.

C. The diagnosis of AFE is one of exclusion.[3] Approach systematically any episode of cardiopulmonary compromise or massive hemorrhage in the peripartum period. The differential diagnosis includes thrombotic or venous air embolism; aspiration of gastric contents; eclampsia; toxic reaction to local anesthetic; total spinal; hemorrhagic, septic, or anaphylactic shock; cardiomyopathy; and intracranial hemorrhage.

D. There is no specific laboratory test for AFE. Patients are usually acutely unstable and it may be difficult to obtain diagnostic tests in a timely fashion. Examine the ECG for signs of cor pulmonale and changes in the T waves and ST segments. Consider a chest x-ray (CXR) to look for evidence of pulmonary edema. A lung V/Q scan may show nonspecific perfusion defects. Echocardiography (echo) can confirm LV failure. A recent report described the use of transesophageal echocardiography (TEE) to aid in the diagnosis of AFE in a patient with cardiovascular collapse during cesarean section.[5] TEE showed a severely dilated, akinetic right ventricle (RV) and an empty left ventricle consistent with dramatic pulmonary vasoconstriction. Aspirate blood from the pulmonary artery (PA) and examine for fetal debris, lanugo, and meconium; all are supportive of AFE. Because AFE resembles anaphylaxis, tryptase has been evaluated as a diagnostic tool, but results are still controversial.[6,7]

E. Provide supportive treatment. Maintain communication with the obstetrician and call for help. Ensure adequate oxygenation and ventilation; most patients require intubation. Add PEEP if the patient is hypoxic despite high FiO_2. Support the circulation by securing two large-bore IV catheters and infusing volume. Insert invasive monitors. Send a blood specimen for ABG, mixed venous gas, type and cross-match, complete blood count (CBC), and coagulation profile. Treat bleeding with blood components (RBC, FFP, cryoprecipitate, platelets) as dictated by lab results. Treat uterine atony. Administer vasopressors and inotropes as required to maintain BP and cardiac output (CO), vasodilators for afterload reduction, and diuretics to treat pulmonary edema as indicated by the clinical circumstance.

REFERENCES

1. Gei AF, Vadhera RB, Hankins GD: Embolism during pregnancy: thrombus, air, and amniotic fluid, *Anesthesiol Clin North Am* 21 (1):165–182, 2003.
2. Pereira A, Krieger BP: Pulmonary complications of pregnancy, *Clin Chest Med* 25 (2):299–310, 2004.
3. Davies S: Amniotic fluid embolus: a review of the literature, *Can J Anaesth* 48 (1):88–98, 2001.
4. Clark SL, Hankins GDV, Dudley DA, et al. Amniotic fluid embolism: analysis of the national registry, *Am J Obstet Gynecol* 172:1158–1167, 1995.
5. Stanten RD, Iverson LI, Daugharty TM, et al.: Amniotic fluid embolism causing catastrophic pulmonary vasoconstriction: diagnosis by transesophageal echocardiogram and treatment by cardiopulmonary bypass, *Obstet Gynecol* 102:496–498, 2003.
6. Farrar SC, Gherman RB: Serum tryptase analysis in a woman with amniotic fluid embolism. A case report, *J Reprod Med* 46:926–928, 2001.
7. Benson MD, Lindberg RE: Amniotic fluid embolism, anaphylaxis, and tryptase, *Am J Obstet Gynecol* 175:737, 1996.

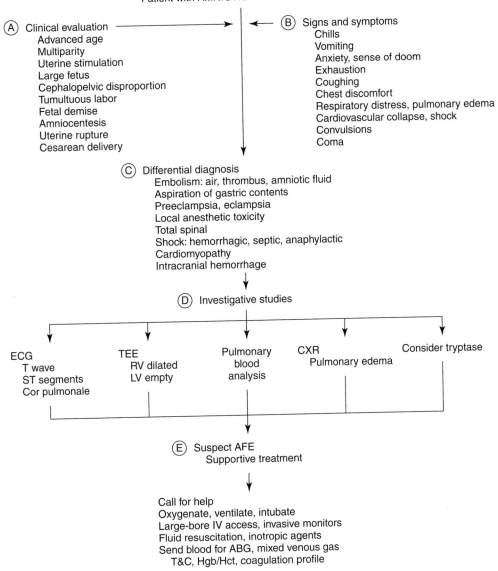

Patient with AMNIOTIC FLUID EMBOLISM

Ⓐ Clinical evaluation
    Advanced age
    Multiparity
    Uterine stimulation
    Large fetus
    Cephalopelvic disproportion
    Tumultuous labor
    Fetal demise
    Amniocentesis
    Uterine rupture
    Cesarean delivery

Ⓑ Signs and symptoms
    Chills
    Vomiting
    Anxiety, sense of doom
    Exhaustion
    Coughing
    Chest discomfort
    Respiratory distress, pulmonary edema
    Cardiovascular collapse, shock
    Convulsions
    Coma

Ⓒ Differential diagnosis
    Embolism: air, thrombus, amniotic fluid
    Aspiration of gastric contents
    Preeclampsia, eclampsia
    Local anesthetic toxicity
    Total spinal
    Shock: hemorrhagic, septic, anaphylactic
    Cardiomyopathy
    Intracranial hemorrhage

Ⓓ Investigative studies

ECG
  T wave
  ST segments
  Cor pulmonale

TEE
  RV dilated
  LV empty

Pulmonary
blood
analysis

CXR
  Pulmonary edema

Consider tryptase

Ⓔ Suspect AFE
  Supportive treatment

Call for help
Oxygenate, ventilate, intubate
Large-bore IV access, invasive monitors
Fluid resuscitation, inotropic agents
Send blood for ABG, mixed venous gas
    T&C, Hgb/Hct, coagulation profile

Morbidly Obese Parturient

MOHAMED TIOURIRINE, M.D.

The combination of obesity and pregnancy presents a major health care dilemma for both the anesthesiologist and the obstetrician.[1,2] The morbidly obese parturient is at increased risk for antepartum, intrapartum, and postpartum complications. These include preeclampsia, gestational hypertension (HTN), gestational diabetes, fetal macrosomia, preterm labor and delivery, postpartum hemorrhage, and an increased incidence of instrumental vaginal delivery and cesarean section. In the midst of such obstetrical misfortune, the anesthesiologist is also faced with a myriad of challenges including IV access, BP measurement, neuraxial anesthesia, aspiration risk, and airway management. Early knowledge of the obstetrical management plan is crucial to developing a safe anesthetic plan.

A. Establish good communication with the obstetrician to determine if maternal complications exist and to learn details of the obstetrical plan (e.g., vaginal versus cesarean delivery, active management of labor, and induction). Perform a thorough history and physical examination. Discuss the anesthetic management plan and any issues related to it with the obstetrician. Include airway management plans in the event of an emergency.[3–5] The cesarean delivery rate in the morbidly obese parturient is approximately 60%; 48% are emergent. The most commonly reported complications are failed intubation, difficult ventilation, hypoxemia, and aspiration. Therefore, avoid general anesthesia whenever possible. Give regional anesthesia the highest priority.

B. If vaginal delivery is expected, place an epidural catheter early. Expect technical difficulties such as inability to identify landmarks, need for special equipment (e.g., long Tuohy needle), false loss-of-resistance, and suboptimal positioning. After epidural catheter placement, confirm proper position by testing and dosing the catheter. Carefully secure the catheter in place; dislodgement is not an uncommon occurrence.[6]

C. Consider other modalities of labor analgesia including continuous low-dose spinal anesthesia. The advantages of this technique are quick onset of analgesia, better control of block spread, low rate of motor blockade, and rapid establishment of surgical anesthesia when cesarean section is necessary. Disadvantages include risks of postdural puncture headache (PDPH), infection, and inadvertent subarachnoid administration of large doses of local anesthetic.

D. Single-shot spinal anesthesia for cesarean section is an option; however, consider the potential risk of a high or total spinal anesthesia which can lead to an airway emergency. If this technique is chosen, dose cautiously.

E. In certain emergency circumstances (e.g., massive maternal bleeding, acute fetal distress, or prolapsed umbilical cord), time does not permit the performance of regional anesthesia. In such cases, emergently inducing general anesthesia to save the baby can place the mother at great risk due to potential difficulties in airway management. Employ the American Society of Anesthesiologists (ASA) Difficult Airway Algorithm. The laryngeal mask airway (LMA) may provide be lifesaving by itself or as a conduit through which tracheal intubation can be accomplished.[4,5]

REFERENCES

1. Saravanakumar K, Rao SG, Cooper GM: Obesity and obstetric anaesthesia, *Anaesthesia* 61 (1):36–48, 2006.
2. Kuczkowski KM: Labor analgesia for the morbidly obese parturient: an old problem—new solution, *Arch Gynecol Obstet* 271 (4): 302–303, 2005.
3. Munnur U, de Boisblanc B, Suresh MS: Airway problems in pregnancy, *Crit Care Med* 33 (10 Suppl):S259–S268, 2005.
4. Bailey SG, Kitching AJ: The laryngeal mask airway in failed obstetric tracheal intubation, *Int J Obstet Anesth* 14 (3):270–271, 2005.
5. Cook TM, Nolan JP: Failed obstetric tracheal intubation and postoperative respiratory support with the proseal laryngeal mask airway, *Anesth Analg* 100 (1):290, 2005.
6. Hamilton CL, Riley ET, Cohen SE: Changes in the position of epidural catheters associated with patient movement, *Anesthesiology* 86:778–784, 1997.

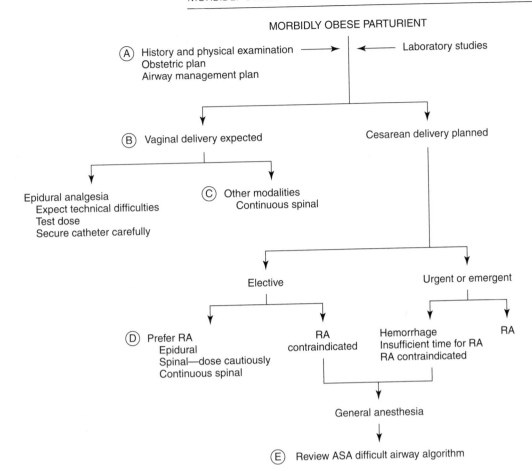

MORBIDLY OBESE PARTURIENT

Ⓐ History and physical examination ⟶ ⟵ Laboratory studies
   Obstetric plan
   Airway management plan

Ⓑ Vaginal delivery expected   Cesarean delivery planned

Epidural analgesia   Ⓒ Other modalities
   Expect technical difficulties   Continuous spinal
Test dose
Secure catheter carefully

Elective   Urgent or emergent

Ⓓ Prefer RA   RA   Hemorrhage   RA
   Epidural   contraindicated   Insufficient time for RA
   Spinal—dose cautiously   RA contraindicated
   Continuous spinal

General anesthesia

Ⓔ Review ASA difficult airway algorithm

Anesthesia for the Patient with Multiple Gestation

HECTOR LaCASSIE, M.D.

CATHERINE K. LINEBERGER, M.D.

Multiple gestation accounts for more than 3% of births in the United States. The twin birth rate is 31.5 per 1,000 live births; the birth rate for triplets/+ is 187.4 per 100,000 births.[1] This is an increase over the last 15 years mainly because of a greater access to fertility therapies and older age of childbearing.[1] Physiological changes occurring in multiple pregnancy are more dramatic than in the singleton state (especially for cardiovascular and pulmonary changes), largely because of increased uterine size, blood volume, and cardiac output (CO).[2] Multiple gestation patients are more likely to develop pregnancy complications including premature labor and fetal and maternal death.[2,3]

A. *Modes of delivery:* Consider all twin presentations as one of the following: vertex A-vertex B; vertex A-nonvertex B; or first twin is nonvertex (Figure 1). Most obstetricians accept vaginal delivery for the first two scenarios, but there is always the possibility of a difficult delivery, particularly for a second twin for whom it may be necessary to deliver abdominally if an external cephalic version or an internal podalic version is not possible.[4] In fact, 9.5% of second twins are delivered by cesarean section; this increases fourfold in the presence of breech or other malpresentations.[5] Cesarean section is almost always the method of delivery for the third scenario and for higher order gestations (triplets or higher).[2]

B. *Anesthesia for labor and vaginal delivery:* Establish adequate IV access and send a blood specimen for type and screen in anticipation of maternal hemorrhage. Administer nonparticulate antacid prior to administration of an anesthetic. Regional anesthesia provides a superior level of pain relief during labor when compared to systemic opioids.[6,7] Epidural and combined spinal-epidural (CSE) analgesia are the preferred techniques of pain relief for multiple gestation, providing the greatest flexibility for maternal analgesia and anesthesia when an operative intervention is required. Minimal exposure of the fetuses to drugs is especially important in the setting of premature delivery. Anticipate possible intrapartum need to provide rapid extension of the epidural for forceps delivery or cesarean section if it becomes necessary (double setup). At times, either external cephalic version or internal breech version with breech extraction of the second twin may be attempted. This will require excellent uterine relaxation; consider administration of halogenated agents or IV nitroglycerine (50 to 100 μg increments).[8]

C. *Anesthesia for cesarean delivery:* Most of the recommendations for regional analgesia in vaginal delivery apply for abdominal delivery as well. Regional anesthesia is the preferred form of anesthesia. Spinal anesthesia is as safe as epidural anesthesia but requires administration of more volume and vasopressors to maintain adequate hemodynamics.[9] For epidural anesthesia, administer local anesthetics incrementally through the catheter to allow a more gradual onset of block and its associated sympathectomy. Provide general anesthesia when maternal refusal or medical problems preclude regional anesthetic techniques. Avoid aortocaval compression, provide adequate prehydration, and minimize uterine incision-to-delivery time. All of the usual concerns regarding general anesthesia in the parturient are applicable, with the additional consideration that FRC is likely to be even smaller than with singleton pregnancy. Be sure to denitrogenate adequately before induction.

D. *Postpartum considerations:* Multiple gestation patients are more likely than their singleton counterparts to experience uterine atony and are at much higher risk for postpartum hemorrhage. Therefore, continue to monitor uterine tone and blood loss postoperatively. Maintain adequate IV access for fluid resuscitation and blood transfusion. The infants from multiple births are often delivered prematurely and may require resuscitation. Obstetric anesthesiologists are often called upon to assist with this task.

Mode of delivery

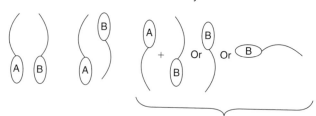

Vaginal   Vaginal or   Cesarean section
              vaginal + cesarean

FIGURE 1   Mode of delivery.

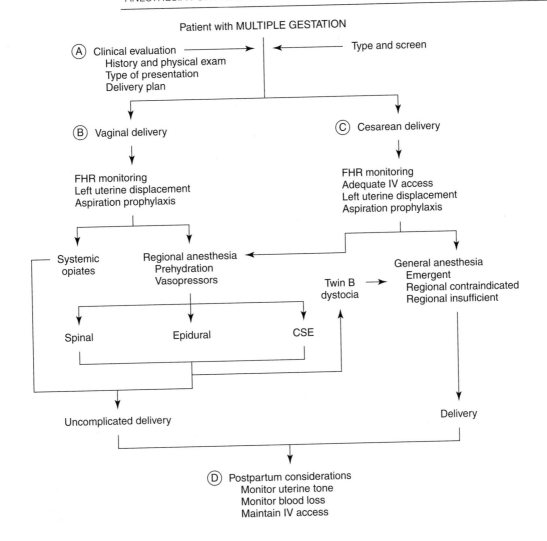

REFERENCES

1. Martin JA, Hamilton BE, Sutton PD, et al.: Births: final data for 2003, *Natl Vital Stat Rep* 54:1–116, 2005.
2. Gorman Maloney SR, Levinson G: Anesthesia for abnormal positions and presentations, shoulder distocia, and multiple births. In: Hughes SC, Levinson G, Rosen MA, editors: *Shnider and Levinson's anesthesia for obstetrics*, ed 4, Philadelphia, 2002, Lippincott Williams & Wilkins.
3. The ESHRE Capri Workshop Group: Multiple gestation pregnancy, *Hum Reprod* 15 (8):1856–1864, 2000.
4. Persad VL, Baskett TF, O'Connell CM, et al.: Combined vaginal-cesarean delivery of twin pregnancies, *Obstet Gynecol* 98 (6): 1032–1037, 2001.
5. Wen SW, Fung KF, Oppenheimer L, et al.: Occurrence and predictors of cesarean delivery for the second twin after vaginal delivery of the first twin, *Obstet Gynecol* 103 (3):413–419, 2004.
6. American College of Obstetrics and Gynecology ACOG Practice bulletin: obstetric analgesia and anesthesia, *Int J Gynaecol Obstet* 78 (3):321–335, 2002.
7. Rosen MA, Hughes SC, Levinson G: Regional anesthesia for labor and delivery. In: Hughes SC, Levinson G, Rosen MA, editors: *Shnider and Levinson's anesthesia for obstetrics*, ed 4, Philadelphia, 2002, Lippincott Williams & Wilkins.
8. American Society of Anesthesiologists Task Force on Obstetrical Anesthesia: Practice guidelines for obstetrical anesthesia: a report by the American Society of Anesthesiologists Task Force on Obstetrical Anesthesia, *Anesthesiology* 90 (2):600–611, 1999.
9. Marino T, Goudas LC, Steinbok V, et al.: The anesthetic management of triplet cesarean delivery: a retrospective case series of maternal outcomes, *Anesth Analg* 93 (4):991–995, 2001.

Fetal Monitoring

STEPHEN DONAHUE, M.D.

Fetal monitoring is performed to assess fetal well-being. The fetal heart rate (FHR) is observed in relation to uterine activity. This can be accomplished via periodic auscultation or by intermittent or continuous electronic means.[1] Electronic fetal monitoring can be performed with internal or external devices. The internal device is a fetal scalp electrode; the external device is a phonocardiographic monitor. Uterine tone is measured internally with an intrauterine pressure catheter or externally with a tocodynamometer applied to the mother's abdominal wall. FHR and uterine tone trends are recorded on a continuous strip of paper for analysis. Chart speed is usually 3 cm/min. Units for FHR are in beats per minute (bpm); units for uterine tone are centimeters of water pressure (cm H_2O). The anesthesiologist should be familiar with the basic fetal cardiac patterns and their causes. Vigilance is especially important when initiating or adjusting labor analgesia.[2] Other types of fetal monitoring are under investigation (e.g., fetal pulse oximetry) but will not be discussed here.[3]

A. Perform a thorough history and physical examination, paying particular attention to the airway evaluation. Anticipate that any women in labor may require a general anesthetic for delivery.

B. Formulate a plan for labor analgesia and a backup plan for emergency cesarean section.

C. Monitor baseline FHR for rate and variability. A normal baseline FHR is 120 to 160 bpm. Bradycardia (FHR < 120 bpm) may indicate hypothermia, structural cardiac defects, or maternal use of beta-adrenergic blockers. Tachycardia (FHR > 160 bpm) may indicate prematurity, thyrotoxicosis, maternal of fetal infection (especially chorioamnionitis), maternal use of beta-sympathomimetic drugs or parasympathetic blocking drugs, or fetal supraventricular tachycardia (SVT).[4] Direct therapy to treat the underlying disease. Ultrasound may help confirm the diagnosis of SVT or structural cardiac disease.[4] Normal variability, represented by an irregular pattern in the baseline FHR, suggests an intact fetal central nervous system (CNS) and cardiac conduction system.[4] The absence of variability may be an indicator of fetal acidosis, hypoxia, anencephaly, fetal drug effects (e.g., morphine, meperidine, diazepam, magnesium sulfate, atropine, or scopolamine), or an abnormal cardiac conduction system.[4,5] Provide therapy to relieve fetal hypoxia. This might include supplemental oxygen for the mother or changing maternal position to relieve aortocaval compression by the uterus.

D. Observe for acceleration and deceleration of the FHR with uterine contractions. Acceleration indicates fetal well-being. Decelerations are divided into three broad categories: early, late, and variable. (The mnemonic "HELP VC" is a good way to remember the most common causes for decelerations: Head-Early, Late-Placenta, and Variable-Cord.) Early decelerations begin at the onset of uterine contraction and return to baseline at the end of the contraction. They are a result of elevated vagal tone from fetal head compression during contraction, are not dangerous, and do not require intervention.[5] Late decelerations begin after the peak of uterine contraction. They suggest decreased placental perfusion, fetal hypoxia, and consequent fetal myocardial depression. Placental hypoperfusion may be a result of maternal hypotension or excessive oxytocin administration. Treat late decelerations with supplemental oxygen, maternal position change, an intravenous (IV) fluid bolus, vasopressor (e.g., ephedrine), or reduction or discontinuation of the oxytocin infusion.[6] Variable decelerations have variable onset and appearance and are caused by occlusion of the umbilical cord. Umbilical cord compression results in fetal hypotension and myocardial hypoxia.[5] Variable decelerations can also occur with head compression, uterine tetany, and severe maternal hypotension.[6] Treat variable decelerations with supplemental oxygen, maternal position change, an IV fluid bolus, or vasopressor. When variable decelerations are caused by head compression, discourage pushing or ballottement of the head during contractions, which may correct the problem.[6]

E. Ominous FHR patterns, such as persistent fetal bradycardia with late or variable decelerations, may indicate the need for urgent or emergency cesarean section. When the patient arrives in the operating room, continue fetal monitoring. If the critical FHR pattern resolves, there may be time for a regional anesthetic. Monitor FHR patterns closely during initiation or redosing of regional anesthesia because of the risk of maternal hypotension.

REFERENCES

1. Thacker SB, Stroup DF, Peterson HB: Efficacy and safety of intrapartum electronic fetal monitoring: an update, *Obstet Gynecol* 86:613–620, 1995.
2. Chestnut DH: Fetal monitoring and anaesthesia for fetal distress, *Can J Anaesth* 40:R74–R80, 1993.
3. Dildy GA: Intrapartum assessment of the fetus: historical and evidence-based practice, *Obstet Gynecol Clin N Am* 32:255–271, 2005.
4. Datta S: Fetal monitoring. In: Datta S, *Obstetric anesthesia handbook*, ed 4, New York, 2006, Springer.
5. Cusick W, Smulian JC, Vintzileos AM: Intrapartum use of fetal heart rate monitoring, contraction monitoring, and amnioinfusion, *Clin Perinatol* 22:875–906, 1995.
6. Schifrin BS: The ABCs of electronic fetal monitoring, *J Perinatol* 14:396–402, 1994.

FETAL MONITORING

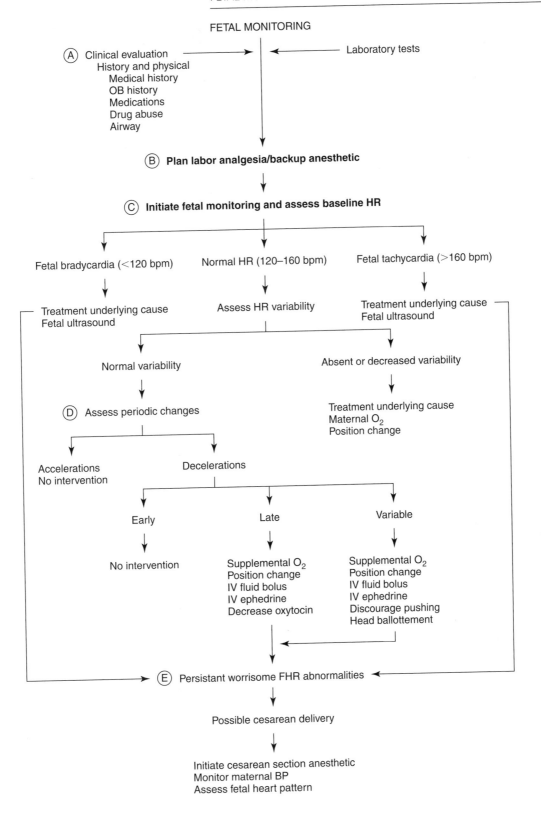

Ⓐ Clinical evaluation → ← Laboratory tests
    History and physical
        Medical history
        OB history
        Medications
        Drug abuse
        Airway

Ⓑ **Plan labor analgesia/backup anesthetic**

Ⓒ **Initiate fetal monitoring and assess baseline HR**

Fetal bradycardia (<120 bpm)   Normal HR (120–160 bpm)   Fetal tachycardia (>160 bpm)

Treatment underlying cause   Assess HR variability   Treatment underlying cause
Fetal ultrasound   Fetal ultrasound

Normal variability   Absent or decreased variability

Ⓓ Assess periodic changes   Treatment underlying cause
                                Maternal O$_2$
                                Position change

Accelerations   Decelerations
No intervention

Early   Late   Variable

No intervention   Supplemental O$_2$ Supplemental O$_2$
                    Position change   Position change
                    IV fluid bolus   IV fluid bolus
                    IV ephedrine   IV ephedrine
                    Decrease oxytocin   Discourage pushing
                                            Head ballottement

Ⓔ Persistant worrisome FHR abnormalities

Possible cesarean delivery

Initiate cesarean section anesthetic
Monitor maternal BP
Assess fetal heart pattern

Postpartum Tubal Ligation (PPTL)

MOHAMED TIOURIRINE, M.D.

Tubal sterilization is considered by many women to be the method of choice for contraception. The preferred time for postpartum tubal ligation (PPTL) is during the early postpartum period, most commonly within the first 8 hours following a vaginal delivery or at the time of a cesarean section because of easy access to the fallopian tubes, shorter hospital stay, and convenience for both patient and obstetrician. Despite its apparent simplicity, complications, such as bowel injury, intraoperative bleeding, and wound infection may occur. An understanding of the early postpartum physiological changes is necessary to provide the patient with optimal care. *Practice Guidelines for Obstetric Anesthesia* revealed that PPTL can be performed safely during the first 8 hours following delivery and that spinal, epidural, or general anesthesia can be provided without increased maternal complications.[1]

A. Perform a thorough preanesthetic evaluation to optimize patient care. Note factors such as pregnancy course; duration of labor; complications of labor or delivery; hemodynamic stability; and maternal risk factors, such as severe preeclampsia, gestational hypertension, and diabetes. Although some data suggest that patients with preexisting disorders may be high risk for PPTL, there have been reports of the safety of PPTL in pregnancies complicated with hypertension.[2]

B. There are no additional maternal risks if PPTL is performed within 8 hours postdelivery. Choose the anesthetic technique taking into account several factors, such as food ingestion, presence of a working epidural catheter, and use of narcotic during labor. Ultrasound examination of the stomach has demonstrated the presence of food particles and delayed gastric emptying during the postpartum period.[3] The use of narcotic during labor may also delay gastric emptying time.

C. Use general anesthesia (GA) when a patient refuses or there is contraindication to regional anesthesia; consider GA when unable to reactivate a previously functional epidural catheter. In these circumstances, consider aspiration prophylaxis and provide a thorough airway examination. Perform a rapid sequence induction (RSI) and intubation and minimize the amount of inhaled anesthetic to avoid uterine relaxation. Apply a BIS monitor if available. Although breastfeeding is of concern, induction agents, such as thiopental and propofol, are safe to use. Narcotics are Class III drugs and compatible with breast feeding.

D. Regional anesthetic techniques are preferred for PPTL. If a previously functioning epidural catheter is in place, attempt reactivation. The time interval from delivery is an important factor in successful catheter reactivation. A success rate of 92% when the catheter was reactivated within the first 24 hours following delivery has been reported, and it fell to 80% afterward.[4] If reactivation fails, consider replacement of the catheter or induction of GA; results after spinal anesthesia in such cases are unpredictable (i.e., high spinal or erratic spread).

E. Spinal anesthesia is an excellent choice as a primary technique for PPTL. It offers rapid onset of motor and sensory block, as well as reduced OR time and cost. Consider the dose and type of local anesthetic to prevent long recovery times. A dose of 7.5 mg of marcaine has been used successfully.[5] Ropivacaine 1% and lidocaine 5% have also been used.

F. Local anesthesia with intraperitoneal lidocaine and IV sedation is possible; however one must consider the risk/benefit ratio of this technique, especially in postpartum patients.

G. Pain after PPTL is minimal. Consider issues related to breastfeeding prior to initiating any pain management protocol. Attempt to minimize those side effects (e.g., drowsiness, nausea, and vomiting) that limit maternal-to-baby interaction. Options for pain control may include intrathecal morphine,[6] epidural morphine, and ibuprofen or ketorolac.

REFERENCES

1. American Society of Anesthesiologists Task Force on Obstetrical Anesthesia: Practice guidelines for obstetrical anesthesia: a report by the American Society of Anesthesiologists Task Force on Obstetrical Anesthesia, *Anesthesiology* 90:600–611, 1999.
2. Suelto MD, Vincent RD Jr., Larmon JE, et al.: Spinal anesthesia for postpartum tubal ligation after pregnancy complicated by preeclampsia or gestational hypertension, *Reg Anesth Pain Med* 25 (2):170–173, 2000.
3. Jayaram A, Bowen MP, Deshpande S, et al.: Ultrasound examination of the stomach contents of women in the postpartum period, *Anesth Analg* 84 (3):522–526, 1997.
4. Goodman EJ, Dumas SD: The rate of successful reactivation of labor epidural catheters for postpartum tubal ligation surgery, *Reg Anesth Pain Med* 23 (3):258–261, 1998.
5. Huffnagle SL, Norris MC, Huffnagle HJ, et al.: Intrathecal hyperbaric bupivacaine dose response in postpartum tubal ligation patients, *Reg Anesth Pain Med* 27 (3):284–288, 2002.
6. Campbell DC, Riben CM, Rooney ME, et al.: Intrathecal morphine for postpartum tubal ligation postoperative analgesia, *Anesth Analg* 93:1006–1011, 2001.

POSTPARTUM TUBAL LIGATION

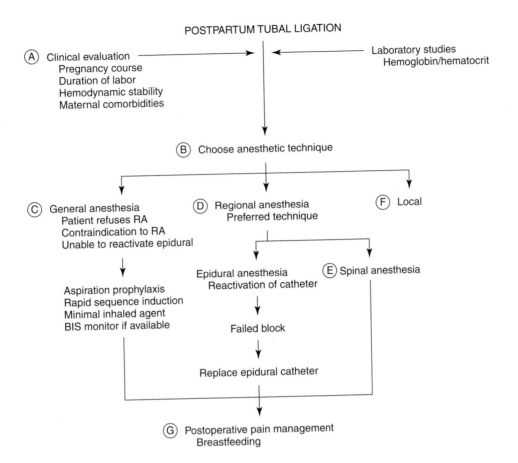

(A) Clinical evaluation
    Pregnancy course
    Duration of labor
    Hemodynamic stability
    Maternal comorbidities

Laboratory studies
    Hemoglobin/hematocrit

(B) Choose anesthetic technique

(C) General anesthesia
    Patient refuses RA
    Contraindication to RA
    Unable to reactivate epidural

(D) Regional anesthesia
    Preferred technique

(F) Local

Aspiration prophylaxis
Rapid sequence induction
Minimal inhaled agent
BIS monitor if available

Epidural anesthesia
Reactivation of catheter

(E) Spinal anesthesia

Failed block

Replace epidural catheter

(G) Postoperative pain management
    Breastfeeding

Fetal Surgery

MARK A. ROSEN, M.D.

Some fetuses with malformations that have harmful developmental consequences may benefit from surgical correction before birth. Over the past two decades, multidisciplinary teams at a handful of institutions (University of California San Francisco, Children's Hospital Pennsylvania, and Vanderbilt University) have developed innovative surgical and anesthetic approaches for fetal surgery.[1-4] Fetal surgery requires anesthesia and monitoring for the mother and the fetus. Uterine incision inevitably induces uterine contractions. Maternal safety remains of primary importance.

A. Fetal surgery is performed only for fetal anomalies that progress in utero and cause harm to the fetus before fetal lungs mature and for which postnatal surgical success is less likely. Most malformations diagnosed in utero are not suitable for prenatal intervention. For each procedure, antenatal surgical intervention warrants controlled clinical trials to establish their efficacy and substantiate safety. Currently, a multicenter trial of myelomeningocele repair is ongoing at the three institutions named previously.

B. Only healthy women are eligible for fetal surgery. Families are counseled about potential fetal benefits and risks, maternal risks, and alternatives. Procedures that involve hysterotomies can be performed between 20 and 30 weeks' gestation. Owing to the required classical uterine incision for fetal surgery, the present gestation and all future gestations must end with cesarean deliveries.

C. Anesthetic management is fundamentally similar to that for nonobstetric surgery during pregnancy. Avoid asphyxia, exposure to potentially teratogenic drugs, and preterm labor. Ensure maternal safety by recognizing the anesthetic implications of maternal physiological changes. Administer oral antacids preoperatively. Minimize other premedicants or adjuvant anesthetic agents, because high doses of halogenated anesthesia are necessary to sustain intraoperative uterine atony. Place an epidural catheter preoperatively for both intraoperative and postoperative use. Induce general anesthesia with a rapid sequence induction (RSI) using cricoid pressure. Displace the uterus to the left. Monitor volume status carefully to reduce risk of pulmonary edema associated with tocolytic administration. Endoscopic procedures can be performed under regional anesthesia, using nitroglycerin (NTG) if needed for uterine tone; however, general anesthesia is preferred.

D. Fetal surgery requires fetal anesthesia, fetal monitoring, and intraoperative uterine atony. Effective fetal monitoring is essential. Surgery may be performed by hysterotomy or endoscopy. For hysterotomy, monitor the fetal heart rate (FHR) and, when possible, SpO_2; and perform intermittent sonography. For endoscopic procedures, monitor intraoperative FHR and assess the quality of fetal cardiac contractility by sonography.

E. Preoperatively, administer rectal indomethacin as a prophylactic tocolytic. Intraoperatively, induce and sustain uterine atony with halogenated agents at relatively high doses (end-tidal 2–3 MAC). For supplemental tocolytic effects, administer boluses of nitroglycerin, 50–200 µg. The dose of halogenated agent is limited by maternal cardiovascular stability; administer vasopressor agents to support maternal blood pressure. As the uterus is closed, administer a loading dose of magnesium sulfate followed by a continuous infusion.

F. As the uterus is closed, discontinue the halogenated agent, administer N20/opioids, and dose the epidural catheter with local anesthetic. This regimen facilitates wake up by allowing time for excretion of the high concentrations of halogenated agent; prevents coughing or straining during a fully awake extubation; and provides exceptional postoperative analgesia, which is sustained by patient controlled epidural analgesia using low dose bupivacaine and fentanyl.

G. Continue fetal monitoring. Continue magnesium infusion for postoperative tocolysis. Supplement with rectal indomethacin for several days and wean tocolytics to oral agents to allow discharge from the hospital.

H. For the fetus with a compromised airway (fetal cystic hygroma, cervical teratoma, large goiter, etc.), cesarean section is modified to allow ex utero intrapartum treatment (EXIT) to inspect and secure the fetal airway (bronchoscopy, laryngoscopy, and intubation) while the fetus remains on placental support. We successfully allowed more than 2 hours of intrapartum surgical time for a fetus in whom an attempted bronchoscopy and laryngoscopy failed. Fetal tracheotomy and central line placement were performed while uterine atony was maintained and the "almost newborn" was monitored with pulse oximetry while still connected to the placenta.

REFERENCES

1. Harrison MR, Anderson J, Rosen MA, et al.: Fetal surgery in the primate I. Anesthetic, surgical, and tocolytic management to maximize fetal-neonatal survival, J Pediatr Surg 17:115–122, 1982.
2. Rosen MA: Anesthesia for fetal surgery and other intrauterine procedures. In: Chestnut D, editor: Obstetric anesthesia: principles and practice, ed 3, St. Louis, 2004, Mosby.
3. Harrison MR: The unborn patient. The art and science of fetal therapy, ed 3, Philadelphia, 2001, Saunders.
4. Mychaliska GB, Bealer JF, Graf JL, et al.: Operating on placental support: the ex utero intrapartum treatment procedure, J Pediatr Surg 32 (2):227–231, 1997.

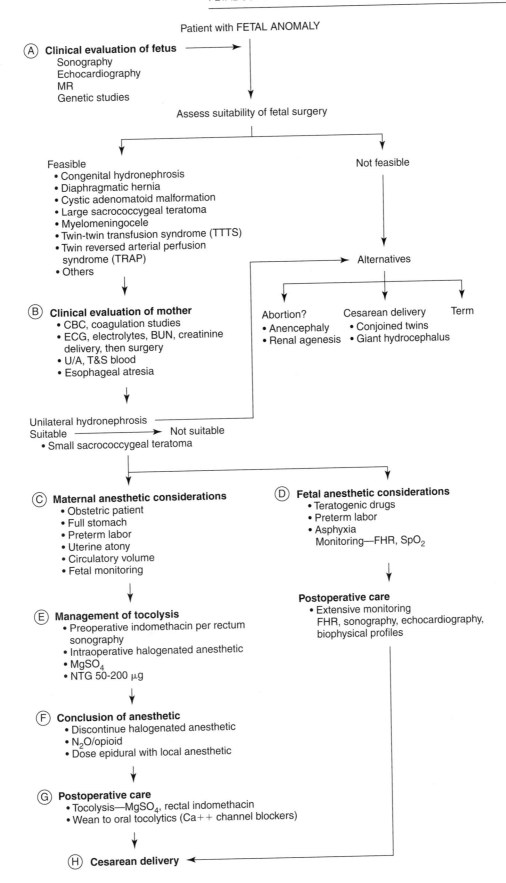

Patient with FETAL ANOMALY

Ⓐ **Clinical evaluation of fetus** ⟶
   Sonography
   Echocardiography
   MR
   Genetic studies

Assess suitability of fetal surgery

Feasible
• Congenital hydronephrosis
• Diaphragmatic hernia
• Cystic adenomatoid malformation
• Large sacrococcygeal teratoma
• Myelomeningocele
• Twin-twin transfusion syndrome (TTTS)
• Twin reversed arterial perfusion
  syndrome (TRAP)
• Others

Not feasible

Alternatives

Abortion?   Cesarean delivery   Term
• Anencephaly   • Conjoined twins
• Renal agenesis   • Giant hydrocephalus

Ⓑ **Clinical evaluation of mother**
• CBC, coagulation studies
• ECG, electrolytes, BUN, creatinine
  delivery, then surgery
• U/A, T&S blood
• Esophageal atresia

Unilateral hydronephrosis
Suitable ⟶ Not suitable
• Small sacrococcygeal teratoma

Ⓒ **Maternal anesthetic considerations**
• Obstetric patient
• Full stomach
• Preterm labor
• Uterine atony
• Circulatory volume
• Fetal monitoring

Ⓓ **Fetal anesthetic considerations**
• Teratogenic drugs
• Preterm labor
• Asphyxia
  Monitoring—FHR, SpO₂

Postoperative care
• Extensive monitoring
  FHR, sonography, echocardiography,
  biophysical profiles

Ⓔ **Management of tocolysis**
• Preoperative indomethacin per rectum
  sonography
• Intraoperative halogenated anesthetic
• MgSO₄
• NTG 50-200 μg

Ⓕ **Conclusion of anesthetic**
• Discontinue halogenated anesthetic
• N₂O/opioid
• Dose epidural with local anesthetic

Ⓖ **Postoperative care**
• Tocolysis—MgSO₄, rectal indomethacin
• Wean to oral tocolytics (Ca++ channel blockers)

Ⓗ **Cesarean delivery** ⟵

Neonatal Resuscitation

MARY ANN GURKOWSKI, M.D.

Respiratory arrest in the neonate may be caused by airway obstruction, depression from maternal drugs or anesthetics, immaturity of lung function or respiratory regulation, CNS hemorrhage, congenital anomalies, infection, metabolic causes, or hypovolemic shock. Any neonate who experiences cardiac or respiratory arrest must be admitted to a neonatal ICU for treatment and monitoring.

A. Anticipate the need for neonatal resuscitation when obstetric complications are present (hemorrhage, abruption, infection, hypertension [HTN], drug dependency, or meconium-stained amniotic fluid) or if the neonate's heart rate (HR) is <100 beats/min (bpm), poor respiratory activity is noted, neuromuscular tone is depressed, or central cyanosis is present.

B. Dry the neonate's body, then discard the wet towels. Place the neonate under a preheated radiant warmer to avoid cold stress (hypothermia, hypoglycemia, and acidosis). If a radiant warmer is unavailable, warm the room and use prewarmed towels. Place the neonate's head in a position optimal for spontaneous or controlled ventilation (folded or rolled cloth under the shoulders with the neck *slightly* extended). This position is known as the sniffing position and will align the posterior pharynx, larynx, and trachea.

C. Gently suction the mouth and then the nares. Excessive catheter suctioning may cause bradycardia and laryngospasm.[1] Provide tactile stimulation by rubbing the back, gently slapping the foot, or flicking the heel.

TABLE 1
Tracheal Tube Size

Tube size (ID mm)	Weight	Gestational age
2.5	Below 1000 g	Below 28 weeks
3.0	1000–2000g	28–34 weeks
3.5	2000–3000 g	34–38 weeks
3.5–4.0	Above 3000 g	Above 38 weeks

Modified from the American Heart Association: *Textbook of Neonatal Resuscitation*, Dallas: American Heart Association/American Academy of Pediatrics, 2000.

D. If the amniotic fluid is meconium stained, suction the mouth, nose, and posterior pharynx after the head is delivered from the vaginal vault but before delivery of the shoulders. After full delivery of the body evaluate the neonate to determine if he or she is vigorous (strong respiratory effort, good muscle tone, HR > 100 bpm). If the neonate is vigorous there is no need to suction the trachea, just proceed with the steps of resuscitation.[2] If the neonate is not vigorous intubate the trachea, attach the endotracheal tube (ETT) to wall suction using a meconium aspirator, and apply suction as the ETT is removed (Table 1). Monitor the HR. Repeat this procedure until the HR falls below 100 or meconium is cleared from the trachea.

TABLE 2
Neonatal Resuscitation Fluids and Medications

Medication	Concentration to administer	Preparation	Dosage/route	Rate/precautions
Epinephrine	1:10,000	1 ml	0.1–0.3 ml/kg IV or ETT	Give rapidly May dilute 1:1 with normal saline if given into the ETT
Volume expanders	0 negative blood Normal saline Ringer's lactate	40 ml	10 ml/mg IV	Give over 5–10 min Give by syringe or IV
Sodium bicarbonate	0.5 mEq/ml (4.2% solution)	20 ml or 2–10 ml prefilled syringes	2 mEq/kg IV or 4 ml/kg or 4.2% solution	Give slowly no faster than a rate of 1 mEq/kg/min Give only if infant is being effectively ventilated
Naloxone	1.0 mg/ml rapidly	1 ml	0.1 mg/kg (0.1 ml/kg) IV, ETT, IM, SQ	Give rapidly IV, ETT preferred IM, SQ acceptable

IV = intravenous; ETT = endotracheal tube; IM = intramuscular; SQ = subcutaneous
Modified from the American Heart Association: *Textbook of neonatal resuscitation*, Dallas, 2000, American Heart Association/American Academy of Pediatrics.

NEONATAL RESUSCITATION

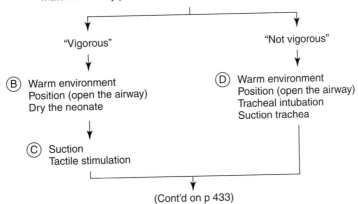

(A) **Clinical evaluation**
  Maternal history
  Obstetrical complications

Maternal history positive for or evidence at delivery of meconium

"Vigorous"

"Not vigorous"

(B) Warm environment
  Position (open the airway)
  Dry the neonate

(D) Warm environment
  Position (open the airway)
  Tracheal intubation
  Suction trachea

(C) Suction
  Tactile stimulation

(Cont'd on p 433)

E. Determine the HR by listening to the left precordium with a stethoscope or by palpating the umbilical stump. Count the HR for 6 seconds and then multiply by 10 to calculate the estimated beats per minute.[2] A normal neonatal HR is 120 to 160 bpm. If the HR is <100 bpm or the infant is gasping or apneic, begin bag or mask positive-pressure ventilations (PPV) with 100% oxygen (O_2) at 40–60 breaths/min. A manometer should be attached to the ventilation circuit. A neonate's first 2 to 3 breaths may require a peak ventilation pressure as high as 40 cm H_2O. Subsequent breaths are usually at a pressure of 20–30 cm H_2O. Relieve gastric distention by passing an oral gastric tube.

F. If after 30 seconds of PPV with 100% O_2 the HR is <60 bpm, start external chest compressions in a ratio of 3:1 so that in 1 minute the neonate receives 90 chest compressions and 30 ventilations.[2-4] Use both thumbs or two fingers placed one finger-breadth below the nipple line but above the xyphoid.[2-4] The usual compression depth is one half to three quarters of an inch.

G. When external cardiac compression is necessary, tracheal intubation allows better airway control.[3] If after 30 seconds of PPV and chest compressions, the HR is <60 bpm, epinephrine may be given and repeated every 3 to 5 minutes if needed. If the HR increases to above 60 bpm, discontinue chest compressions. Epinephrine can be given intravenously or through the ETT.[5]

H. If the HR is still <60 bpm after one dose of epinephrine, consider hypovolemia and give a volume expander or repeat the epinephrine dose. If there is a documented or assumed metabolic acidosis, $NaHCO_3$ can be given (Table 2).[3,5] If after medication is given there is no improvement, always consider these special conditions: pneumothorax, diaphragmatic hernia, and congenital heart disease.

I. If the HR is absent after 15 minutes of efficient CPR, consider cessation of CPR.[2]

REFERENCES

1. Cordero L Jr, Hon EH: Neonatal bradycardia following nasopharyngeal stimulation, *J Pediatr* 78 (3):441–447, 1971.
2. American Heart Association: *Textbook of neonatal resuscitation,* Dallas: American Heart Association/American Academy of Pediatrics, 2000.
3. American Heart Association: 2005 American Heart Association guidelines for cardiopulmonary resuscitation and emergency cardiac care. Part 13: Neonatal resuscitation guidelines, *Circulation* 112:IV-188–IV-195, 2005.
4. Schleien CL, Todres DI: Cardiopulmonary resuscitation. In: Todres Cote, Ryan G, eds. *A practice of anesthesia for infants and children,* ed 3, Philadelphia, 2001, W.B. Saunders.
5. Shaffner DH, Schleien CL, Rogers MC: Cardiopulmonary resuscitation. In: Gregory GA, ed. *Pediatric anesthesia,* ed 4, Philadelphia: Churchill Livingstone, 2002.

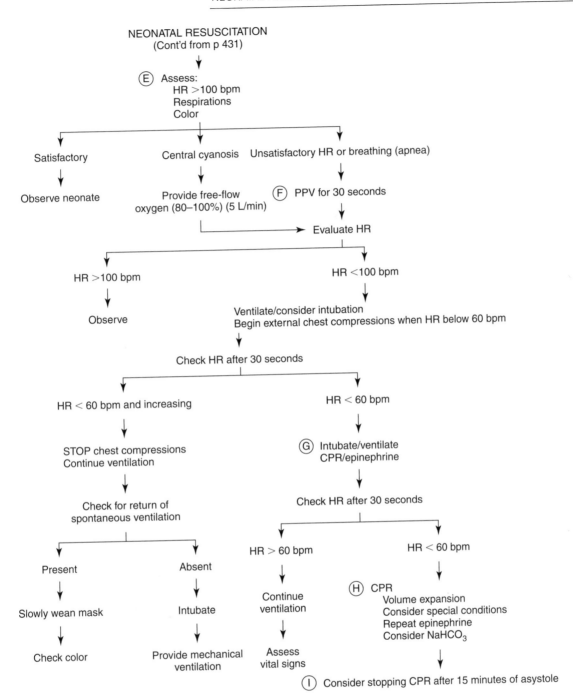

NEONATAL RESUSCITATION
(Cont'd from p 431)

E Assess:
    HR >100 bpm
    Respirations
    Color

Satisfactory   Central cyanosis   Unsatisfactory HR or breathing (apnea)

Observe neonate   Provide free-flow   F PPV for 30 seconds
                      oxygen (80–100%) (5 L/min)

                                    Evaluate HR

HR >100 bpm   HR <100 bpm

Observe   Ventilate/consider intubation
                                     Begin external chest compressions when HR below 60 bpm

                      Check HR after 30 seconds

HR < 60 bpm and increasing   HR < 60 bpm

STOP chest compressions   G Intubate/ventilate
Continue ventilation   CPR/epinephrine

Check for return of   Check HR after 30 seconds
spontaneous ventilation

                                  HR > 60 bpm   HR < 60 bpm

Present   Absent   Continue   H CPR
                                   ventilation   Volume expansion
Slowly wean   Intubate   Consider special conditions
mask   Repeat epinephrine
                                   Assess   Consider NaHCO$_3$
Check color   Provide mechanical vital signs
               ventilation
                                              I Consider stopping CPR after 15 minutes of asystole

ANESTHESIA FOR GENERAL SURGERY

LAPAROSCOPIC SURGERY
BARIATRIC SURGERY
SURGERY OF THE ACUTE ABDOMEN

Laparoscopic Surgery

T. PHILIP MALAN, JR., M.D., PH.D.

Laparoscopic surgery involves insertion of a laparoscope through a small incision in the abdominal wall, allowing visualization of abdominal contents. Insertion of instruments through other small abdominal incisions allows a variety of diagnostic and therapeutic procedures to be performed. Laparoscopic surgery leads to more rapid postoperative recovery and less impairment of postoperative respiratory function compared with laparotomy,[1] but it is not risk free. Published complication rates range from 0.6 to 2.4% and mortality rates from 0.004 to 0.2%.[2] As the complexity and variety of laparoscopic procedures increase and as laparoscopic procedures are performed on more fragile patients, concern over operative and physiological complications has grown. The operative procedure consists of patient positioning (typically supine with head-down tilt for lower abdominal [e.g., gynecologic] procedures and supine with no tilt or head-up tilt for middle and upper abdominal procedures), insertion of a needle into the peritoneal cavity, insufflation with carbon dioxide (CO_2), insertion of trocars and operative instruments, and completion of the required surgical manipulations. Extraperitoneal laparoscopy has been used for procedures on pelvic and flank organs. Extraperitoneal approaches may lessen the risk of some surgical complications and generally require lower insufflation pressures. However, extraperitoneal laparoscopy may result in greater vascular CO_2 absorption than intraperitoneal insufflation and a greater risk of dissection of gas into the mediastinum or pleural cavity.[3]

A. Consider local anesthesia with IV sedation in selected cases.[4] For this technique to be successful, the laparoscopist must be able to perform the procedure with low insufflating pressures (generally less than 10 mm Hg), and the patient must be able to tolerate minor discomforts (usually shoulder discomfort).

B. Consider spinal or epidural anesthesia when low insufflating pressures are used.[4] Some authors have expressed concern over impairment of chest wall muscle function resulting from regional anesthesia in the face of the increased resistance to ventilation and increased CO_2 load associated with laparoscopy.

C. Select general anesthesia for most laparoscopic surgeries.[4] Intubate the trachea to protect from aspiration of gastric contents and to provide for controlled ventilation. The concern over aspiration results from increased intraabdominal pressure due to insufflated gas. Ventilation is typically controlled to prevent respiratory acidosis resulting from the CO_2 load presented by peritoneal insufflation. Consider neuromuscular blockade to prevent respiratory motions, coughing, or patient movement. Place a gastric tube to decompress the stomach. The use of nitrous oxide is controversial.

D. Cardiac dysrhythmias may be a result of sympathetic stimulation (hypercapnia or light anesthesia) or vagal stimulation (peritoneal distention or manipulation of intraabdominal structures).[2] Treat by correcting the underlying cause and administering appropriate antiarrhythmic drugs (e.g., beta-adrenoreceptor antagonists for tachycardia or atropine for bradycardia).

E. Hypotension may occur for a variety of reasons.[2] Increased intraabdominal pressure from gas insufflation does not significantly decrease venous return until pressures above 40 mm Hg are used. However, cardiovascular responses to increased intraabdominal pressure may be exaggerated in hypovolemic patients, patients with cardiovascular disease, and patients rendered relatively hypovolemic by use of the head-up position. Treat hypotension by decreasing the insufflation pressure or releasing the pneumoperitoneum while administering IV fluids or vasoactive drugs.

F. Hypercapnia results from uptake of CO_2 from the pneumoperitoneum (14 to 48 ml CO_2/min) and impaired elimination of CO_2 (preexisting lung disease or impaired ventilation from increased intraabdominal pressure).[2] Treat by increasing minute ventilation.

G. Gas may dissect into extraperitoneal locations, causing subcutaneous emphysema, pneumothorax, pneumomediastinum, or pneumopericardium. Gas in these locations can cause increased vascular uptake of CO_2 and cardiovascular or respiratory compromise.

H. The incidence of clinically evident venous gas embolism during laparoscopy is between 0.002 and 0.02%. Clinical features of this potentially fatal complication are similar to those resulting from other causes. An important factor suggesting venous gas embolism during laparoscopy is onset during abdominal insufflation. Treat by releasing the pneumoperitoneum, administering 100% oxygen (O_2), and supporting the cardiovascular system. Placing the patient in a head-down, left lateral position and attempting to aspirate gas through a central venous catheter are controversial therapeutic maneuvers.

I. Laceration of major blood vessels (including the aorta) may lead to hemorrhage, hypovolemic shock, and cardiovascular collapse. Surgical repair with an open procedure may be required. Resuscitate the patient with volume infusion, including transfusion of blood products.

J. Perforation of a viscus (usually the stomach) may occur during insertion of the insufflation needle or trocar. To minimize this risk, consider administering neuromuscular blockers to prevent patient coughing or movement. A perforated viscus usually requires laparotomy for surgical repair.

K. Pneumoperitoneum may result in oliguria.[5] Causes include vascular and parenchymal compression and systemic hormonal effects. The changes in urine output are pressure dependent and typically not apparent until intraabdominal pressures reach 15 mm Hg or more. Renal function and urine output return to normal, even in patients with preexisting renal disease, once the pneumoperitoneum is released.

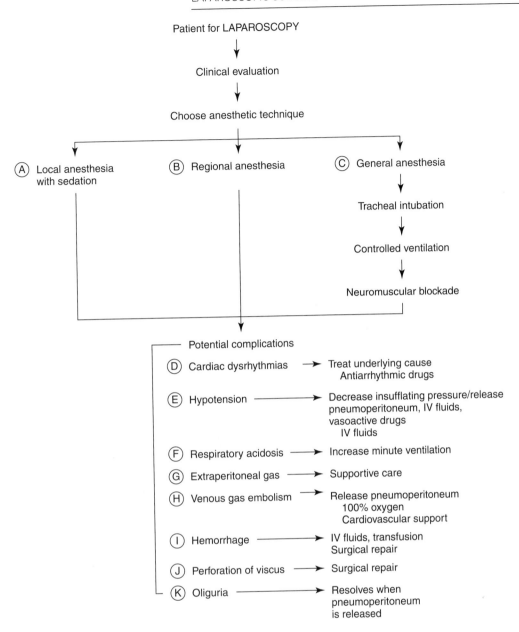

Patient for LAPAROSCOPY

Clinical evaluation

Choose anesthetic technique

(A) Local anesthesia with sedation

(B) Regional anesthesia

(C) General anesthesia

Tracheal intubation

Controlled ventilation

Neuromuscular blockade

Potential complications

(D) Cardiac dysrhythmias → Treat underlying cause
Antiarrhythmic drugs

(E) Hypotension → Decrease insufflating pressure/release pneumoperitoneum, IV fluids, vasoactive drugs
IV fluids

(F) Respiratory acidosis → Increase minute ventilation

(G) Extraperitoneal gas → Supportive care

(H) Venous gas embolism → Release pneumoperitoneum
100% oxygen
Cardiovascular support

(I) Hemorrhage → IV fluids, transfusion
Surgical repair

(J) Perforation of viscus → Surgical repair

(K) Oliguria → Resolves when pneumoperitoneum is released

REFERENCES

1. Putensen-Himmer G, Putensen C, Lammer H, et al.: Comparison of postoperative respiratory function after laparoscopy or open laparotomy for cholecystectomy, *Anesthesiology* 77:675-680, 1992.
2. Wolf JS Jr., Stoller ML: The physiology of laparoscopy: basic principles, complications and other considerations, *J Urol* 152:294-302, 1994.
3. Mullett CE, Viale JP, Sagnard PE, et al.: Pulmonary CO_2 elimination during surgical procedures using intra- or extraperitoneal CO_2 insufflation, *Anesth Analg* 76:622-626, 1993.
4. Hanley ES: Anesthesia for laparoscopic surgery, *Surg Clin North Am* 72:1013-1019, 1992.
5. Dunn MD, McDougall EM: Renal physiology. Laparoscopic considerations, *Urol Clin North Am* 27 (4):609-614, 2000.

Bariatric Surgery

JENNIFER F. VOOKLES, M.D.

DAVID V. NELSON, PH.D.

Bariatric surgeries (gastric banding, Roux-en-Y gastric bypass, and duodenal switch) are increasingly performed as treatment for obesity. Smaller patients without multiple prior abdominal surgeries may be candidates for laparoscopic approaches. Comorbidities related to obesity produce a number of anesthetic challenges perioperatively.[1]

A. Evaluate the airway. Anticipate reduced cardiac reserve, and evaluate for ischemic heart disease, cardiomegaly, and left-sided ventricular or right-sided ventricular failure. Cardiac output (CO) is elevated, and hypertension (HTN) is common. Review a preoperative ECG. FRC is decreased, and decreases are exacerbated by supine position and mechanical ventilation. FRC may be lower than closing volume, increasing dead space. Patients may have obesity hypoventilation ("Pickwickian") syndrome, defined by alveolar hypoventilation, CO_2 retention, hypoxemia, secondary polycythemia, somnolence, and right-sided heart failure. These patients need complete cardiac and pulmonary evaluation including resting blood gas.

B. Position the patient with elevation of the head and shoulders to facilitate airway management. Preoxygenation is essential. Consider awake intubation if there is obstructive sleep apnea or the airway appears particularly difficult. After induction, position with care to avoid pressure sores and nerve injuries (more common in morbidly obese patients). Special operative tables may be needed. The patient should be securely strapped to the table to lessen risk of displacement with change of table position. Bean bags molded to the patient and then vacuum locked into position may prevent shifting.

C. Routine monitoring is tailored to the extent of the planned surgery and the patient's comorbid condition. Good peripheral IV access might be difficult and necessitate placement of central lines. Ultrasound probes can be of assistance in locating the internal jugular vein. Anticipate the need for a large BP cuff size to obtain accurate pressures. The upper arm may have a conical shape that interferes with cuff placement; an arterial line may be needed for adequate BP monitoring if a good fit cannot be achieved.

D. Employ reflux precaution prior to induction of anesthesia. If true gastroesophageal reflux disease (GERD) is present, premedicate with an H_2 blocker, nonparticulate antacid, or metoclopramide, and plan RSI with cricoid pressure. Minimize sedation until the airway is secure.

E. Select anesthetic agents with more rapid onset and elimination. Sevoflurane allows more rapid recovery of mental and physical function, good hemodynamic control, infrequent nausea and vomiting, and early discharge from hospital, compared with isoflurane.[3] Desflurane has also been suggested for use with morbidly obese patients due to its rapid recovery profile.[4] Muscle relaxation is necessary for laparoscopic procedures. Reverse muscle relaxants at completion of the procedure to ensure no residual weakness. Epidural placement is strongly recommended for open bariatric surgeries and may be desirable for laparoscopic procedures (high probability of conversion to open, patients with preoperative pain or opioid tolerance). A thoracic epidural facilitates postoperative analgesia with less sedation and respiratory depression, and a combined general and epidural anesthetic permits lower total doses of anesthetic agents, better muscle relaxation, and higher oxygen concentrations.[5] Anticipate need for placement of a nasogastric (NG) tube and possibly an intragastric balloon. Tests of anastomotic integrity are performed by injection of methylene blue in saline via the NG tube. With laparoscopy, watch for mainstem intubation (cephalad displacement of the diaphragm). Absorption of carbon dioxide (CO_2) can worsen hypercarbia and acidosis. Increased intraabdominal pressure raises systemic vascular resistance. With increases greater than 20 mm Hg, the inferior vena cava is compressed causing decreased venous return. Other potential complications include vasovagal reflex, hemorrhage, venous gas embolus, and perforation of viscus.

F. Postoperative respiratory complications correlate directly with weight. Maintain elevation of the head of the bed and administer supplemental oxygen. Morbid obesity is an independent risk factor for death secondary to acute postoperative pulmonary thromboembolus.[6] Patients typically will have deep vein thrombosis (DVT) prophylaxis, follow current American Society of Anesthesiologists (ASA) guidelines in timing removal of the epidural.

BARIATRIC SURGERY

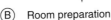 **Clinical evaluation**
- Cardiac:
  Coronary artery disease
  Congestive heart failure
- Respiratory:
  Airway anatomy
  Pulmonary hypertension
  Obstructive sleep apnea
  Obesity hypoventilation syndrome
- Gastrointestinal:
  Gastroesophageal reflux
- Endocrine:
  Diabetes mellitus
- Labs/studies:
  ECG
  CBC
  Bun/Cr
  Glucose
  Possible ABG

 Room preparation
- OR bed
  Positioning with ramp,
  Difficult airway provisions
- Padding

 IV access and monitoring
- Routine monitors
  Large BP cuff
- Possible central line
  Arterial line
- CVP or PA catheter if indicated
  by co-morbid condition

 Premedication and induction
- Reflux prophylaxis
- Light sedation (if indicated)
- Place epidural prior to induction if elected
- Possible rapid sequence induction
- Possible difficult airway

 Maintenance of anesthesia for
open or laparoscopic surgery
- Use insoluble volatile anesthetics
- Muscle relaxation with reversal
  prior to extubation
- If epidural present, use intra-op
  to decrease opioid and anesthetic
  requirements

(F) Postoperative considerations
- Monitor for hypoxemia
- DVT prophylaxis
- Psychological-behavioral
  assistance as needed

REFERENCES

1. Ogunnaike BO, Jones SB, Jones DB, et al.: Anesthetic considerations for bariatric surgery. *Anesth Analg* 95:1793-1805, 2002.
2. Sollazzi L, Perilli V, Modesti C, et al.: Volatile anesthesia in bariatric surgery. *Obes Surg* 11:623-626, 2001.
3. Torri G, Casati A, Albertin A, et al.: Randomized comparison of isoflurane and sevoflurane for laparoscopic gastric banding in morbidly obese patients, *J Clin Anesth* 13:565-570, 2001.
4. Juvin P, Vadam C, Malek L et al.: Postoperative recovery after desflurane, propofol, or isoflurane anesthesia among morbidly obese patients: A prospective, randomized study, *Anesth Analg* 91:714-719, 2000.
5. Buckley FP, Robinson NB, Simonowitz DA, et al.: Anaesthesia in the morbidly obese: A comparison of anaesthetic and analgesic regimens for upper abdominal surgery, *Anaesthesia* 38:840-851, 1983.
6. Blaszyk H, Wollan PC, Witkiewicz AK, et al.: Death from pulmonary thromboembolism in severe obesity: lack of association with established genetic and clinical risk factors, *Virchows Arch* 434:529-532, 1999.

Surgery of the Acute Abdomen

ROBERT H. OVERBAUGH, M.D.

Patients presenting for surgical management of an acute abdomen carry unique challenges for the anesthetist. Significant alterations in physiology and comorbidities accompany acute abdominal pathology.

A. Obtain a complete history and physical examination. Evaluate for cardiac, GI, and pulmonary disease, as over 33 % of these patients are over 65.[1] Expect significant volume shifts and concomitant electrolyte and acid-base perturbations notably hypokalemic, hyponatremic metabolic alkalosis with obstructive bowel pathology (small bowel obstruction or volvulus). Evaluate volume status (orthostatic hypotension, decreased skin turgor, and dry mucous membranes). Consider complete blood count (CBC) in patients with known GI bleeding as evidenced by melena or hematochezia, presumed ruptured viscous or ectopic pregnancy. Serum blood urea nitrogen (BUN)/creatinine (Cr) ratios above 20:1 suggest hypovolemia. Review medications, patients with ulcerative colitis or Crohn's disease may require stress dose of corticosteroids perioperatively. Check transaminases and coagulation parameters if there is hepatic disease.

B. Whenever possible, attempt to restore volume and electrolyte balance. Consider use of GI prophylactic agents (H_2 receptor antagonists, proton pump inhibitors [PPIs], and nonparticulate oral sodium citrate); all patients presenting with acute abdominal pathology should be considered a "full stomach." Combining H_2 antagonists (ranitidine) or PPIs (omeprazole) with oral sodium bicitrate may be superior to each of these agents alone in increasing gastric pH in patients undergoing emergent surgery.[2,3] Promotility agents (metoclopramide) must be used with caution in patients with known intestinal obstruction. Consider type and screen and cross-match blood products when appropriate.

C. Monitor NBP, pulse oximetry, 5 lead ECG (II, V3), and temperature. Consider intraarteriaal blood pressure monitoring and central venous access for patients prone to significant perioperative volume shifts, electrolyte abnormalities, and hemodynamic instability. Consider nasogastric (NG) suction to decompress the stomach prior to induction. Large-bore IV access, fluid warming, and heating blankets are also recommended.

D. Anesthetic technique should take into consideration the presumed etiology of the acute abdominal pathology, patient comorbidity, site of surgery (upper versus lower abdomen), and type of operation (laparoscopic versus open). Regional anesthesia may be a reasonable choice in hemodynamically stable patients presenting for lower abdominal pathology, such as incarcerated inguinal or femoral hernia. When general anesthesia is necessary, airway management is of utmost concern. Weigh risks and benefits of RSI against securing the airway by an awake technique. Regardless, preoxygenation/denitrogenation is recommended prior to induction. In patients with a NG tube in place, suction prior to proceeding with induction, and leave open to drain. The presence of a NG tube does not make cricoid pressure ineffective.[4] Select an induction agent with consideration of the patient's volume status and hemodynamic stability. Etomidate and ketamine may afford less perturbation in BP and HR. Unless specifically contraindicated, succinylcholine (SCC) is the muscle relaxant of choice during induction, given its rapidity of onset. Apply cricoid pressure to prevent passive regurgitation; in an actively retching patient it can lead to severe esophageal injury. Patient stability and comorbidity dictates maintenance technique. Although many practitioners avoid the use of nitrous oxide during abdominal surgery, studies have failed to show that concentrations below 70% lead to increased bowel distention or impaired operating conditions in elective abdominal surgery.[5,6] Animal data reveals nitrous oxide has no negative effects on the intestines in the presence of bowel obstruction.[7] Continue volume replacement intraoperatively to address fluid sequestration, evaporative loss, and third spacing. Continue abdominal relaxation with a nondepolarizing muscle relaxant (NDMR) to facilitate abdominal closure.

E. Extubate patients when they are completely awake with return of airway reflexes. During the postoperative period, monitor the patient for hypoxemia, hypercarbia, hypovolemia, acidosis, and electrolyte abnormalities. Anticipate the need for ongoing volume. Consider regional technique (epidural or paravertebral blockade) to augment postoperative pain control for large incisions. Nausea and vomiting prophylaxis with use of 5-HT3 antagonists, droperidol, or metoclopramide is usually indicated. Patients with evidence of persistent hypovolemia, sepsis, or acute respiratory distress syndrome (ARDS) should be monitored postoperatively in the ICU.

Patient with ACUTE ABDOMINAL PATHOLOGY

Obstructive:
Small bowel obstruction, incarcerated
hernia, volvulus, cholelithiasis
Traumatic:
Perforated viscus
Perforation:
Gastric/duodenal ulcer,
ruptured diverticulum
Vascular:
Ruptured AAA, mesenteric thrombus
Inflammatory:
Chron's disease, ulcerative colitis,
necrotizing pancreatitis, abscess
Gynecologic:
Ectopic pregnancy, ovarian torsion,
ruptured ovarian cyst

(A) **Preoperative evaluation**
History:
GERD, cardio-pulmonary
disease, hiatal hernia
Physical exam:
Airway, volume status: R/O
orthostasis, dry mucous
membranes, decreased
skin turgor
Labs:
Lytes, BUN/Cr, ABG, LFT's,
CBC, ECG, B-HCG,
coagulation, amylase

(B) **Preoperative preparation**
GI prophylaxis: sodium bicitrate
Consider: H_2 blocker, proton pump
inhibitor, metoclopramide
Electrolyte replacement: K^+, Mg^{++}
Volume resuscitation
Antibiotics if indicated
Stress dose steroids if indicated
Blood products available

(C) **Monitors**
ECG leads II/V3, pulse ox,
NBP, large bore IV access,
heated IV fluids, warming
blanket, nasogastric tube
Consider: Intra-arterial BP,
CVP/PA catheter, TEE

(D) **Anesthetic technique**

General anesthesia
Pre-oxygenation/de-nitrogenation
Induction: +/− rapid sequence
induction/intubation with cricoid
pressure vs awake technique
Volatile based vs TIVA +/− N_2O
Continued volume replacement:
Third space loss may exceed 10 cc/kg/hr
Abdominal relaxation: non-depolarizing MR

Regional anesthesia
SAB/epidural: appropriate if no
evidence of hemodynamic
instability or hypovolemia, for
lower abdominal procedures
Para vertebral blockade:
unilateral hernia repair
Ilioinguinal block: inguinal
hernia repair

(E) **Post-operative period**
Monitor for: persistant hypovolemia/ongoing
third space loss, hypoxia, hypercarbia,
metabolic acidosis/alkalosis, electrolyte
abnormality, sepsis/ARDS, poor respiratory
effort due to inadequate pain control
Consider PONV prophylaxis

REFERENCES

1. Doherty GM: The acute abdomen. In: Way L, editor: *Lange current surgical diagnosis and treatment*, ed 12, New York, 2006 McGraw-Hill.
2. Ng A, Smith G: Gastroesophageal reflux and aspiration of gastric contents in anesthesia practice, *Anesth Analg* 93 (2):494-513, 2001.
3. Stuart JC, Kan AF, Rowbottom SJ, et al.: Acid aspiration prophylaxis for emergency caesarean section, *Anaesthesia* 51 (5):415-421, 1996.
4. Salem MR, Joseph NJ, Heyman HJ, et al.: Cricoid compression is effective in obliterating the esophageal lumen in the presence of a nasogastric tube, *Anesthesiology* 63 (4):443-446, 1985.
5. Taylor E, Feinstein R, White P, et al.: Anesthesia for laparoscopic cholecystectomy. Is nitrous oxide contraindicated? *Anesthesiology* 76 (4):541-543, 1992.
6. Karlsten R, Kristensen JD: Nitrous oxide does not influence the surgeon's rating of operating conditions in lower abdominal surgery, *European J Anaesth* 10 (3):215-217, 1993.
7. Pittner A, Nalos M, Theisen M, et al.: Inhaling nitrous oxide or xenon does not influence bowel wall energy during porcine bowel obstruction, *Anesth Analg* 94 (6):1510-1516, 2002.

UROLOGIC ANESTHESIA

TRANSURETHRAL RESECTION OF THE
PROSTATE (TURP)

EXTRACORPOREAL SHOCK WAVE
LITHOTRIPSY (ESWL)

PERCUTANEOUS NEPHROLITHOTRIPSY
(PCNL)

Transurethral Resection of the Prostate (TURP)

VINOD MALHOTRA, M.D.

VIJAYENDRA SUDHEENDRA, M.D.

Transurethral resection of the prostate (TURP) is performed for benign prostatic hypertrophy (BPH). Nonionized irrigation solution (glycine, Cytal, mannitol, urea, or glucose) is infused transurethrally to distend and allow visualization of the bladder and to wash away blood and tissue fragments. If venous sinuses are opened, irrigation fluid may enter the circulation in significant volume. Factors affecting the volume entrained include the size of the prostate gland, resection time, infection, the surgeon's experience, and pressure of irrigating fluid.[1]

A. Patients may be elderly and frequently have comorbidities. Evaluate cardiovascular and volume status and preoperative electrolytes. The patient receiving digitalis should be normokalemic because of the rare risk of dilutional hypokalemia resulting in acute digitalis toxicity.[2] Dilutional hyponatremia is a more common complication.

B. Monitor ECG, indirect BP, pulse oximetry, and temperature in all patients. Avoid heavy sedation to enable communication with the patient and evaluation of mental status during regional anesthesia. The patient with severe cardiorespiratory disease may require invasive monitors to follow ABGs, electrolytes, intravascular volume, and cardiac output (CO) closely.

C. Subarachnoid block to a T10 sensory level is the anesthetic technique of choice, because the awake patient may describe changing sensorium (dilutional hyponatremia or ammonia intoxication) or abdominal pain (bladder perforation). Treat spinal hypotension with vasoconstrictors rather than with large volumes of IV fluid. General anesthesia may be chosen for patients who refuse or have contraindication to regional anesthesia. Mortality, morbidity, and outcomes remain similar for general anesthesia and regional anesthesia in patients undergoing TURP. Incidence of deep venous thrombosis (DVT) is lower with regional anesthesia.

D. TURP syndrome is a constellation of symptoms resulting from circulatory overload, water intoxication, hyponatremia, glycine toxicity, ammonia toxicity, hemolysis, coagulopathy (primary fibrinolysis or DIC), bacteremia, septicemia, or toxemia.[3,4] Suspect intravascular volume overload if systolic, diastolic, and CVPs increase, and watch for pulmonary edema and cardiac failure. Dilutional hyponatremia (serum Na+ <100 to 120 mEq/L) is suggested in the awake patient by changes in mental status (lethargy, agitation, or seizures), nausea and vomiting, and visual changes. Patients undergoing general anesthesia may show no abnormality until hypotension and dysrhythmias develop. Because hypervolemia and hyponatremia frequently coexist, establish a brisk diuresis with furosemide before beginning hypertonic saline infusion. Because glycine is hepatically metabolized to ammonia, investigations have addressed the possible role of ammonia toxicity in the cause of TURP syndrome. Hemolysis occurs most often when sterile water is used for bladder irrigation, although it may also occur with glycine. Induce diuresis with mannitol and furosemide to protect the renal tubules from free hemoglobin deposition. Persistent bleeding may be caused by fibrinolysis (tissue factors released from the prostate activate plasminogen), DIC, or pre-existing coagulopathy (e.g., recent aspirin ingestion). Abdominal pain, a rigid abdomen, or a swollen scrotum may result from bladder perforation, which generally requires surgical repair. Persistent penile erection makes instrumentation technically difficult and increases the risk of trauma. None of the numerous recommended measures work universally. Electrical stimulation of the obturator nerve may cause adduction of the ipsilateral leg. Reduction in electrical current usually solves this problem. Warm irrigating solutions and opioids (systemic and intrathecal) decrease postoperative shivering. Instrumentation of an infected urinary tract may lead to sepsis with fever, chills, tachycardia, and hypotension. Transient bacteremia is common. Septicemia with fever, chills, and hypotension occurs in 6% of patients (mortality rates 25% to 75%). Aggressively treat with broad-spectrum antibiotics and cardiovascular support. Laser prostatectomy is the recent concept being performed at many centers, which usually involves laser (ND-YAG) and avoids TURP syndrome. The advantages are minimal fluid absorption and minimal blood loss. However, coagulation through the prostatic fossa, prostatic debris causing postoperative urinary retention, and fire are some of the other problems with laser use in the OR.[5] Thirty-day mortality from TURP is 0.1% to 0.3%. Preoperative renal failure predicts poor outcome. Blood transfusion is required in 2.5% of patients and 1% of patients end up with capsule perforation.[1]

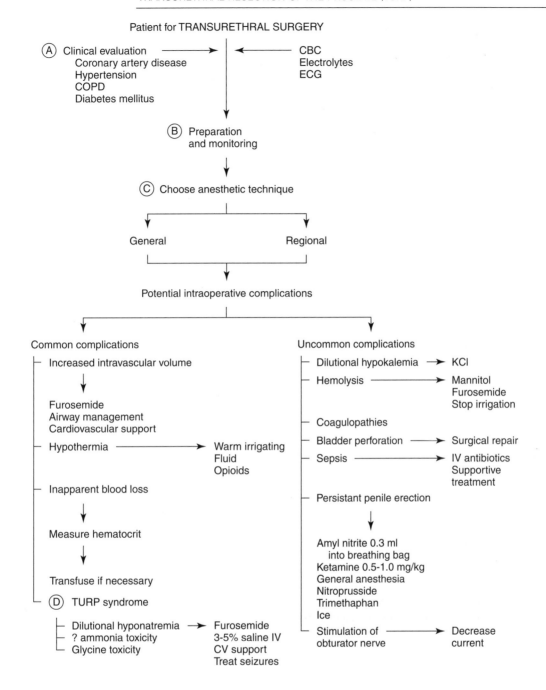

Patient for TRANSURETHRAL SURGERY

(A) Clinical evaluation
    Coronary artery disease
    Hypertension
    COPD
    Diabetes mellitus

CBC
Electrolytes
ECG

(B) Preparation and monitoring

(C) Choose anesthetic technique

General   Regional

Potential intraoperative complications

Common complications
- Increased intravascular volume

Furosemide
Airway management
Cardiovascular support

- Hypothermia ———→ Warm irrigating Fluid Opioids

- Inapparent blood loss

Measure hematocrit

Transfuse if necessary

- (D) TURP syndrome
    - Dilutional hyponatremia ——→ Furosemide
    - ? ammonia toxicity   3-5% saline IV
    - Glycine toxicity   CV support
    Treat seizures

Uncommon complications
- Dilutional hypokalemia ——→ KCl
- Hemolysis ——→ Mannitol Furosemide Stop irrigation
- Coagulopathies
- Bladder perforation ——→ Surgical repair
- Sepsis ——→ IV antibiotics Supportive treatment
- Persistant penile erection

Amyl nitrite 0.3 ml
   into breathing bag
Ketamine 0.5-1.0 mg/kg
General anesthesia
Nitroprusside
Trimethaphan
Ice

- Stimulation of ——→ Decrease obturator nerve current

REFERENCES

1. Malhotra V: Transurethral resection of the prostate, *Anesthesiol Clin North Am* 18:883-897, 2000.
2. Bready LL, Hoff BH, Boyd RC: Acute digitalis toxicity during TURP, *Urology* 25:316-317, 1985.
3. Gravenstein D: Transurethral resection of the prostate (TURP) syndrome: a review of pathophysiology and management, *Anesth Analg* 84:438-446, 1997.
4. Mebust WK, Holtgrewe HL, Cockett AT, et al.: Transurethral prostatectomy: immediate and postoperative complications. A cooperative study of 13 participating institutions evaluating 3,885 patients, *J Urol* 141:243-247, 1989.
5. Malhotra V, Perlmutter A: Caudal anesthesia provides effective anesthesia for laser prostatectomy, *Reg Anesth* 22 (2S):93, 1997.

Extracorporeal Shock Wave Lithotripsy (ESWL)

VINOD MALHOTRA, M.D.

VIJAYENDRA SUDHEENDRA, M.D.

Extracorporeal shock wave lithotripsy (ESWL) uses shock waves to fracture renal stones, resulting in lower morbidity than open pyelolithotomy. The Dornier lithotripter employs a water bath; newer lithotripters do not require patient immersion. The Dornier lithotripter requires special patient management and thus is discussed here in detail. Shock waves are produced by an electrode to which high energy (18–24 kV) is applied. The patient is strapped into a gantry chair and transferred into the tub so that the kidney stone lies at the focus of the shock waves. Normally the shock waves pass through the flank and kidney without causing significant tissue damage. However, shock waves may injure the lung (parenchymal disruption, alveolar rupture, contusion, and hemoptysis).[1,2] Shock waves are triggered by ECG and synchronized (applied in the refractory phase to minimize dysrhythmias, such as atrial and ventricular premature complexes, and rarely, supraventricular tachycardias). Cessation of shock wave application usually terminates dysrhythmias, but some patients require medical therapy. Because ECG is used as a trigger, a good ECG tracing with sufficient voltage is necessary.

Immersion in the water bath produces significant physiological effects. The hydrostatic force of water on the peripheral venous system redistributes blood centrally, increasing CVP and pulmonary artery (PA) pressure. The patient with cardiovascular compromise may develop cardiac failure; in such patients, partial, gradual immersion is recommended. Respiratory changes caused by immersion include decreases in FRC, vital capacity, and expiratory lung volume. Pulmonary blood flow increases. Patients tend to take shallow, rapid breaths. All these changes predispose the spontaneously breathing, sedated patient to hypoxemia; supplemental oxygen (O_2) is advised. Heat transfer is enhanced because of the large surface area and vasodilation induced by anesthesia. Hypothermia and hyperthermia have been reported;[2] the water should be kept thermoneutral (35°C to 37°C).

The newer lithotripters offer many advantages: there is no water bath; hence all problems of immersion are avoided; most use multifunctional tables so that other procedures, such as cystoscopy and stent placement, can be accomplished without moving the patient off the table; the shock waves are focused, so that they cause less pain at the entry site. However, even with piezoelectric lithotripters and low shock wave energy lithotripters, ESWL is a painful procedure requiring anesthesia. Additional interventions performed, such as cystoscopy, stone manipulation, or stent placement, will affect anesthetic requirements. Because many of the newer lithotripters have a smaller focal zone for the shock waves, it is imperative that adequate analgesia and sedation be provided so that the stone excursions with respirations are limited to the focal zone.

A. Pregnancy is a contraindication to lithotripsy; perform a pregnancy test in women with childbearing potential. Rule out bleeding disorders by obtaining coagulation tests.

Patient for LITHOTRIPSY

(A) Clinical evaluation ⟶   ⟵ Urinalysis, hematocrit, ECG (if indicated)
    Assess renal function   Pregnancy test (must be negative)
    Cardiac history of dysrhythmias,   Prothrombin time, partial thromboplastin time (if indicated)
        CHF, pacemaker, AICD   X-ray films to locate the stone
    Pregnancy, obesity, bleeding
        disorders

(Cont'd on p 449)

B. Children are more prone to lung injury than adults because of the close proximity of the lung bases to the kidneys; consider shielding the lungs with a Styrofoam sheet.[3] Obese patients are challenging. Prior to induction, attempt to simulate the procedure in the tub or on the treatment table to ensure that the stone can be brought into focus. For patients with pectoral pacemakers, have a pacemaker programmer and alternative means of cardiac pacing available, because the pacemaker may dysfunction as a result of shock waves.[5] Lithotripsy in contraindicated in patients with abdominal pacemakers. For patients with automatic implantable cardiac defibrillators (AICDs), have the device interrogated and deactivated. Have an external defibrillator available and ready. Reactivate the AICD after the lithotripsy.[4,5] Patients with chronic congestive heart failure (CHF) need preload reduction; minimize the depth of their immersion.

C. For immersion, set up 12-foot tubing for the anesthesia breathing circuit and long monitor cables to allow movement of the patient in the gantry chair. Monitor ECG, automated BP, SpO_2, temperature, and $ETCO_2$ with illuminated monitors. Position ECG leads so that sufficient QRS amplitude is available to trigger the lithotripter; protect leads from water with adhesive tape. Use care in positioning the patient in the frame of the gantry chair to avoid scraping against metal and pressure or stretch injury of the brachial plexus. The sitting position predisposes to hypotension during GETA or epidural anesthesia. Follow the manufacturer's guidelines for the use of electrodes in terms of the electrical safety of the lithotripter.

D. Several types of anesthesia have been used for ESWL. Select an anesthetic technique to ensure minimal patient and stone movement with respiration.[6,7] IV sedation with monitored anesthesia care is adequate for most lithotripters that do not use a water bath. This anesthetic allows faster preparation and recovery times but is not suitable for all patients. Other options include local infiltration, intercostals blocks, epidural, spinal, and general anesthesia. Most patients do not require narcotics for pain. Hematuria is expected; maintain adequate IV hydration to prevent clot retention.

REFERENCES

1. Malhotra V, Rosen RJ, Slepian RL: Life-threatening hypoxemia after lithotripsy in an adult due to shock-wave-induced pulmonary contusion, *Anesthesiology* 75:529-531, 1991.
2. Malhotra V: Hyperthermia and hypothermia as complications of extracorporeal shock wave lithotripsy, *Anesthesiology* 67:448, 1987.
3. Malhotra V, Gomillion MC, Artusio JF Jr: Hemoptysis in a child during extracorporeal shock wave lithotripsy, *Anesth Analg* 69:526-528, 1989.
4. American Society of Anesthesiologists Task Force on Perioperative Management of Patients with Cardiac Rhythm Management Devices: Practice advisory for the perioperative management of patients with cardiac rhythm management devices: pacemakers and implantable cardioverter-defibrillators. A report by the American Society of Anesthesiologists Task Force on Perioperative Management of Patients with Cardiac Rhythm Management Devices, *Anesthesiology* 103:186-198, 2005.
5. Vassolas G, Roth RA, Venditti FJ Jr: Effect of extracorporeal shock wave lithotripsy on implantable cardioverter defibrillator, *Pacing Clin Electrophysiol* 16:1245-1248, 1993.
6. Cicek M, Koroglu A, Demirbilek S, et al.: Comparison of propofol-alfentanil and propofol -remifentanil anaesthesia in percutaneous nephrolithotripsy, *Eur J Anaesthesiol* 22 (9):683-688, 2005.
7. Ugur G, Erhan E, Kocabas S, et al.: Anaesthetic/analgesic management of extracorporeal shock wave lithotripsy in paediatric patients, *Paediatr Anaesth* 13 (1):85-87, 2003.

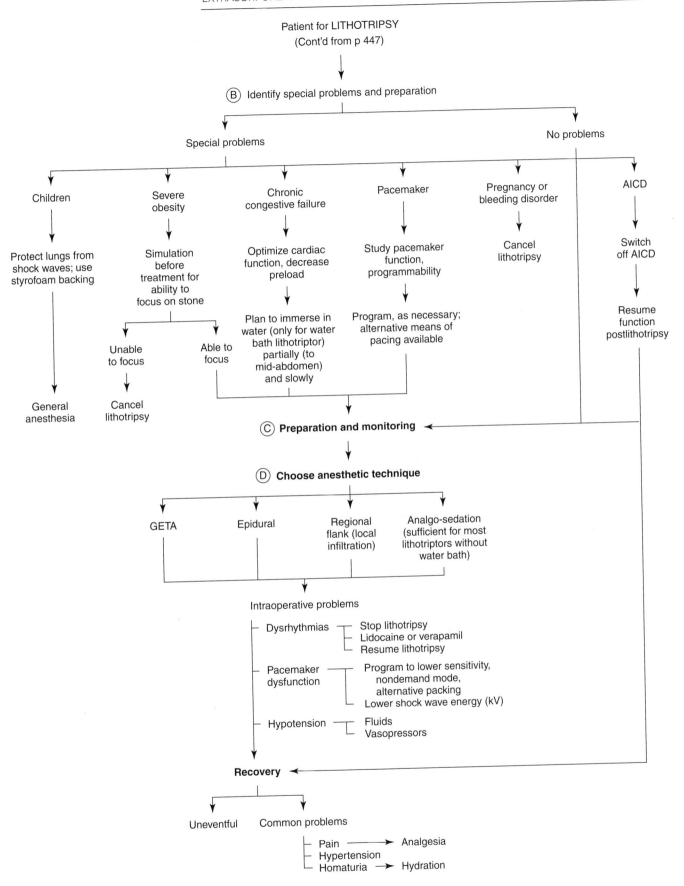

Percutaneous Nephrolithotripsy (PCNL)

KERRI M. ROBERTSON, M.D.

Percutaneous nephrolithotripsy (PCNL) is an essential procedure for treating complex urinary calculi with a success rate of greater than 90% for renal stones and 68% to 94% for ureteral stones.[1,2] PCNL requires percutaneous access to the collecting system of the kidney with fluoroscopy or ultrasonic guidance, creation of a nephrostomy tract, rapid tract dilation for insertion of the nephroscopic sheath, stone fragmentation by pneumatic, laser, or ultrasonic lithotripsy and stone removal.[3] Successful placement of a percutaneous nephrostomy tube can be achieved in more than 95% of cases with mortality rates <0.2% and incidence of 4% and 15% for major and minor complications, respectively. Complication rates may be higher in the morbidly obese patient (37%).[4] Outcomes (less cost, minimal blood loss, and reduced postoperative pain), hospital stay and recovery time are more favorable than with open nephrolithotomy.

A. Evaluate the patient for coexisting disorders and obtain appropriate laboratory values. Many patients require prophylactic antibiotics IV immediately before the procedure and for 24 to 48 hours postoperatively. Those patients at high risk for gram-negative bacteremia include immunosuppressed renal transplant recipients, those with positive urinalysis or urine culture, suspected infectious stones or a urinary ostomy.

B. Anesthetize and intubate the patient in the lithotomy position for insertion of a retrograde ureteral catheter and injection of contrast dye to delineate the collecting system, followed by repositioning to prone or prone oblique. Chest rolls are used to ensure abdominal decompression and optimal ventilation. This positioning facilitates percutaneous puncture of a peripheral renal calyx through a posterolateral subcostal approach. A supracostal approach introduces the risk of pneumothorax or hemothorax, laceration of the lung, liver, or spleen and possible extravasation of irrigating solution or urine into the chest.[5] A lateral decubitus or flank position is feasible in the morbidly obese patient who is difficult to ventilate prone. General anesthesia is preferred to local anesthesia with supplemental analgesia and sedation for management of pain caused by instrumentation within the kidney and distension of the renal capsule with irrigating solutions. Intercostal and epidural anesthetic techniques have also been described. Ample padding and support rolls are needed for positioning. Hypothermia may be a problem due to the use of cool irrigation solutions and a cold OR environment. Use prewarmed irrigation solutions, a forced-air warming unit and cover the patient well using a waterproof drape.

Monitor temperature and inspiratory pressure, along with standard American Society of Anesthesiologists (ASA) monitors. Lead protection is necessary during fluoroscopy. As the use of diathermy is not required, physiological normal saline is the irrigation fluid of choice.

C. Facilitate localization and puncture of the kidney by limiting the patient's tidal volume or providing an expiratory pause. Avoid catheter obstruction to reduce the incidence of intratubular reflux and pyelonephritis. Induce a diuresis before intrarenal manipulation to reduce the possibility of extrarenal extravasation of fluid due to tears in the collecting system. Stone disintegration is completed with ultrasonic lithotripsy. Transparenchymal puncture of the renal collecting system transverses psoas major, quadratus lumborum, arcuate ligaments, fascia, perirenal fat, and capsule and parenchyma of the kidney. Injury to the adjacent pleura, colon, liver and spleen, duodenum, bile duct, and gallbladder has been reported. In theory the pancreas, adrenal glands, and large abdominal vessels are also at risk. Observe peak inspiratory pressure; an increase may indicate development of hydrothorax or pneumothorax.

D. Complications of PNT placement include acute and late bleeding (atrioventricular [AV] fistula or pseudoaneurysm), injury to structures interposed between the posterior aspect of the kidney and abdominal wall, dislodgement of the nephrostomy tube, perforation of the renal parenchyma or collecting system, loss of the nephrostomy tract, sepsis, and air embolism.[6,7] Most acute overt septic events present with fever, chills, or septic shock during the procedure or within 4 to 6 hours of the procedure. Bleeding is one of the most frequent major complications and is caused by injury to the segmental or interlobar renal arteries or veins. Severe bleeding usually stops spontaneously with hydration, forced diuresis with mannitol (12.5 g IV), closure of the PNT or insertion of a large catheter to tamponade the tract. Transfusion rates are estimated at 5% to 6% in nonanemic patients. Continuous or recurrent bleeding and deterioration of renal function requires superselective arterial embolization. Provided the patient remains hemodynamically stable, open surgical exploration for segmental artery ligation is to be avoided because inspection of the kidney rarely results in identification of the bleeding vessel. Fluid absorption and volume overload may occur in patients with compromised cardiopulmonary or renal status and procedures complicated by excessive bleeding and large perforations.

Patient for PERCUTANEOUS NEPHROLITHOTRIPSY

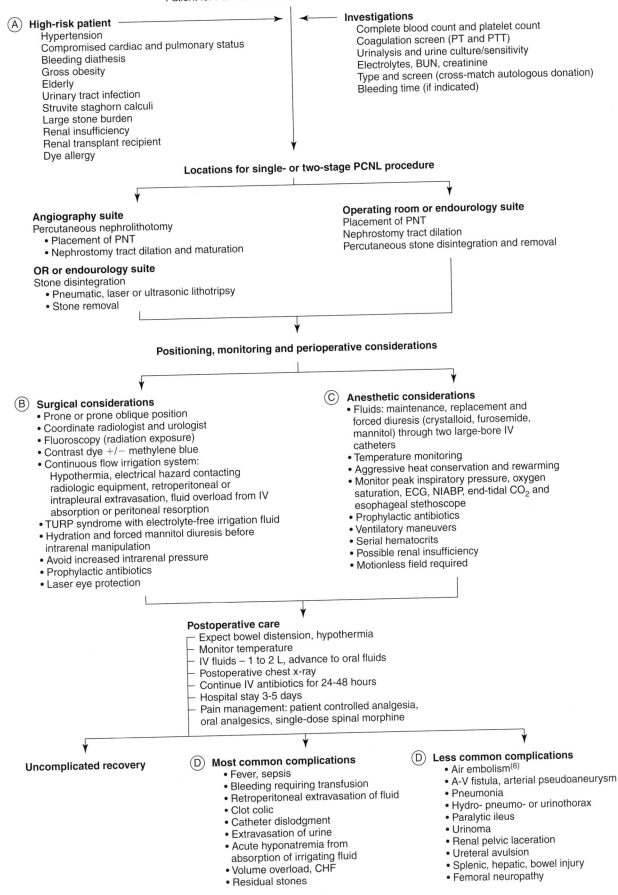

Ⓐ **High-risk patient**
  Hypertension
  Compromised cardiac and pulmonary status
  Bleeding diathesis
  Gross obesity
  Elderly
  Urinary tract infection
  Struvite staghorn calculi
  Large stone burden
  Renal insufficiency
  Renal transplant recipient
  Dye allergy

Investigations
  Complete blood count and platelet count
  Coagulation screen (PT and PTT)
  Urinalysis and urine culture/sensitivity
  Electrolytes, BUN, creatinine
  Type and screen (cross-match autologous donation)
  Bleeding time (if indicated)

Locations for single- or two-stage PCNL procedure

Angiography suite
Percutaneous nephrolithotomy
  • Placement of PNT
  • Nephrostomy tract dilation and maturation

OR or endourology suite
Stone disintegration
  • Pneumatic, laser or ultrasonic lithotripsy
  • Stone removal

Operating room or endourology suite
Placement of PNT
Nephrostomy tract dilation
Percutaneous stone disintegration and removal

Positioning, monitoring and perioperative considerations

Ⓑ **Surgical considerations**
  • Prone or prone oblique position
  • Coordinate radiologist and urologist
  • Fluoroscopy (radiation exposure)
  • Contrast dye +/− methylene blue
  • Continuous flow irrigation system:
    Hypothermia, electrical hazard contacting
    radiologic equipment, retroperitoneal or
    intrapleural extravasation, fluid overload from IV
    absorption or peritoneal resorption
  • TURP syndrome with electrolyte-free irrigation fluid
  • Hydration and forced mannitol diuresis before
    intrarenal manipulation
  • Avoid increased intrarenal pressure
  • Prophylactic antibiotics
  • Laser eye protection

Ⓒ **Anesthetic considerations**
  • Fluids: maintenance, replacement and
    forced diuresis (crystalloid, furosemide,
    mannitol) through two large-bore IV
    catheters
  • Temperature monitoring
  • Aggressive heat conservation and rewarming
  • Monitor peak inspiratory pressure, oxygen
    saturation, ECG, NIABP, end-tidal CO_2 and
    esophageal stethoscope
  • Prophylactic antibiotics
  • Ventilatory maneuvers
  • Serial hematocrits
  • Possible renal insufficiency
  • Motionless field required

Postoperative care
  — Expect bowel distension, hypothermia
  — Monitor temperature
  — IV fluids – 1 to 2 L, advance to oral fluids
  — Postoperative chest x-ray
  — Continue IV antibiotics for 24-48 hours
  — Hospital stay 3-5 days
  — Pain management: patient controlled analgesia,
    oral analgesics, single-dose spinal morphine

Uncomplicated recovery

Ⓓ **Most common complications**
  • Fever, sepsis
  • Bleeding requiring transfusion
  • Retroperitoneal extravasation of fluid
  • Clot colic
  • Catheter dislodgment
  • Extravasation of urine
  • Acute hyponatremia from
    absorption of irrigating fluid
  • Volume overload, CHF
  • Residual stones

Ⓓ **Less common complications**
  • Air embolism[6]
  • A-V fistula, arterial pseudoaneurysm
  • Pneumonia
  • Hydro- pneumo- or urinothorax
  • Paralytic ileus
  • Urinoma
  • Renal pelvic laceration
  • Ureteral avulsion
  • Splenic, hepatic, bowel injury
  • Femoral neuropathy

REFERENCES

1. Faerber GJ, Goh M: Percutaneous nephrolithotripsy in the morbidly obese patient, *Tech Urol* 3 (2):89-95, 1997.
2. Auge BK, Munver R, Kourambas J, et al.: Endoscopic management of symptomatic caliceal diverticula: a retrospective comparison of percutaneous nephrolithotripsy and ureteroscopy, *J Endourol* 16 (8):557-563, 2002.
3. Gravenstein D: Extracorporeal shock wave lithotripsy and percutaneous nephrolithotomy, *Anesthesiol Clin North Am* 18 (4):953-971, 2000.
4. Clayman RV, Castaneda-Zuniga WR: *Techniques in endourology: a guide to the percutaneous removal of renal and ureteral calculi*, Dallas, 1984, Heritage Press.
5. Radecka E, Brehmer M, Holmgren K, et al.: Complications associated with percutaneous nephrolithotripsy: supra- versus subcostal access. A retrospective study, *Acta Radiol* 44 (4):447-451, 2003.
6. Ferral H, Stackhouse DJ, Bjarnason H, et al.: Complications of percutaneous nephrostomy tube placement, *Semin Intervent Radiol* 11:198, 1994.
7. Usha N: Air embolism—a complication of percutaneous nephrolithotripsy, *Br J Anaesth* 91 (5):760-761; author reply 761, 2003.

ANESTHESIA AND TRANSPLANTATION

Organ Procurement in the Cadaveric Organ Donor

GWENDOLYN L. BOYD, M.D.

MICHAEL G. PHILLIPS, B.HS, PA-C

Patients who have met criteria for brain death continue to comprise the majority of cadaveric organ donors. Brain death is a clinical diagnosis made in the absence of potentially reversible effects on the CNS.[1] Two clinical determinations of brain death are done in accordance with individual state laws. Following the diagnosis of brain death and consent for organ donation, organ preservation begins with the management of the cadaveric organ donor.[2,3] It often helps the anesthesia team to consider that the organs already belong to the potential recipients.[4] A recent resurgence of interest in donation after cardiac death donors (DCD) requires several changes in standardized procurement protocols. In certain severely brain damaged patients who do not meet brain death criteria, withdrawal of life support may become appropriate. The decision to withdraw life support *must* be made prior to any discussion with the patient's family regarding organ donation by the organ procurement organization (OPO).[5] Potential non–heart beating donors must be dependent on life sustaining treatment such that stopping it will lead predictably and quickly to death.[6] Every hospital needs to develop its own standards and policies regarding discontinuation of life support as well as those for DCD donors with their ethics committees. It is estimated that currently 70% of hospital deaths are negotiated, with some kind of explicit discussion on termination of life support with the patient or surrogate. Consistent continuity of palliative care is given during the dying process. Only health care providers with appropriate knowledge, training, and expertise in the withdrawal of life support and comfort care should be involved with the DCD donor. Anesthesiologists are not involved in the care of the DCD donor as their training typically does not include palliative care. In addition, they are part of the transplant team and therefore may not be directly involved with the terminal care and never in the pronouncement of death.[7] Anesthesiologists need to be involved in their hospital standards regarding DCD donor to ensure that they are not involved.[8] One difficulty in developing standards is allowing family members to be present at the time of death which may force a choice between holding their dying loved one and organ donation. To improve the viability of the organs, perfusion cannulae may be placed under local anesthesia prior to withdrawal of life support as in situ preservation must occur rapidly after cardiopulmonary arrest. When the DCD donor procurement is controlled (i.e., cannulae inserted prior to withdrawal of life support) then the viability of the transplanted organs has been shown to be equivalent to the brain death donor.[9]

While it had been hoped to increase the number of transplanted organs by 20% or so, this hoped-for increase has not yet been realized.

A. *Hemodynamic sequelae of brain death:* Hypotension is generally caused by hypovolemia secondary to prior diuresis and dehydration, destruction of pontine and medullary structures that regulate circulation and respiration, brainstem herniation precipitating a C_1 spinal cord shock syndrome, or myocardial dysfunction and low cardiac output (CO) state. The sympathetic nervous system becomes nonfunctional after brain death. Treat hemodynamic instability with volume resuscitation (usually several liters) and dopamine, less than 10 $\mu g/kg^{-1}/min^{-1}$; higher doses may impair graft function and success of the renal transplant and lessen suitability for cardiac, lung, or liver donation. Should the systolic pressure remain low despite dopamine infusion, vasopressin may be instituted. Experimentally, adding norepinephrine to dopamine 5 $\mu g/kg^{-1}/min^{-1}$ preserves the renal salutary effects of dopamine while increasing systemic vascular resistance (SVR), making it possibly preferable to greater than 10 $\mu g/kg^{-1}/min^{-1}$ of dopamine. *Endocrine sequelae of brain death:* Most patients with brain death develop diabetes insipidus with polyuria, dehydration, hypernatremia, serum hyperosmolality, and hypokalemia. Treat diabetes insipidus by replacing fluids using milliliter for milliliter of half-normal saline or a sodium-free solution. Vasopressin, 0.5 to 2 μg every 8 to 12 hours by continuous IV infusion, maintains extracellular homeostasis, increasing the number of transplantable organs. Maintain urinary volume of 100 to 250 ml/hour with vasopressin. *Other pathophysiologic sequelae of brain death:* Hypothermia (absence of hypothalamic temperature regulation possibly compounded by unwarmed IV fluids) may lead to ventricular fibrillation at core temperatures <28°C. Tissue oxygen delivery decreases as the oxygen dissociation curve is shifted to the left. Warm IV fluids as well as increasing the environmental temperature may be required to keep the donor's temperature above 34° C. A convectional warming device, i.e., Bair Hugger® or Warm Touch®, can be used to actively warm cold patients as well as to maintain their temperature. Hypothermia below 32°C potentiates the release of tissue fibrinolytic agent from the necrotic brain. Ninety percent of brain death patients have DIC. Factor replacement may not correct the bleeding diathesis. Epsilon-aminocaproic

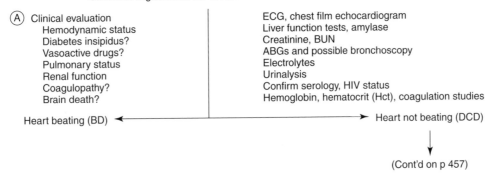

Cadaveric organ donor for ORGAN PROCUREMENT

Ⓐ Clinical evaluation
    Hemodynamic status
    Diabetes insipidus?
    Vasoactive drugs?
    Pulmonary status
    Renal function
    Coagulopathy?
    Brain death?

ECG, chest film echocardiogram
Liver function tests, amylase
Creatinine, BUN
ABGs and possible bronchoscopy
Electrolytes
Urinalysis
Confirm serology, HIV status
Hemoglobin, hematocrit (Hct), coagulation studies

Heart beating (BD) ←   → Heart not beating (DCD)

(Cont'd on p 457)

acid (Amicar®) is not given to reverse the fibrinolysis as it may induce microvascular thrombosis in the donor organs. Coagulopathy conveys a sense of urgency to decrease the total blood loss as well as the need for replacement. Hypokalemia develops in 90% of BD patients while 39% are hyperkalemic sometime during their course. Electrolytes need to be closely monitored before and sometimes during organ procurement.

The PaO_2 should be maintained above 100 while avoiding hyperoxia. Five cm H_2O PEEP helps prevent airway collapse. Production of carbon dioxide (CO_2) decreases after brain death (lowered brain metabolism, hypothermia, and decrease muscle activity). Both hypocarbia and hypercarbia decrease renal blood flow; aim for eucarbia.

B. The hemodynamic status of the donor conveys the relative urgency with which to proceed to the OR for organ procurement.

C. The operating room should be warmed to 70°F or greater depending upon the degree of hypothermia in the brain death donor.

D. Neuromuscular blockade relaxes the abdominal muscles and obscures the various spinal reflexes, including Lazarus's sign, in brain death patients.[9] The increases in HR and BP frequently seen following the incision do not invalidate the diagnosis of brain death.[10]

E. Multiple organ procurement in brain death donors may take several hours and may necessitate blood transfusion. The temperature should be maintained above 32°C. Previously stable donors may herniate and become unstable at any time; anticipate this possibility taking appropriate vasoactive measures to improve post-graft function. Once the incision has been made, the aorta can be cross-clamped below the renal arteries to increase the BP above the level of the clamp. Close communication is to be maintained with the procurement team throughout the procedure. Drugs including heparin, diuretics, and alpha-antagonists, such as chlorpromazine, are routine and given on request. Following aortic cross-clamping in brain death donors, mechanical ventilation is discontinued and monitors turned off.

A_1 Following the decision to withdraw life support, the organ procurement organization may be contacted to determine if the patient is suitable to be considered for DCD donor.

B_1 For the DCD donor, withdrawal of life support may be done either in the ICU or in the OR according to established individual hospital policy and standard. The family's concerns are paramount during the dying process. Vascular cannulas for in situ organ perfusion may be placed under local anesthesia prior to discontinuing life support either in the ICU or in the OR.

C_1 End-of-life care, withdrawal of life support, and pronouncement of death are carried out by the primary care team.

D_1 Anesthesia is not involved in the DCD donor except perhaps to coordinate OR availability.

E_1 Should the potential DCD donor's heart not stop beating during the time frame established by the hospital's organ donation standard, usually 1 to 2 hours, the patient is taken from the OR and returned to an appropriate palliative care area.

REFERENCES

1. Bishop RC, Morawetz RB: Brain death determination. In: Phillips MG, *Organ procurement: preservation and distribution in transplantation*, ed 2, Richmond, VA, 1996, UNOS.
2. Soifer B, Gelb AW: The multiple organ donor: identification and management, *Ann Intern Med* 110:814-823, 1989.
3. Boyd GL, Phillips MG, Henry ML: "Cadaver donor management." In: Hrsg. Philipps MG, editor: *Organ procurement, preservation and distribution in transplantation*, Richmond, VA, 1996, UNOS.
4. Institute of Medicine, committee on non-heart-beating transplantation II: the scientific and ethical basis for practice and protocols: *Non-heart-beating organ transplantation: practice and protocols*. Washington DC, 2000, National Academy Press.
5. Solomon MZ: Donation after cardiac death: non-heart-beating organ donation deserves a green light and hospital oversight, *Anesthesiology* 98:601-602, 2003.
6. Youngner SJ, Arnold RM: Ethical, psychosocial, and public policy implications of procuring organs from non-heart-beating cadaver donors, *JAMA* 269:2769-2774, 1993.
7. Van Norman GA: Another matter of life and death: What every anesthesiologist should know about the ethical, legal and policy implications of the non-heart-beating cadaver organ donor, *Anesthesiology* 98:763-773, 2003.
8. Truog RD: Organ donation after cardiac death: What role for anesthesiologists? *Anesthesiology* 98:599-600, 2003.
9. Cho YW, Terasaki PI, Cecka JM, et al.: Transplantation of kidneys from donors whose hearts have stopped beating, *N Engl J Med* 338:221-225, 1998.
10. Varner PD, McKay RD: Brain death and management of the cadaveric donor. In: Graybar GB, Bready LL, editors: *Anesthesia for renal transplantation*, Boston, 1987, Martinus Nijoff.

Cadaveric organ donor for ORGAN PROCUREMENT

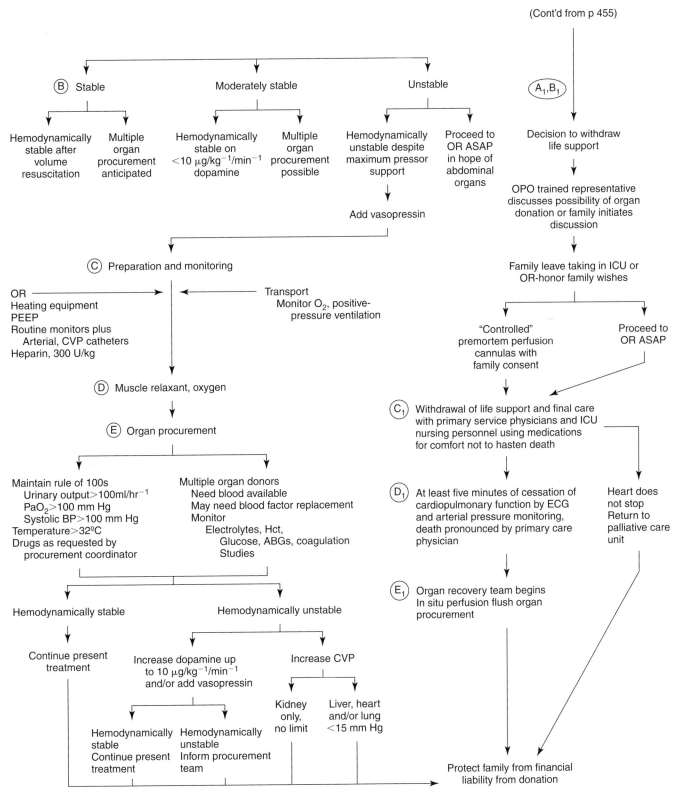

Renal Transplantation

VIVIAN HOU, M.D.

Renal transplantation from a cadaver or living related donor has become the treatment of choice for end-stage renal disease (ESRD).[1] Patients with ESRD have many coexisting problems (e.g., hypertension [HTN], diabetes, ischemic heart disease, pericarditis, hematological abnormalities, and electrolyte disturbances) that can increase perioperative morbidity and mortality during renal transplantation. Perioperative complications can be reduced with meticulous anesthesia care (i.e., adequate preoperative assessment and optimization, smooth anesthetic induction and maintenance, appropriate monitoring and volume replacement, and careful postoperative care).[2,3]

A. Perform a careful history and physical examination. Look for signs and symptoms of ischemic heart disease. Review lab results including complete blood count (CBC), coagulation studies, and chemistries. Treat potassium >5.5 mEq/L. Send a type and screen. Obtain an ECG and chest x-ray (CXR). Consider cardiac noninvasive testing in diabetic patients or those with other cardiac risk factors or symptoms.

B. Ensure that the patient has been NPO for 6 hours (renal transplant does not usually have to be performed urgently) and has had dialysis within 24 to 36 hours of transplant. Continue antihypertensive medications. If the patient has not been taking antihypertensive medications prior to the procedure and the BP is elevated, give perioperative beta-blockers. If the patient is diabetic, hold oral hypoglycemics; give half of the NPH insulin dose and monitor glucose levels. Administer appropriate antibiotics and anxiolytics.

C. Apply standard American Society of Anesthesiologists (ASA) monitors. Place a CVP for volume assessment and drug infusion. Place an arterial line in patients with cardiovascular or pulmonary disease. Observe strict sterile technique during line insertion.

D. Protect any functional dialysis access. Recall that diabetics are prone to nerve injury.

E. Choose induction technique based on volume status, NPO status, and presence of gastroparesis or aspiration risk. The following induction agents have been used safely: thiopental (consider slow administration of smaller dose), propofol (the hypotensive effect can be up to 40%), and etomidate (note adrenal suppressive effects, usually not clinically important). Avoid ketamine. If a RSI is required, it is generally safe to use succinylcholine (SCC) if potassium (K) <5.5 mEq/L in patients without significant neuropathy. SCC induces K increases to the same extent (0.5 to 1 mmol/L) in healthy patients and patients with ESRD without significant neuropathy. Choose rocuronium as an alternative agent for RSI; onset and recovery is unchanged in patients with ESRD. Consider cisatracurium if RSI is not necessary; its metabolism and excretion are not dependent on normal renal function.

F. Maintain anesthesia with volatile anesthetics, being mindful of BP and perfusion pressure (transplanted kidney, atrioventricular [AV] fistula). The volatile agents have no impact on graft function but cause dose-related cardiac depression. Fentanyl, sufentanil, and hydromorphone are all acceptable opioids. Avoid meperidine; its active metabolite can accumulate and cause seizures. Similarly, morphine metabolites can accumulate, resulting in prolonged effects. Maintain adequate relaxation during key anastomoses (renal artery, vein, and ureter).

G. Administer immunosuppressive therapy prior to graft reperfusion. Follow the specific institutional protocol.

H. Consider mannitol or furosemide to promote diuresis in the graft kidney. Administer volume replacement using a combination of colloid and crystalloid to maintain BP and diuresis. Follow CVP; maintain in the range of 10 to 15 mm Hg to improve renal blood flow. Consider dopamine for hypotension refractory to volume therapy. Vasopressors, especially alpha-agonists, can decrease renal perfusion.

I. Postoperatively, obtain a CXR to confirm CVP placement. Maintain normal to slightly elevated blood pressure and CVP to maximize renal perfusion. Observe inputs and outputs; avoid fluid overload and pulmonary edema. If the patient is euvolemic and hypertensive, consider cyclosporine or transplant rejection as etiologies. Provide IV patient controlled analgesia.

REFERENCES

1. Barry JM: Renal transplantation. In: Walsh PC, editor: *Campbell's urology*, ed 8, Philadelphia, 2002, W.B. Saunders.
2. Morris P: *Kidney transplantation: principles and practice*, ed 5, Philadelphia, 2001, W.B. Saunders.
3. Lemmens HJ: Kidney transplantation: recent developments and recommendations for anesthetic management, *Anesthesiol Clin North Am* 22:651-662, 2004.

Patient for RENAL TRANSPLANTATION

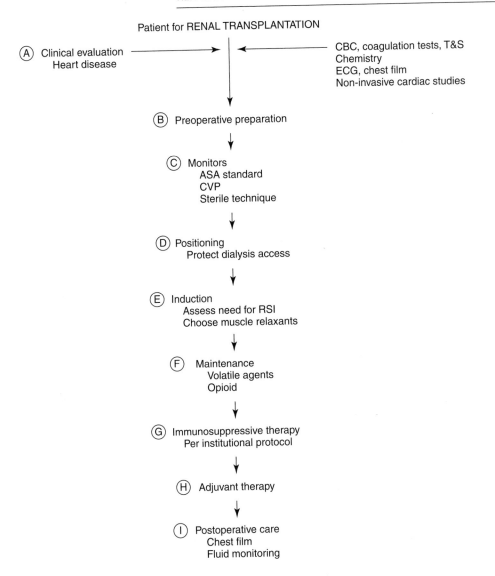

Ⓐ Clinical evaluation
   Heart disease

CBC, coagulation tests, T&S
Chemistry
ECG, chest film
Non-invasive cardiac studies

Ⓑ Preoperative preparation

Ⓒ Monitors
   ASA standard
   CVP
   Sterile technique

Ⓓ Positioning
   Protect dialysis access

Ⓔ Induction
   Assess need for RSI
   Choose muscle relaxants

Ⓕ Maintenance
   Volatile agents
   Opioid

Ⓖ Immunosuppressive therapy
   Per institutional protocol

Ⓗ Adjuvant therapy

Ⓘ Postoperative care
   Chest film
   Fluid monitoring

Living Donor Nephrectomy

GWENDOLYN L. BOYD, M.D.

The outcome of renal transplantation for graft and patient survival remains better with living related donor (LRD) and living unrelated donor (LURD) than with a cadaveric kidney donor, despite improvements in both immunosuppression and treatment of rejection. Cold ischemia time and immunosuppressant requirements are less with living donors than for cadaveric transplantation. Both the living donor's and the recipient's medical status can be optimized compared to cadaveric transplants. Indeed, the number of LURDs has increased because of the newer therapies, such as daclizumab (Zenapax®) and cyclosporine, with resultant increased graft survival. Complications to the living donor are few, with rare serious consequences. Laparoscopic donor nephrectomy minimizes postoperative pain, length of stay, and time to return to function.[4] Laparoscopic nephrectomy has not been shown to have any adverse affects on allograft function or survival compared to open.[5]

A. The LRD or LURD is healthy, with normal renal function. A thorough medical evaluation following the guidelines of the American Society of Transplant Physicians is performed. In addition to assuring that the donor will have adequate renal function after the nephrectomy, the donor's motivation and emotional stability are carefully evaluated. Dual-phase spiral CT with three-dimensional angiography of the living donor patient has been shown to adequately depict renal vasculature when compared to standard angiography. Multiple renal arteries and veins are not a contraindication to laparoscopic donor nephrectomy, but preoperative identification allows the surgeon to anticipate and plan accordingly. The left kidney is generally chosen to transplant as its vein is longer, facilitating transplantation. Donor hydration is usually begun the night prior to surgery. Hydration is particularly important for laparoscopic nephrectomy, as pneumoperitoneum has been shown to significantly decrease renal blood flow. Patients routinely receive 5 to 6 L of crystalloid during donor nephrectomy.

B. The flank position utilized for open donor nephrectomy (Figure 1) results in significant hemodynamic compromise and general discomfort, making general

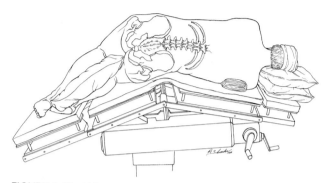

FIGURE 1 The kidney rest is properly placed beneath the down-side iliac crest, offering the least interference with the functions of the down-side lung and diaphragm (From Lawson NW, Meyer DJ: Lateral positions. In: Martin JT, Warner MA, editors: *Positioning in anesthesia and surgery*, ed 3, Philadelphia, 1997, W.B. Saunders.)

anesthesia the technique of choice. A second large-bore IV is started after induction of anesthesia allowing both the treatment of the impaired venous return associated with positioning, as well as the sudden blood loss that occasionally occurs during donor nephrectomy. Flank positioning requires frequent monitoring of BP as the impaired venous return may cause significant hypotension necessitating a light plane of anesthesia, muscle relaxation, and volume loading. Inadequate support of the head and neck may lead to postoperative Horner's syndrome. Evaluate the radial pulse after placement of the axillary roll. Respiration is impaired by the flank position secondary to V/Q mismatching, decreased FRC, decreased vital capacity, and decreased thoracic compliance. Recheck breath sounds, as the endotracheal tube (ETT) may migrate into the mainstem bronchus during positioning. The detrimental effects of flank position on respiration appear to worsen with time, mandating continuous monitoring of end-tidal carbon dioxide (CO_2) and oxygen saturation. The 11th rib is usually removed; pneumothorax is a potential complication. During wound closure, the surgeon may request positive pressure to be maintained while they empty any air from the pleural space.

LIVING DONOR NEPHRECTOMY

(A) Clinical   BUN, creatinine
       General good health   Hemoglobin
       Choice of kidney   Blood type and screen

Overnight hydration to
ensure good urinary output

(B) Preparation and monitoring
       ECG
       Noninvasive BP
       FiO_2
       End-tidal CO_2
       Pulse oximetry

(Cont'd on p 463)

C. The modified flank position (Figure 2) employed for laparoscopic donor nephrectomy is associated with significantly less hemodynamic and respiratory compromise than is the classic flank position.

D. Intraoperatively, maintain eucarbia (both hypocarbia and hypercarbia cause renal vasoconstriction). Maintain good urine output (1 to 2 ml/min) with generous administration of crystalloids and diuretics. Our protocol includes two doses of mannitol (12.5 grams each). Should urinary output decline despite fluid loading and mannitol, furosemide may also be given. Maintain systolic pressure at normal levels. The kidney is rested without manipulation for 15 minutes following its dissection and sectioning of the ureter. Heparin 2500 units is administered to the patient and the kidney then removed. Protamine 25 mg is then given slowly intravenously.

E. Reverse the muscle relaxant and extubate the patient. Check a chest x-ray (CXR) following open donor nephrectomy to rule out pneumothorax or unilateral pulmonary edema. Anticipate significant pain following open nephrectomy and administer appropriately high doses of narcotics or epidural anesthesia. Ketorolac has proven a useful addition in decreasing postoperative pain after donor nephrectomy.

REFERENCES

1. United Network for Organ Sharing (UNOS) and the Division of Transplantation, Bureau of Health Resources and Services Administration: Annual report of the U.S. scientific registry of transplant recipients and organ procurement and transplantation network-transplant data, Rockville, MD, 2005, U.S. Department of Health and Human Services, available at: http://www.ustransplant.org/annual_reports/current/default.htm.
2. Ratner LE, Montgomery RA, Kavoussi LR: Laparoscopic donor nephrectomy. A review of the first 5 years, *Urol Clin North Am* 28 (4):709-719, 2001.
3. Kasiske BL, Ravenscraft M, Ramos EL, et al.: The evaluation of living renal transplant donors: clinical practice guidelines. Ad hoc clinical practice guidelines subcommittee of the patient care and education committee of the American Society of Transplant Physicians, *J Am Soc Nephrol* 7:2288-2313, 1996.
4. Sprung J, Kapural L, Bourke DL, et al: Anesthesia for kidney transplant surgery, *Anesthesiol Clin North Am* 18 (4):919-951, 2000.
5. Conacher ID, Soomro NA, Rix D: Anaesthesia for laparoscopic urological surgery, *Br J Anaesth* 93 (6):859-864, 2004.

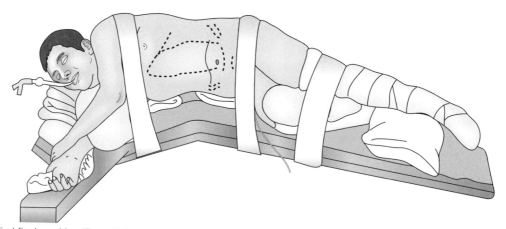

FIGURE 2 Modified flank position (From Bishoff JT, Kavoussi LR: Laparoscopic surgery of the kidney. In: Walsh PC, Retik AB, Vaughn ED Jr, et al., editors: *Campbell's urology*, ed 8, Philadelphia, 2002, W.B. Saunders).

LIVING DONOR NEPHRECTOMY
(Cont'd from p 461)

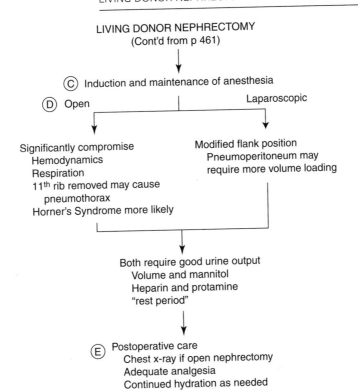

Ⓒ Induction and maintenance of anesthesia

Ⓓ Open   Laparoscopic

Significantly compromise   Modified flank position
Hemodynamics   Pneumoperitoneum may
Respiration   require more volume loading
11th rib removed may cause
    pneumothorax
Horner's Syndrome more likely

Both require good urine output
Volume and mannitol
Heparin and protamine
"rest period"

Ⓔ Postoperative care
    Chest x-ray if open nephrectomy
    Adequate analgesia
    Continued hydration as needed

Cardiac Transplantation

MICHAEL P. HUTCHENS, M.D., M.A.

STEPHEN T. ROBINSON, M.D.

The indications for cardiac transplantation include severe heart failure and congenital heart disease in patients who have failed other therapies. The most common single preoperative diagnosis for cardiac transplant in the early 2000's is ischemic dilated cardiomyopathy. Overall survival at one year is 85% and at three years is 78%.[1]

A. The preoperative status of patients scheduled for cardiac transplant ranges from relatively compensated and living at home to hospitalized with maximal chemical or mechanical support. In some centers patients may arrive from home with inotropic infusions running. Early anesthetic evaluation is useful; once the transplant is scheduled, a donor organ ischemic time of less than 240 minutes is desirable, particularly if the donor is older than 50.[2] Initiate appropriate management for patients with difficult airways, pacemakers, previous cardiac surgery, or other complicating conditions. Assess renal function. Because of the potential for right-sided heart failure, assess hepatic function. Hepatic congestion and ischemic gastropathy may cause delayed gastric emptying; consider full stomach precautions, regardless of NPO status. Assess coagulation status; coagulopathy may be present secondary to hepatic congestion or therapeutic anticoagulation. Note and optimize inotropic infusion, IABP, BiVAD, LVAD, or RVAD settings and plan for safe transport of these devices.

B. Place large-bore IVs, standard monitors, and an arterial line prior to induction. The need for early transplantation precludes full NPO status for many patients. Therefore, consider RSI with maximal reflux precautions (including sodium citrate, metoclopramide, an H_2 blocker, and a PPI). If the patient has a pacemaker or an automatic implantable cardiac defibrillator (AICD), have it interrogated and note its mode, backup mode, and the underlying rhythm. Turn off adaptive rate and tachycardia sensing features and program an asynchronous backup mode to prevent arrhythmia from electrocautery artifact.[3] Continue mechanical and chemical support throughout the preinduction period.

C. Although RSI may be necessary, let the choice of agent be guided by the patient's hemodynamic status.

If RSI is not necessary, a stable induction may be best achieved with slow titration of thiopental or etomidate, although many induction agents have been successfully used, including ketamine, benzodiazepines, and opioids.[4] Pay careful attention to hemodynamic state during induction; be prepared for chemical resuscitation. Long circulation times delay drug onset; avoid giving additional doses of induction medications before initial doses have had time to take effect.

D. Long-term immunosuppression beginning in the perioperative period is a core therapy for transplant patients. Because the immunosuppressive regimen frequently includes high-dose intraoperative steroids, consider glucose management with insulin. Preoperative antibiotics are essential. Give immunosuppressive agents in consultation with the surgical team. Pay careful attention to sterile technique during all perioperative procedures. Full drape, gown, and mask are recommended for central line placement.[5] Anticipate large blood loss volumes in patients with previous sternotomies. In these patients, place additional large-bore access. Aprotinin has been shown to reduce perioperative blood loss in both initial and secondary sternotomy patients,[6] but the risk of anaphylaxis is increased in patients with previous exposure. Maintain muscle relaxation with a nondepolarizing relaxant and anesthesia with opioids, benzodiazepines, or low-dose inhalation agent. N_2O can be used prior to bypass, but it may elevate the pulmonary vascular resistance (PVR), thus exacerbating prebypass right-sided heart failure. Place central venous access before or after induction. In some centers, a left-sided approach is preferred to preserve the right-sided vessels for postoperative cardiac biopsies. If a pulmonary artery (PA) catheter is placed, withdrawn to the central circulation at the onset of cardiopulmonary bypass (CPB) to prevent surgical interference. The catheter may be replaced under direct vision by the surgical team at closure. Transesophageal echocardiography (TEE) is an important modality for analysis of graft function in the postbypass period.

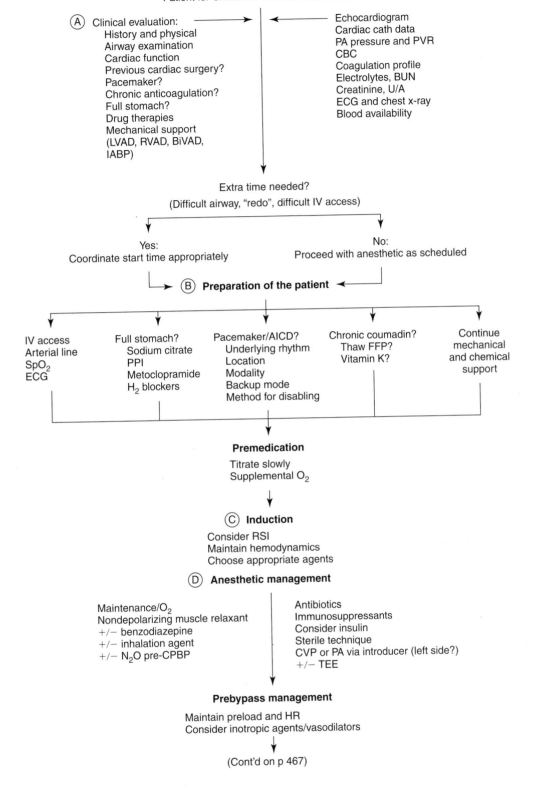

Patient for CARDIAC TRANSPLANTATION

Ⓐ Clinical evaluation:
   History and physical
   Airway examination
   Cardiac function
   Previous cardiac surgery?
   Pacemaker?
   Chronic anticoagulation?
   Full stomach?
   Drug therapies
   Mechanical support
   (LVAD, RVAD, BiVAD,
   IABP)

Echocardiogram
Cardiac cath data
PA pressure and PVR
CBC
Coagulation profile
Electrolytes, BUN
Creatinine, U/A
ECG and chest x-ray
Blood availability

Extra time needed?
(Difficult airway, "redo", difficult IV access)

Yes:
Coordinate start time appropriately

No:
Proceed with anesthetic as scheduled

Ⓑ **Preparation of the patient**

IV access
Arterial line
SpO_2
ECG

Full stomach?
   Sodium citrate
   PPI
   Metoclopramide
   H_2 blockers

Pacemaker/AICD?
   Underlying rhythm
   Location
   Modality
   Backup mode
   Method for disabling

Chronic coumadin?
   Thaw FFP?
   Vitamin K?

Continue
mechanical
and chemical
support

Premedication

Titrate slowly
Supplemental O_2

Ⓒ **Induction**

Consider RSI
Maintain hemodynamics
Choose appropriate agents

Ⓓ **Anesthetic management**

Maintenance/O_2
Nondepolarizing muscle relaxant
+/− benzodiazepine
+/− inhalation agent
+/− N_2O pre-CPBP

Antibiotics
Immunosuppressants
Consider insulin
Sterile technique
CVP or PA via introducer (left side?)
+/− TEE

Prebypass management

Maintain preload and HR
Consider inotropic agents/vasodilators

(Cont'd on p 467)

E. The postbypass donor heart is dependent on optimal end-diastolic ventricular volume and HR to maintain cardiac output (CO). HR is determined by the donor sinoatrial (SA) node, which is denervated, thus atropine, pancuronium, and phenylephrine will no longer affect HR. Therefore, use isoproterenol, other direct acting catecholamines, and pacing (atrial, ventricular, or atrioventricular [AV] sequential) to maintain an elevated HR to optimize CO. Use a PA line or TEE to assess right ventricular (RV) and left ventricular (LV) function. The most common cause of difficulty to wean from bypass is RV failure from exposure of the donor heart to elevated PA pressures. Consider systemic vasodilators, such as nitroglycerin. Other avenues of therapy are intravenous PGE_1, phosphodiesterase inhibitors (PDI), inhaled nitric oxide, and RVAD implantation. Inodilators such as milrinone (a PDI) or dobutamine (a beta agonist) may be especially useful but may require the addition of a vasoconstrictor to maintain SVR and preload. Treat left heart failure with inotropes. If LV failure is due to myocardial ischemia, nitroglycerin may be helpful. If these measures are ineffective, consider IABP or LVAD support. Afterload must be optimal to maintain LV function and preload. Treat low afterload with volume, alpha agonists, or vasopressin. Reduce a high afterload with vasodilators, inodilators, such as dobutamine and milrinone, or by increasing the depth of anesthesia.

F. Continue standard immunosuppression precautions in the immediate postoperative period. Extubate the patient when adequate airway, temperature, hemodynamic, and chest tube output criteria are met. Monitor immunosuppression and graft function. Early postoperative mortality is most frequently due to infection, while late mortality is secondary to graft vasculopathy.[4]

REFERENCES

1. United Network for Organ Sharing. available at: http://www.unos.org.
2. Del Rizzo DF, Menkis AH, Pflugfelder PW, et al.: The role of donor age and ischemic time on survival following orthotopic heart transplantation, *J Heart Lung Transplant* 18 (4):310-319, 1999.
3. Atlee JL, Bernstein AD: Cardiac rhythm management devices (part I): indications, device selection, and function, *Anesthesiology* 95 (5):1265-1280, 2001.
4. Bigham M, Dickstein ML, Hogue Jr, et al.: Cardiac and lung transplantation. In: Estafanous FG, Barash PG, Reves JG, editors: *Cardiac anesthesia: principles and clinical practice*, ed 2, Philadelphia, 2001, Lippincott Williams & Wilkins.
5. O'Grady NP, Alexander M, Dellinger EP, et al.: Guidelines for the prevention of intravascular catheter-related infections. Centers for Disease Control and Prevention, *MMWR Recomm Rep* 51 (RR-10):1-29, 2002.
6. Laupacis A, Fergusson D: Drugs to minimize perioperative blood loss in cardiac surgery: meta-analyses using perioperative blood transfusion as the outcome. The international study of peri-operative transfusion (ISPOT) investigators, *Anesth Analg* 85 (6):1258-1267, 1997.

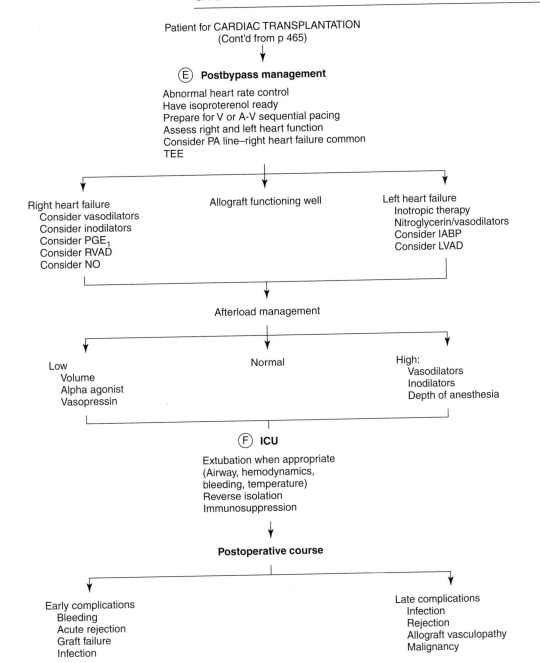

Patient for CARDIAC TRANSPLANTATION
(Cont'd from p 465)

Ⓔ **Postbypass management**

Abnormal heart rate control
Have isoproterenol ready
Prepare for V or A-V sequential pacing
Assess right and left heart function
Consider PA line–right heart failure common
TEE

Right heart failure
    Consider vasodilators
    Consider inodilators
    Consider PGE$_1$
    Consider RVAD
    Consider NO

Allograft functioning well

Left heart failure
    Inotropic therapy
    Nitroglycerin/vasodilators
    Consider IABP
    Consider LVAD

Afterload management

Low
    Volume
    Alpha agonist
    Vasopressin

Normal

High:
    Vasodilators
    Inodilators
    Depth of anesthesia

Ⓕ **ICU**

Extubation when appropriate
(Airway, hemodynamics,
bleeding, temperature)
Reverse isolation
Immunosuppression

Postoperative course

Early complications
    Bleeding
    Acute rejection
    Graft failure
    Infection

Late complications
    Infection
    Rejection
    Allograft vasculopathy
    Malignancy

Cardiac Transplant Recipient Undergoing Noncardiac Surgery

VICTOR NG, M.D

LYDIA CASSORLA, M.D., M.B.A.

Noncardiac surgery in the cardiac transplant recipient occurs in ambulatory, obstetric, and surgical ORs.[1-5] Approximately 2,100 cardiac transplants are performed in the United States annually; over 60,000 have been performed worldwide since the International Society for Heart and Lung Transplantation initiated reporting. One year survival is 85% and 10-year survival is 50%.[6,7] Cholecystitis and pancreatitis occur more frequently than in the general population, and immunosuppression increases infection and malignancy rates.[8]

A. Perform a preoperative assessment of functional status. Ejection fraction and cardiac output (CO) are normal to slightly reduced in the cardiac transplant recipient who is not in rejection. The transplanted heart may have significantly depressed systolic function, either from primary graft failure (rejection) or ischemia (cardiac allograft vasculopathy), a diffuse and concentric form of coronary artery disease (CAD) thought to be immune-related. Vasculopathy is common in patients >1 year post-transplant and is the most frequent reason for retransplantation or death after one year. Because of denervation of the transplanted heart, patients almost never experience chest pain during coronary ischemia.[9,10] Diastolic dysfunction is common in the initial posttransplant period but usually improves. Review posttransplantation echocardiogram (echo) or cardiac catheterization data.

B. Assess heart rhythm; abnormalities are common. If the recipient's native sinoatrial (SA) node is retained, the ECG may demonstrate two sets of P waves; only one is conducted. Ventricular ectopy is common in the first few weeks but usually diminishes. Right bundle branch block is reported in 40% of patients. Up to 20% of patients will have a permanent pacemaker (bradyarrhythmias, heart block). *Atrial* arrhythmias (atrial flutter and fibrillation) are highly associated with rejection and should prompt reassessment of cardiac function.

C. Denervation of the heart is nearly always permanent after transplantation. The sympathetic and parasympathetic influences on resting HR are lost. Resting HR is typically 90 to 100 bpm. The response to stress is both delayed and blunted. Catecholamines will still increase HR and CO; however, endogenous catecholamines take several minutes to peak after an initial stimulus. Therefore, HR and CO do not increase quickly or to a normal extent during hypotension, exercise, stress, or light anesthesia.[11,12] Patients are predominantly dependent on preload to maintain CO (Frank-Starling mechanism). Therefore, anticipate sensitivity to changes in preload (fasting or institution of positive-pressure ventilation).

D. Prepare the patient for the OR. Maintain immunosuppression, which is essential. Use aseptic technique and limit use of invasive lines to specific indications. Administer antibiotics with coverage for staphylococcus prior to placement of any invasive line or surgical incision. Avoid nasal intubation (potential for bacteremia). Review the patient's medications for potential drug interactions with anesthetics.

Important Side Effects of Commonly Used Immunosuppressants

Azathioprine	Myelosuppression, ↓Neuromuscular block
Cyclosporine	Hypertension (HTN), ↓Renal function, ↑K^+, ↓Mg^{++}, ↑Neuromuscular block, ↓Seizure threshold
Mycophenolate mofetil	Myelosuppression, GI bleeding
Prednisone	Hypertension, ↑Glu, Adrenal suppression
Tacrolimus	↓Renal function, ↓Seizure threshold, ↑Glu, ↑K^+, ↓Mg^{++}

HEART TRANSPLANT RECIPIENT FOR NONCARDIAC SURGERY

(A) Clinical evaluation

History and physical exam:
    Functional status
    Medications and interactions
    Infection? rejection?
    Allograft vasculopathy?
    Pacemaker?

ECG/CXR
CBC/electrolytes
BUN/Cr/glucose
Echocardiogram?/cardiac cath?
    New echo if ↓ functional status
Pacemaker information

Transplanted heart: pathology?

Cardiac allograft vasculopathy:
    High incidence after first year
    Diffuse coronary disease
    Coronary ischemia is painless
    Decreased function/prognosis

Diastolic dysfunction: frequent early on
Allograft rejection/failure:
    Supraventricular arrhythmia
    Conduction block
    Fibrosis and myocarditis

(B) Transplanted heart: arrhytmia?

Supraventricular – a flutter or a fib:
    Suspect rejection or graft failure
    Obtain new echocardiogram

Ventricular/PVCs:
    New transplants - should decrease
RBBB: common, not worrisome

(C) Denervated heart: physiology

Reflex tachycardia absent:
    Hypotension/hypovolemia
    Light anesthesia/hypoxia
    Stress/exercise

Cardiac output increased by:
    Increased preload (Frank-Starling)
    Endogenous catecholamines
    Exogenous catecholamines

(D) Patient preparation

Immunosuppression:
    Maintain immunosuppressants/steroids
    Use aseptic technique
    Give antibiotics prior to central line and incision
    Minimize invasive monitoring
Preload dependence:
    Avoid dehydration
    Position patient to maintain preload
    Sensitive to changes w/mechanical ventilation

(Cont'd on p 471)

E. Choose an anesthetic technique. Monitored anesthesia care, regional anesthesia, and general anesthesia have all been employed successfully. Pay strict attention to immunosuppression, volume status, and patient positioning. Design an anesthetic plan appropriate for current cardiac function, control abnormal HR, and ensure adequate preload to maintain CO. Consider spontaneous over mechanical ventilation when appropriate; it has less effect on preload. Due to denervation, tachycardia will not occur with light anesthesia, hypoxia, hypotension, or hypovolemia. Likewise, there is no influence on HR from anticholinergics (atropine, glycopyrrolate, or scopolamine), anticholinesterases (neostigmine or edrophonium), muscle relaxants (pancuronium or succinylcholine), or phenylephrine. Potent vasodilators, such as nifedipine, nitroglycerin, and nitroprusside, may cause an exaggerated decrease in BP due to the lack of baroreceptor-mediated reflex tachycardia.

Maintain hemodynamic control with adequate preload and direct-acting agents (epinephrine, isoproterenol, norepinephrine, dopamine, and dobutamine). Higher doses of alpha$_1$-agonists may be required in patients who had congestive heart failure (CHF) prior to transplant, as altered regulation of receptors may persist many months after the transplant. Vagal maneuvers (carotid sinus massage or Valsalva maneuver) are ineffective. Beta-blockers are effective for HR control; however, caution is advised (negative inotropic effect is preserved).[12] Avoid excess monitoring if cardiac function is good. Keep dilute epinephrine and isoproterenol at hand when administering all anesthetics.

REFERENCES

1. Branch KR, Wagoner LE, McGrory CH, et al.: Risks of subsequent pregnancies on mother and newborn in female heart transplant recipients, *J Heart Lung Transplant* 17:698-702, 1998.
2. Kostopanagiotou G, Smyrniotis V, Arkadopoulos N, et al.: Anesthetic and perioperative management of adult transplant recipients in nontransplant surgery, *Anesth Analg* 89:613-622, 1999.
3. Shaw IH, Kirk AJ, Conacher ID. Anaesthesia for patients with transplanted hearts and lungs undergoing non-cardiac surgery, *Br J Anaesth* 67:772-778, 1991.
4. Cheng DC, Ong DD: Anaesthesia for non-cardiac surgery in heart-transplanted patients, *Can J Anaesth* 40:981-986, 1993.
5. Sharpe MD: Anaesthesia and the transplanted patient, *Can J Anaesth* 43:R89-R98, 1996.
6. Organ Procurement and Transplant Network Database. Available at: http://www.optn.org/data/.
7. Taylor DO, Edwards LB, Boucek MM, et al.: Registry of the International Society for Heart and Lung Transplantation: twenty-second official adult heart transplant report—2005, *J Heart Lung Transplant* 24 (8):945-955, 2005.
8. Yee J, Petsikas D, Ricci MA, et al.: General surgical procedures after heart transplantation, *Can J Surg* 33:185-188, 1990.
9. Dong C, Redenbach D, Wood S, et al.: The pathogenesis of cardiac allograft vasculopathy, *Curr Opin Cardiol* 11:183-190, 1996.
10. Stark RP, McGinn AL, Wilson RF: Chest pain in cardiac-transplant recipients. Evidence of sensory reinnervation after cardiac transplantation, *N Engl J Med* 324:1791-1794, 1991.
11. Ashary N, Kaye AD, Hegazi AR, et al.: Anesthetic considerations in the patient with a heart transplant, *Heart Dis* 4 (3):191-198, 2002.
12. Verani MS, Nishimura S, Mahmarian JJ, et al.: Cardiac function after orthotopic heart transplantation: response to postural changes, exercise, and beta-adrenergic blockade, *J Heart Lung Transplant* 13:181-193, 1994.

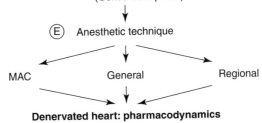

HEART TRANSPLANT RECIPIENT FOR NONCARDIAC SURGERY
(Cont'd from p 469)

(E) Anesthetic technique

MAC   General   Regional

Denervated heart: pharmacodynamics

No change in HR:
  Atropine/glycopyrrolate
  Edrophonium/neostigmine
  Pancuronium
  Succinylcholine
  Phenylephrine

Exaggerated BP decrease:
  Nifedipine
  NTG/nitroprusside
Decreased response:
  Ephedrine
  Alpha$_1$-agonists

Effective:
  Isoproterenol
  Epinephrine/norepinephrine
  Dobutamine/dopamine
  Phenylephrine (BP)
  Beta-blockers

Recovery and discharge: normal criteria

Single-Lung Transplantation

KATHERINE R. McGUIRE, M.D.

RALPH F. ERIAN, M.D., M.SC., FRCP(C)

Transplantation is a therapeutic alternative for patients with end-stage parenchymal or vascular lung disease. Common diagnoses in this patient population include chronic obstructive pulmonary disease (COPD) and idiopathic pulmonary fibrosis (IPF), for which single-lung transplantation (SLT) is commonly performed and cystic fibrosis and primary pulmonary hypertension (HTN), for which double-lung transplantation is often performed.[1]

A. Lung transplantation is considered in patients under age 65 with end-stage lung disease who have exhausted medical therapy and have a life expectancy of less than 24 to 36 months. Additional criteria include absence of significant comorbidities, good nutritional status, ability to tolerate postoperative rehabilitation and immunosuppression, and compliance with therapy.[2] COPD patients typically have an FEV_1 less than 25% to 30% of predicted along with hypoxemia, hypercarbia, and secondary pulmonary HTN. IPF patients are hypoxemic at rest with a vital capacity under 60% to 65% of predicted.[3] Lung size and ABO compatibility determine the match of potential donor and recipient. Previous thoracic surgeries and preoperative V/Q studies are considered in determining the operative side. Usually, the native lung with poorer function is replaced. Because of limited allowable ischemic time (4 to 6 hours) for the allograft lung, preoperative evaluation occurs, at most, a few hours before surgery. Review pulmonary function tests as well as cardiac catheterization and echocardiography (echo) studies.

B. Because of minimal pulmonary reserve, titrate sedative premedication slowly under monitored conditions. Preoperative antibiotics and steroids are indicated. In addition to routine monitors, arterial and CVP monitoring are essential. If a pulmonary artery (PA) catheter is placed, withdraw it before the PA is clamped. Transesophageal echocardiography (TEE) is useful in evaluating right ventricular (RV) function and the presence of pulmonary vein anastomotic obstruction.

C. Begin induction after notification by the transplant surgeon. Use full stomach precautions. Preoxygenate for at least 3 minutes. Opioids, etomidate, propofol, ketamine, and thiopental have all been used successfully. For maintenance, a balanced technique incorporating narcotic, volatile anesthetic, and muscle relaxant is recommended. Avoid nitrous oxide. In COPD patients, the ventilatory mode should allow ample time for exhalation.

D. A double-lumen endobronchial tube (DLT) provides superior lung separation compared to bronchial blockers. Verify proper tube placement both clinically and with fiberoptic bronchoscopy. Reconfirm after placing the patient in the lateral decubitus position.

E. Surgery is usually performed via a posterolateral thoracotomy incision and less frequently via anterior thoracotomy with partial sternotomy. If cardiopulmonary bypass (CPB) seems likely, position the patient to allow ready access to the aorta and right atrium or the femoral artery and vein. Single-lung transplantation is frequently performed without CPB, but occasionally CPB may be planned or may become necessary intraoperatively. Aortic and right atrial cannulation are easier in right-sided single-lung transplant. Femoral artery-to-vein bypass can be easily instituted on either side if necessary.

F. Although most single-lung transplant patients tolerate institution of one-lung ventilation (OLV), hypoxemia, hypercarbia, or hemodynamic instability may occur. Hypoxemia often improves with PA clamping. COPD patients are at risk for carbon dioxide (CO_2) retention, but most patients tolerate an elevated $PaCO_2$ as long as oxygenation is maintained. Attempt to correct hypercarbia by modifying ventilatory parameters or using high-frequency jet ventilation. Hemodynamic compromise occurs from hypoxemia or from attempts to ventilate beyond the capacity of the single ventilated lung. During OLV, pulmonary HTN and dysfunction of the right ventricle (RV) may occur. Support with a vasodilator or inotrope may be necessary to improve RV function. PA clamping may not be well tolerated in patients with severe pulmonary HTN at baseline. If trial PA clamping causes a dramatic rise in PA pressure and reduction in cardiac output (CO), begin pharmacological intervention with pulmonary vasodilators (such as nitroglycerin or nitroprusside) or inodilators (such as isoproterenol or milrinone). Consider the use of inhaled nitric oxide to lower pulmonary vascular resistance and improve oxygenation.[4] RV afterload reduction, enhancement of myocardial contractility, and preload augmentation may enable a patient to tolerate OLV. If, however, successful OLV is not possible due to inadequate oxygenation and ventilation or the development of RV dysfunction and pulmonary HTN, resume two-lung ventilation and prepare for CPB.

SINGLE LUNG TRANSPLANT CANDIDATE

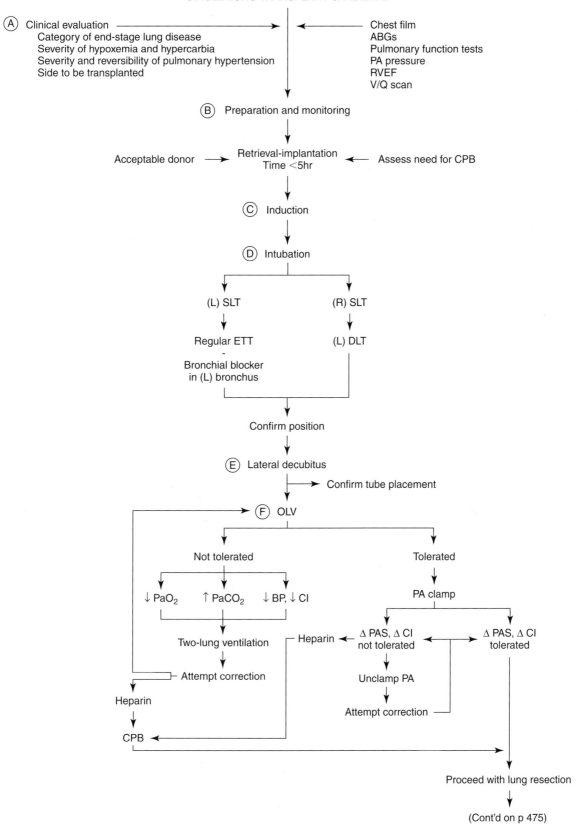

A Clinical evaluation
  Category of end-stage lung disease
  Severity of hypoxemia and hypercarbia
  Severity and reversibility of pulmonary hypertension
  Side to be transplanted

Chest film
ABGs
Pulmonary function tests
PA pressure
RVEF
V/Q scan

B Preparation and monitoring

Acceptable donor → Retrieval-implantation Time <5hr ← Assess need for CPB

C Induction

D Intubation

(L) SLT   (R) SLT

Regular ETT   (L) DLT
-
Bronchial blocker
in (L) bronchus

Confirm position

E Lateral decubitus
                    → Confirm tube placement

F OLV

Not tolerated   Tolerated

↓ PaO₂   ↑ PaCO₂   ↓ BP, ↓ CI   PA clamp

Two-lung ventilation   Heparin ← Δ PAS, Δ CI   Δ PAS, Δ CI
                                not tolerated   tolerated

Attempt correction   Unclamp PA

Heparin   Attempt correction

CPB ←

Proceed with lung resection

(Cont'd on p 475)

G. After pneumonectomy, the sequence of anastomosis of lung structures is pulmonary vein, mainstem bronchus, and PA. The transplanted lung is kept cold until reperfusion. Once circulation is restored, hemostasis is assured and ventilation begins. The lung is inflated and the bronchial anastomosis is tested for leaks at a pressure of 40 cm H_2O. Systemic BP may drop during reperfusion. Bronchoscopy is performed to suction blood and secretions and to examine anastomotic suture lines. At the conclusion of surgery, replace the DLT with a standard single-lumen endotracheal tube (8.0 mm ID or larger). Continue muscle relaxation and sedation. Maintain mechanical ventilation with PEEP to minimize reperfusion pulmonary edema.[5]

REFERENCES

1. Csete M, Glas K: Anesthesia for organ transplantation. In: Barash PG, Cullen BF, Stoelting RK, editors: *Clinical anesthesia*, ed 5, Philadelphia, 2006, Lippincott Williams & Wilkins.
2. Levine SM: Transplant/immunology network of the American College of Chest Physicians: A survey of clinical practice of lung transplantation in North America, *Chest* 125:1224, 2004.
3. Levine SM: Lung transplantation: An overview, *Compr Ther* 23:789, 1997.
4. Cornfield DN, Milla CE, Haddad IY et al: Safety of inhaled nitric oxide after lung transplantation, *J Heart Lung Transplant* 22:903, 2003.
5. Calhoon JH, Grover FL, Gibbons WJ, et al.: Single lung transplantation: Alternative indications and technique, *J Thorac Cardiovasc Surg* 101:816, 1991.

SINGLE LUNG TRANSPLANT CANDIDATE

(Cont'd from p 473)
↓

Expansion of new lung ◄─────────────── Ⓖ Anastomosis of new lung
        ↓   ├─ PV
     ICU   ├─ Bronchus
                                             └─ PA

Liver Failure and Orthotopic Liver Transplantation

JUDITH A. FREEMAN, M.D.

One-year survival for orthotopic liver transplantation is now close to 90%. Hepatic function in patients presenting for orthotopic liver transplantation ranges from normal (neoplasm) to severe hepatocellular disease with associated portal hypertension (HTN) and multisystem organ failure. Anesthetic management involves maintenance of homeostasis in the face of physiologic derangements induced by the vascular and metabolic effects of the anhepatic phase and moderate to massive hemorrhage.

A. Physiological derangements include circulatory disturbances (increased cardiac output [CO], low systemic vascular resistance [SVR]), pulmonary dysfunction (hypoxemia caused by V/Q mismatch, hepatopulmonary syndrome, pleural effusions, or adult respiratory distress syndrome [ARDS]), renal failure, and electrolyte imbalance, coagulopathy, and poor nutritional status. Portopulmonary HTN with pulmonary artery pressure > 35 mm Hg and PVR > 250 dynes/s/cm^{-5} is associated with high mortality. CNS dysfunction (encephalopathy) and impaired glucose homeostasis leading to hypoglycemia result from impaired metabolic function. Associated renal dysfunction (prerenal, ATN, hepatorenal syndrome) leads to fluid and electrolyte imbalances. Lack of synthetic function results in hypoalbuminemia with poor nutritional status and coagulopathy from inadequate coagulation factor synthesis. Look for coexisting cardiac disease (alcoholic cirrhosis and hemochromatosis). Exercise tolerance is a poor indicator of function (chronic fatigue and ascites). A dobutamine stress echocardiogram (Echo) is essential for cardiac assessment. If this is abnormal, cardiac catheterization may be necessary. Pulmonary artery pressure (PAP) may also be estimated from Echo. Attempt to correct preoperative abnormalities (e.g., drainage of large pleural effusions). Ensure availability of PRBCs, FFP, and platelets.

B. In addition to standard monitors, insert arterial (radial or femoral) and pulmonary artery (PA) catheters. Insert one or two 8.5F IV catheters or their equivalent in the arms or jugular veins for rapid transfusion. If planning percutaneous venovenous bypass (VVB) an additional large-bore catheter may be necessary. Plan for prolonged anesthesia paying special attention to positioning, padding pressure points, and minimizing heat loss (1 to 2 forced-air heating blankets). Previous remote orthotopic liver transplantation or other abdominal surgery increases risk of hemorrhage. A cell-saving device and a rapid transfusion device (RIS Haemonetics, FMS 2000 Belmont, or Level 1 high flow blood warmer) should always be available.

C. Perform an RSI with standard induction agents and succinylcholine (SCC) to facilitate endotracheal intubation. Institute mechanical ventilation with room air or 100% oxygen (O_2) to maintain normocapnia. Maintain anesthesia with fentanyl (5 to 20 μg/kg), isoflurane, benzodiazepine for amnesia, and muscle relaxant. Titrate all drugs carefully. Disturbances in volume of distribution, protein binding, hepatic and renal clearance, and rapid blood loss all affect drug pharmacokinetics and dynamics.

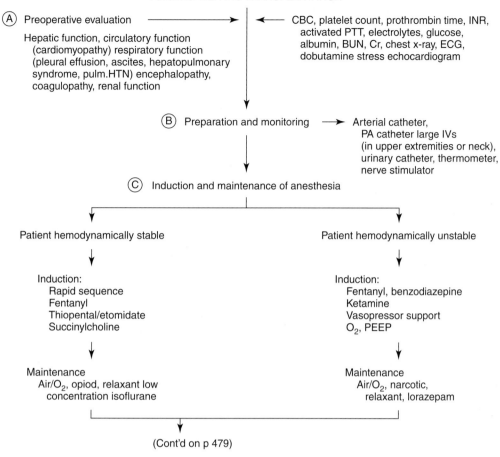

Patient for HEPATIC TRANSPLANTATION

Ⓐ Preoperative evaluation ⟶ ← CBC, platelet count, prothrombin time, INR, activated PTT, electrolytes, glucose, albumin, BUN, Cr, chest x-ray, ECG, dobutamine stress echocardiogram

Hepatic function, circulatory function (cardiomyopathy) respiratory function (pleural effusion, ascites, hepatopulmonary syndrome, pulm.HTN) encephalopathy, coagulopathy, renal function

Ⓑ Preparation and monitoring ⟶ Arterial catheter, PA catheter large IVs (in upper extremities or neck), urinary catheter, thermometer, nerve stimulator

Ⓒ Induction and maintenance of anesthesia

Patient hemodynamically stable

Induction:
Rapid sequence
Fentanyl
Thiopental/etomidate
Succinylcholine

Maintenance
Air/O₂, opiod, relaxant low concentration isoflurane

Patient hemodynamically unstable

Induction:
Fentanyl, benzodiazepine
Ketamine
Vasopressor support
O₂, PEEP

Maintenance
Air/O₂, narcotic, relaxant, lorazepam

(Cont'd on p 479)

D. Stage 1 consists of dissection of hepatic vessels and ligaments. Stage 2, the anhepatic stage follows clamping of the portal vein hepatic artery and suprahepatic and infrahepatic inferior vena cava (IVC). With the classical approach, the liver is removed together with the intrahepatic portion of the IVC. Cross-clamping the IVC leads to an abrupt decrease in venous return, CO, and systemic BP. Compensate for these derangements by administering fluids and vasopressors (dopamine and epinephrine.) A trial of cross-clamping may be performed to test for adequate volume replacement. Extreme changes may be circumvented with VVB in adults. Heparin-bonded cannulae are inserted into the femoral and portal veins. Drained blood is diverted through a centrifugal pump and returned to the upper part of the body either via a cut-down in the axillary vein or via additional percutaneous cannulae previously inserted by the anesthesiologist. Minimum flows of 1 L/min are required to prevent clotting. In the alternative piggy-back approach, a recipient hepatic vein is isolated for anastomosis with the donor suprahepatic IVC. The recipient IVC remains intact with a side clamp placed during the anastomoses.

E. After anastomoses of the donor and recipient IVCs and portal veins, graft reperfusion occurs. Stage 3, the neohepatic stage, begins here. Abrupt transient hemodynamic changes consisting of hypotension (possibly leading to cardiac arrest), bradycardia, high filling pressures, and decreased SVR occur in a small number of cases. These changes result from the cold, acidotic, hyperkalemic donor liver perfusate, containing vasoactive substances and small air emboli, reaching the recipient circulation. Treat aggressively with epinephrine boluses (10 to 20 μg initially), $CaCl_2$ (1 g), and $NaHCO_3$ (50 mEq). The remainder of the procedure (hepatic artery anastomosis and biliary reconstruction) usually proceeds uneventfully. Major bleeding may occur as a result of difficult dissection, adhesions from previous surgery, portal HTN, preexisting coagulopathy, or increased fibrinolysis. A poorly functioning graft will produce sustained fibrinolysis. Monitor coagulation closely using either routine tests (international normalized ratio [INR], partial thromboplastin time [PTT], platelet count, D-dimer) or thromboelastography. Use platelets, FFP, and cryoprecipitate aggressively during stage 3. Counter primary fibrinolysis with aminocaproic acid. Hypocalcemia and less frequently hypomagnesemia can occur as a result of citrate toxicity especially during massive transfusion during the anhepatic phase. Treat with frequent boluses of $CaCl_2$. 0.5 to 1 g, and $MgSO_4$ 1 to 3 g. Hyperkalemia may be preexistent or result from massive transfusion. Treat this aggressively, especially before reperfusion, with $NaHCO_3$, hyperventilation, glucose, and insulin, and wash all banked blood in the cell saver. Mannitol and possible furosemide may help to maintain urinary output and help to prevent postoperative oliguric renal failure. Metabolic acidosis and increased lactate levels occur during the anhepatic phase and are accentuated during reperfusion. Treat base deficits >5 mEq/L with $NaHCO_3$ or THAM.

F. Persistent hypocalcemia, lactic acidosis, hyperglycemia, hypotension, oliguria, and coagulopathy indicate poor graft function.

REFERENCES

1. Carton EG, Rettke SR, Plevak DJ, et al.: Perioperative care of the liver transplant patient, *Anesth Analg* 78 (Part 1):120–133, 1994.
2. Carton EG, Rettke SR, Plevak DJ, et al.: Perioperative care of the liver transplant patient, *Anesth Analg* 78 (Part 2):382–399, 1994.
3. Rand EB, Olthoff KM: Overview of pediatric liver transplantation, *Gastroenterol Clin North Am* 32:913–929, 2003.
4. Kramer D, Mazariegos G, Fung J: Intensive care of liver transplant recipients In: Grenvik A, Shoemaker WC, Ayres SM, editors: *Textbook of critical care*, ed 4, Philadelphia, 2000, W.B. Saunders.

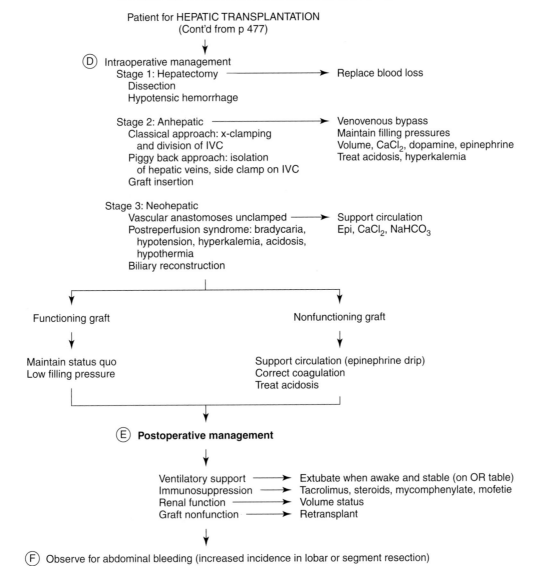

Patient for HEPATIC TRANSPLANTATION
(Cont'd from p 477)

D Intraoperative management
    Stage 1: Hepatectomy ⟶ Replace blood loss
        Dissection
        Hypotensic hemorrhage

    Stage 2: Anhepatic ⟶ Venovenous bypass
        Classical approach: x-clamping   Maintain filling pressures
            and division of IVC   Volume, $CaCl_2$, dopamine, epinephrine
        Piggy back approach: isolation   Treat acidosis, hyperkalemia
            of hepatic veins, side clamp on IVC
        Graft insertion

    Stage 3: Neohepatic
        Vascular anastomoses unclamped ⟶ Support circulation
        Postreperfusion syndrome: bradycaria,   Epi, $CaCl_2$, $NaHCO_3$
            hypotension, hyperkalemia, acidosis,
            hypothermia
        Biliary reconstruction

Functioning graft   Nonfunctioning graft

Maintain status quo   Support circulation (epinephrine drip)
Low filling pressure   Correct coagulation
                                           Treat acidosis

E **Postoperative management**

    Ventilatory support ⟶ Extubate when awake and stable (on OR table)
    Immunosuppression ⟶ Tacrolimus, steroids, mycomphenylate, mofetie
    Renal function ⟶ Volume status
    Graft nonfunction ⟶ Retransplant

F Observe for abdominal bleeding (increased incidence in lobar or segment resection)

Pancreatic Transplantation

GWENDOLYN L. BOYD, M.D.

The first three editions of *Decision Making in Anesthesiology* indicated that "until a cure is found for type I diabetes mellitus, pancreatic transplantation offers the best chance of treatment and possibly the best means of preventing the progression of its multiorgan complications." At this time, islet cell transplantation is anticipated as an alternative technique, to be performed transhepatically by interventional radiologists. Because islet cell transplantation is still in its infancy with essentially unknown long-term results, it will not supplant whole organ pancreas transplantation for selected patients in the foreseeable future.[1]

Most pancreas transplants are performed concurrently with a renal transplant in type I diabetics who also have renal failure (simultaneous pancreas/kidney transplant [SPK]) The second most common group includes patients receiving a pancreas after a prior kidney transplant (pancreas after kidney [PAK]). The last group includes patients who have no renal failure and receive a whole pancreas transplant alone (pancreas transplant alone [PTA]). The PTA group has 1-year pancreas graft survival rates of 70 to 75% compared to 80 to 85% for SPK and PAK recipients. Signs of rejection in SPK recipients usually occur first in the kidney. The addition of a pancreatic graft with the renal graft does not appear to adversely affect either patient or graft survival significantly in type I diabetes mellitus patients undergoing renal transplantation. More than two thirds of patients who have undergone SPK transplantation are no longer dialysis or insulin dependent. Anesthetic management has been described.[2–4]

A. Type I diabetes mellitus affects all organ systems. Atherosclerosis (coronary, cerebral, and peripheral) frequently coexists. Obtain a thorough cardiac workup in all candidates for pancreatic transplantation, including catheterization if indicated by preliminary studies, such as a MIBI scan or thallium exercise testing. Significant coronary artery disease (CAD) is a contraindication to pancreatic transplantation until treated with stenting or coronary artery bypass grafting (CABG). Cardiomyopathy results from thickened basement membranes and increased connective tissue in the myocardium. Diffuse microangiopathy leads to neuropathy, retinopathy, and nephropathy. Cardiac autonomic neuropathy may cause sudden death in the perioperative period. The heart becomes denervated, similar to the transplanted heart, and may not respond to atropine. Therefore, epinephrine may be required for severe bradycardia in diabetic patients. Autonomic neuropathy may lead to gastroparesis; consider these patients as having full stomachs.

Evaluate for evidence of diabetic stiff-joint syndrome (DSJS). Beginning in the joints of the little finger, DSJS can also occur in the atlantooccipital joint, making direct visualization of the vocal cords and intubation impossible.[5]

B. Premedicate with metoclopramide and an H_2 antagonist. Insert a central venous catheter. Consider an arterial line. If DSJS appears to involve the neck, have difficult airway equipment readily available.

C. Preoxygenate the patient. Place routine monitors. Induce anesthesia with RSI or awake fiberoptic intubation, depending on the presence of significant DSJS in the neck.

D. Maintain anesthesia with inhalation agents and narcotics. Cisatracurium may be the muscle relaxant of choice because of its lack of cumulative effects. Perform frequent measurements of blood glucose and potassium. The goal is to have the blood glucose approximately 300 mg/dl^{-1} before revascularization. Maintain the CVP at 10 to 12 mm Hg and the systolic BP near 130 mm Hg with crystalloids and colloids. Blood is infrequently needed; most end-stage renal disease (ESRD) patients receive erythropoietin. Add dopamine (5 to 10 μg/kg^1/min^1) if the systolic BP is low despite adequate volume loading as reflected by the CVP. Maintain eucarbia because both hypocarbia and hypercarbia cause renal vasospasm.

E. The pancreatic graft is usually anastomosed to the right iliac vessels because the anatomy of the left iliac vessel predisposes to portal vein thrombosis. While the pancreas is prepared on the back table for transplantation, the kidney is grafted to the left iliac vessels. The use of UW solution has increased the allowable ischemia time while improving graft function of both the kidney and the pancreas. Some transplant centers anastomose the pancreatic duct to the intestine. This technique is associated with a 5 to 10% incidence of anastomotic leak. Our center grafts the pancreatic duct to the bladder, allowing urinary determinations of amylase. Approximately 5 to 10% of these patients will require enteric conversion due to dehydration, recurrent urinary tract infections, or alkali loss. However, these patients suffer much less morbidity than those with anastomotic leaks. The spleen is removed to avoid graft-versus-host disease (GVHD). Reperfusion of the pancreatic graft is usually associated with several hundred milliliters of blood loss; the anesthesia team must be prepared for rapid volume repletion at that time. The blood glucose should decrease to normal within 6 to 10 hours of revascularization and should remain normal thereafter.

Patient for PANCREATIC/RENAL TRANSPLANT (SPK)

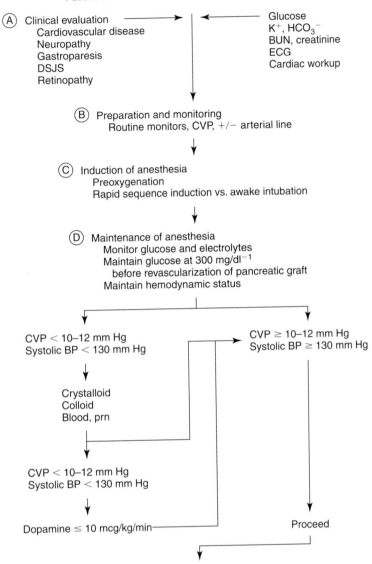

(A) Clinical evaluation ——————→   ←——— Glucose
        Cardiovascular disease K^+, HCO_3^-
        Neuropathy   BUN, creatinine
        Gastroparesis   ECG
        DSJS   Cardiac workup
        Retinopathy

        (B) Preparation and monitoring
                Routine monitors, CVP, $+/-$ arterial line

        (C) Induction of anesthesia
                Preoxygenation
                Rapid sequence induction vs. awake intubation

        (D) Maintenance of anesthesia
                Monitor glucose and electrolytes
                Maintain glucose at 300 mg/dl^{-1}
                    before revascularization of pancreatic graft
                Maintain hemodynamic status

CVP < 10–12 mm Hg   CVP $\geq$ 10–12 mm Hg
Systolic BP < 130 mm Hg   Systolic BP $\geq$ 130 mm Hg

    Crystalloid
    Colloid
    Blood, prn

CVP < 10–12 mm Hg
Systolic BP < 130 mm Hg

Dopamine $\leq$ 10 mcg/kg/min————   Proceed

        (E) Renal transplant/pancreas transplant
                Monitor glucose and electrolytes
                Anticipate 500-ml blood loss with revascularization of pancreatic graft

(Cont'd on p 483)

F. Delay extubation until the patient is fully awake. Reversal of neuromuscular blockade with neostigmine and glycopyrrolate may result in severe bradycardia and even sudden cardiac arrest. Atropine may not be effective; administer epinephrine early.[6] Loss of cholinergic tone in the airways due to autonomic neuropathy predisposes diabetic patients to hypoxemia, especially in the presence of residual anesthetics and analgesics. Therefore, select short-acting agents. Admit patients to the surgical ICU postoperatively for close monitoring of cardiorespiratory status as well as blood chemistries.

REFERENCES

1. Nath DS, Gruessner AC, Kandaswamy R, et al.: Outcomes of pancreas transplants for patients with type 2 diabetes mellitus, *Clin Transplant* 19 (6):792–797, 2005.
2. Graybar GB, Deierhoi MH: Anesthesia and pancreatic transplantation, *Anesth Clin North Am* 7:515, 1989.
3. Larson-Wadd K, Belani KG: Pancreas and islet cell transplantation, *Anesthesiol Clin North Am* 22 (4):663–674, 2004.
4. Halpern H, Miyoshi E, Kataoka LM, et al.: Anesthesia for pancreas transplantation alone or simultaneous with kidney, *Transplant Proc* 36 (10):3105–3106, 2004.
5. Salzarulo HH, Taylor LA: Diabetic "Stiff joint syndrome" as a cause of difficult endotracheal intubation, *Anesthesiology* 64:366–368, 1986.
6. Triantafillou AN, Tsueda K, Berg J, et al.: Refractory bradycardia after reversal of muscle relaxant in a diabetic with vagal neuropathy, *Anesth Analg* 65:1237–1241, 1986.

Patient for PANCREATIC/RENAL TRANSPLANT (SPK)
(Cont'd from p 481)

↓

(F) Postoperative care
   Delay extubation as with other full stomach
      and/or difficult intubation patients
   Monitor glucose, creatinine, and electrolytes
   Replace urine volume with crystalloids per protocol
   Close observation of cardiorespiratory system

ANESTHESIA FOR ENDOSCOPY AND HEAD AND NECK SURGERY

FOREIGN BODY ASPIRATION

ACUTE EPIGLOTTITIS

CLEFT LIP AND PALATE

POST-TONSILLECTOMY BLEEDING (PTB)

VOCAL CORD PAPILLOMAS

UPPER AIRWAY OBSTRUCTION

LASER SURGERY

ENDOSCOPIC SINUS SURGERY

HEAD AND NECK ONCOLOGIC SURGERY

LARYNGOSCOPY

BRONCHOSCOPY

Foreign Body Aspiration

MARY ANN GURKOWSKI, M.D.

CHRISTOPHER A. BRACKEN, M.D., PH.D.

Aspiration of a foreign body is a cause of airway obstruction in children (highest at 1 to 3 years[1]) and adults. Children aspirate both food (hot dogs, nuts) and nonfood objects (coins, beads), but adults aspirate food (meat, fish bones).

A. Determine the onset of the problem, the attempts at relieving it, the presence of respiratory difficulty, the nature of the suspected object, NPO status, and any other medical conditions. Consider foreign body aspiration when there is a history of severe choking, coughing, gagging, or cyanosis.[2,3] Patients usually have wheezing, cough, and shortness of breath. If the foreign body is *distal* to the trachea, physical examination will reveal unequal breath sounds; if the foreign body is at the level of the *larynx or trachea*, expect stridor, hemoptysis, retraction, or use of accessory muscles of breathing. Chest x-rays (CXRs) may not be diagnostic with radiolucent foreign body, but inspiratory and expiratory films may help indicate the presence of atelectasis or obstructive emphysema.[3] Fluoroscopy is diagnostic in approximately 90% of children with foreign body aspiration.[2,4]

B. Have an appropriate sized tracheostomy tray immediately available for the patients with a foreign body of the larynx and upper trachea. When intubation is planned, have a variety of endotracheal tube (ETT) sizes available. Invasive monitors may be indicated by the patient's medical history (e.g., coronary artery disease [CAD], emphysema, congenital heart disease [CHD]).

C. Historically, an inhalational induction with maintenance of spontaneous ventilation has been thought to be the safest method of induction if the foreign body is in the larynx or trachea.[5] Avoid assisting or controlling the respirations as this could theoretically move the foreign body distally and create a total obstruction or worsen pulmonary hyperinflation in the presence of impaired exhalation, although there is no evidence that the use of controlled ventilation influences the occurrence of adverse events.[6] A laryngeal foreign body is usually extracted during laryngoscopy without tracheal intubation. If the foreign body is sharp, use careful manipulation to avoid causing further injury. Once the foreign body is removed, the patient may be allowed to awaken without intubation. If the patient has a full stomach, place an ETT and then suction the stomach before awakening.

D. If the foreign body is in a bronchus, an adult can receive an IV induction. In a child, start with an inhalational induction to avoid the agitation caused by IV placement. Agitation theoretically could dislodge the foreign body into the carina or trachea, worsening the obstruction. A distal tracheal or proximal bronchus foreign body requires ventilation via a small ETT or a ventilating bronchoscope.[1] If a small ETT is used, the bronchoscope is passed alongside. Once ventilation is verified, a muscle relaxant may be used. If the foreign body is organic (nuts, seeds), anticipate swelling of the foreign body as it absorbs moisture. Inhalation of a bronchodilator or a diluted solution of racemic epinephrine may aid removal.[7]

E. If the foreign body is in the distal airway, it is safe to perform an IV induction in adults or children. The potential for dislodgment is small, and even if this happens, the size of the foreign body is such that it should not cause complete obstruction of the larger airways. Give an anti-sialagogue and preoxygenate before induction. If the patient has a full stomach, perform an RSI. Although a fiberoptic bronchoscope can be passed through a large ETT to remove a distal foreign body, it is more common to use a rigid ventilating bronchoscope with other helpful instruments, such as optical forceps, a flexible grasper, or a balloon catheter. Rarely, a thoracotomy must be performed to remove the foreign body.[4]

F. The most common postoperative complication is pneumonia. Other problems include hemoptysis, pneumomediastinum, and lower and upper airway obstruction. The use of IV steroids to reduce the inflammation and edema associated with a foreign body and instrumentation is controversial.[3] Obtain a baseline postoperative CXR. Monitor respiratory function closely.

REFERENCES

1. Reilly JS: Airway foreign bodies: update and analysis, *Int Anesthesiol Clin* 30:49–55, 1992.
2. Wolach B, Raz A, Weinberg J, et al.: Aspirated foreign bodies in the respiratory tract of children: eleven years experience with 127 patients, *Int J Pediatr Otorhinolaryngol* 30:1–10, 1994.
3. Hoeve LJ, Rombout J, Pot DJ: Foreign body aspiration in children. The diagnostic value of signs, symptoms and pre-operative examination, *Clin Otolaryngol Allied Sci* 18:55–57, 1993.
4. Black RE, Johnson DG, Matlak ME: Bronchoscopic removal of aspirated foreign bodies in children, *J Pediatr Surg* 29:682–684, 1994.
5. Tan HK, Tan SS: Inhaled foreign bodies in children-anaesthetic considerations, *Singapore Medical Journal* 41 (10):506–510, 2000.
6. Litman RS, Ponnuri J, Trogan I: Anesthesia for tracheal or bronchial foreign body removal in children: an analysis of ninety-four cases, *Anesth Analg* 91:1389–1391, 2000.
7. Bready LL, Orr MD, Petty C, et al.: Bronchoscopic administration of nebulized racemic epinephrine to facilitate removal of aspirated peanut fragments in pediatric patients: report of three cases, *Anesthesiology* 65:523–525, 1986.

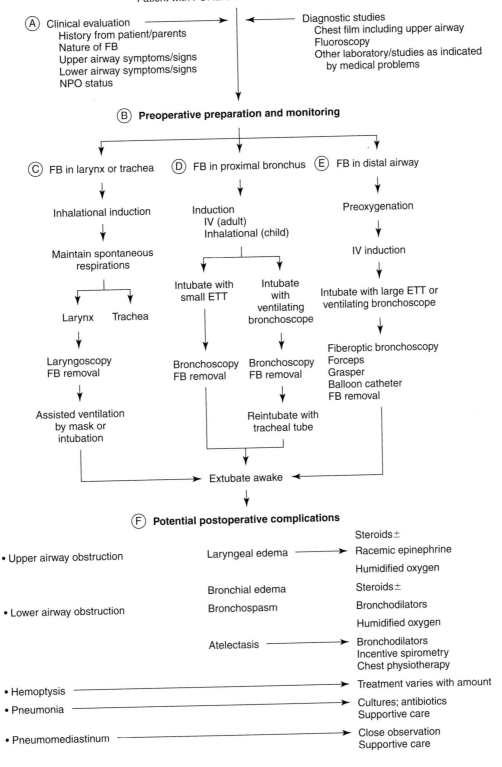

Patient with FOREIGN BODY ASPIRATION

(A) Clinical evaluation
    History from patient/parents
    Nature of FB
    Upper airway symptoms/signs
    Lower airway symptoms/signs
    NPO status

Diagnostic studies
    Chest film including upper airway
    Fluoroscopy
    Other laboratory/studies as indicated
      by medical problems

(B) **Preoperative preparation and monitoring**

(C) FB in larynx or trachea

(D) FB in proximal bronchus

(E) FB in distal airway

Inhalational induction

Induction
IV (adult)
Inhalational (child)

Preoxygenation

Maintain spontaneous respirations

IV induction

Larynx   Trachea

Intubate with small ETT

Intubate with ventilating bronchoscope

Intubate with large ETT or ventilating bronchoscope

Laryngoscopy
FB removal

Bronchoscopy
FB removal

Bronchoscopy
FB removal

Fiberoptic bronchoscopy
Forceps
Grasper
Balloon catheter
FB removal

Assisted ventilation by mask or intubation

Reintubate with tracheal tube

Extubate awake

(F) **Potential postoperative complications**

- Upper airway obstruction   Laryngeal edema → Steroids±
Racemic epinephrine
Humidified oxygen

- Lower airway obstruction

Bronchial edema
Bronchospasm   Steroids±
Bronchodilators
Humidified oxygen

Atelectasis → Bronchodilators
Incentive spirometry
Chest physiotherapy

- Hemoptysis → Treatment varies with amount
- Pneumonia → Cultures; antibiotics
Supportive care

- Pneumomediastinum → Close observation
Supportive care

Acute Epiglottitis

KIRK LALWANI, M.D.

ANGELA ZIMMERMAN, M.D.

Acute epiglottitis, or supraglottitis, is a potentially life-threatening swelling of the supraglottic structures, which may result in sudden, complete upper airway obstruction. Classic signs in children are four D's: drooling, dyspnea, dysphagia, and dysphonia. Patients may assume the tripod posture (upright seated posture, leaning forward, and resting on both hands with neck extension) and may have stridor. Atypical presentations occur commonly, particularly at the extremes of age.[1] Acute epiglottis is usually infectious in origin; incidence of acute epiglottis has declined dramatically[2] following the introduction of a vaccine for *Haemophilus influenzae* type b (Hib) in 1987. Hib is still implicated as a cause of acute epiglottis in unprotected individuals, or following vaccine failure. Noninfectious acute epiglottis is usually due to thermal or corrosive injury (ingestion, inhalation, or mechanical trauma).

A. The child with acute epiglottis typically appears toxic, with high-grade fever, and little or no cough, all of which help differentiate it from croup (laryngotracheobronchitis). Predictors of the need for airway intervention (dyspnea, stridor, drooling, <12 hours duration of symptoms, and enlarged epiglottis on radiography are not always reliable). One report describes successful conservative management in patients with stridor[3]; conversely, sudden fatal airway obstruction may occur with no history of stridor.[4] Concomitant or recent infections (otitis media, cellulitis, pneumonia, or meningitis) may be present in approximately 50%.[5] Lateral neck radiography may reveal the "thumb print" sign (enlarged epiglottis) or the "vallecula sign" (absence of a deep, well-defined vallecula as it is traced inferiorly toward the hyoid bone). Definitive diagnosis may be accomplished by awake nasal fiberoptic laryngoscopy in stable, cooperative adults by an experienced otolaryngologist. The differential diagnosis of acute epiglottis includes croup, retropharyngeal abscess, foreign body aspiration, and bacterial tracheitis. Rapidly assess the airway, respiratory effort, circulatory adequacy, and oxygen saturation to determine whether the patient's condition requires rapid mobilization of the OR team, otolaryngologist, and preparation for emergency airway management in the OR without delay. Oxygen should be administered if necessary. Do not attempt procedures that might upset a child (oral examination, IV placement, and such). An experienced health care provider with airway management skills must accompany the patient at all times. Nebulized racemic epinephrine may decrease swelling and improve breathing, but this should be considered a short-term measure until definitive airway control is established. In adults, the otolaryngologist may also perform flexible fiberoptic nasolaryngoscopy.

B. Adults with a confirmed diagnosis and mild symptoms may be managed conservatively on ICU with antibiotics and supportive treatment, but children with a confirmed diagnosis on radiography should have their airway secured. The OR team must be mobilized and ready for emergency tracheostomy in the event of a lost airway during induction. Have difficult airway equipment, a selection of endotracheal tubes ([ETTs] 0.5 to 1 size smaller than normal), halothane or sevoflurane vaporizers, heliox if available, a cricothyrotomy kit with a jet ventilator, and an experienced assistant. Induce anesthesia by inhalation of halothane or sevoflurane in oxygen, with the child allowed to remain upright in a parent's lap following preoxygenation. Induction may be prolonged, but maintenance of airway patency and spontaneous respiration should be the goal. Application of 5 to 10 cm of CPAP, or a two-handed jaw thrust maneuver may help maintain airway patency. Heliox may be helpful with severe airway narrowing. Following adequate anesthesia, an IV should be placed and a fluid bolus (20 ml/kg) given. Perform direct laryngoscopy and endotracheal intubation when anesthesia is judged to be deep enough; if intubation is not possible with laryngoscopy alone, other devices may be used (i.e., gum elastic bougie or a fiberoptic bronchoscope) while maintaining spontaneous respiration. If control of the airway is lost, or if attempts at intubation are unsuccessful, tracheostomy (or cricothyrotomy) should be performed. In cooperative adults, consider awake fiberoptic intubation with the OR team standing by. An oral tube may be changed to a nasal tube for comfort if intubation is straightforward.

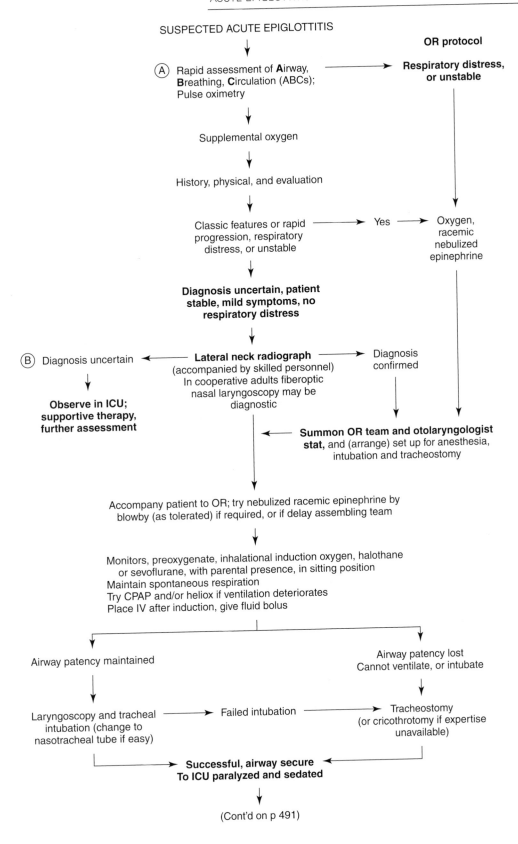

SUSPECTED ACUTE EPIGLOTTITIS

OR protocol

Ⓐ Rapid assessment of **A**irway, **B**reathing, **C**irculation (ABCs); Pulse oximetry → **Respiratory distress, or unstable**

Supplemental oxygen

History, physical, and evaluation

Classic features or rapid progression, respiratory distress, or unstable → Yes → Oxygen, racemic nebulized epinephrine

Diagnosis uncertain, patient stable, mild symptoms, no respiratory distress

Ⓑ Diagnosis uncertain ← **Lateral neck radiograph** (accompanied by skilled personnel) In cooperative adults fiberoptic nasal laryngoscopy may be diagnostic → Diagnosis confirmed

Observe in ICU; supportive therapy, further assessment

Summon OR team and otolaryngologist stat, and (arrange) set up for anesthesia, intubation and tracheostomy

Accompany patient to OR; try nebulized racemic epinephrine by blowby (as tolerated) if required, or if delay assembling team

Monitors, preoxygenate, inhalational induction oxygen, halothane or sevoflurane, with parental presence, in sitting position
Maintain spontaneous respiration
Try CPAP and/or heliox if ventilation deteriorates
Place IV after induction, give fluid bolus

Airway patency maintained

Airway patency lost
Cannot ventilate, or intubate

Laryngoscopy and tracheal intubation (change to nasotracheal tube if easy) → Failed intubation → Tracheostomy (or cricothrotomy if expertise unavailable)

**Successful, airway secure
To ICU paralyzed and sedated**

(Cont'd on p 491)

C. The patient is sedated, paralyzed, and ventilated for transport to the ICU for further management and monitoring. ICU management includes antibiotics (cefotaxime, ceftriaxone) fluids, and supportive therapy until the airway swelling has subsided, typically 24 to 48 hours later. Corticosteroids prior to extubation may decrease postextubation stridor, particularly in children.[6] Airway assessment may be performed by fiberoptic nasoendoscopy, direct laryngoscopy, or the "leak test" to determine airway patency around the ETT.

REFERENCES

1. Singer JI, McCabe JB: Epiglottitis at the extremes of age, *Am J Emerg Med* 6 (3):228–231, 1988.
2. Tanner K, Fitzsimmons G, Carroll ED, et al.: *Haemophilus influenzae* type b epiglottitis as a cause of acute upper airways obstruction in children, *BMJ* 325:1099–1100, 2002.
3. Wolf M, Strauss B, Kronenberg J, et al.: Conservative management of adult epiglottitis, *Laryngoscope* 100 (2 Pt 1):183–185, 1990.
4. Mayo-Smith M: Fatal respiratory arrest in adult epiglottitis in the intensive care unit. Implications for airway management, *Chest* 104:964–965, 1993.
5. Dunham ME, Holinger LD: Stridor, aspiration and cough. In: Bailey BJ, editor: *Head and neck surgery—otolaryngology*, vol 1, ed 2. Philadelphia, 1998 Lippincott-Raven.
6. Markovitz BP, Randolph AG: Corticosteroids for the prevention and treatment of post-extubation stridor in neonates, children and adults (Cochrane Methodology Review). In: *The Cochrane Library*, Issue 4. Chichester, UK, 2003, John Wiley & Sons, Ltd.

SUSPECTED ACUTE EPIGLOTTITIS
(Cont'd from p 489)

↓

 Antibiotics, supportive therapy
Extubate when stable, and leak test/visual inspection
confirm adequate leak around ETT (typically 24–48 hours)

Cleft Lip and Palate

MARY ANN GURKOWSKI, M.D.

CHRISTOPHER A. BRACKEN, M.D., PH.D.

Oral clefts occur in 1.5 per 1,000 live births, with combined cleft lip and palate in 50% of cases. In Caucasians the occurrence is approximately 1 in 1,000 live births; in African Americans it is 0.41 per 1,000 live births. Cleft lip repair is often performed using Musgrave's rule of 10: weight 10 lb, age 10 weeks, hemoglobin 10 g/dl, and WBC count 10,000 or less. Cleft palate repair is performed before speech begins (6 to 12 months of age). Pharyngeal flap procedures are performed in older children.[1–3]

A. Coexisting congenital defects occur in 2 to 11% of patients, with an incidence of congenital heart disease (CHD) of 3 to 7%. There are approximately 150 syndromes associated with oral clefts—Pierre Robin, Goldenhar, Klippel-Feil, and Treacher Collins (mandibular hypoplasia makes intubation difficult; feeding difficulties lead to poor nutritional status). Anemia at the time of planned surgery is common in infants with cleft lip because of nutritional impairment and the "physiologic nadir." Chronic rhinorrhea is common and should be differentiated from an upper respiratory infection. Malignant hyperthermia may occur more commonly in patients with midline defects.

B. Prevent hypothermia (warm OR, warming blanket, and humidifier). Anticipate a difficult airway and ensure the availability of adjunct equipment (including a tracheostomy tray) and personnel. The child's palatal prosthesis or a small, tagged, rolled gauze pad can be inserted into the palatal cleft as needed.

C. Induction may be via IV or inhalational routes. If no IV is present, insert one and give an anticholinergic to lessen secretions and prevent vagal reflex during intubation. If the airway can be maintained by mask, a muscle relaxant may be used to facilitate oral intubation and lessen potential laryngeal trauma. Never give a muscle relaxant if the airway cannot be maintained by mask. Secure the endotracheal tube (ETT) under the lower lip with skin adhesive and tape, or have the surgeon suture it to the alveolar ridge. An alternative anesthetic technique used for infants <6 weeks for cleft lip repair is local anesthesia and IM hydroxyzine or ketamine, thus avoiding intubation.[4]

D. The incidence of failed intubation is 1%, and the incidence of difficult laryngoscopy is 7.38%. Factors associated with difficult laryngoscopy are bilateral cleft lip and alveolus with protruding premaxilla, retrognathia, and age <6 months.[1–3] If a difficult intubation is anticipated, give IV sedation, apply oral topical local anesthesia, and perform awake laryngoscopy. Moderate sedation and topical local anesthesia or a well-controlled inhalation induction is usually needed for older children. In infants, if the glottis is visualized, awake intubation can usually be performed. In infants or children, if the glottis cannot be visualized, the choices for intubation include prone position (infant), blind oral, digital oral, awake fiberoptic (child), retrograde, tracheostomy, or laryngeal mask.[5–8] If the airway is impossible to manage, a percutaneous cricothyrotomy followed by jet ventilation can be performed (exhalation must be possible).

E. Cleft palate and pharyngeal flap procedures require insertion of a mouth gag, which may kink the ETT or force it further into the trachea. Monitor bilateral breath sounds and chest movement. Remove any throat packs before extubation. Neck extension and Trendelenburg position may be used to improve visualization of the posterior pharynx and palate. Be careful to assure the child is securely strapped on the bed.

Patient with CLEFT LIP AND PALATE

Ⓐ Clinical evaluation ⟶   ⟵ Hematocrit, WBC
    Airway   Type and cross-match
    Congenital anomalies   (cleft palate,
        (especially cardiac)   pharyngoplasty)
    Review previous anesthetic records

Ⓑ Preparation and monitoring

Assess likelihood of difficult intubation

Ⓒ No difficulty   Ⓓ Difficult intubation
    anticipated   anticipated

                            Awake laryngoscopy   Inhalational induction

                                                         Maintain spontaneous
                                                             respirations
Induction ⟵   Glottis easily   Glottis not   Attempt intubation
IV   visualized   visualized
Inhalational

Oral intubation ⟵   Awake intubation   Blind oral
with RAE tube   Fiberoptic
                                              Laryngeal mask
                                              Tracheostomy

                                                      Easy   Difficult

Cleft lip   Cleft   Pharyngeal
               palate   flap   Oral intubation   Fiberoptic
                                                     with RAE tube   Blind oral
                         Ⓔ Insertion of   Laryngeal mask
                             throat pack and   Tracheostomy
                             mouth gag
                             Extension of
                             neck/Trendelenburg
                             position

Reevaluate tube position and patency

(cont'd on p 495)

F. Epinephrine is infiltrated into the operative site to reduce blood loss.[9] Halothane, unlike sevoflurane, sensitizes the myocardium to epinephrine. If using halothane, ensure adequate oxygenation and hypocarbia; infants may tolerate up to 10 μg/kg epinephrine in 1% lidocaine without dysrhythmias, although lesser doses (1.5 to 4.5 μcg/kg) have generally been recommended.

G. After cleft lip repair, a Logan bow may be placed to protect the lip and remove tension from the sutures. Consider having the surgeon place a tongue suture so that retraction on the suture will reduce upper airway obstruction postoperatively. Infraorbital nerve block can be used for pain relief after cleft lip repair. Remove throat packs, suction the oropharynx gently under direct vision, and extubate while the patient is awake. Wrap the arms before transport to serve as arm restraints and prevent disruption of repair.

REFERENCES

1. Infosino A: Pediatric upper airway and congenital anomalies, *Anesthesiol Clin North Am* 20 (4):747–766, 2002.
2. Nargozian C: The airway in patients with craniofacial abnormalities, *Paediatr Anaesth* 14 (1):53–59, 2004.
3. Gunawardana RH: Difficult laryngoscopy in cleft lip and palate surgery, *Br J Anaesth* 76:757–759, 1996.
4. Kapetansky D, Warren R, Hawtof D: Cleft lip repair using intramuscular hydroxyzine sedation and local anesthesia, *Cleft Palate Craniofac J* 29:481–483, 1992.
5. Populaire C, Lundi JN, Pinaud M, et al.: Elective tracheal intubation in the prone position for a neonate with Pierre Robin syndrome, *Anesthesiology* 62:214–215, 1985.
6. Sutera PT, Gordon GJ: Digitally assisted tracheal intubation in a neonate with Pierre Robin syndrome, *Anesthesiology* 78:983–985, 1993.
7. Schwartz D, Singh J: Retrograde wire-guided direct laryngoscopy in a 1-month old infant, *Anesthesiology* 77:607–608, 1992.
8. Johnson CM, Sims C: Awake fiberoptic intubation via a laryngeal mask in an infant with Goldenhar's syndrome, *Anaesth Intensive Care* 22:194–197, 1994.
9. Karl HW, Swedlow DB, Lee KW, et al.: Epinephrine-halothane interactions in children, *Anesthesiology* 58:142–145, 1983.

Patient with CLEFT LIP AND PALATE
(Cont'd from p 493)

(F) Infiltration with local
     anesthesic and epinephrine

(G) 1. Place tongue suture
     2. Consider infraorbital nerve block
     3. Remove throat packs
     4. Suction carefully
     5. Extubate awake

Postoperative care

Monitor respiratory function

Uncomplicated recovery

Potential complications
   Laryngeal obstruction
      Edema → Nebulized racemic epinephrine
      Blood or secretions → Suction gently
      Tongue → Retract tongue stitch
   Nasopharyngeal obstruction
      Edema → Phenylephrine nose drops
      Pharyngeal flap → Retract tongue stitch
   Disruption of repair → Surgical evaluation

Post-Tonsillectomy Bleeding (PTB)

KIRK LALWANI, M.D.

Post-tonsillectomy bleeding (PTB) is a surgical emergency with challenging management issues for the anesthesiologist. A recent meta-analysis revealed a PTB rate of 3.3% in patients with normal coagulation studies.[1] Bleeding may be primary (within 24 hours) or secondary (between the 5th and 10th postoperative day (dislodgement or sloughing of the primary eschar).[2] PTB occurs more often in adults and is more likely to present as primary bleeding.[3] If pharyngeal packs and cautery are unsuccessful at controlling bleeding initially, the patient is usually examined and treated under anesthesia in the OR. Multiple surgical procedures may be necessary to control bleeding, including arteriography, ligature of the external carotid artery, or selective embolization.[4] Hemorrhagic shock and airway obstruction due to blood clots may complicate profuse bleeding and may be fatal. Anesthetic concerns include a tendency to underestimate the magnitude of blood loss (due to swallowing), hypovolemia, a full stomach (blood and possibly food) with the risk of pulmonary aspiration during anesthesia, a difficult airway or intubation, and the residual effects of recent anesthesia and related medications (e.g., opiates) in cases of primary hemorrhage.

A. If the airway is compromised or signs of shock are evident, immediately place large-bore IV cannulas, begin fluid resuscitation, blood transfusion, and institute airway control measures, concurrent with obtaining a brief history, chart review, and a rapid assessment of the patient's airway, breathing, and circulation (ABCs). Involve experienced personnel and transfusion services. Prepare equipment for management of a difficult airway.

B. If the patient's condition is stable, obtain a more thorough anesthetic and medical history. Assess volume status (e.g., level of consciousness, urinary output, postural dizziness, and syncope); ask about recent oral intake and witnessed blood loss. If hypovolemia is apparent, begin aggressive fluid resuscitation or blood transfusion. Examine the airway and note any factors complicating airway management (e.g., large tongue, pharyngeal edema, frank bleeding, clots, intermittent airway obstruction, or apnea); modify the anesthetic plan accordingly.

C. Administer oxygen. Monitor BP and SpO2. Place a reliable large-bore IV cannula. Draw blood for an immediate hematocrit (may be falsely high due to hemoconcentration) and venous blood gas measurement. Send blood samples to the laboratory for hemoglobin, coagulation profile, and cross-match. Replace the intravascular fluid deficit; transfuse as necessary. Administer glycopyrrolate to dry oral secretions in preparation for anesthesia. Avoid sedatives and drugs that depress respiration. Assess the adequacy of resuscitation; obtain serial hematocrit measurements if the clinical condition permits. Prepare the OR. Have difficult airway equipment, anesthetic and emergency drugs, two large-bore suction devices (clots can block the line), a rapid-infusion system, blood warmers, and blood for transfusion available, checked, and ready to use.

D. Transport the patient directly to the OR.

E. If the patient is rushed to the OR in extremis, consider an awake intubation following direct laryngoscopy and visualization of the vocal cords. If the patient is stable, perform an RSI with preoxygenation and cricoid pressure. Have alternative plans to secure the airway in the event of unsuspected difficult or failed intubation. Use induction agents that minimize hypotension, such as ketamine (with glycopyrrolate given early) or etomidate. Succinylcholine (SCC) is the muscle relaxant of choice. Administer additional nondepolarizing muscle relaxants (NDMRs) along with a short-acting opioid if necessary. Avoid nonsteroidal anti-inflammatory drugs (NSAIDs).[5] Electrocautery usually is successful in stopping the bleeding. Consider administering desmopressin (DDAVP), particularly in patients with hemophilia A, von Willebrand's disease, and platelet function disorders. DDAVP may cause severe hyponatremia, seizures, and death, particularly in children.[6]

Perform gentle oro-gastric suction with a large-bore tube, followed by gentle oropharyngeal suction to empty the stomach and clear the airway of secretions and blood. Reverse nondepolarizing neuromuscular block and administer antiemetic therapy. A single, large dose of dexamethasone is an effective antiemetic[7] and may decrease postoperative pharyngeal edema. Avoid antiemetics with concurrent sedative effects. Extubate the patient awake, preferably in the lateral Trendelenburg position to facilitate pooling of blood and secretions in the dependent cheek, as opposed to in the lower airway.

F. If the patient is stable and has a patent airway, transport to the PACU with oxygen and monitoring. If the intubation was difficult, traumatic, or there was massive hemorrhage, or if the patient's condition is tenuous in any way (decreased sensorium, intermittent apnea or obstruction, stridor, hypoxemia, hypotension, etc.), admit to the ICU for observation and further management. When the patient is hemodynamically stable, evaluate the airway and extubate.

REFERENCES

1. Krishna P, Lee D: Post-tonsillectomy bleeding: a meta-analysis, *Laryngoscope* 111:1358–1361, 2001.
2. Johnson LB, Elluru RG, Myer CM: Complications of adenotonsillectomy, *Laryngoscope* 112 (8 Pt 2 Suppl 100):35–36, 2002.

Patient for POST-TONSILLECTOMY BLEEDING

(A) **Rapid assessment** ⟶   ⟵ Vital signs
     Airway, **B**reathing, **C**irculation (ABCs) O_2 saturation

Stable condition   **Compromised airway,
                                                     shock, or in extremis**

(B) **History, physical, chart review** O_2
     Previous anesthetic/intubation history   Large-bore IVs
     OSA, bleeding disorders, medications   Cutdown/CVP/intraosseous
     Airway assessment   Aggressive resuscitation
     Assessment of hypovolemia   Summon help
                                                   Equipment for airway control

(C) **Prepare patient for OR**   Consider awake intubation if obtunded
     Administer O_2
     Monitor BP and O_2 saturation
     Large-bore IV access
     Blood for cross-match, Hct, CBC, coagulation profile, VBG
     Fluid and/or blood resuscitation
        (follow serial Hct and clinical signs)
     Glcopyrrolate
     Mobilize OR team
     Set up anesthetic equipment,
        drugs, difficult airway cart, transfusion apparatus
     Check blood products
     Prepare for emergency surgical airway

(D) **Transport to OR**
     O_2, monitoring, resuscitation equipment, drugs

(E) **Anesthetic care**
     Preoxygenation
     Rapid-sequence induction vs. awake intubation
     Avoid NSAIDs and long-acting opiates

Airway secure   **Failed intubation**

Good airway   Tenuous airway   ASA difficult airway algorithm
Stable   Major bleed
                     Unstable   Airway patency lost
                                                   Cannot intubate and cannot ventilate
(F) Awake extubation

To PACU   To ICU intubated ⟵ Tracheotomy/cricothyrotomy

3. Windfuhr JP, Chen YS, Remmert S: Hemorrhage following tonsillectomy and adenoidectomy in 15,218 patients, *Otolaryngol Head Neck Surg* 132:281–286, 2005.
4. Windfuhr JP: Indications for interventional arteriography in post-tonsillectomy hemorrhage, *J Otolaryngol* 31 (1):18–22, 2002.
5. Marret E, Flahault A, Samama CM, et al.: Effects of postoperative, nonsteroidal, antiinflammatory drugs on bleeding risk after tonsillectomy: meta-analysis of randomized, controlled trials, *Anesthesiology* 98:1497–1502, 2003.
6. Smith TJ, Gill JC, Ambruso DR, et al.: Hyponatremia and seizures in young children given DDAVP, *Am J Hematol* 31:199–202, 1989.
7. Steward DL, Welge JA, Myer CM: Steroids for improving recovery following tonsillectomy in children, *Cochrane Database Syst Rev* (1):CD003997, 2003.

Vocal Cord Papillomas

ANGELA KENDRICK, M.D.

STEVEN C. ONSTAD

Papillomas are benign epithelial tumors of the upper respiratory tract that are caused by infection with human papilloma virus (HPV) type 6 or 11. They occur in both children (juvenile onset is at <12 years of age) and adults. Diagnosis is usually made in children between the ages of 2 and 5 and requires inspection of the larynx. Infants and children may present with wheezing, hoarseness, or stridor.[1] Pediatric patients require multiple surgical excisions, most commonly with the carbon dioxide (CO_2) laser, but the 585-nm pulse dye, argon plasma, KTP lasers, and powered micro debridement, can be used in removal of HPV lesions and their reoccurrences.[2] Some children have regression of the lesions with puberty. There is an association between gastroesophageal reflux disease (GERD) and laryngeal papillomas in the pediatric population. Adult disease is often more localized and less severe. Goals of treatment are debulking, improvement of voice, and to promote remission of the papillomas. Surgical therapy may result in iatrogenic airway stenosis secondary to scarring or laryngeal web formation.

A. Patients may have profound airway obstruction secondary to papilloma growth on the vocal cords or epiglottis. Assess the degree of stridor (inspiratory/expiratory), use of accessory muscles, quality of voice (hoarse or silent), respiratory rate, and resting oxygen saturation. Close cooperation and communication among members of the OR team is required. Discuss the plan for induction and airway management with the surgeon preoperatively, as a shared airway is necessary for this surgery. Avoid elective tracheostomy to limit spread of the virus. Prepare the bronchoscope and laser prior to induction.

B. Pediatric patients (if not in profound respiratory distress) may need oral premedication (midazolam 0.5 mg/kg), especially if returning for frequent OR visits. Facilitate IV with topical anesthetic cream. Consider inhalational induction with sevoflurane or halothane prior to the start of the IV in select pediatric patients. Give IV steroids routinely. The surgeon may want to examine the airway of a spontaneously breathing patient; tailor the anesthetic to avoid obstruction or paralysis. Assess the ability to mask ventilate with positive-pressure breaths. If unable to ventilate by mask, promptly intubate the trachea. Have smaller endotracheal tubes (ETTs) available. If intubation is difficult, proceed through the difficult airway algorithm.[1,3]

C. There are many airway management techniques for microsurgery on the larynx. For laser surgery with tracheal intubation, choose a laser safe tube (Xomed, Mallinckrodt, or Bivona); silicon (Xomed, Bivona) is still combustible. Follow strict laser safety precautions (FiO_2 < 0.3, goggles, and laser masks).[4] Consider jet ventilation above or below the vocal cords, which allows adequate ventilation but has a risk of barotrauma, pneumothorax, pneumomediastinum, and gastric insufflation. An apneic technique involving periodic extubation and of the trachea allows an open view of the larynx and avoids ETT combustion. It is important that the vocal cords not move during laser surgery. There are two methods to maintain anesthesia in the nonintubated and spontaneously breathing patient. Volatile anesthetic can be delivered via the side port of the laryngoscope or bronchoscope. However, laryngospasm can occur with this technique and suctioning during laser use can make delivery of volatile anesthetic quite variable. IV maintenance may be more effective. These two techniques do not rule out the possibility of an airway fire.

D. In the event of an airway fire, disconnect the oxygen source and remove any burning material from the airway, including the ETT. Irrigate with sterile water or saline and mask ventilate or reintubate immediately. Evaluate the extent of the injury with laryngoscope or bronchoscope, and closely monitor the patient with pulse oximetry, serial ABGs, and chest x-ray (CXR) for at least 24 hours.[4]

E. At conclusion of the procedure, carefully assess hemostasis and tissue edema. If necessary, reintubate the trachea with a standard ETT. Extubate after the patient is fully awake. Consider administering high humidity and racemic epinephrine in the recovery room. Carefully monitor for several hours prior to discharge; occasionally the patient will require hospital admission for overnight observation.[1]

REFERENCES

1. Derkay CS: Recurrent respiratory papillomatosis, *Laryngoscope* 111:57–69, 2001.
2. Rimell FL: Pediatric laser bronchoscopy, *Intl Anesthesiol Clin* 35:107, 1997.
3. RRP Task Force Guidelines available at: http://www.rrpwebsite.org/#Mission.
4. Pashayan AG, Ehrenwreth J: Lasers and electrical safety in the operating room. In: Ehrenwreth J, Eisenkraft JB, editors: *Anesthesia equipment: principles and applications*, St. Louis, 1993, Mosby.

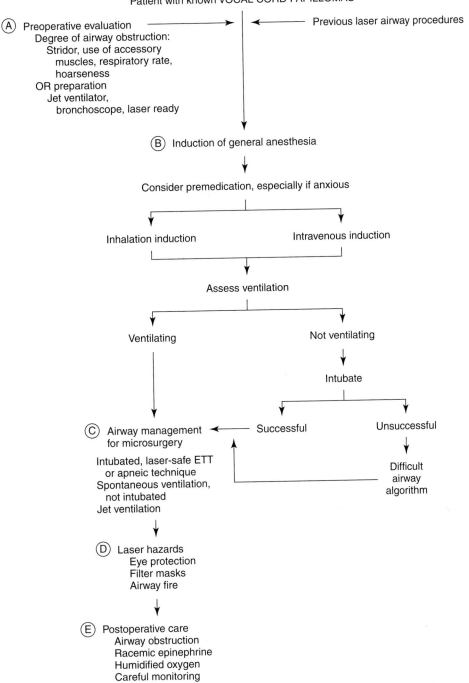

Patient with known VOCAL CORD PAPILLOMAS

(A) Preoperative evaluation ——————————→ ←—————— Previous laser airway procedures
    Degree of airway obstruction:
      Stridor, use of accessory
        muscles, respiratory rate,
        hoarseness
    OR preparation
      Jet ventilator,
        bronchoscope, laser ready

(B) Induction of general anesthesia

Consider premedication, especially if anxious

Inhalation induction   Intravenous induction

Assess ventilation

Ventilating   Not ventilating

                                        Intubate

                            Successful   Unsuccessful

(C) Airway management ←——— Successful   Unsuccessful
    for microsurgery

    Intubated, laser-safe ETT   Difficult
      or apneic technique   airway
    Spontaneous ventilation,   algorithm
      not intubated
    Jet ventilation

(D) Laser hazards
      Eye protection
      Filter masks
      Airway fire

(E) Postoperative care
      Airway obstruction
      Racemic epinephrine
      Humidified oxygen
      Careful monitoring

Upper Airway Obstruction

MARY ANN GURKOWSKI, M.D.

Upper airway obstruction (UAO) can be caused by congenital abnormalities; infection; edema; tumor; trauma; or a foreign body involving the neck, larynx, or pharynx.[1,2] The patient may be hypoxemic, hypercarbic, dehydrated, and maximally stressed. Careful management is needed to avoid precipitating complete airway occlusion.

A. Assess the degree of UAO. Look for intercostal retractions, tachypnea, cyanosis, dyspnea, anxiety, increased work of breathing, sweating, tachycardia, audible wheezing, stridor, and SpO_2.[2] Evaluate mouth opening, using Mallampati classification and neck range of motion. If impending obstruction is not present, consider obtaining chest x-ray (CXR), neck film, CT or magnetic resonance imaging (MRI) scan, and ABG.

B. Newborns and infants may have congenital malformations (laryngeal atresia, stenosis, or web; subglottic stenosis; hemangioma; vocal cord paralysis) or congenital syndromes (Pierre-Robin, Treacher-Collins, Hurlers, or Hunters)[3] that make airway management difficult. Children may have croup; adults or children may have epiglottitis. Patients of all ages may have foreign body aspiration, edema, infection, allergic reaction, or trauma. Neoplasms are most common in adults but may be seen in all ages.

C. Secure a difficulty intubation cart with assorted laryngoscope blades and endotracheal tubes (ETTs), nasal and oral airways, laryngeal mask airways (LMAs),[4] suction catheters, stylets, Magill forceps, fiberoptic bronchoscope, 14-gauge needle or syringe, retrograde wire kit, jet ventilator, tracheostomy tray, and topical anesthetic. Monitor SpO_2 and end-tidal carbon dioxide (CO_2). Omit sedative premedication, but consider IV aspiration prophylaxis and an antisialagogue. Be aware to total doses of topical local anesthesia (seizures, methemoglobinemia).[5]

D. UAO caused by trauma necessitates immediate restoration of the airway. Suspect concomitant cervical spine fracture. Appropriate techniques to secure the airway include direct laryngoscopy followed by intubation; retrograde intubation, fiberoptic intubation (visualization may be poor because of blood and debris); or tracheostomy with local anesthesia. Blind intubation is not recommended, because it may initiate bleeding, is complicated by distorted anatomy, and may create a false passage. In addition, foreign bodies (teeth, tissue) may occlude the ETT. In facial trauma, if the larynx is easily visualized on awake laryngoscopy, an IV induction may be performed. Before intubation, while the airway is being secured, placing the patient in a semi-sitting position may facilitate spontaneous ventilation. If oxygenation by face mask is impossible consider

transtracheal jet oxygenation (TTJO); assess for exhalation with first breath to avoid barotrauma. Occasionally UAO is due to epiglottic hematoma after traumatic intubation.[6]

E. Treat acute allergic airway edema with subcutaneous epinephrine, parenteral steroids, and antihistamines. If medical management is failing, opt for early intubation (i.e., awake sedated versus asleep) before the need for emergent airway management occurs. If edema is severe, tracheostomy under local anesthesia is performed. Smoke inhalation can also lead to acute UAO from laryngeal edema. Give the patient 100% oxygen (O_2). Perform an examination of the oral pharynx and larynx (nasal fiberoptic); soot, burns, or erythema dictates elective intubation because pharyngeal edema and eventual UAO can develop within 24 hours.

F. Most infections affecting the airway originate in the tonsillar region, tongue, or hypopharynx. When limited mouth opening is a problem, the patient can be sedated, if not in respiratory distress, and with topical or local anesthesia, laryngoscopy or fiberoptic intubation is performed. If the vocal cords are visualized, awake intubation or an IV induction followed by intubation can be done. If no vocal cords are seen, awake tracheostomy is the safest way to secure the airway.

G. Delineate the location and extent of neoplasm-induced UAO. Options include awake intubation by direct laryngoscopy, fiberoptic laryngoscopy, or tracheostomy. Tailor the approach to the severity of obstruction and the experience of the anesthesiologist.

H. Maintain intubation and ventilation as necessary until either the UAO has resolved medically or surgically, or until a surgical airway bypasses the obstruction.

REFERENCES

1. Deem S, Bishop MJ: Evaluation and management of the difficult airway, *Crit Care Clin* 11:1–27, 1995.
2. Heidegger T, Gerig HJ, Henderson JJ: Strategies and algorithms for management of the difficult airway, *Best Pract Res Clin Anaesthesiol* 19 (4):661–674, 2005.
3. Walker RW: Management of the difficult airway in children, *J R Soc Med* 94:341–344, 2001.
4. ASA Task Force on Difficult Airway Management: Guidelines for management of the difficult airway. An updated report by the ASA Task Force on Management of the Difficult Airway, *Anesthesiology* 98:1269–1277, 2003.
5. Kern K, Langevin PB, Dunn BM: Methemoglobinemia after topical anesthesia with lidocaine and benzocaine for a difficult intubation, *J Clin Anesth* 12:167–172, 2000.
6. Brown I, Kleinman B: Epiglottic hematoma leading to airway obstruction after general anesthesia, *J Clinic Anesth* 14 (1):34–35, 2002.

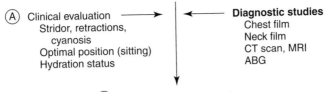

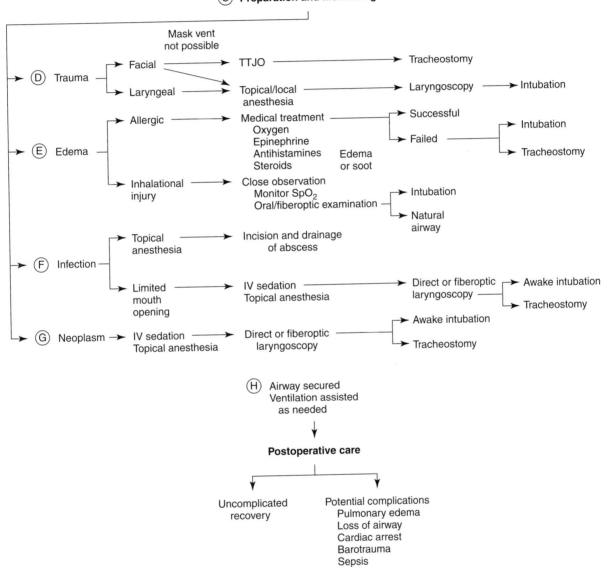

Laser Surgery

LOUIS A. STOOL, M.D.

KEVIN K. KLEIN, M.D.

Many surgical specialties perform laser surgery in close proximity to the airway. Neoplasms, papillomas, vascular malformations, stenoses of the aero-digestive tract, as well as various otologic, ophthalmological, and dermatological lesions are subject to laser treatment. Types of lasers include the carbon dioxide (CO_2), Nd-YAG, Nd-YAG-KTP, argon, and krypton, each with a unique wavelength, thermal effect, tissue penetration, and specific medical use. Careful anesthetic technique and planning are essential because the laser beam may cause burn injury or ignite flammable materials, causing thermal and chemical injury.[1-3]

A. Begin with a careful history and physical examination. Look for signs of possible difficult laryngoscopy or airway obstruction. Preview x-rays, CTs, magnetic resonance images (MRIs), and laryngeal tomograms. Review previous laryngoscopy results, which may define existing pathology and help predict airway difficulties. Communicate with the surgeon preoperatively to obtain information regarding lesion pathology, surgical field exposure requirements, the expected length of the procedure, and the type of laser to be used. Premedicate lightly; consider a benzodiazepine and antisialagogue.

B. Laser surgery requires special preparation and safety precautions because of the potential of tissue damage, combustion, and exposure to the laser plume (smoke). OR personnel must be familiar with laser safety and a laser safety officer must be present. Close all OR doors, cover windows, and place warning signs to identify that a laser is in use. Protect the patient's eyes and all tissues adjacent to the surgical field with moist gauze or towels. Use water-based lubricants and flame-resistant drapes. Outfit OR personnel with protective eyewear designed specifically for the laser wavelength in use as well as an appropriate face mask to protect from the potentially toxic or infectious laser plume, which should be aggressively suctioned. Choose instruments that are not combustible or reflective.

C. Employ general anesthesia for airway lesions using IV or inhaled agent for induction. Consider preemptive analgesia with 4% topical lidocaine. For dermatological procedures, use IV sedation with local anesthetic infiltration or nerve block. Always communicate closely with the surgeon to ensure patient safety.

Patient for LASER SURGERY

(A) Preoperative evaluation ⟶ ⟵ Special studies/evaluations
    History and physical   Direct/indirect laryngoscopy
    History of difficult airway   CT
    Signs of obstruction   MRI
    Nature of lesion   Tomograms
    Intended procedure

(B) **Preparation**
    Talk to surgeon
    Premedication
    Safety measures
        Doors and windows secured
        Laser on stand-by
        Safety officer present
        Safety goggles/face mask on
        Eyes and skin protected
        Field identified

(C) **Anesthetic technique**

General anesthesia   IV sedation with
                                       local anesthesia

IV induction   Inhalation induction

For airway procedures consider preemptive
    analgesia with 4% lidocaine

(Cont'd on p 505)

D. Select the method of ventilation after discussing the nature of the patient's pathology and intended procedure with the surgeon. Intermittent positive-pressure ventilation (IPPV) through a laser-safe endotracheal tube (ETT) allows use of a potent inhalational agent or IV anesthetic with neuromuscular blockade. This technique is useful for supraglottic and laryngeal lesions. Many laser-safe ETTs are available (e.g., Xomed Laser Shield II, Sheridan Laser-Trach, Torre-CUF, and the Mallinckrodt Laser-Flex). Only metal ETTs are nonflammable. PVC, red rubber, and silicone will ignite and may release toxic fumes that can damage the airway. Wrapping a nonmetal ETT with reflective metal tape (aluminum or copper) may create rough surfaces on the ETT, increase the external diameter, and decrease tube flexibility. Fill the ETT cuff with saline and methylene blue, both to act as a heat sink and help detect cuff perforation should it occur. Wrap the ETT cuff with saline soaked cottonoids to protect from direct laser contact. Maintain an $FiO_2 < 0.30$ as tolerated; dilute the oxygen (O_2) with nitrogen, helium, or air while the laser is in use. Helium may offer some advantages because of its higher thermal capacity and lower density, which may improve gas flow through narrow airways.[4]

IPPV via mask is an alternative for brief procedures. A technique using propofol, succinylcholine, and 100% O_2 will allow the surgeon several minutes of operating time during apneic periods. Monitor O_2 saturation with pulse oximetry. Flammable materials must not be in the laser path.

Jet ventilation is the best technique for subglottic procedures requiring an unobstructed view of the larynx or trachea. Maintain anesthesia with propofol, muscle relaxant, and topical anesthesia (4% lidocaine) of the larynx and trachea. Jet ventilate with 100% O_2 directed through a suspension laryngoscope or through a catheter placed within the tracheal lumen.

Spontaneous ventilation techniques are best suited for procedures that are superficial and require only IV sedation with local anesthesia. In selected circumstances a laryngeal mask airway (LMA) may be used, but it is also flammable and must have appropriate shielding.[5] When using open breathing systems, take care to avoid the combination of a flammable substance (plastic, paper, cloth), a high O_2 concentration, and a source of ignition (laser).

E. Postoperative care requires vigilance and careful monitoring of the patient's vital signs. Complete recovery from anesthesia is critical to avoid airway mishaps. Consider applying topical anesthesia after laser surgery of the airway. This allows the patient to recover more fully before removal of the ETT and may prevent laryngospasm secondary to pain. Extubate only when the patient is awake and alert with recovery of airway reflexes. Potential complications include laryngospasm, airway edema, bleeding, pneumothorax, trauma to adjacent tissue, and ocular or dental injury.

F. Airway fire is a disastrous complication of laser surgery. Severe thermal and chemical injury can occur within seconds. In case of airway fire, remove ignition source, stop ventilation, remove the ETT, and douse the fire with saline. Mask ventilate and reintubate the trachea. Perform laryngoscopy and bronchoscopy to evaluate the injury. Obtain chest x-ray (CXR) and consider short-term steroid therapy to minimize edema. Further support and therapy depends on the degree of injury and the patient's clinical status.

REFERENCES

1. Van Der Spek AFL, Spargo PM, Norton ML: The physics of lasers and implications for their use during airway surgery, *Br J Anaesth* 60:709–729, 1988.
2. Pashayan AG: *Anesthesia for laser surgery. ASA 1994 Annual Refresher Course Lectures*, San Francisco, 1994, American Society of Anesthesiologists.
3. Rampil IJ: Anesthetic considerations for laser surgery, *Anesth Analg* 74:424–435, 1992.
4. Pashayan AG, Gravenstein JS, Cassisi NJ, et al.: The helium protocol for laryngotracheal operations with CO2 laser: a retrospective review of 523 cases, *Anesthesiology* 68:801–804, 1988.
5. Pennant JH, Gajraj NM, Miller JF: Resistance of the laryngeal mask airway to the CO$_2$ laser. *Anesthesiology* 79:3A, 1993.

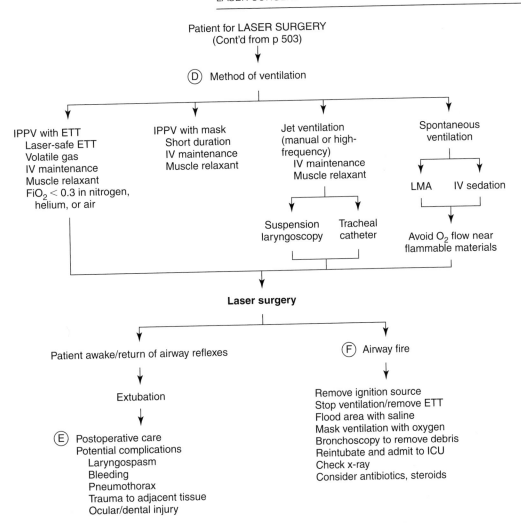

Patient for LASER SURGERY
(Cont'd from p 503)

(D) Method of ventilation

IPPV with ETT
  Laser-safe ETT
  Volatile gas
  IV maintenance
  Muscle relaxant
  $FiO_2 < 0.3$ in nitrogen,
    helium, or air

IPPV with mask
  Short duration
  IV maintenance
  Muscle relaxant

Jet ventilation
(manual or high-
frequency)
  IV maintenance
  Muscle relaxant

Spontaneous
ventilation

LMA   IV sedation

Suspension   Tracheal
laryngoscopy   catheter

Avoid O_2 flow near
flammable materials

Laser surgery

Patient awake/return of airway reflexes

Extubation

(E) Postoperative care
  Potential complications
    Laryngospasm
    Bleeding
    Pneumothorax
    Trauma to adjacent tissue
    Ocular/dental injury

(F) Airway fire

Remove ignition source
Stop ventilation/remove ETT
Flood area with saline
Mask ventilation with oxygen
Bronchoscopy to remove debris
Reintubate and admit to ICU
Check x-ray
Consider antibiotics, steroids

Endoscopic Sinus Surgery

JEFFERY E. TERRELL, M.D.

ALLAN C.D. BROWN, M.D.

Functional endoscopic sinus surgery (FESS) is performed on patients with chronic sinusitis refractory to medical treatment. Patients with chronic sinusitis present with purulent nasal discharge, facial pressure headaches, congestion, postnasal drip, hyposmia, and (less frequently) cough, asthma, and ear complaints. Less common indications for FESS include recurrent acute sinusitis, symptomatic nasal polyps, mucoceles, foreign bodies, recurrent epistaxis, repair of CSF leaks, biopsy of nasal masses, orbital decompression, and pituitary surgery. FESS offers two advantages over the Caldwell Luc procedure and more traditional sinus operations. The normal mucosa of the sinuses is left intact to preserve function, and the natural ostia of the sinuses through which the mucociliary flow occurs are preserved, maintaining a more functional opening into the sinuses.[1]

A. Patients with nasal polyps and asthma have a high incidence of triad asthma, which is characterized by sensitivity to aspirin or nonsteroidal anti-inflammatory drugs (NSAIDs). Triad patients tend to have worse asthma, worse polyps, worse intraoperative bleeding, and higher rates of recurrence for nasal polyposis and symptoms. Treat these patients with preoperative systemic steroids for 4 to 5 days to reduce the polypoid mass and decrease bleeding at operation. Optimize all patients with asthma preoperatively. Cystic fibrosis patients may require an IV antibiotic clean out before surgery.

Preoperative treatment of active infectious and inflammatory processes can reduce operative bleeding. Preoperative decongestant nasal sprays (e.g., oxymetazoline), preoperative control of hypertension (HTN), and anesthetic techniques that minimize vasocongestion (with or without the judicious use of deliberate hypotension) all may contribute to a decreased intraoperative blood loss.

B. Combined topical and infiltration local anesthesia has the advantages of shorter induction and recovery times, less bleeding from vasodilation, and an awake patient who may be able to warn the surgeon of trauma to the orbital periosteum or dura (this warning may not be reliable). Topical anesthesia can be achieved with cocaine solution or crystals (be aware of cocaine risks) or 4% lidocaine solution on nasal pledgets, with special attention to the middle meatus region and the sphenopalatine ganglia. A 1% solution of lidocaine with 1:100,000 epinephrine is used for infiltration in the middle meatus and near the sphenoid rostrum (if the sphenoid sinus will be opened).

Intraoperatively, hemostasis is important and may require intermittent packing with vasoconstrictor-soaked pledgets. Bleeding into the pharynx may limit the amount of narcotic and sedative drugs that may be given (risk of aspiration or laryngospasm) and can limit the extent of the procedure. During a local anesthetic procedure, monitor the patient for signs of mental status changes, restlessness, or confusion, which may be caused by oversedation or hypoxia, drug toxicity or reactions, and intracranial penetration. Provide supplemental oxygen (O_2); beware of fire risk.

C. General anesthesia is required for patients with extensive sinus disease, large polyps, or when there is concern about blood triggering airway hyperreactivity. Place a cuffed oral endotracheal tube (ETT). Apply topical lidocaine to the vocal cords and trachea during laryngoscopy to reduce reactivity. An intraoperative throat pack may be used, and postoperative nasal packing may be placed to minimize the risk of blood triggering laryngospasm after extubation. Muscle relaxants are unnecessary for the operation; a single inhalation agent will suffice (with or without controlled ventilation) unless a balanced technique is indicated for medical reasons. Keep in mind the risk of cardiac dysrhythmia when using epinephrine-containing solutions for infiltration in the presence of halogenated anesthetics. Consider deep extubation in the tonsil position when not contraindicated to minimize the amount of coughing or Valsalva-induced bleeding. There is a risk of negative pressure pulmonary edema.

D. Detect and treat intracranial and intraorbital complications of FESS early. Treat postoperative plain adequately. Even with nasal packing in place, some blood will be swallowed. Anticipate nausea and treat with an antiemetic drug. The major postoperative anesthetic risks are associated with continued postnasal bleeding, which may lead to hypovolemia, airway obstruction from blood or laryngospasm, and hematemesis. If the patient becomes restless, the cause is most likely pain, hypovolemia, or hypoxia (in order of frequency), but hypoxia must be excluded first.

REFERENCES

1. Stammberger H: *Functional endoscopic sinus surgery*, St. Louis, 1991, Mosby.

Patient requiring FUNCTIONAL ENDOSCOPIC SINUS SURGERY

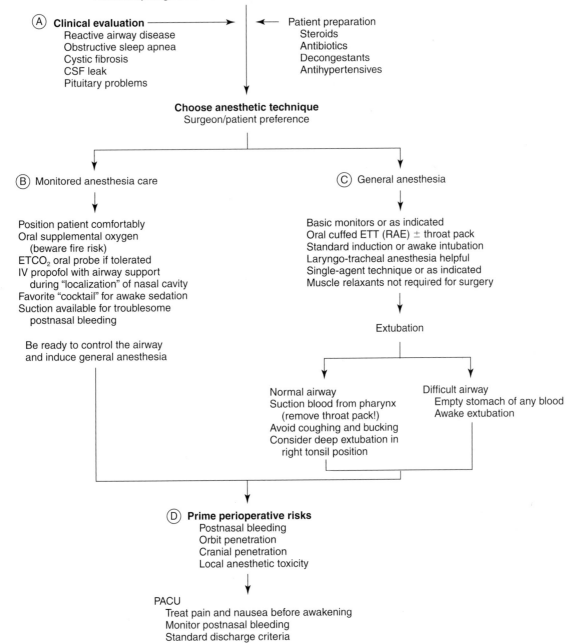

(A) **Clinical evaluation**
   Reactive airway disease
   Obstructive sleep apnea
   Cystic fibrosis
   CSF leak
   Pituitary problems

Patient preparation
   Steroids
   Antibiotics
   Decongestants
   Antihypertensives

Choose anesthetic technique
Surgeon/patient preference

(B) Monitored anesthesia care

Position patient comfortably
Oral supplemental oxygen
   (beware fire risk)
ETCO₂ oral probe if tolerated
IV propofol with airway support
   during "localization" of nasal cavity
Favorite "cocktail" for awake sedation
Suction available for troublesome
   postnasal bleeding

Be ready to control the airway
and induce general anesthesia

(C) General anesthesia

Basic monitors or as indicated
Oral cuffed ETT (RAE) ± throat pack
Standard induction or awake intubation
Laryngo-tracheal anesthesia helpful
Single-agent technique or as indicated
Muscle relaxants not required for surgery

Extubation

Normal airway
Suction blood from pharynx
   (remove throat pack!)
Avoid coughing and bucking
Consider deep extubation in
   right tonsil position

Difficult airway
   Empty stomach of any blood
   Awake extubation

(D) **Prime perioperative risks**
   Postnasal bleeding
   Orbit penetration
   Cranial penetration
   Local anesthetic toxicity

PACU
   Treat pain and nausea before awakening
   Monitor postnasal bleeding
   Standard discharge criteria

Head and Neck Oncologic Surgery

ALLAN C.D. BROWN, M.D.

CAROL R. BRADFORD, M.D.

The majority of head and neck cancer operations are for squamous cell carcinoma. The main etiologic factors are tobacco and alcohol. Stage I and II tumors are treated with surgery or radiation therapy. Advanced Stage III and IV tumors are treated with combined surgery and radiation therapy. After initial treatment, patients may return with recurrent tumors and grossly distorted airway anatomy.[1] Several surgical procedures may be required depending on the size and location of the tumor. Initial evaluation usually leads to diagnostic endoscopy with biopsy of any masses. The definitive operation may involve selective or radical neck dissection, composite resection, or laryngectomy. Tracheotomy is often required for preoperative distortion of the upper airway or the risk of postoperative edema interfering with the patient's breathing. Depending on the extent of the resection, closure of the wound may require a range of techniques from split-thickness skin grafting to pedicled flaps or free flaps. Extensive resections and complex wound closures contribute significantly to the length of the operation.[2]

A. Patients may complain of a palpable mass, pain, dysphagia, dyspnea, weight loss, and voice changes. If dysphagia and weight loss are prominent, anticipate malnourishment and dehydration. The etiologic factors for the tumor (tobacco or alcohol) also have serious implications for the cardiovascular and pulmonary systems. The disease frequently involves the upper airway, which can pose problems for standard laryngoscopy and intubation. This may be further complicated by scarring from radiation therapy. A full airway evaluation is mandatory. Determine a management plan (e.g., positioning, airway management, fluids) with the surgeon in advance. Many techniques are available for managing a difficult airway, but if the problems to be overcome are severe, consider an awake tracheotomy under local anesthesia, particularly if one will be required postoperatively.

B. These operations require general anesthesia. The choice of technique is a compromise between conflicting patient and surgical requirements. Significant systemic disease limits anesthetic choices but a single inhalation technique is usually sufficient without initial use of nondepolarizing muscle relaxants (NDMRs). The longer the operation, the greater are the problems associated with fluid management, temperature homeostasis, and patient positioning. (Procedure length ranges from 6 to 24 hours.) When possible, place standard monitors, arterial pressure, and any central lines on the dominant side (flap donor sites are usually on the nondominant side of the patient).

Standard fluid replacement regimens tend to overload these patients over time; patients do better when fluid is restricted as vital signs permit. Monitor core temperature (a temperature-sensing Foley catheter works well). Actively warm the patient with forced-air warming blankets. Securing the blanket is difficult because of the extent of the surgical preparation area, but warming one leg, the lower part of the abdomen, and the patient breathing circuit has proved adequate for homeostasis. Carefully position the patient to avoid decubitus ulcers, particularly when the patient is in a lateral position for trapezius and latissimus dorsi flaps and scapular-free flaps.[3] The requirements for BP control change throughout the operation. An appropriate degree of deliberate hypotension facilitates dissection. However, during flap creation and wound closure, flap perfusion must be maintained. Use fluid volume, inotropic agents, chronotropic agents, and topical vasodilators rather than vasopressors. Somatosensory-evoked potential monitoring may require suppression of background muscle noise, but surgical motor nerve stimulation requires some twitch response. A continuous infusion of a short-acting nondepolarizer, maintaining a two-twitch response to train-of-four stimulation is a practical compromise if required.[4]

C. The same principles govern the management of fluids and BP in the postoperative period. Promptly control hypertension (HTN) to avoid wound hematoma. Administer supplemental humidified oxygen (O_2) as dictated by blood gas analysis. Maintain a secure airway; mechanical ventilation may be required. Administer IV narcotics for pain relief. Continue deep venous thrombosis (DVT) prophylaxis. Carefully monitor flap perfusion, and take immediate action if deterioration occurs. Patients with extensive resections are best nursed in an ICU after discharge from the PACU.

REFERENCES

1. American Joint Committee on Cancer: Head and neck sites. In: *AJCC cancer staging manual*, ed 6, 2002, AJCC.
2. Silver CE, Rubin JS: *Atlas of head and neck surgery*, ed 2, New York, 1999, Churchill Livingstone.
3. Brown ACD: Anesthesia for ear, nose and throat surgery. In: Cohen TEJ, Healy PJ, editors: *Churchill Davidson's a practice of anaesthesia*, ed 6, London, 1995, E Arnold.
4. Urken ML, Cheney ML, Sullivan MJ, editors: *Atlas of regional and free flaps for head and neck reconstruction*, New York, 1995, Raven Press.
5. Perel A: Assessing fluid responsiveness by the systolic pressure variation in mechanically ventilated patients, *Anesthesiology* 89: 1309–1310, 1998.

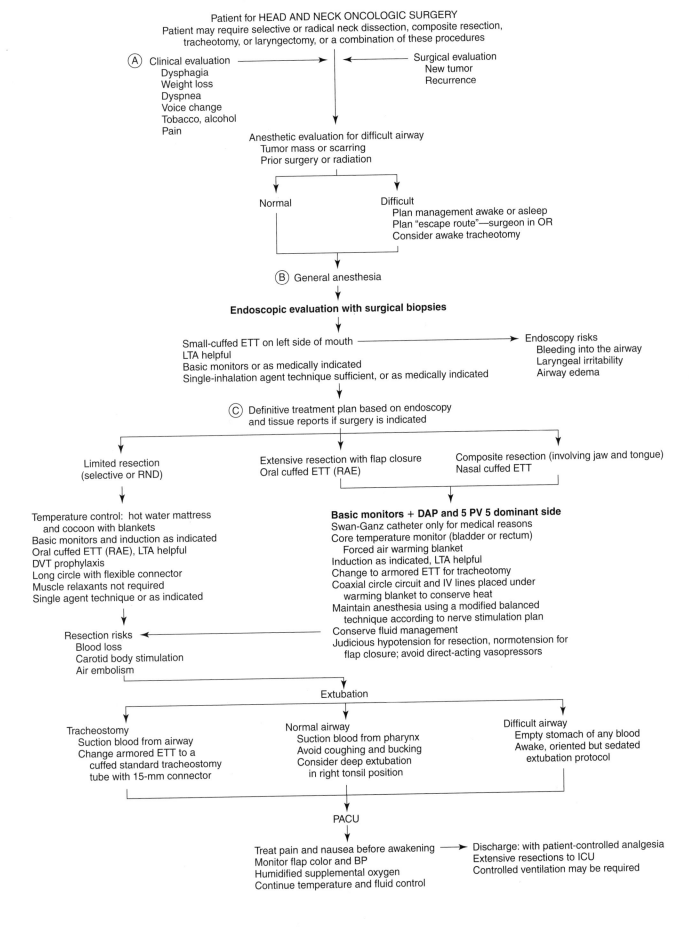

Patient for HEAD AND NECK ONCOLOGIC SURGERY
Patient may require selective or radical neck dissection, composite resection,
tracheotomy, or laryngectomy, or a combination of these procedures

Ⓐ Clinical evaluation ─────────────▶   ◀───────── Surgical evaluation
        Dysphagia   New tumor
        Weight loss   Recurrence
        Dyspnea
        Voice change
        Tobacco, alcohol
        Pain
                            Anesthetic evaluation for difficult airway
                                Tumor mass or scarring
                                Prior surgery or radiation

                Normal   Difficult
                                                    Plan management awake or asleep
                                                    Plan "escape route"—surgeon in OR
                                                    Consider awake tracheotomy

                        Ⓑ General anesthesia

                Endoscopic evaluation with surgical biopsies

Small-cuffed ETT on left side of mouth ──────────────▶ Endoscopy risks
LTA helpful   Bleeding into the airway
Basic monitors or as medically indicated   Laryngeal irritability
Single-inhalation agent technique sufficient, or as medically indicated   Airway edema

                Ⓒ Definitive treatment plan based on endoscopy
                    and tissue reports if surgery is indicated

Limited resection   Extensive resection with flap closure   Composite resection (involving jaw and tongue)
(selective or RND)   Oral cuffed ETT (RAE)   Nasal cuffed ETT

Temperature control: hot water mattress   **Basic monitors + DAP and 5 PV 5 dominant side**
    and cocoon with blankets   Swan-Ganz catheter only for medical reasons
Basic monitors and induction as indicated   Core temperature monitor (bladder or rectum)
Oral cuffed ETT (RAE), LTA helpful   Forced air warming blanket
DVT prophylaxis   Induction as indicated, LTA helpful
Long circle with flexible connector   Change to armored ETT for tracheotomy
Muscle relaxants not required   Coaxial circle circuit and IV lines placed under
Single agent technique or as indicated   warming blanket to conserve heat
                                                 Maintain anesthesia using a modified balanced
                                                    technique according to nerve stimulation plan
                                                 Conserve fluid management
    Resection risks ◀───────────────────────── Judicious hypotension for resection, normotension for
        Blood loss   flap closure; avoid direct-acting vasopressors
        Carotid body stimulation
        Air embolism

                            Extubation

Tracheostomy   Normal airway   Difficult airway
Suction blood from airway   Suction blood from pharynx   Empty stomach of any blood
Change armored ETT to a   Avoid coughing and bucking   Awake, oriented but sedated
    cuffed standard tracheostomy Consider deep extubation   extubation protocol
    tube with 15-mm connector   in right tonsil position

                            PACU

Treat pain and nausea before awakening ──────▶ Discharge: with patient-controlled analgesia
Monitor flap color and BP   Extensive resections to ICU
Humidified supplemental oxygen   Controlled ventilation may be required
Continue temperature and fluid control

Laryngoscopy

GARY D. SKRIVANEK, M.D.

KEVIN K. KLEIN, M.D.

Laryngoscopy is routinely performed by anesthesiologists for tracheal intubation. In panendoscopy and microlaryngoscopy the airway is shared by the anesthesiologist and surgeon. In these surgical cases, laryngoscopy is performed to allow visualization of the oropharynx or larynx for diagnostic (vocal cord function, biopsies) or therapeutic benefits (removal of foreign bodies, excision of tumor or abnormal tissue growths).

A. Perform a thorough history and physical examination. Focus particular attention on the airway examination (Mallampati classification)[1] for prediction of ease of intubation. Note signs of airway distress, such as shortness of breath, stridor, hoarseness, drooling, tracheal deviation, or limited mouth opening. These patients frequently have a significant tobacco history with associated pulmonary and cardiac risks. Obtain necessary laboratory tests and other studies (e.g., chest x-ray [CXR], pulmonary function tests [PFTs], ABGs, ECG, stress test, echocardiogram [echo]) based on the preoperative assessment. Many patients will have a history of alcohol abuse and may require adjustment of anesthetic doses or monitoring for alcohol withdrawal. Frequently these patients present with a prior history of cancer and radiation treatment which may make intubation or ventilation more difficult.

B. Formulate an anesthetic plan based on the type of laryngoscopy (indirect, direct, suspension, flexible, or rigid), the nature of the procedure (biopsies, excision, dilation, or laser), and the duration of the procedure. Consider premedication with an antisialagogue (glycopyrrolate, 0.1 mg), bronchodilator to optimize pulmonary function, steroid (dexamethasone, 8 mg) to reduce edema or swelling, and aspiration prophylaxis (sodium citrate or H_2 blockers and metoclopramide). Use sedating drugs (benzodiazepines or opiates) carefully and only with continuous monitoring because of the risks of respiratory depression and obstruction.

C. For brief procedures on cooperative patients, direct laryngoscopy and flexible fiberoptic laryngoscopy may be performed with IV sedation and local anesthesia. There are a variety of approaches. Anesthetize the nasal mucosa with topical cocaine (4%) or oxymetazoline plus 4% lidocaine to provide anesthesia and vasoconstriction, allowing visualization of the vocal cords via the nares with a flexible fiberoptic scope. (Use of cocaine for this purpose has declined.) Anesthetize the oropharynx with nebulized anesthetics or gargled viscous 2% lidocaine. Block the superior laryngeal nerve by injection, bilaterally, as it passes through the thyrohyoid membrane. Spray topical 4% lidocaine into the vocal cords through the flexible fiberoptic laryngoscope or via laryngotracheal anesthesia (LTA) kit. Block the recurrent laryngeal nerve by injection of 4 ml of 4% lidocaine transtracheally via the cricothyroid membrane. Provide sedation with small doses of propofol, benzodiazepines, or narcotics; titrate judiciously to assist in the performance of these procedures. Continuously monitor the adequacy of ventilation by visualization, auscultation, capnography, and pulse oximetry. Local anesthetics may cause methemoglobinemia; monitor for this condition while performing these blocks.[2,3]

D. For procedures that require laryngoscopy of significant duration or in pediatric or uncooperative patients, general anesthesia is the best choice. After IV induction and muscle relaxation, intubate the trachea with a small diameter endotracheal tube. Provide a sufficient depth of anesthesia to avoid movement or hemodynamic response, yet allow a rapid recovery to baseline status.[4,5] For quick examinations, consider an induction with propofol, succinylcholine (SCC), and 4 ml of 4% lidocaine via an LTA. In patients with severe or impending airway obstruction, spontaneous ventilation with sevoflurane may be useful. For longer duration cases, use small doses of an intermediate duration nondepolarizing muscle relaxant (NDMR) with IV anesthetics (e.g., propofol, remifentanil) or inhalational agents. In some patients, consider jet ventilation to allow the best view of the larynx to the surgeon.[6,7] Total IV anesthesia (TIVA) with good neuromuscular blockade is usually required in such cases. Ask the surgeon to apply topical lidocaine at the end of the procedure to facilitate emergence by lessening the chance of laryngospasm.

E. Complications of laryngoscopy include inadequate ventilation, loss of airway, aspiration, hypertension (HTN), dysrhythmias, eye trauma, dental trauma, laryngospasm, bronchospasm, perforation of the airway or esophagus, bleeding, edema, and airway obstruction. The anesthesiologist must remain vigilant for the occurrence of these complications intraoperatively and in the postoperative recovery period.

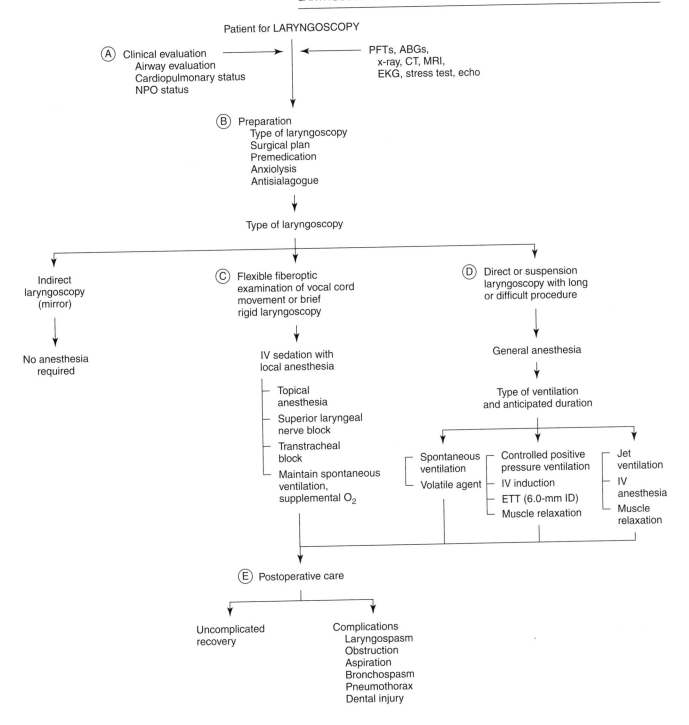

Patient for LARYNGOSCOPY

Ⓐ Clinical evaluation
   Airway evaluation
   Cardiopulmonary status
   NPO status

PFTs, ABGs,
   x-ray, CT, MRI,
   EKG, stress test, echo

Ⓑ Preparation
   Type of laryngoscopy
   Surgical plan
   Premedication
   Anxiolysis
   Antisialagogue

Type of laryngoscopy

Indirect
laryngoscopy
(mirror)

No anesthesia
required

Ⓒ Flexible fiberoptic
   examination of vocal cord
   movement or brief
   rigid laryngoscopy

IV sedation with
local anesthesia

— Topical
   anesthesia
— Superior laryngeal
   nerve block
— Transtracheal
   block
— Maintain spontaneous
   ventilation,
   supplemental O_2

Ⓓ Direct or suspension
   laryngoscopy with long
   or difficult procedure

General anesthesia

Type of ventilation
and anticipated duration

┌ Spontaneous
│ ventilation
└ Volatile agent

┌ Controlled positive
│ pressure ventilation
├ IV induction
├ ETT (6.0-mm ID)
└ Muscle relaxation

┌ Jet
│ ventilation
├ IV
│ anesthesia
└ Muscle
   relaxation

Ⓔ Postoperative care

Uncomplicated
recovery

Complications
   Laryngospasm
   Obstruction
   Aspiration
   Bronchospasm
   Pneumothorax
   Dental injury

REFERENCES

1. Mallampati SR, Gatt SP, Gugino LD, et al.: A clinical sign to predict difficult tracheal intubation: a prospective study, *Can Anaesth Soc J* 32:429–434, 1985.
2. Nguyen ST, Cabrales RE, Bashour CA, et al.: Benzocaine-induced methemoglobinemia, *Anesth Analg* 90:369–371, 2000.
3. Karim A, Ahmed S, Siddiqui R, et al.: Methemoglobinemia complicating topical lidocaine use during endoscopic procedures, *Am J Med* 111:150–153, 2001.
4. Chung KS, Sinatra RS, Chung JH: The effect of an intermediate dose of labetalol on heart rate and blood pressure responses to laryngoscopy and intubation, *J Clin Anesth* 4:11–15, 1992.
5. Smith RB: Anesthesia for endoscopy, *Trans Pa Acad Ophthalmol Otolaryngol* 28:167–173, 1975.
6. Oulton JL, Donald DM: A ventilating laryngoscope, *Anesthesiology* 35:540–542, 1971.
7. Smith RB, Babinski M, Petruscak J: A method for ventilating patients during laryngoscopy, *Laryngoscope* 84:553–559, 1974.

Bronchoscopy

JAMES D. GRIFFIN, M.D.

KEVIN K. KLEIN, M.D.

Bronchoscopy is usually performed as a diagnostic procedure for patients with real or potential pulmonary pathology or foreign body aspiration. Flexible fiberoptic bronchoscopy may be performed with topical anesthesia and IV sedation or with general anesthesia. Rigid bronchoscopy usually requires general anesthesia and neuromuscular blockade. Diagnostic bronchoscopy often precedes a planned surgical procedure, such as excision of a head and neck cancer or thoracotomy.[1-3]

A. Perform a complete history and physical examination. Direct attention to the airway and respiratory system for evidence of disease or obstruction and adequacy of pulmonary function. Consider obtaining a chest x-ray (CXR), ECG, ABG, and pulmonary function tests (PFTs)(FEV_1). Premedicate with an antisialagogue and bronchodilator (as needed). Consider the need for aspiration prophylaxis. Sedate the patient with a small dose of benzodiazepine, using caution to avoid respiratory depression. Avoid opioids in most cases.

B. Have an appropriate endotracheal tube (ETT) available. A tube of at least 8.0 mm inside diameter (ID) is best for passing a flexible fiberoptic bronchoscopy. A Portex adapter with diaphragm is useful to allow uninterrupted ventilation. A small (6.0 mm ID) reinforced ETT is desirable for panendoscopy or when a bronchoscope is passed beside the ETT. Routinely monitor pulse oximetry, ECG, temperature, noninvasive BP, and end-tidal carbon dioxide (CO_2). ST segment monitoring is useful to detect myocardial ischemia. Have drugs readily available to treat bronchospasm, swings in BP and pulse, and myocardial ischemia.

C. Plan the anesthetic, taking into account the surgical procedure and type of bronchoscopy. Consult with the surgeon to determine if an obstruction, foreign body, or tumor is present or if a biopsy planned. Provide topical anesthesia of the larynx to reduce anesthetic requirements and avoid excessive autonomic stimulation. Consider using an IV anesthetic technique, which may include short-acting agents given by bolus or continuous infusion (e.g., propofol, remifentanil, mivacurium, or succinylcholine).

D. For flexible, fiberoptic bronchoscopy, choose either local anesthesia with IV sedation or general anesthesia. Local anesthesia is accomplished by a variety of techniques, including application of topical anesthetics to the nasal and oropharyngeal mucosa. The superior laryngeal nerve, which provides sensory innervation to the lower pharynx and upper pharynx, may be blocked directly where it transverses the thyrohyoid muscle. The recurrent laryngeal nerve provides sensory innervation to the trachea and may be anesthetized by injection of 4 ml of 4% lidocaine, either through the glottic opening or by cricothyroid puncture. For general anesthesia, consider using an ETT of at least 8.0 mm ID and a Portex adapter with diaphragm. Alternatively, place a small ETT (6.0 mm ID) to allow passage of a bronchoscope beside the ETT. Both of these techniques allow uninterrupted ventilation and use of volatile anesthetic agents.

E. For rigid bronchoscopy, administer general anesthesia. Although spontaneous ventilation is possible, controlled positive-pressure ventilation with neuromuscular blockade is usually preferred. There are two basic types of bronchoscopes: the rigid ventilating bronchoscope with a sideport to connect to the breathing circuit and a glass eyepiece to close the system and an open Venturi bronchoscope designed to use with a high pressure (50 pound per square inch [psi]) source of oxygen for jet ventilation. The ventilating bronchoscope will leak around the distal end but, with the glass eyepiece in place, will allow the use of volatile agent and a high fresh gas flow (10 L/min). This technique may lead to significant anesthetic gas pollution; an IV technique may be preferred. Administer a high FiO_2 prior to opening the glass eyepiece to allow apneic oxygenation and monitor oxygen saturation with a pulse oximeter. For jet ventilation, use IV anesthesia and neuromuscular blockade. Take care not to induce barotrauma from the high pressure jet.[4-6]

F. Observe for the following complications which may occur during or after bronchoscopy: cardiac dysrhythmia, myocardial ischemia, aspiration, hemorrhage, barotrauma, laceration, pneumothorax, and bronchospasm.

REFERENCES

1. Roberts JT, editor: Fiberoptics in anesthesia, *Anesthesiol Clin North Am* 9 (1), 1991.
2. Kaplan JA, Slinger PD: *Thoracic anesthesia*, ed 3, New York, 2003, Churchill Livingstone.
3. Benumof JL: *Anesthesia for thoracic surgery*, ed 2, Philadelphia, 1995, W.B. Saunders.
4. Fraioli RL, Sheffer LA, Steffenson JL: Pulmonary and cardiovascular effects of apneic oxygenation in man, *Anesthesiology* 39:588–596, 1973.
5. Giesecke AH, Gerbershagen HU, Dortman C, et al.: Comparison of the ventilating and injection bronchoscopes, *Anesthesiology* 38:298–303, 1973.
6. Smith RB, Lindholm CE, Klain M: Jet ventilation for fiberoptic bronchoscopy under general anesthesia, *Acta Anaesthesiol Scand* 20:111–116, 1976.

Patient for BRONCHOSCOPY

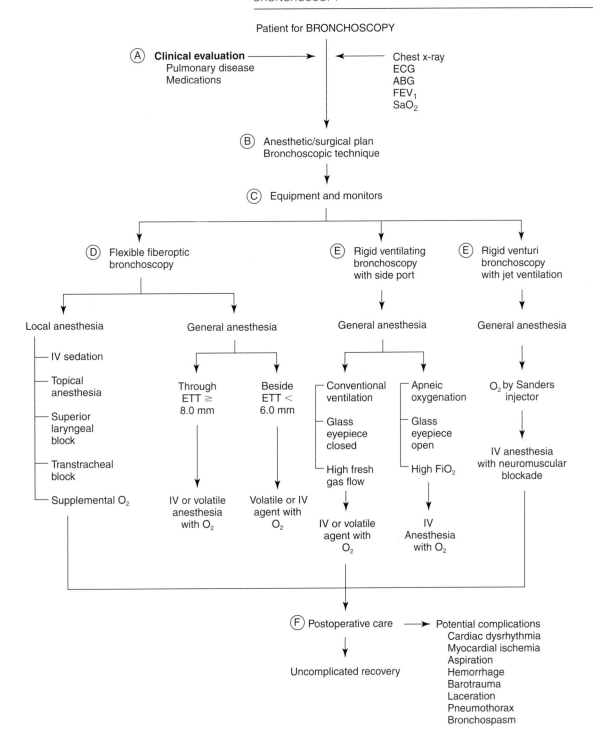

Ⓐ **Clinical evaluation** ⟶ ⟵ Chest x-ray
   Pulmonary disease   ECG
   Medications   ABG
                                  FEV_1
                                  SaO_2

Ⓑ Anesthetic/surgical plan
   Bronchoscopic technique

Ⓒ Equipment and monitors

Ⓓ Flexible fiberoptic   Ⓔ Rigid ventilating   Ⓔ Rigid venturi
   bronchoscopy   bronchoscopy   bronchoscopy
                                  with side port   with jet ventilation

Local anesthesia   General anesthesia   General anesthesia   General anesthesia

— IV sedation

— Topical
  anesthesia   Through   Beside
                            ETT ≥   ETT <
— Superior   8.0 mm   6.0 mm
  laryngeal
  block

— Transtracheal
  block

— Supplemental O_2 IV or volatile   Volatile or IV
                            anesthesia   agent with
                            with O_2 O_2

— Conventional   — Apneic O_2 by Sanders
  ventilation   oxygenation   injector

— Glass   — Glass
  eyepiece   eyepiece
  closed   open   IV anesthesia
                                            with neuromuscular
— High fresh   — High FiO_2 blockade
  gas flow

IV or volatile   IV
agent with   Anesthesia
O_2 with O_2

Ⓕ Postoperative care ⟶ Potential complications
                          Cardiac dysrhythmia
                          Myocardial ischemia
                          Aspiration
Uncomplicated recovery   Hemorrhage
                          Barotrauma
                          Laceration
                          Pneumothorax
                          Bronchospasm

OPHTHALMOLOGIC ANESTHESIA

OPEN GLOBE

CATARACT EXTRACTION

RETINAL DETACHMENT

ANESTHESIA FOR STRABISMUS SURGERY IN
CHILDREN

Open Globe

KATHRYN E. McGOLDRICK, M.D.

Penetrating injuries of the eye usually demand urgent repair to ensure an optimal visual result. Most experts agree on the intraoperative maintenance of patients with an open eye and a full stomach, but controversy has focused for decades on induction techniques, specifically the selection of neuromuscular blocking agents to facilitate intubation. The goal is prevention of increases in intraocular, venous, and arterial pressures while simultaneously maintaining oxygenation and preventing aspiration. Because laryngoscopy and endotracheal intubation increase BP and IOP more than any drug, anesthetic induction must be smooth and rapid. Adequate depth of anesthesia and stable IOP must be maintained intraoperatively, and extubation and emergence must be safe and nontumultuous.

A. Ascertain the time since the patient's last oral intake and determine any concomitant medical problems.

B. IOP is increased by coughing, straining, vomiting, venous congestion, crying, acute arterial hypertension (HTN), pressure of a too tightly applied face mask, hypercarbia, and (slightly and transiently) the use of succinylcholine (SCC).

C. GETA is selected for almost all open eye cases, because retrobulbar injection causes an increase in IOP, which is capable of producing extrusion of intraocular contents through a large wound. Nonetheless, come case reports of successful use of ophthalmic blocks in selected patients with an open globe have been published.[1,2] General anesthesia, however, is a prudent choice for most patients. Choice of induction technique depends on whether the patient had recently ingested food before the injury.

D. Awake intubation may trigger coughing and straining and should be considered only if an extremely difficult intubation is anticipated; flexible fiberoptic endoscopy skillfully performed with topical anesthesia and judicious sedation is less stimulating than rigid laryngoscopy. If difficulty is not anticipated, management of an eye trauma patient with a full stomach requires preoxygenation via a gently applied facemask followed by a RSI with cricoid pressure. Administer H_2 blockers, metoclopramide, and nonparticulate antacids preoperatively as prophylaxis against aspiration. Additionally, premedication with drugs such as acetazolamide, alfentanil[3] and other narcotics, propranolol, nitroglycerin, clonidine, and defasciculating doses of nondepolarizing muscle relaxant (NDMR) may prevent or attenuate increases in IOP caused by laryngoscopy, intubation, and the use of SCC. Perform RSI with generous doses of either propofol (2 to 2.5 mg/kg IV), thiopental (4 to 7 mg/kg), or, if hypotension is a concern, etomidate (0.3 mg/kg) followed by SCC (1.5 mg/kg). The rapid, reliable onset of SCC permits a swift, smooth intubation without coughing on the endotracheal tube (ETT), a detrimental response that can elevate IOP by more than 40 mm Hg. Currently available NDMRs, even when given synergistically to prime onset or given in extremely large doses to accelerate onset, do not reliably provide these ideal intubating conditions as rapidly. Insufficient data are available to recommend the use of high-dose rocuronium (1.2 mg/kg) in this setting. The rapid return of spontaneous ventilation can be invaluable when managing an unexpectedly difficult intubation. The use of large intubating doses of NDMRs eliminates this option. The search for a NDMR with the rapid onset of SCC, reliability, and brief duration continues. At present, unless contraindicated (e.g., hyperkalemia or malignant hyperthermia susceptibility), the use of SCC after pretreatment is a rational solution to the open eye–full stomach challenge.[4,5] After induction and intubation, place a gastric tube to decompress the stomach.

E. Anesthetic induction in the fasted patient without risk factors for reflux can be accomplished with similar induction agents and a conventional intubating dose of a NDMR. Ensure adequate depth of anesthesia before performing laryngoscopy. (Use of a peripheral nerve stimulator to predict intubating conditions can be unreliable, because muscle groups vary in their response to relaxants.) Lidocaine given via IV before laryngoscopy to attenuate intubation-associated arterial HTN does not reliably prevent increases in IOP; narcotics given via IV are recommended.

F. The inhalation agents lower IOP in a dose-dependent fashion, along with IV narcotics and hyperventilation. Keep the patient paralyzed until the wound is surgically closed. Administer an antiemetic to prevent postoperative nausea and vomiting. Surgical manipulation of the eye may trigger the oculocardiac reflex. Any residual neuromuscular blockade must be reversed before extubation. Lidocaine administered via IV may facilitate smooth extubation, but the patient with a full stomach must be awake before extubation.

REFERENCES

1. Scott IU, McCabe CM, Flynn HW Jr, et al.: Local anesthesia with intravenous sedation for surgical repair of selected open globe injuries, Am J Ophthalmol 134:707, 2002.
2. Boscia F, LaTegola MG, Colombo G, et al.: Combined topical anesthesia and sedation for open-globe injuries in selected patients, Ophthalmology 110:1555, 2003.
3. Zimmerman AA, Funk KJ, Tidwell JL: Propofol and alfentanil prevent the increase in intraocular pressure caused by succinylcholine and endotracheal intubation during a rapid sequence induction of anesthesia, Anesth Analg 83:814, 1996.
4. McGoldrick KE: The open globe: is an alternative to succinylcholine necessary? J Clin Anesth 5:1, 1993.
5. Moreno RJ, Kloess P, Carlson DW: Effect of succinylcholine on the intraocular contents of open globes, Ophthalmology 98:636, 1991.

Patient with AN OPEN GLOBE

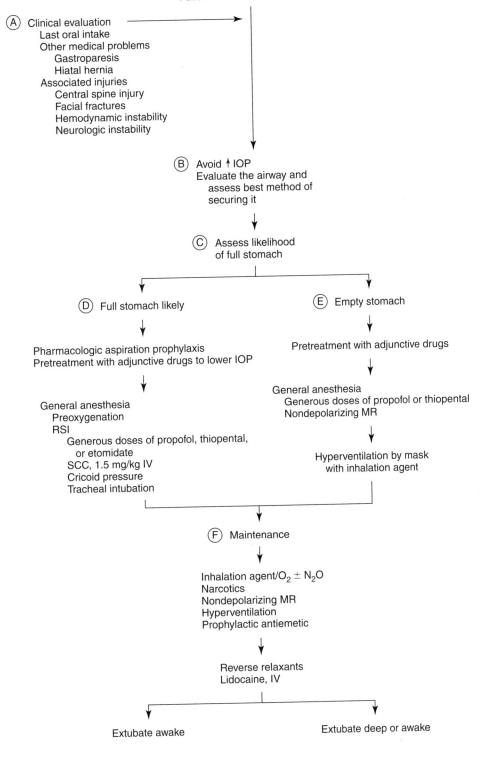

(A) Clinical evaluation
   Last oral intake
   Other medical problems
      Gastroparesis
      Hiatal hernia
   Associated injuries
      Central spine injury
      Facial fractures
      Hemodynamic instability
      Neurologic instability

(B) Avoid ↑ IOP
   Evaluate the airway and
      assess best method of
      securing it

(C) Assess likelihood
   of full stomach

(D) Full stomach likely

Pharmacologic aspiration prophylaxis
Pretreatment with adjunctive drugs to lower IOP

General anesthesia
   Preoxygenation
   RSI
      Generous doses of propofol, thiopental,
         or etomidate
      SCC, 1.5 mg/kg IV
      Cricoid pressure
      Tracheal intubation

(E) Empty stomach

Pretreatment with adjunctive drugs

General anesthesia
   Generous doses of propofol or thiopental
   Nondepolarizing MR

Hyperventilation by mask
   with inhalation agent

(F) Maintenance

Inhalation agent/$O_2 \pm N_2O$
Narcotics
Nondepolarizing MR
Hyperventilation
Prophylactic antiemetic

Reverse relaxants
Lidocaine, IV

Extubate awake

Extubate deep or awake

Cataract Extraction

KATHRYN E. McGOLDRICK, M.D.

A rapidly growing elderly population, development of the intraocular lens implant, and the widespread availability of surgical techniques employing operating microscopes, phacoemulsification, and allied devices have increased the demand for cataract surgery.[1] Moreover, cataract surgery is almost always performed as an outpatient procedure. Cataract extraction is a delicate intraocular operation; maintaining akinesia and a stable intraocular pressure (IOP) is critical. Failure to meet these requirements can result in lens dislocation, loss of vitreous, retinal detachment, macular edema, expulsive hemorrhage, and other complications that are ultimately capable of producing blindness in the operated eye.

A. The cataract patient is typically elderly and may be afflicted with a variety of medical problems. The patient may have other ocular conditions, including glaucoma. Obtain a thorough drug history; topical and systemic medication for glaucoma may have important anesthetic implications.[2] Because intraoperative immobility is important, assess the patient for chronic coughing, inability to lie flat, and impaired ability to follow instructions and remain motionless because of excessive anxiety, arthritis, claustrophobia, deafness, tremors, or senility. In these patients, GETA is indicated. Cataracts are not confined to the geriatric age group. Cataracts in pediatric patients can be idiopathic or associated with chromosomal disorders, inborn errors of metabolism, intrauterine infections, trauma, or steroid therapy.

B. Historically, GETA was popular for cataract extraction. Since the 1970s, however, regional anesthesia (retrobulbar or peribulbar block) or various other less invasive techniques, such as subconjunctival (perilimbal) or sub-Tenon's injection[3] or topical corneoconjunctival analgesia, has gradually replaced GETA in most cases. Indeed, a recent survey disclosed that 59% of responding ophthalmologists in the United States use topical analgesia for cataract surgery.[4] Because topical analgesia does not provide ocular akinesia, it is imperative that these patients be able to control their eye movement. The complications of retrobulbar block include retrobulbar hemorrhage,[5] perforation of the globe, central spread of local anesthetic that may affect the brainstem and cause respiratory arrest,[6] intraarterial injection with immediate seizures, and optic nerve injury. Moreover, many of these complications have also been associated with peribulbar and sub-Tenon's anesthesia.[7]

C. When GETA is selected, choose propofol, thiopental, or etomidate as induction agents (these will lower IOP). Propofol is strongly recommended because of its antiemetic properties. Nondepolarizing neuromuscular blockers do not elevate IOP. Select a neuromuscular blocker based on the agent's hemodynamic profile and the anticipated duration of surgery. Succinylcholine (SCC) is an acceptable alternative to facilitate intubation, because the small, transient increase in IOP associated with SCC will be dissipated before the cornea is incised. Narcotics, beta-blockers, and acetazolamide are useful adjuncts to reduce IOP. Lidocaine administered via IV is inconsistent in preventing the increase in IOP associated with SCC and intubation. The laryngeal mask airway (LMA) is gaining popularity, especially in the United Kingdom, for ophthalmic surgery. The LMA is generally easy to insert and affords a smooth emergence without coughing. The LMA does not protect against regurgitation. Furthermore, vigilance must be maintained to detect initial misplacement or intraoperative displacement of the LMA. Additionally, intraoperative laryngospasm in neonates and infants is not uncommon with an LMA.

D. All inhalation agents cause a dose-dependent reduction in IOP. Administer any volatile agent in combination with N_2O and oxygen (O_2). Alternatively, a total IV technique with propofol can be selected. Maintain a sufficiently deep level of anesthesia until the incision is closed; administer a nondepolarizing muscle relaxant (NDMR) and use peripheral nerve monitoring. If the patient moves unexpectedly during intraocular surgery, immediately give thiopental (IV), propofol, or a similar, fast-acting drug that lowers IOP. SCC is contraindicated after the eye has been surgically opened. Control and monitor ventilation using an end-tidal carbon dioxide (CO_2) measurement to avoid hypercarbia and its deleterious effect on IOP. Administer a prophylactic antiemetic (e.g., droperidol, 10 to 20 µg/kg IV or ondansetron 4 mg/kg IV). After completion of surgery, reverse any residual neuromuscular blockade.

E. Smooth extubation is desirable. Lidocaine, 1 to 1.5 mg/kg IV, can be given a few minutes before extubation to prevent or attenuate periextubation bucking and coughing. Although mild to moderate coughing should not compromise any suture lines, try to prevent severe coughing.

F. Recovery is typically associated with minimal postoperative pain. Patients are instructed to avoid bending, lifting, and straining in the postoperative period to protect the surgical result.

Patient for CATARACT EXTRACTION

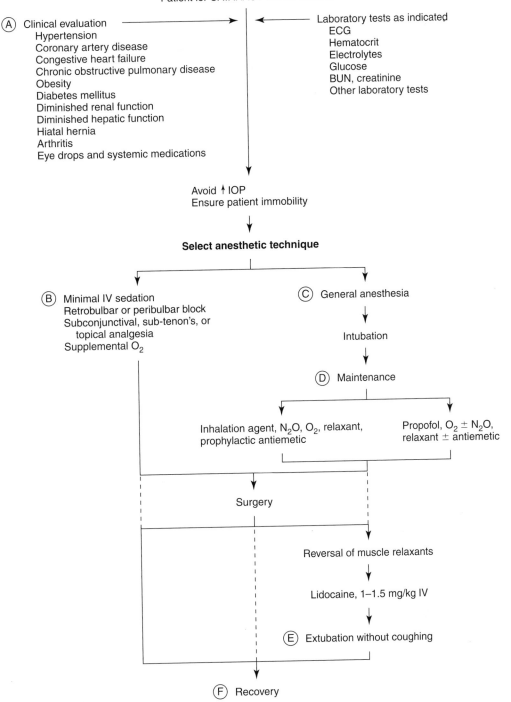

Ⓐ Clinical evaluation
    Hypertension
    Coronary artery disease
    Congestive heart failure
    Chronic obstructive pulmonary disease
    Obesity
    Diabetes mellitus
    Diminished renal function
    Diminished hepatic function
    Hiatal hernia
    Arthritis
    Eye drops and systemic medications

Laboratory tests as indicated
    ECG
    Hematocrit
    Electrolytes
    Glucose
    BUN, creatinine
    Other laboratory tests

Avoid ↑ IOP
Ensure patient immobility

Select anesthetic technique

Ⓑ Minimal IV sedation
    Retrobulbar or peribulbar block
    Subconjunctival, sub-tenon's, or
        topical analgesia
    Supplemental O$_2$

Ⓒ General anesthesia

Intubation

Ⓓ Maintenance

Inhalation agent, N$_2$O, O$_2$, relaxant,
prophylactic antiemetic

Propofol, O$_2$ ± N$_2$O,
relaxant ± antiemetic

Surgery

Reversal of muscle relaxants

Lidocaine, 1–1.5 mg/kg IV

Ⓔ Extubation without coughing

Ⓕ Recovery

REFERENCES

1. Solomon R, Donnenfeld ED: Recent advances and future frontiers in treating age-related cataracts, *JAMA* 290:248, 2003.
2. McGoldrick KE: Anesthetic ramifications of ophthalmic drugs. In: McGoldrick KE, editor: *Anesthesia for ophthalmic and otolaryngologic surgery*, Philadelphia, 1992, W.B. Saunders.
3. Guise PA: Sub-Tenon anesthesia: A prospective study of 6,000 blocks, *Anesthesiology* 98:964, 2003.
4. Leaming DV: Practice styles and preferences of ASCRS members: 2002 survey, *J Cataract Refract Surg* 29:1412, 2003.
5. Edge KR, Nicoll JMV: Retrobulbar hemorrhage after 12,500 retrobulbar blocks, *Anesth Analg* 76:1019, 1993.
6. Hamilton RC: Brain-stem anesthesia as a complication of regional anesthesia for ophthalmic surgery, *Can J Ophthalmol* 27:323, 1992.
7. Ruschen H, Bremmer FD, Carr C: Complications after sub-Tenon's eye block, *Anesth Analg* 96:273, 2003.

Retinal Detachment

KATHRYN E. McGOLDRICK, M.D.

Most patients with retinal detachment (RD) are >55 years old and may have significant coexisting diseases. RDs are classified according to their type: rhegmatogenous or nonrhegmatogenous (traction or exudative). Traction RDs are frequently encountered with proliferative diabetic retinopathy or sickle cell retinopathy. Exudative RDs are seen with a variety of diseases, including tumors (metastases from breast or lung, retinoblastoma, primary melanoma), certain ocular inflammatory conditions, choroidal hemangioma, and severe pediatric renal disease. Rhegmatogenous (traction) RDs, caused by retinal tears, are common in myopic adults and may also occur in adults following cataract surgery or ocular trauma. Rhegmatogenous RDs are uncommon in children, usually secondary to trauma, myopia, aphakia, Marfan's syndrome, or retinopathy of prematurity. Rhegmatogenous RDs are preceded by a tiny hole or tear in the retina, which becomes detached if the vitreous lifts the retina off from the pigment epithelium. Symptoms associated with retinal tears include floaters and flashes. Therapy for tears includes cryotherapy or laser photocoagulation. When retinal tears progress to RD, peripheral visual field defects occur that may progress to include loss of central vision, and scleral buckling is indicated. Occasionally, complex R require vitrectomy with or without scleral buckling to treat giant retinal tears or proliferative vitreoretinopathy.

A. Surgical repair is usually not an emergency unless the macula is threatened. Thus, obtain medical consultation as needed and optimize the patient's medical condition before surgery.

B. Although a simple, primary RD may be repaired in an hour, retinal surgery is often lengthy and complex, lasting >3 hours; prepare for a prolonged procedure. Position the patient comfortably, ensuring adequate padding of bony prominences. Place a pillow under the knees to minimize back pain. Use standard monitors and a peripheral nerve stimulator, and possibly a urinary catheter (see D). Depending on the patient's medical condition, more invasive monitoring may be indicated.

C. Regional anesthesia[1] (retrobulbar or peribulbar block) is an option in appropriate cases. However, a long-acting local anesthetic agent, such as bupivacaine, should be used or some technique that allows "topping up." Immobilize the head. The airway must be perfectly patent.[2] Administer minimal sedation; the goal is a calm, cooperative, comfortable, conscious patient.

D. When extensive surgery is required, administer GETA. Use an IV induction (propofol is excellent because of its antiemetic properties). Unless RSI is indicated, facilitate intubation with a nondepolarizing muscle relaxant (NDMR) after topical laryngotracheal anesthesia (LTA) 4% lidocaine to prevent coughing. Select the NDMR based on hemodynamic considerations and the anticipated surgical duration. Administer a prophylactic antiemetic. During RD repair a soft eye is desirable; anticipate a request for IV acetazolamide or mannitol to reduce IOP.

E. Keep the patient immobile. RD surgery is extremely delicate; the thin scleral layer can rupture if the patient coughs. Globe rotation with traction on the extraocular muscles is needed to position the scleral buckle; watch for oculocardiac reflex. Carefully monitor and, if necessary, treat associated dysrhythmias. The surgeon may inject sulfur hexafluoride (SF_6) or a perfluorocarbon bubble to mechanically facilitate reattachment. N_2O diffuses into the bubble, causing expansion of the bubble and increased IOP that could compromise retinal perfusion; discontinue N_2O >15 minutes before gas injection.[3] Extubate the patient with the goal of minimal coughing.

F. If a patient who recently had an ocular gas injection requires anesthesia, he or she should not be given N_2O during the postoperative period (>5 days after an air injection and for 10 days after SF_6 injection; possibly >30 days with perfluoropropane).[4-7] It is prudent to use air during general anesthesia for any patient who has undergone vitreoretinal surgery within the preceding 3 months.

REFERENCES

1. Troll GF: Regional ophthalmic anesthesia: safe techniques and avoidance of complications, *J Clin Anesth* 7:163, 1995.
2. McGoldrick KE, Mardirossian J: Ophthalmic surgery. In: McGoldrick KE, editor: *Ambulatory anesthesiology: a problem-oriented approach*, Baltimore, 1995, Williams & Wilkins.
3. Stinson TW, Donlon JV, Jr: Interaction of intraocular air and sulfur hexafluoride with nitrous oxide: a computer simulation, *Anesthesiology* 56:385, 1982.
4. McGoldrick KE, Anesthesia and the eye. In: Barash PG, Cullen BF, Stoelting RK, editors: *Clinical anesthesia*, ed 4, Philadelphia, 2001, Lippincott Williams & Wilkins.
5. Vote BJ, Hart R, Worsley DR, et al.: Visual loss after use of nitrous oxide gas with general anesthetic in patients with intraocular gas still persistent up to 30 days after vitrectomy, *Anesthesiology* 97:1305, 2002.
6. Hart RH, Vote BJ, Borthwick JH, et al.: Loss of vision caused by expansion of intraocular perfluoropropane (C_3F_8) gas during nitrous oxide anesthesia, *Am J Ophthalmol* 134:761, 2002.
7. Lee EJ: Use of nitrous oxide causing severe visual loss 37 days after retinal surgery, *Br J Anaesth* 93:464, 2004.

Patient with RETINAL DETACHMENT

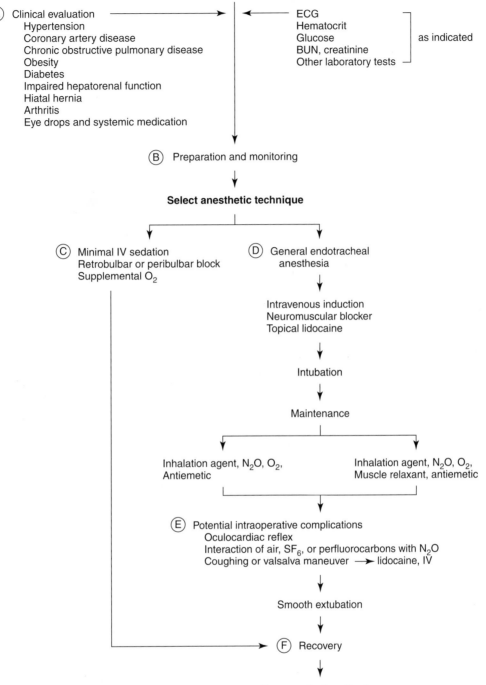

(A) Clinical evaluation ──────────────→   ←──── ECG
        Hypertension   Hematocrit
        Coronary artery disease   Glucose   as indicated
        Chronic obstructive pulmonary disease   BUN, creatinine
        Obesity   Other laboratory tests ┘
        Diabetes
        Impaired hepatorenal function
        Hiatal hernia
        Arthritis
        Eye drops and systemic medication

(B) Preparation and monitoring

Select anesthetic technique

(C) Minimal IV sedation   (D) General endotracheal
     Retrobulbar or peribulbar block   anesthesia
     Supplemental O$_2$

                                              Intravenous induction
                                              Neuromuscular blocker
                                              Topical lidocaine

                                              Intubation

                                              Maintenance

Inhalation agent, N$_2$O, O$_2$,   Inhalation agent, N$_2$O, O$_2$,
Antiemetic   Muscle relaxant, antiemetic

(E) Potential intraoperative complications
     Oculocardiac reflex
     Interaction of air, SF$_6$, or perfluorocarbons with N$_2$O
     Coughing or valsalva maneuver ──→ lidocaine, IV

Smooth extubation

(F) Recovery

Proper patient positioning

Anesthesia for Strabismus Surgery in Children

JAMIE McELRATH SCHWARTZ, M.D.

EUGENIE HEITMILLER, M.D.

Strabismus is the misalignment of the visual axes of the eyes. Realignment of the deviated eye(s) is important for binocular vision as well as to maintain the cosmetic and communication role of the eyes. There are several issues that are of particular interest to the anesthesiologist when preparing for strabismus surgery: increased risk for malignant hyperthermia, high incidence of postoperative nausea and vomiting (PONV), possibility of triggering the oculocardiac reflex, and possible need for additional postoperative muscle manipulation by the surgeon.

A. Obtain a thorough history, including the routine questions regarding muscle disorders, family history of anesthetic problems, asthma, heart problems, recent upper respiratory infections, and last oral intake. Evaluate for preexisting medical conditions and take their specific anesthetic considerations into account. Examine the child, with particular attention to respiratory system and discuss the anesthetic plan with the family.
B. Premedication is commonly used in toddlers and young children, and in older children who seem particularly anxious. Midazolam 0.5 to 1 mg/kg via the oral, rectal, or intranasal route provides a smooth transition into the operative environment. Each route has it disadvantages: the oral preparation has a bitter taste, the nasal route causing a burning sensation in the nares and the rectal route is typically used only for infants and toddlers. In some cases, the surgeon may want to examine the child before the sedation is given.
C. General anesthesia is the usual choice for strabismus surgery in children because of the need for a motionless operative field. Inhalation induction with sevoflurane or halothane is most commonly used in younger patients. Older children may prefer IV induction. A laryngeal mask airway (LMA) is often utilized in appropriate patients, but because the head of the patient is turned 90 degrees away from the anesthesiologist, there will be limited access to the airway during the procedure if adjustments are needed.

There have been several case reports in the literature of patients developing masseter spasm and symptoms of malignant hyperthermia.[1] Acquired strabismus may represent an underlying subclinical myopathy in some patients. Patients should therefore have temperature and end-tidal carbon dioxide ($ETCO_2$) carefully monitored throughout the case.

The oculocardiac reflex (OCR) can be elicited during strabismus surgery from traction on extraocular muscles. The OCR has an afferent loop through the trigeminal nerve and an efferent loop through the vagus nerve, resulting in bradycardia, ventricular dysrhythmias, or in extreme cases, asystole. The immediate treatment for this reflex is the release of the muscle tension by the surgeon. Studies have shown decreased incidence of OCR with pretreatment with IV or intraglossal atropine.[2] The reflex will fatigue over time and gradually increasing traction strength will also decrease OCR incidence. Some authors have looked at various anesthetic techniques to decrease OCR. The use of propofol or propofol/nitrous oxide as maintenance agent increases risk of OCR.[3,4]

PONV can be a significant problem in strabismus surgery. Ondansetron has been shown in many studies to decrease the PONV associated with strabismus. Intraoperative anticholinergics and benzodiazepines have also been used with success. Using nonsteroidal anti-inflammatory pain relievers rather than opiates may also be helpful.

D. Postoperative adjustment of sutures in selected patients has significantly decreased the re-operation rate for strabismus. In older children, this can be done in the recovery room area with topical anesthesia after the patient has recovered from the surgical anesthetic and can be cooperative with this short procedure. At our institution, younger or uncooperative children are re-anesthetized in the recovery room with a bolus of propofol (2 to 4 mg/kg) after the surgeon has assessed the patient. The patient is then monitored in the recovery room until discharge criteria are met.

REFERENCES

1. Carroll JB: Increased incidence of masseter spasm in children with strabismus anesthetized with halothane and succinylcholine, *Anesthesiology* 67:559, 1987.
2. Arnold RW, Farah RF, Monroe G: The attenuating effect of intraglossal atropine on the oculocardiac reflex, *Binocul Vis Strabismus Q* 17:313–318, 2002.
3. Tramer MR, Sansonetti A, Fuchs-Buder T, et al.: Oculocardiac reflex and postoperative vomiting in paediatric strabismus surgery. A randomised controlled trial comparing four anaesthetic techniques, *Acta Anaesthesiol Scand* 42:117–123, 1998.
4. Hahnenkamp K, Honemann CW, Fischer LG, et al.: Effect of different anaesthetic regimes on the oculocardiac reflex during paediatric strabismus surgery, *Paediatr Anaesth* 10:601–608, 2000.

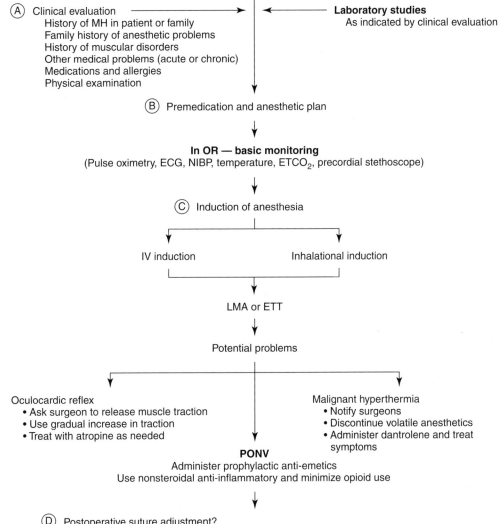

Pediatric patient with STRABISMUS

(A) Clinical evaluation ──────────→ ←────── **Laboratory studies**
    History of MH in patient or family   As indicated by clinical evaluation
    Family history of anesthetic problems
    History of muscular disorders
    Other medical problems (acute or chronic)
    Medications and allergies
    Physical examination

(B) Premedication and anesthetic plan

In OR — basic monitoring
(Pulse oximetry, ECG, NIBP, temperature, $ETCO_2$, precordial stethoscope)

(C) Induction of anesthesia

IV induction   Inhalational induction

LMA or ETT

Potential problems

Oculocardic reflex
 • Ask surgeon to release muscle traction
 • Use gradual increase in traction
 • Treat with atropine as needed

Malignant hyperthermia
 • Notify surgeons
 • Discontinue volatile anesthetics
 • Administer dantrolene and treat symptoms

PONV
Administer prophylactic anti-emetics
Use nonsteroidal anti-inflammatory and minimize opioid use

(D) Postoperative suture adjustment?
    Administration of topical anesthesia and short-acting anesthetic (propofol) if needed

ANESTHESIA FOR SPINAL AND ORTHOPEDIC PROCEDURES

SCOLIOSIS
TOTAL HIP REPLACEMENT (THR)
KNEE ARTHROSCOPY
TOTAL KNEE REPLACEMENT (TKR)
SHOULDER SURGERY
ISOVOLEMIC HEMODILUTION (IVH)

Scoliosis

TOD B. SLOAN, M.D., PH.D.

―――

Scoliosis is a common condition involving lateral and rotational changes in the spine (up to 4% of population) that may require major spine corrective surgery to improve appearance and prevent later sequelae (e.g., restrictive lung disease, pulmonary hypertension [HTN], cor pulmonale, pain, and neurological impairment, which can be fatal by age 50).[1,2] Intraoperative problems include major blood loss (15 to 60% of blood volume), venous air embolism (VAE), and spinal cord injury (SCI). Surgical approaches include posterior instrumentation (Harrington distraction, Wisconsin or Lugue [segmental wiring], combined distraction and wiring [Cotrel-Dubousset]), and mechanical fixation using pedicle screws but occasionally involve anterior release or instrumentation requiring thoracotomy or thoracoabdominal incision (Dwyer, Weiss springs).[3] Patients are graded by the degrees of angle of curvature based on the Cobb method and surgery is usually indicated when this angle exceeds 50 degrees.

A. Determine the cause of scoliosis. Although 70 to 80% of patients have idiopathic scoliosis (genetic, multifactorial, sex-linked), identifiable neural, muscular, or orthopedic causes with associated problems or specific risk factors are noted in some.[2,5] Muscle disorders may carry an increased risk of malignant hyperthermia or cardiac decompensation and often are associated with poor pulmonary function. Other etiologies are associated with neuromuscular disease (notably muscular dystrophy and cerebral palsy), mesenchymal disorders, such as Marfan's syndrome, structural anomalies (myelodysplasia), primary or secondary malignancies of the spine, and trauma. Evaluate associated medical conditions with these diagnoses. Congenital scoliosis is associated with coarctation of the aorta and cyanotic congenital heart disease. Seizure disorders are common; patients taking valproic acid may develop coagulation disorders. Cardiac failure occurs from cardiomyopathy, arrhythmias, and cor pulmonale. Back pain in pediatric patients suggests infection, tumor, trauma, or Scheuermann's kyphosis.[1]

B. Assess the airway and the pulmonary, cardiovascular, and neurological changes associated with the scoliosis. Restrictive lung disease is directly related to Cobb angle and worse with kyphosis.[1] Pulmonary function tests (PFTs, predicted volumes based on arm span not height) usually show a restrictive defect with vital capacity (VC) and forced vital capacity (FVC) reduced proportionally to curvature (especially at $>50°$ Cobb[6]). VC is a good predictor of respiratory embarrassment; significant reduction may require postoperative ventilation. Alveolar hypoventilation and V/Q mismatching lead to hypoxemia and right-sided heart failure. Increased V_D to V_T ratio and reduced compliance are common. Optimize preoperative pulmonary function (e.g., bronchodilators if needed). Discuss the wake-up test (see G) and reduce its psychological impact. Consider endocarditis antibiotic prophylaxis for the 25 to 28% of patients with mitral valve prolapse (MVP). Use premedication with caution in patients with cardiac and pulmonary problems. Document all neurological abnormalities that mark an increase in neurological risk with surgery (especially bulbar involvement with muscular dystrophy).

C. Place two large-bore IV catheters. Plan a nasogastric (NG) tube for postoperative ileus (common). Warm fluids, gases, and the patient to avoid hypothermia and associated problems. Watch for latex allergy in patients with myelomeningocele. Note that intraoperative positioning may limit pulmonary function.

D. Plan for general anesthesia by endotracheal tube (ETT) in most cases (consider nasotracheal tube if postoperative ventilation is probable); epidural and spinal anesthesia have been used. A double-lumen ETT (DLT) may be needed for anterior procedures. Maintain normal $PaCO_2$ for normal spinal cord blood flow. Watch for dysrhythmias if epinephrine is injected into the incision site. Avoid succinylcholine (SCC) and titrate nondepolarizing muscle relaxants (NDMB) in patients with paraplegia, muscular dystrophy, or other neuromuscular disease, and myotonic dystrophy (see G). Narcotic-based anesthesia may be preferable for wake-up tests or to monitor neurological function (sensory or motor evoked potentials). Muscle relaxant metabolism may be increased by antiepileptic medications.

E. Position is usually prone; pad bony prominences and position the patient to have the abdomen free to avoid ventilatory difficulty and vena caval obstruction (increased epidural vein bleeding). Watch for VAE with the Relton-Hall or CHOP frame. For anterior procedures in the lateral decubitus position, carefully pad the axilla and monitor the down arm radial pulse.

F. Plan for large blood loss during bone removal and stripping of muscle from spine. Consider preoperative autologous transfusion, intraoperative normovolemic hemodilution (i.e., blood removal to hematocrit 20 to 30 with retransfusion at conclusion), and cell salvaging (may recover 50 to 70% estimated blood loss [EBL]). Deliberate hypotension (MAP 60 to 70) reduces EBL and OR time but is controversial due to risks of SCI. Use heating methods as possible, especially if neurological compromise is present (loss of sympathetic tone)

Patient with SCOLIOSIS

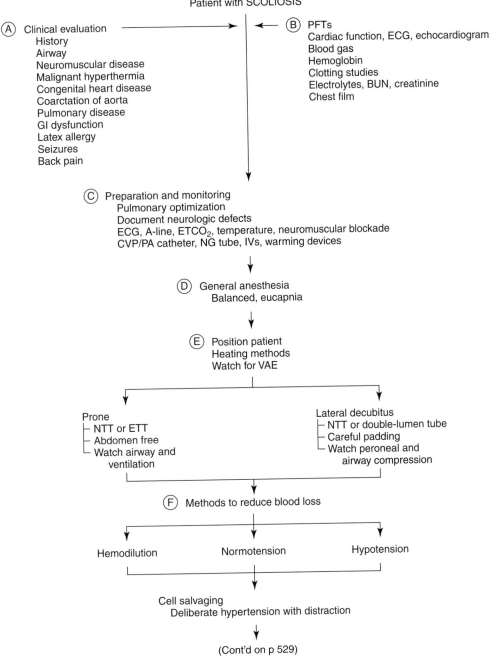

(A) Clinical evaluation
    History
    Airway
    Neuromuscular disease
    Malignant hyperthermia
    Congenital heart disease
    Coarctation of aorta
    Pulmonary disease
    GI dysfunction
    Latex allergy
    Seizures
    Back pain

(B) PFTs
    Cardiac function, ECG, echocardiogram
    Blood gas
    Hemoglobin
    Clotting studies
    Electrolytes, BUN, creatinine
    Chest film

(C) Preparation and monitoring
    Pulmonary optimization
    Document neurologic defects
    ECG, A-line, ETCO$_2$, temperature, neuromuscular blockade
    CVP/PA catheter, NG tube, IVs, warming devices

(D) General anesthesia
    Balanced, eucapnia

(E) Position patient
    Heating methods
    Watch for VAE

Prone
 ├ NTT or ETT
 ├ Abdomen free
 └ Watch airway and
   ventilation

Lateral decubitus
 ├ NTT or double-lumen tube
 ├ Careful padding
 └ Watch peroneal and
   airway compression

(F) Methods to reduce blood loss

Hemodilution   Normotension   Hypotension

Cell salvaging
Deliberate hypertension with distraction

(Cont'd on p 529)

G. Neurological monitoring is now a standard of care.[7] One option is a wake-up test (performed by reducing the anesthetic concentrations; partial neuromuscular, or narcotic reversal may be needed) looking for ability to move the feet or evoked responses on command. More commonly, continuous monitoring with somatosensory evoked potentials or motor evoked potentials will be used. Limited doses of inhalational agents (<0.5 MAC) may be acceptable or may need to be eliminated. Muscle relaxation may need to be severely restricted with motor evoked potentials or EMG recording for neural irritation or stimulation (notably with pedicle screws).

H. Postoperatively, awaken the patient promptly to identify neurological problems requiring immediate surgical reexploration. Extubate when appropriate or use postoperative ventilation for patients with poor PFTs (usually required if preoperative VC is less than 30 to 35% of predicted), neuromuscular disease, or diaphragmatic transection during anterior procedures. Controversy exists whether pulmonary function is improved by surgery. Look for atelectasis, pleural effusion, and respiratory failure with the anterior procedure. Watch for thromboembolic complications.

Postoperative pain is severe for 3 to 4 days; consider intraspinal narcotics. Consider nutritional support between staged surgeries or with ileus. Consider methylprednisolone (as with acute spinal cord injury) if neurological injury occurs.

REFERENCES

1. Boachie-Adjei O, Lonner B: Spinal deformity, *Pediatr Clin North Am* 43:883–897, 1996.
2. Raw DA, Beattie JK, Hunter JM, Anaesthesia for spinal surgery in adults, *Br J Anaesth* 91:886–904, 2003.
3. Troll GF: Anesthesia for surgical correction of idiopathic scoliosis, *Curr Rev Clin Anesth* 3:166, 1983.
4. Youngman PM, Edgar MA: Posterior spinal fusion and instrumentation in the treatment of adolescent idiopathic scoliosis, *Ann R Coll Surg Engl* 67:313–317, 1985.
5. Engler GL: Preoperative and intraoperative considerations in adolescent idiopathic scoliosis, *Instr Course Lect* 38:137–141, 1989.
6. Winter S: Preoperative assessment of the child with neuromuscular scoliosis, *Orthop Clin North Am* 25:239–245, 1995.
7. Kafer ER: Respiratory and cardiovascular functions in scoliosis and the principles of anesthetic management, *Anesthesiology* 52:339–351, 1980.
8. Sloan TB: Anesthesia effects and evoked potentials, In: Reisen R, Nuwer M, Hallett M, editors: *Advances in clinical neurophysiology*, vol 54 (Suppl): 325–328, 2002.

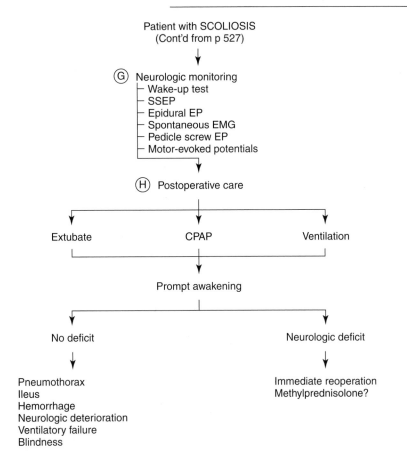

Patient with SCOLIOSIS
(Cont'd from p 527)

Ⓖ Neurologic monitoring
├ Wake-up test
├ SSEP
├ Epidural EP
├ Spontaneous EMG
├ Pedicle screw EP
├ Motor-evoked potentials

Ⓗ Postoperative care

Extubate   CPAP   Ventilation

Prompt awakening

No deficit   Neurologic deficit

Pneumothorax   Immediate reoperation
Ileus   Methylprednisolone?
Hemorrhage
Neurologic deterioration
Ventilatory failure
Blindness

Total Hip Replacement (THR)

JOHN E. TETZLAFF, M.D.

JOHN A. DILGER, M.D.

Total hip replacement (THR) is indicated when congenital defects, arthritis, trauma, or malignancy destroys the hip joint. Pain, abnormal gait, or fractures of the proximal femur or acetabulum are the presenting symptoms. Whether to choose THR or more conservative surgical procedures for acute or pathological fractures is partially determined by the health of the patient.

A. Perform a preoperative evaluation. Younger patients often have accelerated arthritis, pathological fracture, or trauma. Patients with rheumatoid arthritis (RA) may have airway pathology, an unstable cervical spine, or impaired cardiopulmonary function. Avascular necrosis of the femoral head can be secondary to chronic steroid use, alcoholism, or IV drug abuse. Patients with pathological fractures may have other consequences of malignancy, including hepatic or renal insufficiency, superior vena cava syndrome, or toxicity from chemotherapy. After trauma, THR is indicated when hip fracture is an isolated injury; visceral disruption, CNS trauma, and thoracic injury must be ruled out. When acetabular fracture is the presenting indication, intrapelvic hemorrhage or pelvic organ injury is possible. Evaluate geriatric patients for hypertension (HTN), coronary artery disease (CAD), valvular heart disease, and pulmonary disease. Hip pain can severely restrict activity; consider functional testing in the sedentary patient (e.g., pulmonary function tests [PFTs], pharmacological cardiac stress testing, and cardiac catheterization). Antiplatelet medications may impact anesthetic choice (i.e., safety of regional anesthesia) as well as intraoperative blood loss. Anticipate major blood loss, especially for revision THR. Consider predonation of autologous blood and intraoperative and postoperative cell salvage.

B. Choose monitors based on the surgical indication (primary, revision, or fracture), comorbid disease, and estimated blood loss. Standard monitors may be adequate for routine THR in a healthy adult. Consider an arterial line in patients with proximal femoral fracture, acetabular fracture, or revision of a previously cemented or long stem THR (frequent blood samples and control of massive transfusion). Certain diseases with hip pathology (Paget's disease, metastatic renal cell carcinoma, multiple myeloma) are known to greatly increase blood loss. For such patients, consider arterial and CVP catheters and generous IV access. Monitor urine output if large blood loss is expected. Patients with pathological fracture or aseptic necrosis secondary to alcoholism may have diminished myocardial reserves; consider invasive monitoring with arterial line, CVP, and pulmonary artery (PA) catheter. THRs that have been revised

several times often require multiple blood volume transfusions (scarring, difficult instrumentation, and removal of methylmethacrylate).

C. Select an anesthetic technique. For general anesthesia, intubate the trachea. Although a laryngeal mask airway (LMA) could be used, the vigorous activity of a hip replacement (reaming, femoral stem placement) could displace the LMA when the patient is in the lateral position. Place an axillary roll to prevent injury of the dependent brachial plexus. Protect the dependent face, eye, and ear to prevent injury. Keep the head and neck in a neutral position; severe positioning can cause vision defects. Complete neuromuscular blockade is not required, but active muscle tone will interfere with the surgery. Prolonged intervals in the lateral position can induce edema of the head, neck, and airway. Use caution when extubating in the OR. If there is any doubt, defer extubation when there is no detectable air leakage around the deflated endotracheal tube (ETT) cuff at 20 mm Hg positive pressure or less.

If regional anesthesia is selected, choose the technique based on the anticipated duration of the surgery and pain control plans. Complete anesthesia of the hip is possible with peripheral conduction block if a sciatic nerve block is combined with a psoas compartment block of the lumbosacral plexus. If the psoas compartment block is performed with a catheter, it can be used postoperatively to achieve excellent pain control. However, patient discomfort, incomplete block of the gluteal muscles, and proximity of the sciatic block to the surgical field make this an infrequent choice. Spinal anesthesia is a common choice because of technical ease, profound anesthesia, and low total dose of local anesthetic required. Use tetracaine or bupivacaine; add epinephrine to prolong the duration of tetracaine or improve the quality of block with bupivacaine. Add opiates to extend analgesia into the postoperative period. Lipophilic opioids, such as fentanyl, extend analgesia for 4 to 6 hours. Morphine 0.1 mg provides analgesia for 12 to 18 hours after surgery; there is a risk of delayed respiratory depression, accentuated by advancing age. Consider epidural anesthesia with a catheter. Advantages include a slowly achieved block, flexibility in duration, and availability for postoperative pain control. Both epidural and spinal anesthesia reduce perioperative blood loss compared to general anesthesia and reduce the incidence of postoperative thromboembolic events.[1] Consider combined spinal/epidural (CSE) anesthesia to achieve the advantages of both techniques (rapid onset of dense block, the option to redose for longer procedures, and use for postoperative pain management).

Patient for TOTAL HIP REPLACEMENT

Ⓐ Preoperative evaluation ⟶ ⟵ EKG
HTN　　　　　　　　　　　　　　　　Echo
CAD　　　　　　　　　　　　　　　　Stress test
COPD　　　　　　　　　　　　　　　PFTs
RA, OA　　　　　　　　　　　　　　ABG
Paget's　　　　　　　　　　　　　　C-spine
　malignancy　　　　　　　　　　　Airway
　trauma
　　　　　Ⓑ Monitoring

Primary THR　　　　　Hip fracture　　　　　Revision THR

Routine ASA monitors　　　　　　Urinary catheter
　(invasive per patient health)　　Arterial line
Autologous blood　　　　　　　　CVP (volume, pressure)
　　　　　　　　　　　　　　　　Temperature support
　　　　　　　　　　　　　　　　PA catheter—severe CAD
　　　　　　　　　　　　　　　　Autologous blood
　　　　　　　　　　　　　　　　Cell salvage

Ⓒ Anesthetic technique

General endotracheal anesthesia　　　　　　Regional anesthesia

Sciatic-psoas blocks　　　SAB　　　Epidural　　Combined spinal epidural (CSE)

(Cont'd on p 533)

D. The decision to use methylmethacrylate is determined by age, patient prognosis, and bone quality. Younger patients with good bone usually receive porous-coated prostheses, which do not require methylmethacrylate. Older patients and those with pathological fracture or poor bone quality from prior hip surgery may require methylmethacrylate and are most at risk from its hemodynamic consequences. Blood levels of the monomeric form of methylmethacrylate result in vasodilation, histamine release, and negative inotropy.[2] These effects are worsened by hypovolemia, decreased left ventricular (LV) function, and deep levels of myocardial depressant anesthetics. Large doses of methylmethacrylate or use of the liquid form accentuate the effects, especially if high pressure is used during prosthesis insertion. Pressurized insertion can also cause embolism of air, fat, or marrow. Rarely, massive embolism can cause cardiovascular collapse.[3] Massive fat embolism has been reported during THR. Fat is universally[4] found in the central circulation during femoral reaming and femoral stem insertion. Confusion and hypoxia are clinical signs of fat embolism during regional anesthesia. Hypoxia, reduced pulmonary compliance, and cardiovascular collapse can be manifestations of massive fat embolism during general anesthesia. Massive blood loss during THR can be difficult to detect because blood loss onto drapes, floor, and instruments may not be obvious.

E. Postoperatively, treat pain, maintain volume status, and provide prophylaxis for deep venous thrombosis (DVT). Achieve pain control with on-demand opiates, patient–controlled analgesia (PCA), intrathecal opiates, epidural analgesia, and combinations. Consider ketorolac for multimodal analgesia (some surgeons avoid ketorolac due to concern for wound hematoma, impaired bone healing, or acute renal injury).

Assess volume status in the PACU. Wound salvage from the OR and from drains can contribute to red cell conservation. Delay in the use of autologous blood until the PACU also contributes to red cell conservation. Case reports of vasodilatation, hypotension, bronchospasm, or airway edema during infusion of wound salvage blood have been attributed to vasoactive intracellular substances in the blood.[5] DVT is the leading cause of major morbidity.[6] Provide pneumatic compression stockings (PCSs). Anticoagulation with warfarin, subcutaneous heparin, or low molecular weight heparin (LMWH) has been established as effective DVT prophylaxis.[7] The strong preference of surgeons for LMWH has reduced the use of epidural catheters for acute pain control. It appears to be acceptable to use continuous peripheral blocks in the presence of LMWH.

REFERENCES

1. Modig J, Borg T, Karlstrom G, et al.: Thromboembolism after total hip replacement: role of epidural and general anesthesia, *Anesth Analg* 62:174–180, 1983.
2. Learned DW, Hantler CB: Lethal progression of heart block after prosthesis cementing with methylmethacrylate, *Anesthesiology* 77:1044–1046, 1992.
3. Renne J, Wuthier R, House E, et al.: Fat macroglobulinemia caused by fractures or total hip replacement, *J Bone Joint Surg Am* 60:613–618, 1978.
4. Lafont ND, Kalonji MK, Barre J, et al.: Clinical features and echocardiography of embolism during cemented hip arthroplasty, *Can J Anaesth* 44:112–117, 1997.
5. Woda R, Tetzlaff JE: Upper airway oedema following autologous blood transfusion from a wound drainage system, *Can J Anaesth* 39:290–292, 1992.
6. Sharrock NE, Cazan MG, Hargett MJ, et al.: Changes in mortality after total hip and knee arthroplasty over a ten-year period, *Anesth Analg* 80:242–248, 1995.
7. Harris WH, Salzman EW, Athanasoulis C, et al.: Comparison of warfarin, low-molecular-weight dextran, aspirin, and subcutaneous heparin in the prevention of venous thromboembolism following total hip replacement, *J Bone Joint Surg Am* 56:1552–1562, 1974.

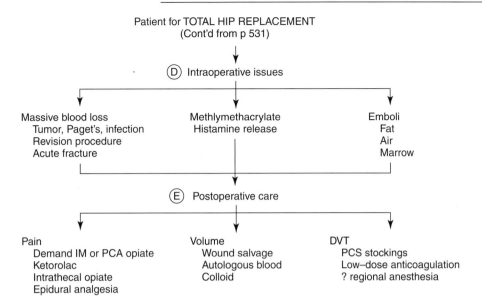

Patient for TOTAL HIP REPLACEMENT
(Cont'd from p 531)

Ⓓ Intraoperative issues

Massive blood loss
  Tumor, Paget's, infection
  Revision procedure
  Acute fracture

Methlymethacrylate
  Histamine release

Emboli
  Fat
  Air
  Marrow

Ⓔ Postoperative care

Pain
  Demand IM or PCA opiate
  Ketorolac
  Intrathecal opiate
  Epidural analgesia

Volume
  Wound salvage
  Autologous blood
  Colloid

DVT
  PCS stockings
  Low–dose anticoagulation
  ? regional anesthesia

Knee Arthroscopy

JEFFREY M. RICHMAN, M.D.

Knee arthroscopy is a common orthopedic surgical technique for the diagnosis and treatment of various knee pathologies, performed most frequently as an outpatient procedure on healthy American Society of Anesthesiologists (ASA) I and II patients. A variety of anesthetic techniques (including general anesthesia, neuraxial block, peripheral nerve block, and local anesthesia) have been successfully employed to safely manage patients undergoing this procedure. The surgical procedure involves the placement of two or more portals adjacent to the patellar tendon in the anteromedial, anterolateral, or supermedial aspects of the knee joint. Irrigating fluid is administered continuously through these portals to enhance visualization of structures and wash away blood and debris. Knee arthroscopy can be used to aid diagnosis, perform meniscal repairs, debridement, synovectomy, loose body removal, ligament reconstruction, and lateral release along with other procedures. A thigh tourniquet is often used to reduce bleeding, but may contribute to intraoperative pain, nerve damage, and hypertension (HTN).

A. Perform a routine preoperative history and directed physical examination, including evaluation of airway, NPO status, medical conditions, and medications. The majority of patients receiving knee arthroscopy are young and healthy, and therefore do not require laboratory tests or ECG unless indicated by age or a medical condition expected to alter these tests. Patients with neurological injury, lumbar disease, severe gastroesophageal reflux, or severe arthritis may not be appropriate candidates for regional anesthesia and sedation. Choose the anesthetic technique after informed consent and a presentation of risks and benefits, considering patient feedback (e.g., preferring being awake or asleep intraoperatively), comorbidites, and the surgeon and anesthesiologist preferences.

B. A well-conducted preoperative interview may provide adequate anxiolysis, but in appropriate situations, consider the administration of midazolam or opioids. Administer reflux prophylaxis (e.g., a nonparticulate antacid, such as sodium citrate) to patients with moderate-to-severe reflux or with diabetic gastroparesis. Consider antibiotic (e.g., first-generation cephalosporin) to provide prophylaxis against common skin flora. If neuraxial anesthesia is planned, provide adequate IV hydration to minimize the risk of bradycardia and cardiac arrest.

C. No one technique is perfect for all cases, therefore consider the benefits and detriments of each. General anesthesia can be performed with laryngeal mask airway (LMA) or endotracheal intubation and is well-suited for anxious patients and children. Isoflurane may result in slow recovery; sevoflurane may be associated with increased nausea and vomiting when compared with propofol.[1] A propofol-nitrous oxide technique has facilitated recovery times and is associated with a high rate of patient satisfaction.[1] Neuraxial anesthesia provides motor blockade and analgesia with the advantage of an awake or lightly sedated patient. Small–gauge, pencil–point needles minimize the risk of postdural puncture headache (PDPH). Intrathecal opioids may allow lower doses of local anesthetic and provide postoperative analgesia. Epidural 3% 2-chloroprocaine compares favorably with general anesthesia and small-dose lidocaine spinal anesthesia and has minimal side effects.[1–3] Peripheral nerve blockade can provide excellent analgesia, shorten PACU stays, and have a low incidence of side effects. Such nerve blocks may be more time consuming, have a decreased patient satisfaction, and result in prolonged motor blockade, placing certain patients at higher risk for a fall.[4] Femoral nerve block may be adequate but is often combined with obturator, lateral femoral cutaneous, and occasionally, sciatic block to provide a more complete anesthetic that does not require supplementation. The use of intraarticular local anesthetics (20 to 40 ml bupivacaine 0.25 to 0.5% with 1:200,000 epinephrine) and subcutaneous infiltration allows adequate analgesia, a rapid recovery, minimal side effects, and may be the ideal choice for nonanxious patients.[5] A small percentage of patients will require supplemental analgesia or sedation. Local anesthesia is not ideal when lateral port placement through the vastus lateralis will be performed or long tourniquet times are expected. Combined techniques involving general anesthesia with local anesthesia or peripheral nerve block may be used but do not necessarily provide a benefit for diagnostic procedures since pain is usually well-controlled with nonsteroidal anti-inflammatory drugs (NSAIDs) and oral opioids.

D. Apply routine ASA standard monitors. Add additional monitors as needed based on the medical condition of the patient. The majority of patients are healthy and will not require additional monitoring. Positioning is always a concern due to the risk of nerve injury. Pad pressure points in both upper and lower extremities. Most procedures are performed in semilithotomy with the back of the table slightly flexed. Tourniquet pain may be an issue with nerve blocks or local anesthesia; provide IV opioid or sedation and reassurance. Propofol, midazolam, and fentanyl have a relatively short duration of action. Fluid losses are generally minimal and a single IV is generally adequate.

Patient for KNEE ARTHROSCOPY

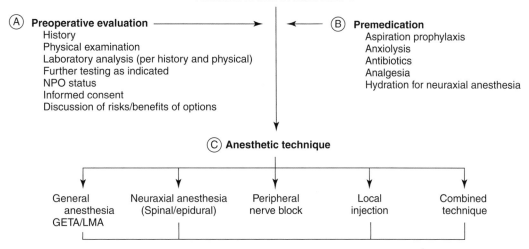

(A) **Preoperative evaluation**
   History
   Physical examination
   Laboratory analysis (per history and physical)
   Further testing as indicated
   NPO status
   Informed consent
   Discussion of risks/benefits of options

(B) **Premedication**
   Aspiration prophylaxis
   Anxiolysis
   Antibiotics
   Analgesia
   Hydration for neuraxial anesthesia

(C) **Anesthetic technique**

General anesthesia GETA/LMA   Neuraxial anesthesia (Spinal/epidural)   Peripheral nerve block   Local injection   Combined technique

(D) **Intraoperative management**
   Routine noninvasive ASA monitoring
   Invasive monitoring as needed
   Positioning with prevention of neuropathy
   Tourniquet pain
   Additional anxiolysis or pain control
   Fluid management

(Cont'd on p 537)

E. The majority of patients are unlikely to have complications; however, nausea and vomiting, sedation, back pain, PDPH, neuropathy, transient neurological syndrome, urinary retention, and hypotension may occur. Surgical complications include pain, neuropathy, bleeding, infection, hemarthrosis, and the need for further surgery. Pain may be managed postoperatively with intrarticular bupivacaine or peripheral nerve block (which may last 24 hours), NSAIDs (e.g., ketorolac, ibuprofen), oral opioids, and rarely cryotherapy or transcutaneous electrical nerve stimulation (TENS).

REFERENCES

1. Horlocker TT, Hebl JR: Anesthesia for outpatient knee arthroscopy: is there an optimal technique? *Reg Anesth Pain Med* 28:58–63, 2003.

2. Pollock JE, Mulroy MF, Bent E, et al.: A comparison of two regional anesthetic techniques for outpatient knee arthroscopy, *Anesth Analg* 97:397–401, 2003.

3. Mulroy MF, Larkin KL, Hodgson PS, et al.: A comparison of spinal, epidural, and general anesthesia for outpatient knee arthroscopy, *Anesth Analg* 91:860–864, 2000.

4. Casati A, Cappelleri G, Berti M, et al.: Randomized comparison of remifentanil-propofol with a sciatic-femoral nerve block for outpatient knee arthroscopy, *Eur J Anaesthesiol* 19:109–114, 2002.

5. Jacobson E, Forssblad M, Rosenberg J, et al.: Can local anesthesia be recommended for routine use in elective knee arthroscopy? A comparison between local, spinal, and general anesthesia, *Arthroscopy* 16:183–190, 2000.

Patient for KNEE ARTHROSCOPY
(Cont'd from p 535)

(E) **Postoperative management**

No complications
Discharge
Pain management

Surgical complications
Bleeding
Infection
Nerve damage
Hemarthrosis
Chronic pain
Need for further surgery

Anesthetic complications
Nausea/vomiting
Pain
Neuropathy
Transient neurologic syndrome
Post dural puncture headache
Urinary retention
Hypotension
Sedation

Total Knee Replacement (TKR)

JOHN A. DILGER, M.D.

JOHN E. TETZLAFF, M.D.

Total knee replacement (TKR) is indicated when conservative management of degeneration of the knee joint fails. Pain, deformity, and alteration of gait are the presenting symptoms. Patient suitability is related to age, weight, and general health.[1]

A. TKR is considered to be an intermediate risk procedure. Evaluate the patient for comorbid disease. Hypertension (HTN) is common; antihypertensive treatment can contribute to hemodynamic lability during anesthesia. Coronary artery disease (CAD) may be asymptomatic in the sedentary patient. A stress test, cardiac catheterization with intervention, and coronary revascularization may be required preoperatively. Patients with pulmonary disease may need pulmonary function tests (PFTs) and aggressive treatment to ensure pulmonary reserve for rehabilitation. A patient with a loose or infected TKR may require an urgent procedure. Patients should be encouraged to donate autologous blood. The advantage of autologous blood donation is reduced if the starting hematocrit is greater than 37% and perioperative blood salvage is used because the risk of allogenic transfusion is 1.2%.

B. Select monitors based on the general health of the patient. Bilateral TKR requires additional monitoring because of the extended surgical time and increased blood loss. An arterial line, a second large-bore IV catheter, and a urinary catheter may be necessary. Active temperature support and red cell salvage are indicated.

C. For general anesthesia, the airway can be managed via endotracheal intubation, laryngeal mask airway (LMA), or mask ventilation. Select an induction agent based on the health of the patient. If intubation is planned, a nondepolarizing muscle relaxant (NDMR) combined with volatile anesthesia may improve surgical conditions. Full neuromuscular block is unnecessary, but active muscle tone can interfere with geometric osteotomies. Spinal anesthesia, epidural anesthesia, or peripheral nerve block techniques offer alternatives. Neuraxial blocks have been favored, because they decrease the risk of early deep vein thrombosis (DVT). Perform spinal anesthesia with tetracaine or bupivacaine (isobaric or hyperbaric). Lidocaine may not have a sufficient duration and may cause transient neurological syndrome. Add epinephrine to extend the duration of tetracaine or improve the quality of the block with bupivacaine. Add opiates to extend analgesia into the postoperative period. Lipophilic agents such as fentanyl extend analgesia 6 to 8 hours into the postoperative period with little risk of respiratory depression. Intrathecal morphine doses as low as 0.1 mg extend analgesia for 14 to 24 hours, although the risk of delayed respiratory depression is greater, especially in the elderly. Epidural anesthesia includes placement of a catheter, with the option to redose being a distinct advantage. Lidocaine, mepivacaine, and bupivacaine are the most common agents selected. Shorter acting agents resolve more quickly and shorten the time in PACU. Alkalinization of lidocaine or mepivacaine will accelerate the onset and improve the quality of the block.[2] Epinephrine and opiates in the epidural space have the same advantages and risks as in spinal anesthesia.

Peripheral nerve blocks provide good perioperative anesthesia and analgesia and do not result in major hemodynamic changes. The lumbar plexus (LP) innervates the anterior knee and the sciatic nerve (S) innervates the posterior knee; LP block combined with S block achieves complete anesthesia of the leg. Psoas (P) block is the preferred approach to the LP, because it blocks all three branches (femoral, lateral femoral cutaneous, and obturator). The femoral (F) or three-in-one block, another LP approach, is less optimal because it may miss the obturator and lateral femoral cutaneous nerves. The S nerve block is required for surgical anesthesia but may be omitted when an LP block is performed solely for postoperative analgesia. Local anesthetics used include bupivacaine or ropivacaine; dilute solutions are infused postoperatively. The LP block is popular for TKR analgesia. It results in significantly lower pain scores and greater range of motion of the knee joint postoperatively when compared to IV opioids.[3]

D. During the course of the operation a tourniquet is placed on the leg. The response under general anesthesia is a sympathetically mediated hyperdynamic state.[4] Under regional anesthesia, HTN and tachycardia do not occur,[5] but visceral pain ("tourniquet pain") can develop and is difficult to treat.[6] Deflation of the tourniquet can cause hemodynamic instability. Lactic acid, carbon dioxide, and by-products of anaerobic metabolism are released, resulting in direct vasodilation, release of histamine from mast cells, and negative inotropy leading to hypotension. Hypovolemia and decreased cardiovascular reserve increase this risk. Rarely, tourniquet deflation can result in embolism of fat, air, or clot, and hemodynamic and respiratory compromise.[7] Intraoperative use of methylmethacrylate can cause vasodilation and histamine release, although to a lesser extent than during total hip surgery as a result of the inflated pneumatic tourniquet.[8]

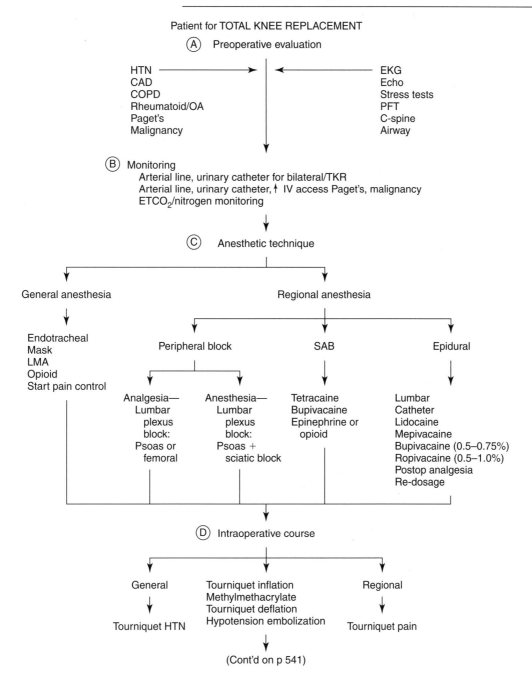

Patient for TOTAL KNEE REPLACEMENT

(A) Preoperative evaluation

HTN	EKG
CAD	Echo
COPD	Stress tests
Rheumatoid/OA	PFT
Paget's	C-spine
Malignancy	Airway

(B) Monitoring
  Arterial line, urinary catheter for bilateral/TKR
  Arterial line, urinary catheter, ↑ IV access Paget's, malignancy
  ETCO$_2$/nitrogen monitoring

(C) Anesthetic technique

General anesthesia   Regional anesthesia

General anesthesia:
Endotracheal
Mask
LMA
Opioid
Start pain control

Peripheral block   SAB   Epidural

Analgesia—   Anesthesia—   Tetracaine   Lumbar
Lumbar   Lumbar   Bupivacaine   Catheter
plexus   plexus   Epinephrine or   Lidocaine
block: block: opioid   Mepivacaine
Psoas or   Psoas +   Bupivacaine (0.5–0.75%)
femoral   sciatic block   Ropivacaine (0.5–1.0%)
                                                               Postop analgesia
                                                               Re-dosage

(D) Intraoperative course

General   Tourniquet inflation   Regional
                 Methylmethacrylate
Tourniquet HTN   Tourniquet deflation   Tourniquet pain
                 Hypotension embolization

(Cont'd on p 541)

E. Postoperative pain control can be achieved with patient controlled analgesia (PCA), epidural analgesia, or continuous LP blocks combined with opioids. Multimodal analgesia, achieved with the addition of acetaminophen and cyclooxygenase-inhibiting drugs, improves pain control and decreases opioid side effects. Patient volume status requires attention. Delay administration of autologous blood or salvaged red cells until the patient is taken to PACU. Deep vein thrombus (DVT) prophylaxis after TKR is important; 30 to 40% of patients will form DVT without prophylaxis. The consequences of DVT are the leading cause of major morbidity.[9] Sequential compression devices (SCDs) should be applied perioperatively to the help prevent DVT formation. Management of anticoagulants in the perioperative period is discussed in another chapter.

REFERENCES

1. Harris WH, Sledge CB: Total hip and knee replacement (part two), *N Engl J Med* 323:801–806, 1990.
2. Tetzlaff JE, Yoon HJ, Brems J, et al.: Alkalinization of mepivacaine improves the quality of motor block associated with interscalene brachial plexus anesthesia for shoulder surgery, *Reg Anesth* 20:128–132, 1995.
3. Singelyn FJ, Deyaert M, Joris D, et al.: Effects of intravenous patient-controlled analgesia with morphine, continuous epidural analgesia, and continuous three-in-one block on postoperative pain and knee rehabilitation after unilateral total knee arthroplasty, *Anesth Analg* 87 (1):88–92, 1998.
4. Gielen MJM, Stienstra R, Tourniquet hypertension and its prevention: a review, *Reg Anesth* 16:191–194, 1991.
5. Kahn RL, Marino V, Urquhart B, et al.: Hemodynamic changes associated with tourniquet use under epidural anesthesia for total knee arthroplasty, *Reg Anesth* 17:228–232, 1992.
6. Bridenbaugh PO, Hagenouw RR, Gielen MJ, et al.: Addition of glucose to bupivacaine in spinal anesthesia increases the incidence of tourniquet pain, *Anesth Analg* 65:1181–1185, 1986.
7. Cohen JD, Keslin JS, Nili M, et al.: Massive pulmonary embolism and tourniquet deflation. *Anesth Analg* 79:583–585, 1994.
8. Byrick RJ, Forbes D, Waddell JP: A monitored cardiovascular collapse during cemented total knee replacement, *Anesthesiology* 65:213–216, 1986.
9. Lotke PA, Ecker ML, Alavi A, et al.: Indications for the treatment of deep venous thrombosis following total knee replacement, *J Bone Joint Surg* 66:202–208, 1984.

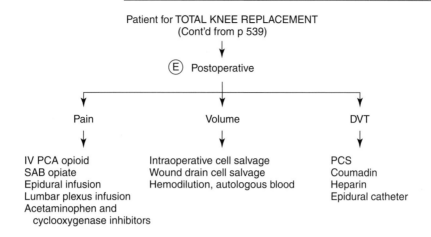

Patient for TOTAL KNEE REPLACEMENT
(Cont'd from p 539)

Ⓔ Postoperative

Pain	Volume	DVT
IV PCA opioid	Intraoperative cell salvage	PCS
SAB opiate	Wound drain cell salvage	Coumadin
Epidural infusion	Hemodilution, autologous blood	Heparin
Lumbar plexus infusion		Epidural catheter
Acetaminophen and		
cyclooxygenase inhibitors		

Shoulder Surgery

JOHN E. TETZLAFF, M.D.

JOHN A. DILGER, M.D.

Shoulder surgery is performed for a wide variety of indications, including congenital defects, degenerative arthritis, and injuries. Anesthetic management is determined by the health of the patient and the surgical plan.

A. Many shoulder procedures start with an arthroscopic examination of the shoulder joint. Shoulder arthroscopy requires anesthesia for port placement and muscle relaxation for capsular expansion so that structures can be visualized with less risk to the joint surface. Inferior ports may be outside the innervation of the brachial plexus; if an interscalene block is planned, local anesthetic infiltration may be required. A rotator cuff tear decreases the stability of the shoulder, leading to inflammation, pain, and decreased mobility. Surgical treatment requires repair of the tear and alteration of irregular surfaces of the acromion. Other procedures are designed to correct congenital or traumatic laxity of the shoulder capsule. Capsulorrhaphy is achieved by a variety of techniques. Inferior and posterior capsular surgery can go outside the limits of the brachial plexus. The most complex shoulder procedure involves replacement of one or both of the bony components of the shoulder joint to treat degenerative arthritis or a complex fracture. Hemiarthroplasty involves replacement of the humeral head; total shoulder replacement (TSR) involves a prosthetic replacement of the glenoid and the humeral head. Significant blood loss may be encountered. Complete muscle relaxation is mandatory because of the need for geometric osteotomy. The surgical incision extends distally on the medial surface of the upper arm and can involve dermatomes outside the brachial plexus. Supplemental local anesthesia in the subcutaneous tissue or paravertebral block of T_1 and T_2 may be required.

B. The patient will be placed in the supine, beach chair, or lateral position. When supine, the patient is placed near the edge of the bed. The beach chair position uses gravity to tighten structures and optimize their identification. This increases the risk for injuries and requires stabilization of the head. The beach chair position may also cause hypotension from decreased preload; volume support and vasopressors may be required. The lateral position requires an axillary roll to avoid injury to the dependent brachial plexus, and protection of the dependent eye and ear.

C. Select monitors based on the health of the patient. Invasive monitoring for shoulder surgery is uncommon.

D. Most shoulder procedures are performed under general anesthesia, but regional anesthesia with an interscalene block is an alternative.[1] Transverse or posterior incisions require supplemental local infiltration.

Incisions that extend to the pectoral prominence require the somatic block of the first and second intercostal nerves, best achieved with a paravertebral block. For anxious or claustrophobic patients, consider general anesthesia because the sterile field will cover the patient's face. For TSR or hemiarthroplasty, consider combined regional and general anesthesia to provide excellent muscle relaxation and pain control.

E. If general anesthesia is chosen, consider muscle relaxation. Complete neuromuscular blockade is not mandatory but facilitates visualization of the shoulder capsule. Opioids may contribute to a stable intraoperative course. The primary regional technique is interscalene brachial plexus block. Use appropriate concentrations of local anesthetic to achieve complete relaxation of the shoulder girdle. The volume required is 40 ml. Common agents are lidocaine, mepivacaine, ropivacaine, and bupivacaine. Mepivacaine, 1.4 to 1.5%, achieves excellent motor block, good sensory anesthesia, and has a low toxic potential if used with epinephrine.[2] Bupivacaine, 0.5%, may not provide the motor block needed; 0.75% bupivacaine may result in a toxic dose. Ropivacaine and levobupivacaine are excellent alternatives to bupivacaine and have a reduced risk of cardiac toxicity. When interscalene block is combined with general anesthesia, bupivacaine provides prolonged postoperative analgesia. Superficial cervical plexus block can add to the sensory anesthesia over the anterior deltoid and neck region. Paravertebral blocks of the first and second intercostal nerves provide sensory anesthesia over the medial upper arm and the axillary region.

F. If general anesthesia is selected, intubate and secure the airway. For regional techniques, establish excellent anesthesia of a sufficient duration; emergent airway management is difficult and may require violation of the surgical field. Regional anesthesia complications include dyspnea and ventilatory compromise from phrenic nerve block.[3] Avoid extremes of positioning. In a small wound, bleeding can limit visualization; control the BP to decrease bleeding. If the surgeon plans to place a full shoulder spica cast, the patient may need to be sitting or standing; a rapid emergence technique is advantageous (e.g., propofol). Orthostasis can occur. Volume expansion and vasopressors may be necessary. Regional anesthesia works well when a standing cast is planned as long as heavy sedation is avoided. Sudden bradycardia occurring in patients in the beach chair position during shoulder surgery using interscalene block has been reported and attributed to the Bezold-Jarisch reflex.[4]

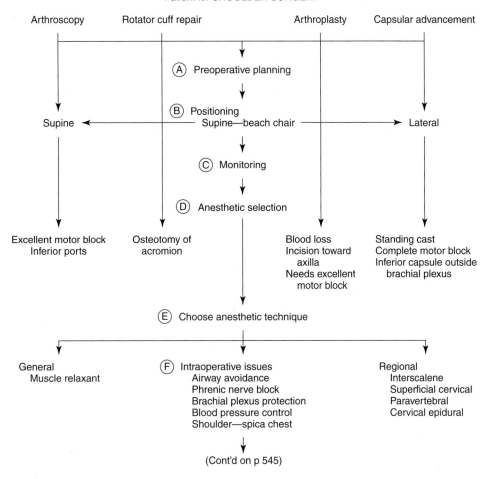

Patient for SHOULDER SURGERY

Arthroscopy   Rotator cuff repair   Arthroplasty   Capsular advancement

(A) Preoperative planning

(B) Positioning
Supine ←   Supine—beach chair   → Lateral

(C) Monitoring

(D) Anesthetic selection

Supine
Excellent motor block   Osteotomy of   Blood loss   Standing cast
Inferior ports   acromion   Incision toward   Complete motor block
                                                         axilla   Inferior capsule outside
                                                    Needs excellent   brachial plexus
                                                      motor block

(E) Choose anesthetic technique

General   (F) Intraoperative issues   Regional
Muscle relaxant   Airway avoidance   Interscalene
                               Phrenic nerve block   Superficial cervical
                               Brachial plexus protection   Paravertebral
                               Blood pressure control   Cervical epidural
                               Shoulder—spica chest

(Cont'd on p 545)

G. Postoperatively, verify the integrity of the brachial plexus before discharge from the PACU. Recurrent neurological deficit is an indication to look for compressive hematoma or dislocation of a prosthesis. Plan postoperative pain management; patient-controlled analgesia (PCA) with opiates is a common choice. Ketorolac is useful when preoperative frozen shoulder mandates early postoperative movement of a painful shoulder. Intraarticular and wound injection of local anesthetics, perhaps mixed with opiates, is another option.[5] Consider continuous infusion of local anesthetic; home pain control has been achieved with elastomeric or spring-driven reservoirs.[6] Continuous interscalene analgesia provides excellent pain control, but placement and maintenance of the catheter are technically difficult. Excellent pain control, full neurological function, and ambulation without disequilibrium are minimum standards for outpatient release because one upper limb will not be available for protection in a fall.

REFERENCES

1. Tetzlaff JE, Yoon HJ, Brems J: Interscalene brachial plexus block for shoulder surgery, *Reg Anesth* 19:339–343, 1994.
2. Tetzlaff JE, Yoon HJ, O'Hara J, et al.: Alkalinization of mepivacaine accelerates onset of interscalene block for shoulder surgery, *Reg Anesth* 15:242–244, 1990.
3. Urmey WF, Talts KH, Sharrock NE: One hundred percent incidence of hemidiaphragmatic paresis associated with interscalene brachial plexus anesthesia as demonstrated by ultrasonography, *Anesth Analg* 72:489–503, 1991.
4. D'Alessio JG, Weller RS, Rosenblum M: Activation of the Bezold-Jarisch reflex in the sitting position for shoulder arthroscopy using interscalene block, *Anesth Analg* 80:1158–1162, 1995.
5. Tetzlaff JE, Brems J, Dilger J: Intraarticular morphine and bupivacaine reduces postoperative pain after rotator cuff repair, *Reg Anesth Pain Med* 25 (6):611–614, 2000.
6. Klein SM, Grant SA, Greengrass RA, et al.: Interscalene brachial plexus block with a continuous catheter insertion system and a disposable infusion pump, *Anesth Analg* 91:1473–1478, 2000.

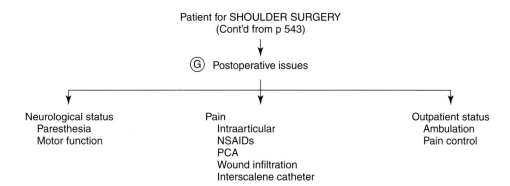

Patient for SHOULDER SURGERY
(Cont'd from p 543)

Ⓖ Postoperative issues

Neurological status
Paresthesia
Motor function

Pain
Intraarticular
NSAIDs
PCA
Wound infiltration
Interscalene catheter

Outpatient status
Ambulation
Pain control

Isovolemic Hemodilution (IVH)

GAELAN B. LUHN, M.D.

Isovolemic (normovolemic, intentional) hemodilution (IVH) is a technique in which a portion of a patient's blood volume is withdrawn and stored in the immediate presurgical period and reinfused during or after surgery. As blood is removed, it is replaced with a sanguinous fluid; the hematocrit (Hct) declines, but blood volume is maintained. IVH reduces transfusion requirements by dilution of intraoperative blood loss. Decreased blood viscosity decreases systemic vascular resistance (SVR), which increases cardiac output (CO) and venous return. In addition, increased oxygen extraction allows maintenance of tissue oxygen consumption.[1] Another advantage of IVH is it provides additional plasma and platelets at the end of surgery for hemostasis. IVH has also been used in combination with cell saver and was found to offer better transfusion avoidance than either technique alone.[2] The relatively new technique of hypervolemic hemodilution (the purposeful dilution of Hct without blood withdrawal) has shown promise for decreasing transfusion requirements in healthy patients, but further study is necessary.[3]

A. Suitable candidates for IVH are patients with adequate Hct and normal cardiac reserve who are expected to lose at least 1000 mL of blood or 20 to 30% of their blood volume. Typical procedures include total joint replacement, coronary artery bypass grafting (CABG), hepatic resection, and spine, pelvic, and cancer surgeries. IVH is acceptable to many Jehovah's Witnesses.[4] Relative contraindications include preoperative anemia (hemoglobin < 12 g/dL), coronary and cerebral vascular disease, myocardial dysfunction, pulmonary disease, hypertension (HTN), liver cirrhosis, coagulopathy, diabetes, advanced age, and prior administration of myocardial depressant drugs. However, IVH has been used safely in patients with known coronary artery disease (CAD).[5] Patients with questionable cardiac reserve may benefit from invasive monitoring to ensure maintenance of euvolemia, cardiac filling pressures, oxygen transport, and mixed venous oxygen saturation during IVH. Patients should be euvolemic before beginning the procedure.

B. Calculate the amount of blood that can be withdrawn using this formula:

$$ABL = \frac{EBV \times (Hct_s - Hct_f)}{Hct_{avg}}$$

where ABL = allowable blood loss, EBV = estimated blood volume, Hct_s = starting Hct, Hct_f = final desired Hct, and Hct_{avg} = the average of the starting and desired Hct. Blood should be diluted to an Hct of 27 to 30, or lower.[6]

C. Using strict aseptic techniques, draw arterial or venous blood from the patient before induction of anesthesia or between induction and the start of significant blood loss into standard citrate-phosphate-dextrose-adenine (CDP-A) blood bags obtained from the blood bank. Frequently agitate the blood as it flows into the bag to ensure adequate dispersal of the anticoagulant. Place a stopcock and syringe between the vascular access and the blood bag to facilitate rapid transfer of the blood through the length of tubing. Place the bag on a scale to allow estimation of the volume of blood removed. Standard blood bags will contain 450 mL of blood, or as labeled otherwise. Label the bags clearly with the patient's name and hospital number, and the date, time, and volume of the collection. As blood is withdrawn, replace it with crystalloid at a 3:1 ratio or colloid at a 1:1 ratio of the volume of blood removed. When applicable, use invasive monitoring to maintain the baseline CVP or pulmonary artery wedge pressure.

D. Blood can be stored in CDP-A bags for up to 4 hours without refrigeration to maintain immediate platelet activity. If longer storage is required, refrigerate the blood for up to 12 hours. Most blood banks will not store blood collected in the OR.

E. Indications for reinfusion of autologous blood are similar to, but not as stringent as, those for allogeneic blood. Blood that has left the OR is still subject to the same risk of clerical error that causes transfusion reactions. For blood that has remained in the OR, the main danger is bacterial growth.

F. When there are indications for transfusion, reinfuse the stored blood in the reverse order from which it was withdrawn: blood with the highest concentration of RBCs and serum protein, which was obtained first, is infused last. Unless special arrangements are made with the blood bank, blood not reinfused in the immediate perioperative period cannot be stored for later usage.

REFERENCES

1. Spahn D, Leone BJ, Reves JG, et al.: Cardiovascular and coronary physiology of acute isovolemic hemodilution: a review of non-oxygen-carrying and oxygen-carrying solutions, Anesth Analg 78:1000–1021, 1994.
2. Waters JH, Lee JS, Karafa MT: A mathematical model of cell salvage compared and combined with normovolemic hemodilution, Transfusion 44:1412–1416, 2004.

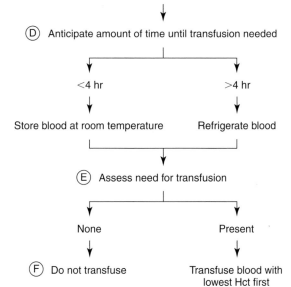

ISOVOLEMIC HEMODILUTION

(A) Identify patient who may benefit from IVH
├─ Obtain consent
├─ Determine level of patient monitoring needed
└─ Collect needed materials to perform IVH
   Intravascular catheters
   Tubing, blood bags
   Syringes and stopcocks
   Sponge scale

(B) Calculate amount of blood to be removed as

$$\text{Removed blood} = \text{patient's estimated blood volume} = \frac{Hct_{start} - Hct_{final}}{Hct_{average}}$$

(C) Transfer blood aseptically into labeled CPD-A blood bags with frequent agitation
Replace blood with 3:1 ratio of crystalloid or 1:1 ratio of colloid solution
Maintain constant central venous or pulmonary artery wedge pressure

(D) Anticipate amount of time until transfusion needed

<4 hr   >4 hr

Store blood at room temperature   Refrigerate blood

(E) Assess need for transfusion

None   Present

(F) Do not transfuse   Transfuse blood with
                            lowest Hct first

3. Kumar R, Chakraborty I, Sehgal R: A prospective randomized study comparing two techniques of perioperative blood conservation: isovolemic hemodilution and hypervolemic hemodilution, *Anesth Analg* 95:1154–1161, 2002.
4. Khine HH, Naidu R, Cowell H, et al.: A method of blood conservation in Jehovah's Witnesses: incirculation diversion and refusion, *Anesth Analg* 57:279–280, 1978.
5. Spahn DR, Schmid ER, Seifert B, et al.: Hemodilution tolerance in patients with coronary disease who are receiving chronic beta-adrenergic blocker therapy, *Anesth Analg* 82:687–694, 1996.
6. Fontana JL, Welborn L, Mongan PD, et al.: Oxygen consumption and cardiovascular function in children during profound intraoperative normovolemic hemodilution, *Anesth Analg* 80:219–225, 1995.

TRAUMA ANESTHESIA

Evaluation of the Trauma Patient

DAVID I. SHAPIRO, M.D.

The evaluation of the trauma patient is an ongoing process performed throughout the trauma care continuum. The nature and evolution of physiological derangements and their impact on oxygen (O_2) delivery in the multitraumatized patient will dictate management priorities. Closely observing the patient's response to resuscitation and anesthesia will provide valuable feedback.

A. Perform the initial anesthetic assessment as early as possible. While the trauma team is following the ATLS protocol, quickly assess the patient's airway, breathing, circulation (ABCs). Confirmation of a patent airway and adequate breathing is performed by observation, auscultation, and pulse oximetry. Perform immediate tracheal intubation in cases of hypoxia, hypercarbia, Glasgow Coma Scale (GCS) <9, airway obstruction caused by maxillofacial injuries or expanding neck lesions, apparent airway burn injury, or shock unresponsive to initial resuscitation.[1] Consider prophylactic early intubation when the extent of injury, mechanism of injury, or previous medical condition raises the index of suspicion for future decompensation. Intubation may also be required in an intoxicated or combative patient to facilitate diagnostic studies. Provide supplemental oxygen to those trauma patients not requiring intubation. Traumatically injured patients should be considered to have full stomachs and be at risk for aspiration, as gastric emptying ceases at the moment of injury. Except those with isolated limb injuries, all trauma patients are at risk for cervical spine injuries. Evaluate circulation; determine whether the patient is in shock. Level of consciousness, vital signs, and skin color are gross indicators of end-organ tissue perfusion and oxygenation. Remember that a supine young patient may still have a normal BP and HR even after losing more than 20% of blood volume.[2] Closely monitor urine output, serial hemoglobins (Hgb), acid-base status, and ongoing blood loss. Measure the patient's core temperature early and often. Hypothermia may be an iatrogenic occurrence in the traumatized patient but can also relate to the severity of injury. The patient's response to an initial bolus of warm crystalloid provides critical information about the degree of hypovolemia.

B. A more comprehensive assessment follows. Review the patient's ECG, chest x-ray (CXR), and initial blood work. If possible, query the patient or family about past medical history, allergies, and current medications. Alcohol and illicit drug use are common. Toxicology screens may prove valuable. Order a urine HCG in all females of childbearing age. Pregnant patients carrying a viable fetus require fetal monitoring intraoperatively and for the first 24 hours postoperatively. Determine the mechanisms, extent, location, and kinetics of the injury as these correlate with specific injury patterns, and with morbidity and mortality. Long bone fractures may cause fat emboli syndrome. A detailed trauma workup includes radiographic studies of the bony elements; intravenous pyelograms (IVPs); CT scans of the head, neck, and abdomen; and comprehensive blood tests. For patients in shock unresponsive to resuscitative efforts, there may only be time for an ultrasound in the emergency department. Focused assessment by sonography for trauma (FAST) can provide immediate information about the presence of intraabdominal or intrathoracic hemorrhage.[3]

C. Multitraumatized patients arrive in the OR at varying stages of the evaluative process. Intraoperatively, continue the ongoing assessment of O_2 delivery. Monitor breath sounds, pulmonary compliance, PaO_2/FiO_2 ratios, and A-a gradients to give early indications of previously undiagnosed pulmonary processes. Arterial BP, urine output, serial hemoglobins, coagulation profiles, and pH analysis are helpful in estimating perfusion. The degree of hemodynamic deterioration following anesthetic induction may indicate adequacy of volume resuscitation or pump function. Evaluate the patient's perfusion status intraoperatively for early diagnosis of inadequate resuscitation, cardiac contusion, pericardial tamponade, occult bleeding, and coagulopathic states. In patients with closed-head injuries, consider the potential for development of intracranial hypertension (HTN). Intracranial pressure monitoring may be required to ensure adequate cerebral perfusion pressure.

D. Continue the evaluation of the trauma patient in the postoperative period. Persistent metabolic acidosis, hypothermia, and coagulopathy, despite aggressive resuscitation and surgical intervention, are poor prognostic indicators. Ongoing vigilance for the onset of acute respiratory distress syndrome (ARDS) and multisystem organ failure is prudent in the severely traumatized patient.

REFERENCES

1. Dunham CM, Barraco RD, Clark DE, et al.: Guidelines for emergency tracheal intubation immediately after traumatic injury, *J Trauma* 55 (1):162–179, 2003.
2. Barker SJ: Anesthesia for trauma, IARS 2002 review course lectures.
3. Melanson SW, Heller M: The emerging role of bedside ultrasonography in trauma care, *Emerg Med Clin North Am* 16 (1):165–189, 1998.

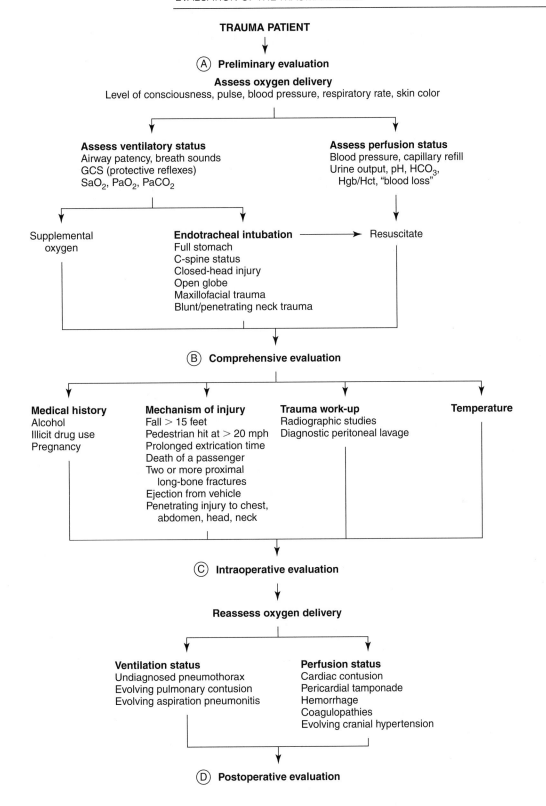

Anesthesia for the Trauma Patient

DAVID I. SHAPIRO, M.D.

Ideally, an anesthesiologist is involved in the initial evaluation and resuscitation of any multitrauma patient. Once the initial evaluation is accomplished, provisions are made for rapid airway control and resuscitation. Rapid surgical control of traumatic bleeding is essential.

A. Perform a preliminary patient evaluation, assessing ABCs (oxygen [O_2] delivery, ventilation, and perfusion). Provide supplementary O_2 or intubate the patient and begin fluid resuscitation. Prepare the OR. A properly equipped and set up trauma OR saves precious time. Prepare standard equipment, monitors, and drugs in advance. Have available a high-flow fluid warmer, forced-air blanket, and invasive pressure monitoring equipment. Warm the room prior to patient arrival to prevent worsening of hypothermia.

B. If time permits, perform a more comprehensive evaluation.

C. Bring the patient to the OR. Begin preoxygenation while monitors are applied. If the patient arrives without adequate IV access (minimum of two large peripheral catheters), place a large caliber central venous catheter prior to induction. If the patient has a palpable radial or brachial pulse, insert an arterial catheter prior to induction (it may be impossible later). An arterial line is critical not only for monitoring BP but also for allowing frequent measurements of pH, hematocrit (Hct), and electrolytes. Assume all trauma patients to be hypovolemic, even when vital signs are normal. Begin fluid resuscitation prior to induction. Perform an awake fiberoptic intubation or awake cricothyroidotomy in trauma patients with deformities of the face or neck. Perform a RSI if a normal airway is anticipated, with one assistant providing manual in-line stabilization of the cervical spine and another providing cricoid pressure. Consider ketamine and midazolam for induction; patients in shock may require only muscle relaxation. Succinylcholine (SCC) provides the most reliable, rapid intubating conditions and is safe within 24 hours of burns or spinal injuries. Oral tracheal intubation can be accomplished safely in the vast majority of patients. Have adjuvant airway equipment (e.g., intubating laryngeal mask airway [LMA], bougie, glide scope, etc.) immediately available in case of an unanticipated difficult airway. Personnel and equipment for a surgical airway should always be present at induction.

Note the patient's hemodynamic response to induction, which will provide information about volume status. Use low-dose inhaled agents for anesthetic maintenance, if tolerated. Opioids are useful adjuncts, because they have minimal cardiovascular effects. Avoid N_2O; it has few indications in trauma care. N_2O is a myocardial depressant, expands trapped gases, elevates ICP, and limits FiO_2. Continue fluid resuscitation throughout the intraoperative period. Choose warmed isotonic crystalloids for initial trauma resuscitation; studies have shown no improved outcomes from more expensive colloids.[1] Hypertonic saline is only indicated in military and disaster situations where its portability is an advantage.[2] There is a growing belief that excessive fluid resuscitation early in trauma may lead to increased bleeding and poorer outcomes.[3] Prior to surgical control of hemorrhage, aim for a systolic blood pressure of only 80 to 90 mm Hg (higher in the elderly or those with brain injury, in whom cerebral perfusion is paramount). Blood losses will usually eventually require transfusion of PRBCs; the target hemoglobin (Hgb) will depend on the patient's underlying medical condition and the rate of ongoing blood loss. The most common coagulopathy associated with massive transfusion is dilutional thrombocytopenia. Transfuse platelets to maintain a count of at least 50,000 to 70,000. Give FFP based on results of coagulation studies. Monitor calcium levels; the citrate in PRBCs binds calcium. Calcium replacement will treat the coagulopathy and hypotension associated with hypocalcemia. In trauma patients with severe coagulopathies unresponsive to transfusion of platelets, FFP, and cryoprecipitate, consider administration of factor VIIa (50 to 100 μg/kg).[4] If trauma patients have continued unexplained hypotension after surgical control of bleeding, consider transesophageal echocardiography (TEE) to rapidly differentiate between hypovolemia, ischemia, and tamponade. Throughout the intraoperative period, communicate with the surgical team and keep them informed of the patient's BP, arterial pH, urine output, and Hgb. Current trauma surgery guidelines promote damage control only in severe trauma and it may be best to leave the OR once the main sources of bleeding are controlled.

D. In the absence of major trauma to the airway or chest, it may be possible to extubate some trauma patients at the end of surgery. Keep the patient intubated if there is uncorrected hypothermia, acidosis, hypotension, or intoxication. Major trauma patients will usually require ICU care and may have hemodynamic instability in the immediate postoperative period. At this point they may benefit from pulmonary artery (PA) catheterization.

REFERENCES

1. Boldt J: Fluid choice for resuscitation of the trauma patient: a review of the physiological, pharmacological, and clinical evidence, *Can J Anaesth* 51 (5):500–513, 2004.
2. Smith JE, Hall MJ. Hypertonic saline. *J R Army Med Corps* 150 (4):239–243, 2004.
3. Revell M, Greaves I, Porter K: Endpoints for fluid resuscitation in hemorrhagic shock, *J Trauma* 54:S63–S67, 2003.
4. Dutton RP, McCunn M, Hyder M, et al.: Factor VIIa for correction of traumatic coagulopathy, *J Trauma* 57 (4):709–718, 2004.

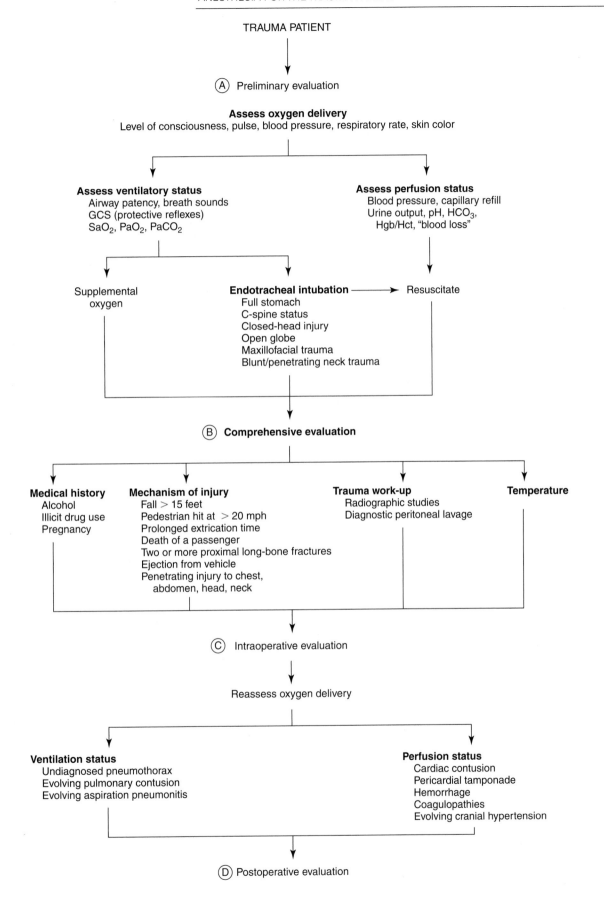

TRAUMA PATIENT

Ⓐ Preliminary evaluation

Assess oxygen delivery
Level of consciousness, pulse, blood pressure, respiratory rate, skin color

Assess ventilatory status
   Airway patency, breath sounds
   GCS (protective reflexes)
   SaO_2, PaO_2, $PaCO_2$

Assess perfusion status
   Blood pressure, capillary refill
   Urine output, pH, HCO_3,
      Hgb/Hct, "blood loss"

Supplemental
oxygen

Endotracheal intubation ⟶ Resuscitate
   Full stomach
   C-spine status
   Closed-head injury
   Open globe
   Maxillofacial trauma
   Blunt/penetrating neck trauma

Ⓑ **Comprehensive evaluation**

Medical history
Alcohol
Illicit drug use
Pregnancy

Mechanism of injury
Fall > 15 feet
Pedestrian hit at > 20 mph
Prolonged extrication time
Death of a passenger
Two or more proximal long-bone fractures
Ejection from vehicle
Penetrating injury to chest,
   abdomen, head, neck

Trauma work-up
   Radiographic studies
   Diagnostic peritoneal lavage

Temperature

Ⓒ Intraoperative evaluation

Reassess oxygen delivery

Ventilation status
   Undiagnosed pneumothorax
   Evolving pulmonary contusion
   Evolving aspiration pneumonitis

Perfusion status
   Cardiac contusion
   Pericardial tamponade
   Hemorrhage
   Coagulopathies
   Evolving cranial hypertension

Ⓓ Postoperative evaluation

Massive Blood Transfusion

MALCOLM D. ORR, M.D., PH.D.

Massive exsanguination is lethal unless resuscitation is undertaken promptly. Initial treatment includes placement of multiple large-bore vascular access catheters and infusion of fluids. Invasive monitoring devices may be extremely helpful in determining the need for further fluid replacement, particularly when the patient has sustained most of the blood loss before arrival at hospital.

A. Some patients at risk for massive bleeding (thoracic aneurysms, repeat valve replacements) may benefit from sequestration of platelet-rich plasma before cardiopulmonary bypass (CPB). This has resulted in a significant decrease in homologous blood usage when platelets and WBCs are protected from the extracorporeal circuit.[1] As increasing percentages of circulating blood volume (CBV) are lost, peripheral perfusion decreases (cold, pale, pulseless extremities), renal perfusion drops (oliguria), and CNS perfusion is compromised (confusion, loss of consciousness). Estimate the degree of blood loss already incurred, as well as further losses to be expected, so that appropriate transfusion may be given. In the multitrauma patient, diagnosis of injuries may have to proceed concomitant with treatment; hypotension that does not respond to vigorous volume infusion may be secondary to other disease processes (e.g., spinal shock, myocardial dysfunction, sepsis). Attempt to keep the patient warm during the resuscitation.

B. The greatest resistance to flow of an IV line is the IV catheter. Place the largest caliber catheters possible for massive transfusion. Pulmonary artery (PA) catheter introducers (8F) may be placed in neck, saphenous, or other accessible veins. IV tubing may be placed directly into the vena cava or right atrium.

C. The composition of fluids used for volume restoration depends on the needs of each patient, but may be estimated according to the degree of blood loss (Table 1). During loss of the first 0.5 CBV, it is most important to maintain the CBV to prevent stasis and provide a vehicle for oxygen (O_2) transport and carbon dioxide (CO_2) excretion. The peak O_2 delivery may occur at a hematocrit (Hct) of 30%;[2] many anesthetists infuse only crystalloids and/or colloids (no RBCs) until the Hct falls to <24%. Reduced blood viscosity may enhance tissue flow by reducing sludging and microaggregate formation. IV crystalloid is distributed between the plasma and interstitial fluid (in a ratio of 1:4), so that if volume resuscitation is performed with crystalloid alone, tissue edema (including cerebral and pulmonary edema) results. However, crystalloid is considerably less expensive than colloids, and most anesthetists give some combination of the two. If there is a decrease in mixed venous O_2 saturation or other evidence of O_2 deprivation, transfuse more RBCs as needed. During the replacement of the second 0.5 CBV, dilutional coagulopathy frequently occurs.[3] Give thawed FFP as needed to keep the international normalized ratio (INR) or prothrombin time (PT) and partial thromboplastin time (PTT) in a functional range. Observe the surgical field, which may give information about clotting or its absence. When a complete CBV has been replaced, dilutional thrombocytopenia occurs. Administer platelet infusions to raise the circulating platelet count to >50,000/mm^2. The RBCs, FFP, and platelets administered are essentially reconstituted whole blood. (Whole blood would be preferable, in that exposure to antigens and viral infections is reduced, but it is not generally available.)

D. Rapid-infusion pumps facilitate transfusion. Autologous transfusion of shed blood is economical when large volumes of clean blood are lost. Collection, filtration, purification, and reinfusion of RBCs reduce the risk of transfusion reaction or acquisition of blood-borne disease.

E. Treat profound vasoconstriction (secondary to shock) to improve tissue microcirculation. Observe patients for signs and symptoms of transfusion-related lung injury (TRALI), usually occurring during or within 6 hours of transfusion. TRALI is a leading cause of transfusion-related morbidity and mortality. Steroid treatment is controversial (reports are anecdotal).[4]

REFERENCES

1. Giordano GF, Rivers SL, Chung GK, et al.: Autologous platelet-rich plasma in cardiac surgery: effect on intraoperative and postoperative transfusion requirements, *Ann Thorac Surg* 46:416–419, 1988.
2. Messmer K, Sunder-Plassman L, Klovekorn WP, et al.: Circulatory significance of hemodilution: rheological changes and limitations, *Adv Microcirc* 4:1–77, 1972.
3. DeLoughery TG. Coagulation defects in trauma patients: etiology, recognition, and therapy, *Crit Care Clin* 20:13–24, 2004.
4. Moore SB: Transfusion-related acute lung injury (TRALI): clinical presentation, treatment, and prognosis, *Crit Care Med* 34 (5 Suppl): S114–S117, 2006.

TABLE 1
Estimated Circulating Blood Volume by Age

Patient	Blood volume (ml/kg)
Adult	60
Child	60–70
Infant	70–80
Neonate	80–100

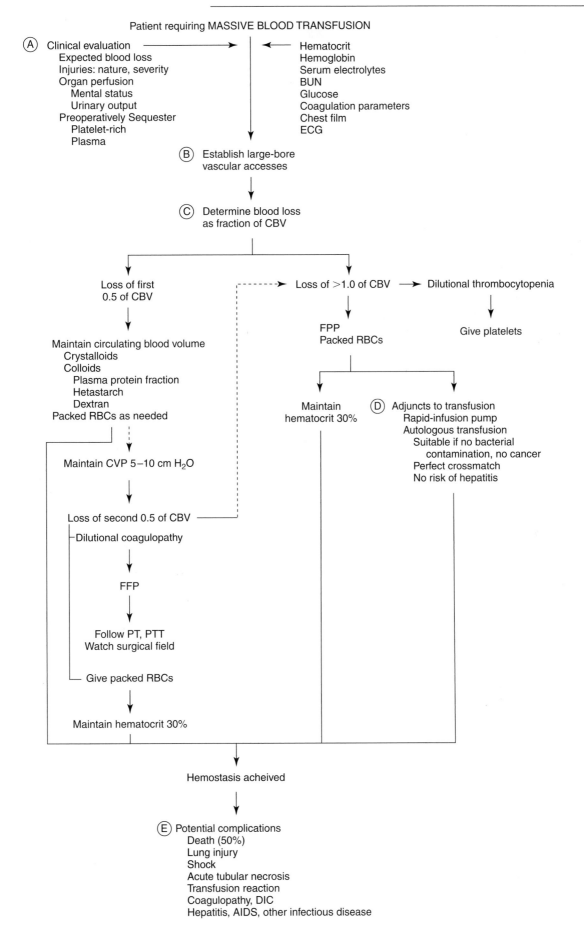

Patient requiring MASSIVE BLOOD TRANSFUSION

Ⓐ Clinical evaluation
- Expected blood loss
- Injuries: nature, severity
- Organ perfusion
  - Mental status
  - Urinary output
- Preoperatively Sequester
  - Platelet-rich
  - Plasma

Hematocrit
Hemoglobin
Serum electrolytes
BUN
Glucose
Coagulation parameters
Chest film
ECG

Ⓑ Establish large-bore vascular accesses

Ⓒ Determine blood loss as fraction of CBV

Loss of first 0.5 of CBV

Loss of >1.0 of CBV → Dilutional thrombocytopenia

FPP
Packed RBCs

Give platelets

Maintain circulating blood volume
- Crystalloids
- Colloids
  - Plasma protein fraction
  - Hetastarch
  - Dextran
- Packed RBCs as needed

Maintain hematocrit 30%

Ⓓ Adjuncts to transfusion
- Rapid-infusion pump
- Autologous transfusion
  - Suitable if no bacterial contamination, no cancer
- Perfect crossmatch
- No risk of hepatitis

Maintain CVP 5–10 cm H$_2$O

Loss of second 0.5 of CBV
- Dilutional coagulopathy

FFP

Follow PT, PTT
Watch surgical field

- Give packed RBCs

Maintain hematocrit 30%

Hemostasis acheived

Ⓔ Potential complications
- Death (50%)
- Lung injury
- Shock
- Acute tubular necrosis
- Transfusion reaction
- Coagulopathy, DIC
- Hepatitis, AIDS, other infectious disease

Shock

MALCOLM D. ORR, M.D., PH.D.

SUSAN H. NOORILY, M.D.

Shock is defined as any pathological state that leads to hypoperfusion of the tissues and inadequate oxygen (O_2) delivery to meet metabolic needs.[1-3] It is a complex phenomenon involving both hemodynamic and inflammatory components. Shock is classified as cardiogenic (pump failure) or due to decreased venous return (as a result of hypovolemia or vasodilation). Cardiogenic shock occurs with left ventricular (LV) and right ventricular (RV) failure (possibly due to myocardial infarction or ischemia), arrhythmia, valvular dysfunction, pericardial tamponade, and pulmonary embolism. Hypovolemia is a result of hemorrhage or dehydration. Vasodilation can be caused by sepsis, anaphylaxis, neurogenic insult, and burn injury. Other causes of shock include adrenal insufficiency, carbon monoxide poisoning, and severe thyroid disease. Early treatment of shock is necessary to prevent multisystem organ failure.

A. Perform a history and physical examination with attention focused on airway, breathing, and circulation (advanced cardiac life support [ACLS]/ATLS protocols). Intubate and mechanically ventilate the patient who has signs of hypoxemia, inability to protect the airway, or ventilatory failure, including respiratory muscle fatigue.

B. Assess the adequacy of the cardiac output (CO) by checking the pulse, skin temperature, and capillary refill. If CO appears to be increased, the systemic vascular resistance (SVR) is likely decreased. If the CO appears to be decreased, determine volume status. Ensure adequate IV access and begin to resuscitate with IV fluids to restore volume. Give blood products as needed through a blood warmer. The risk of death increases with the number of units of blood transfused; when more than one blood volume is replaced, mortality rate approaches 50%. Place routine monitors. Insert an arterial line and send blood samples for analysis. Use special monitors to obtain objective data (e.g., urinary catheter, echocardiogram [echo], central venous or pulmonary artery [PA] catheter, mixed venous O_2 saturation, pulse contour analysis, and esophageal Doppler) to allow goal-directed therapy.

C. Determine the cause of the shock state. It may be obvious (gunshot wound with massive blood loss) or obscure (hypoglycemia or transfusion reaction under general anesthesia). Management will often require simultaneous diagnosis and treatment. Consider administering vasoactive drugs after instituting volume resuscitation. If the CO is low and filling pressures high, provide inotropic support. If the CO is high, administer pressors to treat hypotension. Titrate to signs of end-organ perfusion. Continue to assess BP, temperature, urine output, and acid-base status. Do not treat acidosis with sodium bicarbonate.

D. Attempt to correct the underlying disorder. Continually reassess the patient during the course of treatment. Definitive management of hemorrhagic shock usually requires operative intervention. Consult with a cardiologist in cases of cardiogenic shock, which may require angiography and revascularization. Although septic shock has an inflammatory component, steroid administration is controversial. High-dose steroid therapy may worsen outcomes but low-dose treatment may be beneficial in cases where there is accompanying adrenal insufficiency. Perform an adrenocorticotropic hormone (ACTH) stimulation test to evaluate adrenal insufficiency.

REFERENCES

1. Holmes CL, Walley KR: The evaluation and management of shock, *Clin Chest Med* 24:775–789, 2003.
2. Kress JP: Shock. In: Hall JB, Freid EB, editors: *SCCM ACCP 4th Combined Critical Care Course*, 2002, American College of Chest Physicians and the Society of Critical Care Medicine.
3. Rosenthal MH: Management of cardiogenic, hyperdynamic and hypovolemic shock. In: American Society of Anesthesiologists, *Annual refresher course lectures* 112, 1999.

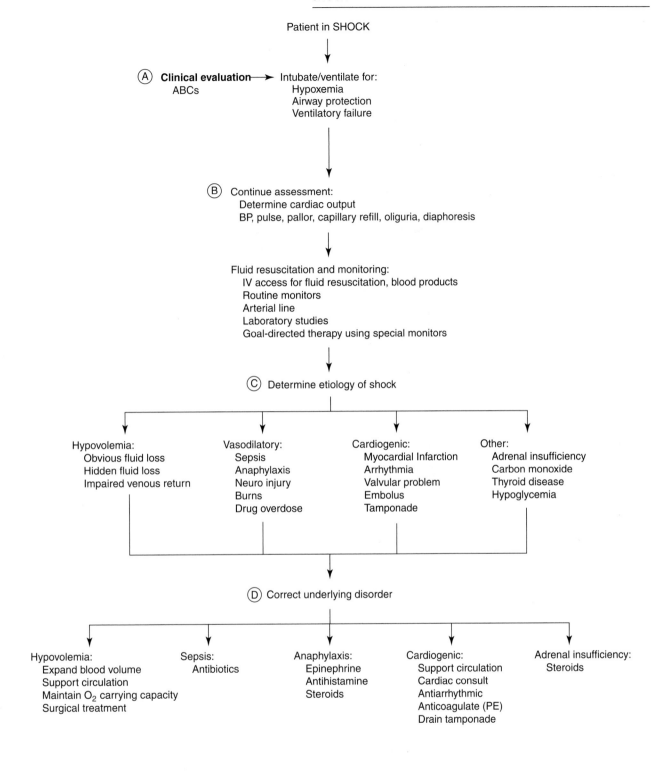

Patient in SHOCK

(A) **Clinical evaluation** ⟶ Intubate/ventilate for:
ABCs   Hypoxemia
                                 Airway protection
                                 Ventilatory failure

(B) Continue assessment:
     Determine cardiac output
     BP, pulse, pallor, capillary refill, oliguria, diaphoresis

Fluid resuscitation and monitoring:
     IV access for fluid resuscitation, blood products
     Routine monitors
     Arterial line
     Laboratory studies
     Goal-directed therapy using special monitors

(C) Determine etiology of shock

Hypovolemia:
     Obvious fluid loss
     Hidden fluid loss
     Impaired venous return

Vasodilatory:
     Sepsis
     Anaphylaxis
     Neuro injury
     Burns
     Drug overdose

Cardiogenic:
     Myocardial Infarction
     Arrhythmia
     Valvular problem
     Embolus
     Tamponade

Other:
     Adrenal insufficiency
     Carbon monoxide
     Thyroid disease
     Hypoglycemia

(D) Correct underlying disorder

Hypovolemia:
     Expand blood volume
     Support circulation
     Maintain O_2 carrying capacity
     Surgical treatment

Sepsis:
     Antibiotics

Anaphylaxis:
     Epinephrine
     Antihistamine
     Steroids

Cardiogenic:
     Support circulation
     Cardiac consult
     Antiarrhythmic
     Anticoagulate (PE)
     Drain tamponade

Adrenal insufficiency:
     Steroids

Hypotension in the Acutely Traumatized Patient

KEVIN B. GEROLD, D.O., J.D.

COLIN F. MACKENZIE, M.B., Ch.B., F.C.C.M.

Symptomatic hypotension in the acutely traumatized patient signals a potentially life-threatening condition and requires immediate intervention. Conduct initial resuscitative efforts in a systematic manner directed to identify and correct the condition, even when the definitive diagnosis is unknown.[1] Hypotension becomes clinically significant when the systolic blood pressure (SBP) falls below 90 torr or is associated with clinical manifestations of inadequate end-organ perfusion. Evidence of end-organ hypoperfusion include alterations in mental status, decreased urine output, myocardial ischemia on ECG or echocardiogram (echo), and delayed capillary refill of the distal extremities. Chronically hypertensive patients and those with preexisting medical conditions may experience symptomatic hypotension with BPs greater than 90 torr and require resuscitation to higher than normal end points to restore perfusion.

A. Ensure a patent airway, confirm the adequacy of ventilation, and control obvious hemorrhage. Insert large-bore venous cannulae (14 gauge IV or 9 Fr introducer sheath) percutaneously or by cut-down to permit the administration of IV fluids and blood products. In all trauma patients, consider the possibility of injury to the cervical spine and, when necessary, immobilize the neck in a neutral position. During the initial resuscitative effort, perform a basic neurological examination that includes a determination of mental status (Glasgow Coma Scale), pupillary responses to light, and motor function of the extremities. To the extent possible, obtain from the patient, prehospital care providers, or bystanders, a brief history to include drug allergies, the regular use of medications, the presence of preexisting medical conditions, the name of the patient's primary care practitioner and location of medical records, and the circumstances and mechanisms surrounding the injury.

HYPOTENSIVE, ACUTELY TRAUMATIZED PATIENT

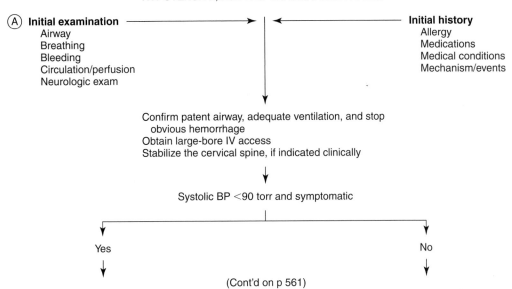

Ⓐ **Initial examination**
Airway
Breathing
Bleeding
Circulation/perfusion
Neurologic exam

Initial history
Allergy
Medications
Medical conditions
Mechanism/events

Confirm patent airway, adequate ventilation, and stop
  obvious hemorrhage
Obtain large-bore IV access
Stabilize the cervical spine, if indicated clinically

Systolic BP <90 torr and symptomatic

Yes

No

(Cont'd on p 561)

B. Disturbances in cardiac rate and rhythm may contribute to symptomatic hypotension in traumatized patient. Identify rhythm disturbances with early ECG monitoring. Bradycardia is associated with severe head trauma and cervical spinal cord injury. Accelerate bradycardias associated with hypotension using atropine, external pacing, epinephrine, dopamine, or isoproterenol. Nonsinus tachydysrhythmias, such as uncontrolled atrial fibrillation, atrial flutter, ventricular tachycardia, or ventricular fibrillation, are seen rarely in acute trauma but may contribute to hypotension. Correct tachydysrhythmias associated with hypotension without delay using electrical or pharmacological cardioversion.

C. Assess for hypovolemia due to external or internal hemorrhage. Minimize ongoing blood loss in hypovolemic shock; delay aggressive restitution of the intravascular volume until major bleeding is under control. If extremity bleeding is uncontrollable by direct pressure alone, consider applying a tourniquet.[2] Consider applying a hemostatic agent (QuickClot®) to control significant ongoing hemorrhage in large truncal or proximal extremity wounds.[3,4] When placed in a wound, these agents rapidly adsorb fluids in and around the wound and concentrate clotting factors. All uncontrollable hemorrhage requires immediate surgical intervention. Attempting to restore the intravascular volume in the face of continued ongoing hemorrhage will increase the blood loss, dilute the number of platelets, coagulation factors and other plasma proteins, and promote hypothermia.[5–8] Therefore, limit volume resuscitation to that necessary to maintain perfusion to vital organs, such as the brain and heart. Once hemorrhage is controlled, aggressively restore the intravascular volume by rapidly delivering a 20 to 40 ml/kg fluid challenge using a dextrose-free isotonic crystalloid (Lactated Ringer's solution, normal saline, or Plasmalyte A). Hypertonic saline, colloid solutions, or hydroxyethyl starch (Hetastarch), alone or in combination with crystalloid, will restore the intravascular volume but the advantage over isotonic crystalloid resuscitation alone remains unproven.[9–12] Administer blood products if the BP fails to improve with the initial volume challenge or if the estimated blood loss (EBL) exceeds 20 to 30 ml/kg (30 to 40% of the patient's estimated blood volume). Type-specific, cross-matched blood is preferred, but type-specific only or type-O blood is an acceptable alternative for emergency use. Women of childbearing age requiring blood transfusion prior to type and cross-match should receive Rh negative blood whenever possible. Anticipate early the need for FFP and platelets. FFP and platelets are often necessary when the blood loss exceeds 40% of the estimated blood volume. In the presence of ongoing hemorrhage and coagulopathy, consider the addition of activated clotting factor VII (VIIa) to reduce the absolute blood loss and facilitate the resuscitative effort.

D. Assess for possible tension pneumothorax or pericardial tamponade if hypotension persists despite an adequate intravascular volume. These conditions physically obstruct the heart or great vessels, causing a reduced stroke volume and compensatory tachycardia. Treat tension pneumothorax by immediate needle decompression followed by a chest tube thoracostomy. To diagnose pericardial tamponade in acute trauma, perform a pericardial window and visualize blood in the pericardial sac. If this procedure is not possible, then perform a pericardiocentesis. In either case, a positive result will require emergency surgery to repair the cardiac injury.

E. It is difficult to assess the extent of blood lost and the adequacy of volume resuscitation in patients with multiple injuries and ongoing blood loss during surgical efforts at hemostasis. Therefore, monitor CVP and observe responses to fluid challenge to more accurately assess intravascular volume and right ventricular performance. There is no evidence that the use of a pulmonary artery (PA) catheter provides information useful during the early phases of resuscitation; its insertion and use may distract caregivers from other more important treatment priorities. A low (<10 torr) CVP in the presence of a low BP suggests intravascular volume depletion or an increased venous capacitance. In these patients, consider additional volume. Suspect cardiac dysfunction when the hypotension persists in the presence of sustained elevations (>15 torr) of CVP. In such cases, consider the need for inotropic support with dopamine, epinephrine, or norepinephrine.

F. Remember that trauma patients may have preexisting medical conditions. When a patient fails to respond to initial resuscitative measures, consider etiologies of hypotension not associated directly with the injury. Continue supportive measures, including volume expansion and pharmacological support of BP while definitive diagnostic and therapeutic measures proceed.

REFERENCES

1. American College of Surgeons: *Advanced trauma life support*, Chicago, 2004, American College of Surgeons.
2. *Prehospital trauma life support*, St Louis, 2005, Mosby.
3. Alam HB, Uy GB, Miller D, et al.: Comparative analysis of hemostatic agents in a swine model of lethal groin injury, *J Trauma* 54:1077–1082, 2003.
4. Alam HB, Chen Z, Jaskeille A, et al.: Application of a zeolite hemostatic agent achieves 100% survival in a lethal model of complex groin injury in swine, *J Trauma* 56:974–983, 2004.
5. Dutton RP, Mackenzie CF, Scalea TM: Hypotensive resuscitation during active hemorrhage: impact on in-hospital mortality, *J Trauma* 52:1141–1146, 2002.
6. Bickell WH, Wall MJ Jr, Pepe PE, et al.: Immediate versus delayed fluid resuscitation for hypotensive patients with penetrating torso injuries, *N Engl J Med* 331:1105–1109, 1994.
7. Kowalenko T, Stern S, Dronen S, et al.: Improved outcome with hypotensive resuscitation of uncontrolled hemorrhagic shock in a swine model, *J Trauma* 33:349–353, 1992.
8. Revell M, Porter K, Greaves I: Fluid resuscitation in prehospital trauma care: a consensus view, *Emerg Med J* 19:494–498, 2002.
9. SAFE Study Investigators: A comparison of albumin and saline for fluid resuscitation in the intensive care unit, *N Engl J Med* 350:2247–2256, 2004.
10. Weil MH, Tang W: Albumin versus crystalloid solutions for the critically ill and injured, *Crit Care Med* 32:2154–2155, 2004.
11. Schierhout G, Roberts I: Fluid resuscitation with colloid or crystalloid solutions in critically ill patients: a systematic review of randomised trials, *Br Med J* 316:961–964, 1998.
12. Rotstein OD: Novel strategies for immunomodulation after trauma: revisiting hypertonic saline as a resuscitation strategy for hemorrhagic shock, *J Trauma* 49:580–583, 2000.

HYPOTENSIVE, ACUTELY TRAUMATIZED PATIENT
(Cont'd from p 559)

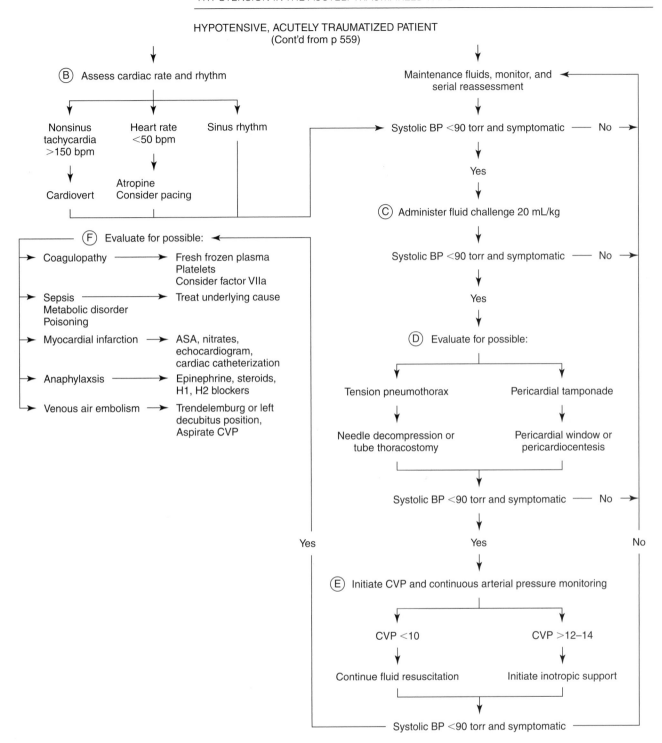

Hypoxemia in the Acutely Traumatized Patient

HAROLD D. CLINE, M.D.

FRED G. PANICO, M.D.

COLIN F. MACKENZIE, M.D., CH.B., F.C.C.M.

Hypoxemia may be caused by hypoxia (low inspired oxygen [O_2]), cardiac failure (stagnant hypoxemia), anemia (anemic hypoxemia), or toxins, such as cyanide or carbon monoxide (histotoxic hypoxemia).[1] There is increased awareness of hypoxemia because pulse oximetry provides a continuous display of O_2 saturation (SpO_2). SpO_2 is related to PaO_2, by the oxyhemoglobin dissociation curve, so that an SpO_2 of 90% is approximately equivalent to PaO_2 of 60 mm Hg under normal physiological conditions.[2] In this algorithm, hypoxemia is arbitrarily defined as a PaO_2 <60 mm Hg, because as PaO_2 decreases below 60 mm Hg, the O_2 dissociation curve is steeper, resulting in a large fall in SpO_2 for a small decrease in PaO_2. Clinical findings suggestive of hypoxemia in the trauma patient include confusion, combativeness, and cyanosis.[3]

A. Assess airway, breathing, and circulation (ABCs) immediately on presentation of the trauma patient. Is the airway patent? Check for the presence and equality of breath sounds. Shallow respirations and diminished respiratory rate require attention. Subcutaneous emphysema suggests airway rupture or pneumothorax. Jugular venous distension (JVD) may indicate a tension pneumothorax, cardiac failure, or pericardial tamponade. With tension pneumothorax, tracheal deviation occurs away from the pneumothorax. Initial assessment and vital signs take <1 minute. SpO_2 is helpful but is no substitute for good clinical acumen; in the presence of hypothermia, vasoconstriction, hypotension, or patient combativeness, the pulse oximeter readings may be unreliable. Order a chest x-ray (CXR), ABG, complete blood count (CBC), and toxicology screen.

B. Airway obstruction or other causes of hypoventilation may be manifest by tracheal tug or respiratory stridor caused by the presence of blood, tissue, vomitus, or a foreign body in the airway. Suspect direct trauma to the trachea if the voice is muffled, the overlying skin is bruised, or there is crepitus on palpation. Acute quadriplegia may result in hypoventilation and hypoxemia. If the level of consciousness is impaired by head injury or CNS depressant drugs, then central hypoventilation occurs, and upper airway reflexes may be blunted. Reversal of CNS depressants (e.g., with naloxone and flumazenil) may prevent the need for intubation. If the patient is already intubated, consider esophageal intubation as the cause of hypoxemia. The presence of a normal end-tidal carbon dioxide ($ETCO_2$) waveform for five consecutive breaths is the gold standard for confirmation of tracheal intubation.

C. Significant hemorrhage results in decreased perfusion to the respiratory center in the CNS. Initially, hyperventilation will occur, but with continued ongoing blood loss, hypoventilation and apnea ensue. Manage the airway and transfuse as needed. Blunt or penetrating chest trauma may also result in a decreased cardiac output (CO) caused by pericardial tamponade, tension pneumothorax, hemothorax, or cardiac contusion. Patients with preexisting coronary artery disease (CAD) may have decreased contractility. Relieve cardiac tamponade and tension pneumothorax and manage decreased CO with fluids and inotropic agents.

D. Intrapulmonary shunting may be caused by endobronchial intubation. After intubation, listen for breath sounds high in the axillae. Diminished breath sounds may indicate a pneumothorax or hemothorax, which may be resolved with chest tube placement. Endobronchial intubation requires withdrawal of the endotracheal tube (ETT). Bowel sounds in the chest may indicate ruptured diaphragm with intestinal herniation. Other causes of shunting include pulmonary edema, pulmonary contusion, or aspiration. All are managed with tracheal intubation and application of positive pressure. Pulmonary embolism is an additional cause of shunting.

E. In cases of house fires or inhalation of fumes from combustion engines or gas furnaces, carbon monoxide toxicity and cyanide poisoning may occur.[4] Beware, pulse oximetry overestimates the SpO_2 by interpreting the carboxy Hb form as OxyHb. Treat with 100% O_2; hyperbaric O_2 (HBO) is preferable when available.

F. The etiology of hypoxemia in the trauma patient is often multifactorial. The decision to treat hypoxemia is usually based on the clinical assessment of the patient within the first few moments of presentation. Laboratory and other tests, while augmenting decisions, are usually available after procedures are performed (e.g., intubation, chest tube placement, blood transfusion, or inotropic support). Even after such initial maneuvers have been performed, hypoxemia may still evolve during critical care management. If intubation, optimal mechanical ventilation, removal of secretions, and exclusion of airway pathology fail to resolve hypoxemia, evaluate for a cardiac cause. If hypoxemia remains resistant after optimization of cardiac function, additional technology, including extracorporeal membrane oxygenation (ECMO), nitric oxide (NO) inhalation, or extracorporeal lung assist (ECLA), may be employed.

HYPOXEMIA IN THE ACUTELY TRAUMATIZED PATIENT

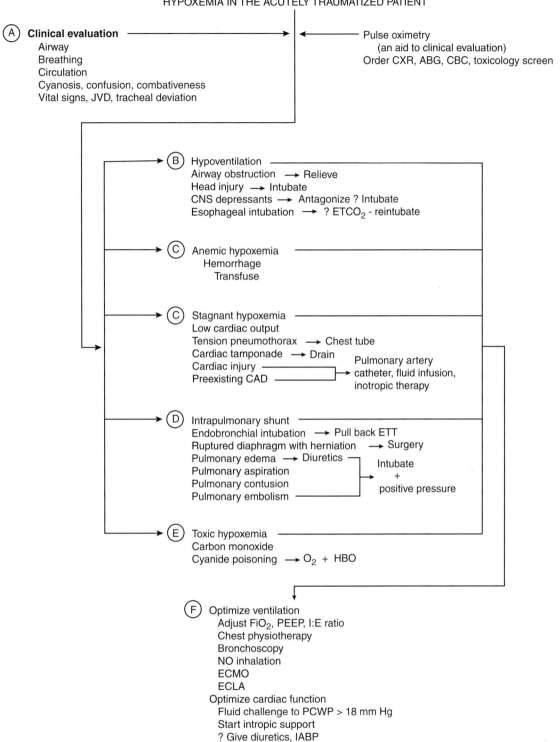

(A) **Clinical evaluation**
Airway
Breathing
Circulation
Cyanosis, confusion, combativeness
Vital signs, JVD, tracheal deviation

Pulse oximetry
(an aid to clinical evaluation)
Order CXR, ABG, CBC, toxicology screen

(B) Hypoventilation
Airway obstruction ⟶ Relieve
Head injury ⟶ Intubate
CNS depressants ⟶ Antagonize ? Intubate
Esophageal intubation ⟶ ? $ETCO_2$ - reintubate

(C) Anemic hypoxemia
Hemorrhage
Transfuse

(C) Stagnant hypoxemia
Low cardiac output
Tension pneumothorax ⟶ Chest tube
Cardiac tamponade ⟶ Drain
Cardiac injury
Preexisting CAD ⟶ Pulmonary artery catheter, fluid infusion, inotropic therapy

(D) Intrapulmonary shunt
Endobronchial intubation ⟶ Pull back ETT
Ruptured diaphragm with herniation ⟶ Surgery
Pulmonary edema ⟶ Diuretics
Pulmonary aspiration
Pulmonary contusion
Pulmonary embolism
Intubate
+
positive pressure

(E) Toxic hypoxemia
Carbon monoxide
Cyanide poisoning ⟶ O_2 + HBO

(F) Optimize ventilation
Adjust FiO_2, PEEP, I:E ratio
Chest physiotherapy
Bronchoscopy
NO inhalation
ECMO
ECLA
Optimize cardiac function
Fluid challenge to PCWP > 18 mm Hg
Start intropic support
? Give diuretics, IABP

REFERENCES

1. Guyton AC: Respiratory insufficiency: pathophysiology, diagnosis, oxygen therapy. In: Guyton AC, editor: *Textbook of medical physiology*, ed 11, Philadelphia, 2005, W.B. Saunders.
2. Lumb A: Oxygen. In: *Nunn's applied respiratory physiology*, ed 5, Oxford, 1999, Butterworth-Heinemann, Linarce House, Jordan Hill.
3. Carmona RM, Trunkey DD: Examination and evaluation of the shock patient. In: Hardaway RM, editor: *Shock: the reversible stage of dying*. Littleton CO, 1988, PSG Publishing.
4. Lambert Y, Carli PA, Cantineau JP: Smoke inhalation injury. In: Grande CM, editor: *Textbook of trauma anesthesia and critical care*, St. Louis, 1993, Mosby-Year Book.

REMOTE LOCATIONS

Anesthesia for Electroconvulsive Therapy (ECT)

General Anesthesia in Dentistry

Magnetic Resonance Imaging (MRI)

Office-Based Anesthesia

Anesthesia for Electroconvulsive Therapy (ECT)

COREY COLLINS, D.O.

Electroconvulsive therapy (ECT) remains an effective but historically maligned therapy with an increasing number of indications.[1,2] Despite increased attention among researchers, the mechanism of action remains elusive, as has the most effective mode and dosage of delivery. Advances in anesthetic management of ECT patients have decreased the incidence of fractures, hyperkalemia, and death, yet morbidity is still significant in up to 50 to 65% of patients.[3] Life-threatening morbidity is usually due to pulmonary or cardiac events (myocardial ischemia, aspiration, or bronchospasm). Confusion, amnesia, headaches, and poorly controlled cardiovascular responses occur much more frequently. Anesthesia goals include minimizing morbidity, airway management, and optimizing seizure duration. Therapy typically includes 9 to 12 ECT sessions delivered two to three times per week as an inpatient, although in many centers outpatient therapy is common. The majority of patients are women over 55, however, increasingly adolescent and young adults patients receive treatment. ECT is effective and considered safe in pregnant patients.

A. Clinical evaluation requires careful consideration of coexisting diseases. As most patients are elderly, the pathophysiologic response to the seizure must be anticipated. Profound parasympathetically induced bradycardia followed by sympathetic discharge and resultant hypertension (HTN) and tachycardia may cause greatly increased myocardial oxygen demands. ECT causes left ventricular (LV) dysfunction and acute ECG changes. Preictal beta blockade ameliorates the catecholaminergic surge but may decrease seizure duration. Pheochromocytoma may be one of the only contraindications to ECT. Intracranial pathology, such as aneurysm, masses, or intracranial hypertension, is a relative contraindication but adequate preparation and tight BP control has been shown to minimize morbidity.

B. Certain medications have been associated with profound hypertension after ECT. monoamine oxidase inhibitors (MAO-I) medications should be withheld for 2 to 3 weeks, although safe ECT courses have been reported without interruption of the medication. Use of narcotics, including meperidine, cocaine, and opioids, should be excluded. Tricyclic antidepressants have intrinsic anticholinergic activity and may contribute to dysrhythmia and hypotension.

C. Airway evaluation is critical as pulmonary and dental morbidity is significant. Mask anesthetics are most common. If there is aspiration risk, consideration of endotracheal intubation is warranted. There are reports of successful ECT series in pregnancy using the laryngeal mask airway (LMA). In one report, the ProSeal® LMA was used for a series of ECT treatments in a parturient.[4] Because the patient's masseter muscles contract strongly with the ECT stimulus, pay particular attention to dental protection; use of standard oral airway devices may result in broken or avulsed incisors.

D. Use standard American Society of Anesthesiologists (ASA) monitors. Many ECT units display EEG information to document the grand mal seizure. Resuscitation equipment and a suction device must be immediately available. Insert an IV line. Premedications to consider include anticholinergics or antisialagogues, usually glycopyrrolate 0.05 mg/kg to minimize secretions and parasympathetically mediated bradycardia, heart block, or sinus arrest. Beta blockade, usually esmolol for its short action, is considered in patients with ischemic heart disease. Nitroglycerine and calcium channel blockers have been shown to minimize HTN. Preoxygenation is necessary as apnea is expected during the seizure. Also, patients may have longer seizures if pretreated with methyxanthines, usually as IV caffeine.

E. Induction can be accomplished with a number of agents. Methohexital provides excellent anesthesia and has long been the agent of choice. Alternate agents are propofol or etomidate. Sodium thiopental and ketamine increase the seizure threshold and should be avoided. Succinylcholine (SCC), unless contraindicated, is the relaxant of choice. An extremity tourniquet permits a visual monitor of tonic-clonic activity. The ultrashort acting opioids remifentanil (1 μg/kg intravenously) and alfentanil (10 μg/kg intravenously) have been shown to permit lower doses of propofol and result in longer seizures. Positive-pressure ventilation is provided until spontaneous respiration resumes. Postictal analgesia with ketorolac, amnesia with midazolam, or antihypertensive and tachycardia therapy with beta blockade may be considered.

F. Confusion, agitation, and headaches are the most common side effects. Patients should be monitored for hemodynamic derangements and treated as necessary.

REFERENCES

1. Ding Z, White PF: Anesthesia for electroconvulsive therapy, *Anesth Analg* 94:1351–1364, 2002.
2. Glass RM: Electroconvulsive therapy: time to bring it out of the shadows, *JAMA* 285:134–1348, 2001.
3. Tecoult E., Nathan N: Morbidity in electroconvulsive therapy, *Eur J Anesth* 18:511–518, 2001.
4. Brown NI, Mack PF, Mitera DM, et al.: Use of the ProSeal™ laryngeal mask airway in a pregnant patient with a difficult airway during electroconvulsive therapy, *Br J Anesth* 91:752–754, 2003.

Patient Scheduled for ELECTROCONVULSIVE THERAPY

(A) **Clinical evaluation** ──────────────→   ←─── ECG, other parameters as indicated
Elevated ICP, IOP
Coronary artery disease
Cardiac pacemaker function
Hypertension
Beta-blockers, antidepressants

(B) MAOIs

Discontinue   No MAOIs ──────────→
MAOIs for
2–3 wk if feasible ──────────────────→

(C) **Assess Airway**

Mask   Intubate

(D) **Premedication,**   ──→ No benzodiazepines
Preparation,
Monitoring
                           ──→ Isolated limb?

(E) **Induction of Anesthesia**
                ┌ O$_2$
                ├ Defasciculate
                ├ Anticholinergic
                ├ Methohexital
                └ Succinylcholine

(F) ECT

No seizure   Seizure ──→ Hypertension

Repeat ECT   Beta-blockers
                                 Nitroglycerin
                                 Calcium channel blockers

Recovery

General Anesthesia in Dentistry

W. CORBETT HOLMGREEN, M.D., D.D.S.

Practitioners of oral and maxillofacial surgery, pediatric dentistry, and adult general restorative dentistry frequently use general anesthesia. In major oral surgery procedures and most restorative procedures, nasotracheal intubation is preferred because it allows best access to the oral cavity and the ability to assess physiological dental occlusion. Some minor procedures may not require tracheal intubation.

A. Evaluate airway patency and determine whether management and intubation of the airway are likely to be difficult. Maxillofacial emergencies, such as orofacial infections (e.g., Ludwig's angina), may require immediate airway evaluation and securing by intubation or tracheostomy. In maxillofacial trauma cases, look also for full stomach, CSF rhinorrhea, and concomitant injuries. Remember that intraoral hemorrhage may result in the patient's swallowing large amounts of blood, which constitutes a full stomach.

B. Once the nasal tube is in place, cut the tube and insert an acute-angle connector (unless a nasal RAE tube is used). Secure the anesthetic delivery tubes to the patient's head with adhesive tape to minimize tracheal trauma caused by frequent movement of the head during a lengthy procedure. Avoid pressure on the nose and ears, which may result in necrosis. An oropharyngeal pack is usually placed by the dentist to prevent debris from collecting in the supraglottic region. It is imperative that the anesthetist witness the removal of this "throat pack," especially if the patient is placed into maxillo-mandibular fixation (MMF). Perform direct laryngoscopy with suctioning if an excessive amount of foreign material appears to be present.

C. Common challenges of major oral and maxillofacial surgical procedures are airway management and excessive blood loss. Suspected difficult intubations may require awake intubation or elective tracheostomy. A slight head-up tilt (which increases venous return) and controlled hypotensive anesthesia can reduce blood loss. Extubate patients in MMF only when they are well recovered from the anesthetic and then only with wire cutters and hemostats present at the bedside. (Should the need arise to release the MMF, remove the cut wires or elastic bands from the oral cavity in their entirety.)

D. Complications are likely to be related to airway compromise. The endotracheal tube (ETT) may be kinked or occluded by clotted blood or mucous secretions. Sublingual emphysema has also been reported.

E. Deep IV sedation or general anesthesia is used for routine oral surgical procedures in dental offices throughout the United States on an outpatient basis.[1] These procedures usually can be accomplished within 15 to 20 minutes, often using a nasal mask and without intubation. The patient is placed in a semisupine position in the dental chair. Once anesthesia has been induced either via inhalation or intravenously, the oral cavity is kept open with a rubber mouth prop (obviating the need for muscle relaxants). Immediately after induction, the dentist administers a local anesthetic agent (usually containing epinephrine) to the surgical site(s). The use of local anesthesia provides a significant analgesic component to the anesthetic as well as reducing the anesthetic requirements and providing pain relief during the immediate postoperative period.[2] The vasoconstrictor assists in providing hemostasis. Be aware of the total dose of local anesthetic and vasoconstrictor. A thin, dry gauze pack is inserted just posterior to the dental arch. This "throat screen" is in contradistinction to the more bulky oropharyngeal pack used in dental patients being intubated.

F. The choice of induction agents and other anesthetic drugs has an increased importance for the outpatient, because a prolonged recovery time is undesirable. In preparing a tooth to receive a crown, dentists occasionally use a gingival retraction cord impregnated with high concentrations of epinephrine. Because the total dose of epinephrine absorbed from this cord is difficult to quantitate, the use of an inhalational agent that sensitizes the myocardium to catecholamines is discouraged.[3]

REFERENCES

1. Allen GD, *Dental anesthesia and analgesia*, ed 3, Toronto, 1984 BC Decker.
2. Brown RS, Rhodus NL: Epinephrine and local anesthesia revisited, *Oral Surg Oral Med Oral Pathol Oral Radiol Endod* 100 (4): 401–408, 2005.
3. Hilley MD, Milam SB, Giesecke AH Jr, et al.: Fatality associated with the combined use of halothane and gingival retraction cord, *Anesthesiology* 60:587, 1984.

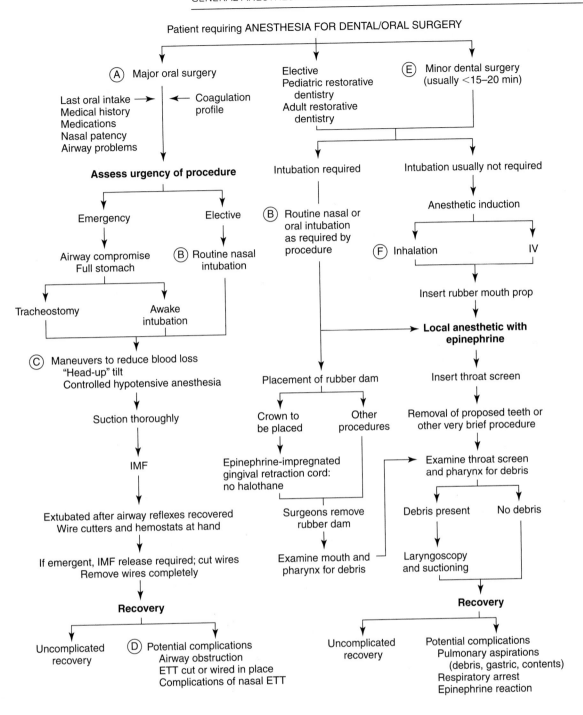

Patient requiring ANESTHESIA FOR DENTAL/ORAL SURGERY

(A) Major oral surgery

Last oral intake → ← Coagulation
Medical history   profile
Medications
Nasal patency
Airway problems

Assess urgency of procedure

Emergency   Elective

Airway compromise   (B) Routine nasal
Full stomach   intubation

Tracheostomy   Awake
                    intubation

(C) Maneuvers to reduce blood loss
     "Head-up" tilt
     Controlled hypotensive anesthesia

Suction thoroughly

IMF

Extubated after airway reflexes recovered
Wire cutters and hemostats at hand

If emergent, IMF release required; cut wires
Remove wires completely

Recovery

Uncomplicated   (D) Potential complications
recovery   Airway obstruction
                      ETT cut or wired in place
                      Complications of nasal ETT

Elective
Pediatric restorative
  dentistry
Adult restorative
  dentistry

Intubation required

(B) Routine nasal or
     oral intubation
     as required by
     procedure

Placement of rubber dam

Crown to   Other
be placed   procedures

Epinephrine-impregnated
gingival retraction cord:
no halothane

Surgeons remove
rubber dam

Examine mouth and
pharynx for debris

(E) Minor dental surgery
     (usually <15–20 min)

Intubation usually not required

Anesthetic induction

(F) Inhalation   IV

Insert rubber mouth prop

**Local anesthetic with
epinephrine**

Insert throat screen

Removal of proposed teeth or
other very brief procedure

Examine throat screen
and pharynx for debris

Debris present   No debris

Laryngoscopy
and suctioning

Recovery

Uncomplicated   Potential complications
recovery   Pulmonary aspirations
                        (debris, gastric, contents)
                      Respiratory arrest
                      Epinephrine reaction

Magnetic Resonance Imaging (MRI)

KIMBERLY D. MILHOAN, M.D.

Magnetic resonance imaging (MRI) combines static and time-varying magnetic fields with radiofrequency pulses to produce detailed images of the body.[1] Given the absence of ionizing radiation, there are no known biological hazards of MRI.[1,2] During MRI, the patient is enclosed in the bore of the magnet, must remain completely still to ensure good image quality, and is inaccessible. Sedation or general anesthesia may be indicated in pediatric patients or critically ill or anxious adults. Unique safety concerns largely relate to the presence of ferromagnetic objects or equipment, noise, and use of contrast agents.[2,3]

A. Access to the MRI control room or scanner magnet room itself is strictly controlled by MRI personnel and granted only after successfully passing a MRI safety screening process.[3] Implanted ferromagnetic devices may move or dislodge during MRI, causing image distortion, or, more importantly, injury or death to the patient.[1–4] Potential hazardous items are too numerous to list but include aneurysmal clips, prosthetic heart valves, tissue expanders with metallic ports, implantable infusion pumps, and cochlear implants. Metallic-based substances, such as permanent make-up or tattoos, can produce local skin irritation.[5,6] Cardiac pacemakers may be switched to a synchronous mode, completely inhibited, or pace the heart at the frequency of the applied imaging pulses.[4] No one with a pacemaker or ICD should be allowed in the magnet room.

B. After the preoperative assessment and MRI safety screening process, decide whether to proceed with sedation or general anesthesia. Fourteen to 20% of adults require sedation due to claustrophobia or anxiety.[2] Most can be managed with oral or IV benzodiazepines, although a propofol infusion can be considered. If there are any concerns regarding potential airway compromise or instability of the patient, general anesthesia, with a secured airway, may be required. Most pediatric patients will require some form of anesthetic. Agents used for pediatric sedation for MRI include oral chloral hydrate; rectal methohexital; IM or IV ketamine; oral, rectal, or IV pentobarbital; and oral and IV midazolam (although this agent alone is not successful). Propofol infusion with maintenance of spontaneous respiration can also be considered. Preterm neonates, neonates, and children with obstructive sleep apnea or adenotonsillar hypertrophy and other upper airway pathology or malformation are likely to need a secured airway. Laryngeal mask airways (LMAs) are a potential alternative to endotracheal intubation in the appropriate patient. Utilizing an anesthesia machine allows for the administration of inhalational agents and permits inhalational inductions in pediatric patients. Anesthesia machines in the MRI suite should be modified to be nonferromagnetic, positioned outside the magnet room and connected to the patient with extension tubing, or securely bolted to the wall in the magnet room to prevent injury. In the absence of an anesthesia machine, total intravenous anesthesia (TIVA) can be provided. Patients with asthma, allergic respiratory histories, prior iodinated or gadolinium-based contrast reactions are at risk for adverse reactions if they are to be given an IV contrast agent.[3] These patients should, at minimum, be monitored more closely. Consideration can be given to premedicating them with corticosteroids or antihistamines.

C. Have a traveling cart stocked with anesthesia equipment. Emergency resuscitation equipment and assistance should be immediately available.

D. A serious and preventable patient risk is projectile ferromagnetic objects. All patients and personnel should be inspected for ferromagnetic objects, such as pens, clamps, scissors, stethoscopes, nonlithium batteries, and standard medical gas cylinders, before entering the magnet room.[2]

E. The throughput of the MRI suite should be minimally affected by the requirement for anesthesia. Sedation or general anesthesia is initiated in a holding area outside the magnet room while the preceding study is still being performed. This practice will also decrease the risk of ferrous objects being brought into the magnet room. Due to the noise produced by the MRI scanner, earplugs should be placed in all patients. MRI-compatible monitors and equipment are preferable. Use of a standard ECG monitor can cause distortion of the image.[2] Wire leads are also an electrical shock and burn risk for the patient. A nonferrous or fiberoptically cabled pulse oximeter should be used. A sidestream capnograph with a long sampling line is important for monitoring of ventilation, anesthetic gas concentration, and circuit disconnection. A rubber precordial or an esophageal stethoscope may be used, but noise generated during the MRI is louder than heart and breath sounds. Oscillometric noninvasive blood pressure monitoring is not affected by magnetic fields. Fiberoptic systems used with invasive BP monitors are also successful.

F. If airway compromise or cardiac instability occurs during the MRI, remove the patient from the scanner for safe resuscitation and accurate monitoring.

G. Transport patients to the PACU in a safe manner (maintain intubated, or awake and extubated with intact airway reflexes). Use appropriate monitoring during transport and have resuscitation drugs and airway equipment available.

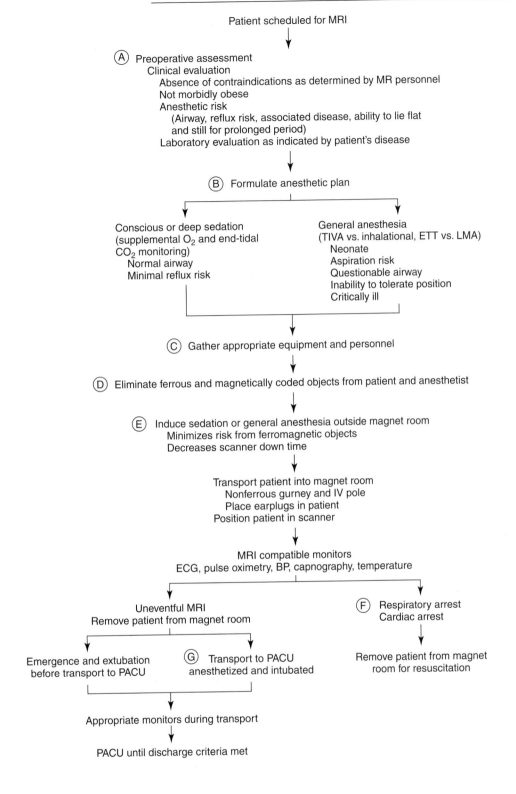

Patient scheduled for MRI

Ⓐ Preoperative assessment
   Clinical evaluation
      Absence of contraindications as determined by MR personnel
   Not morbidly obese
   Anesthetic risk
      (Airway, reflux risk, associated disease, ability to lie flat
      and still for prolonged period)
   Laboratory evaluation as indicated by patient's disease

Ⓑ Formulate anesthetic plan

Conscious or deep sedation   General anesthesia
(supplemental O₂ and end-tidal   (TIVA vs. inhalational, ETT vs. LMA)
CO₂ monitoring)   Neonate
   Normal airway   Aspiration risk
   Minimal reflux risk   Questionable airway
                                      Inability to tolerate position
                                      Critically ill

Ⓒ Gather appropriate equipment and personnel

Ⓓ Eliminate ferrous and magnetically coded objects from patient and anesthetist

Ⓔ Induce sedation or general anesthesia outside magnet room
   Minimizes risk from ferromagnetic objects
   Decreases scanner down time

Transport patient into magnet room
   Nonferrous gurney and IV pole
   Place earplugs in patient
Position patient in scanner

MRI compatible monitors
ECG, pulse oximetry, BP, capnography, temperature

Uneventful MRI   Ⓕ Respiratory arrest
Remove patient from magnet room   Cardiac arrest

Emergence and extubation   Ⓖ Transport to PACU   Remove patient from magnet
before transport to PACU   anesthetized and intubated   room for resuscitation

Appropriate monitors during transport

PACU until discharge criteria met

REFERENCES

1. Berger A: How does it work? Magnetic resonance imaging, *Br Med J* 324:35, 2002.
2. Gooden CK, Dilos B: Anesthesia for magnetic resonance imaging, *Int Anesthesiol Clin* 41:29, 2003.
3. Kanal E, Borgstede JP, Barkovich A, et al.: American College of Radiology white paper on MR safety, *Am J Roentgenol* 178:1335, 2002.
4. Goldschlager N, Epstein A, Friedman P, et al.: Environmental and drug effects on patients with pacemakers and implantable cardioverter/defibrillators: A practical guide to patient treatment, *Arch Intern Med* 161:649, 2001.
5. Wagle WA, Smith M: Tattoo-induced skin burn during MR imaging, *Am J Roentgenol* 174:1795, 2000.
6. Tope WD, Shellock FG: Magnetic resonance imaging and permanent cosmetics (tattoos): survey of complications and adverse events, *J Magn Reson Imaging* 15:180, 2002.

Office-Based Anesthesia

SALLY COMBEST, M.D.

Office-based anesthesia is a rapidly growing segment of anesthesiology practice, comprising 20 to 25% of all outpatient surgery in the United States. The American Society of Anesthesiologists (ASA) published guidelines in 1999, reaffirmed in October 2004, to help anesthesiologists provide safe care in a less familiar environment. Less invasive surgical techniques and improved anesthesia techniques, monitoring, and medication allow greater flexibility and a more rapid recovery. Some third-party payers' payments to surgeons favor office-based practice.[1] Patients prefer increased privacy, shorter stays, and decreased expense. Compared with traditional practice sites, office-based anesthesia may lack peer review, quality assurance mechanisms, risk management, or overnight facilities for postoperative care. Overdose of local anesthesia (especially during tumescent local anesthesia used in plastic surgery), mismanagement of fluid administration, complications of sedation or general anesthesia, use of unqualified personnel in the care of patients, and the lack of adequate monitors, emergent medications, or equipment have been cited as contributing factors to reported serious adverse outcomes. The ASA Closed Claim Project revealed that, as compared to ambulatory surgery claims, office-based anesthesia claims had a higher severity of claims (64% for death), a higher percentage of injuries deemed probably preventable by better monitoring, a higher percentage of the claims judged to be due to substandard care, and the claims resulted in greater payment amounts.[2] Many states regulate office-performed procedures with requirements for accreditation, mandatory reporting of untoward events, credentialing, equipment, medications, and conduct of care. Accreditation organizations for offices include the Joint Commission on the Accreditation of Healthcare Organizations (JCAHO), the American Association for the Accreditation of Ambulatory Surgical Facilities (AAAASF), and the American Association of Ambulatory Health Centers (AAAHC), which also accredits itinerant, office-based anesthesiologists' practices. The American Medical Association's (AMA) "Office-Based Surgery Core Principles"[3] and the Federation of State Medical Boards' "Report of the Special Committee on Outpatient (Office-Based) Surgery"[4] provide guidelines for setting standards for office-based surgery and anesthesia.

A. Before expanding practice into the office arena, investigate the state laws that govern this practice. Will your malpractice carrier cover the provision of care in the office setting?

B. The individual performing the procedure should have privileges for those same procedures in a local hospital or surgery center. The health care provider or dentist's office may range from being a simple medical office to a state-of-the-art, free-standing surgery center with a PACU and expanded staffing. Regardless of the scenario, there should be written policies regarding preoperative laboratory studies, patient selection, NPO status, discharge criteria, care of patients with latex allergy, emergency protocols for cardiopulmonary emergencies, and other internal and external disasters, such as fire. There should be ready access to advanced cardiac life support (ACLS) algorithms and pediatric drug dosages if pediatric cases are to be performed. There must be an adequate supply of oxygen (O_2), suction capability, an apparatus to deliver positive-pressure ventilation (which may consist only of an AMBU apparatus), and at least basic airway management equipment consisting of appropriately sized endotracheal tubes (ETTs), laryngoscopes, and nasal and oral airways. Depending on the type of cases to be done, an anesthesia machine may not be necessary (potential cost savings). One must also consider the support personnel available in the office setting: If cases are to be performed in a simple office setting, there is less likelihood that the support people will be educated in the management of malignant hyperthermia (MH) and thus, of limited help during the crisis. A defibrillator and standard monitoring of ECG, pulse oximetry, and noninvasive BP is required. All equipment must be inspected according to manufacturer's specifications with standard-of-care features and have a backup power source. There should also be a designated hospital for emergency transfers and an emergency medical services (EMS) transfer agreement. The anesthesiologist and health care provider or dentist must have an understanding of who will provide the equipment, supplies, and personnel to meet the obligations of patient care, including postoperative recovery. Again, this can vary from one practice to another, with some anesthesiologists providing a wide-ranging portion of the monitoring equipment, medications, IV supplies, and so on. Record-keeping should also be maintained: anesthesia preoperative evaluation and anesthesia records, meeting discharge criteria, postoperative and home-care instructions, consent forms, and forms to track pharmaceuticals (especially controlled substances).[5]

C. All patients should undergo a history and physical with review of laboratory studies and assignment of an ASA class. The anesthetic plan with its risks and benefits should be discussed with the patient.[6]

Patient considered for OFFICE-BASED ANESTHESIA

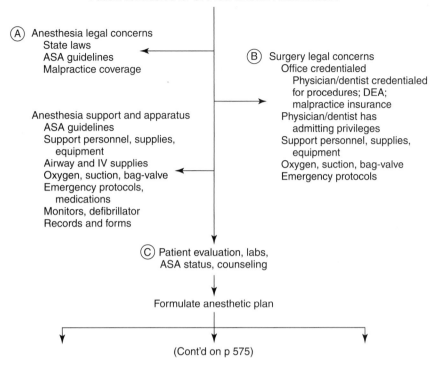

(A) Anesthesia legal concerns
  State laws
  ASA guidelines
  Malpractice coverage

(B) Surgery legal concerns
  Office credentialed
    Physician/dentist credentialed
    for procedures; DEA;
    malpractice insurance
  Physician/dentist has
    admitting privileges
  Support personnel, supplies,
    equipment
  Oxygen, suction, bag-valve
  Emergency protocols

Anesthesia support and apparatus
  ASA guidelines
  Support personnel, supplies,
    equipment
  Airway and IV supplies
  Oxygen, suction, bag-valve
  Emergency protocols,
    medications
  Monitors, defibrillator
  Records and forms

(C) Patient evaluation, labs,
  ASA status, counseling

Formulate anesthetic plan

(Cont'd on p 575)

D. Select a safe technique with goal of prompt recovery. Limit IV fluids; large volumes are not indicated for many healthy, elective procedures, and patients usually can resume oral fluid consumption quickly. Minimize opioid use and use local anesthesia for pain control; opioids increase risk of depressed laryngeal reflexes, respiratory depression necessitating supplemental O_2, and postoperative nausea and vomiting (PONV). General anesthesia can be performed with ventilation by mask, laryngeal mask airway (LMA) or ETT.

E. Spinal and epidural blocks are possibly less desirable due to the risk of delayed recovery of motor, sensory and autonomic functions, and postdural puncture headache (PDPH). Peripheral regional anesthesia techniques provide anesthesia or postoperative pain control after general anesthesia.

F. Often local anesthesia is used with monitored anesthesia care. This allows rapid recovery, postoperative pain relief, and a low incidence of side effects that could delay recovery. Propofol is commonly used because of its favorable recovery profile and low risk of PONV. It also is not a trigger for MH and can be used for varying levels of sedation or general anesthesia. Ketamine in conjunction with versed or propofol facilitates the injection of local anesthesia by providing profound analgesia for 10 to 20 minutes[7]; it also intensifies laryngeal reflexes and is an antagonist of NMDA receptors, an important component of pain processing.

G. Postoperative care of office-based anesthesia patients focuses on hemodynamic stability, return to baseline mental status, pain control, and prevention or treatment of PONV. PONV prophylaxis is based on risk factors (gender, age, and nonsmoker), and surgical procedure, which may have an increased risk of PONV.

H. Discharge to the care of a competent adult with home care instructions, review of potential complications, phone numbers for questions, and the nearest treatment facility in case of emergencies. Consider contacting the patient by phone later in the day or postoperative day 1 to follow recuperative progress.

REFERENCES

1. Chung: Office-based anesthesiology: can it be done safely? European Society of Anesthesiologists Refresher Courses, 2002.
2. Domino KB: Office-based anesthesia: lessons learned from the closed claims project, *ASA Newsletter* 65 (6):9–11, 15, 2001.
3. American Medical Association House of Delegates: Office-based surgery core principles, 2003.
4. Federation of State Medical Boards: Report of the special committee on outpatient (office-based) surgery, 2002.
5. American Society of Anesthesiologists House of Delegates: Guidelines for office-based anesthesia, 2004.
6. American Society of Anesthesiologists House of Delegates: Documentation of anesthesia care, 2003.
7. Friedberg, BL: Profofol-ketamine technique: dissociative anesthesia for office surgery (a five year review of 1264 cases), *Aesthetic Plast Surg*, 23:70–75, 1999.

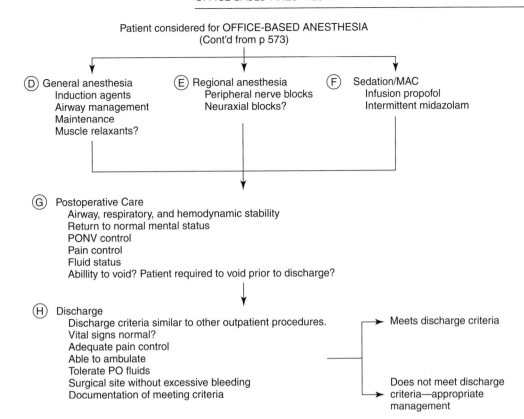

Patient considered for OFFICE-BASED ANESTHESIA
(Cont'd from p 573)

(D) General anesthesia
Induction agents
Airway management
Maintenance
Muscle relaxants?

(E) Regional anesthesia
Peripheral nerve blocks
Neuraxial blocks?

(F) Sedation/MAC
Infusion propofol
Intermittent midazolam

(G) Postoperative Care
Airway, respiratory, and hemodynamic stability
Return to normal mental status
PONV control
Pain control
Fluid status
Abillity to void? Patient required to void prior to discharge?

(H) Discharge
Discharge criteria similar to other outpatient procedures.
Vital signs normal?
Adequate pain control
Able to ambulate
Tolerate PO fluids
Surgical site without excessive bleeding
Documentation of meeting criteria

Meets discharge criteria

Does not meet discharge
criteria—appropriate
management

POSTOPERATIVE MANAGEMENT

ACUTE POSTOPERATIVE ANALGESIC
MANAGEMENT

POSTOPERATIVE NAUSEA AND VOMITING
(PONV)

DELAYED AWAKENING OR DELIRIUM

POSTOPERATIVE HYPOTENSION

POSTOPERATIVE HYPERTENSION (HTN)

PROLONGED POSTOPERATIVE APNEA

WEANING FROM MECHANICAL VENTILATION

NEUROLOGIC SEQUELAE FOLLOWING
REGIONAL ANESTHESIA

PERIOPERATIVE SEIZURES

POSTOPERATIVE OLIGURIA

POSTDURAL PUNCTURE HEADACHE (PDPH)

POSTOPERATIVE HEPATIC DYSFUNCTION
(PHD)

SALIVARY GLAND SWELLING

DENTAL INJURIES ASSOCIATED WITH
GENERAL ANESTHESIA

MANAGEMENT OF A NEEDLESTICK

Acute Postoperative Analgesic Management

LYNDA T. WELLS, M.D.

Over half of postoperative patients report moderate to severe pain. In general, health care providers underprescribe analgesic regimens and nursing staff undermedicate. World Health Organization (WHO) guidelines on pain management recommend oral administration when possible, titration of drug doses to effect, scheduling dosing to maintain a constant level of analgesia with additional medications available for breakthrough pain as needed, dosing intervals customized to each patient's needs (e.g., longer in elderly patients, shorter in young children), and treatment of side effects. These guidelines have been endorsed by the American Pain Society (APS), the United States Department of Health and Human Services (USDHHS), and the Joint Commission on the Accreditation of Healthcare Organizations (JCAHO). Pain is a complex emotion with physical (nociceptive), emotional, psychological, social, and spiritual elements.[1–5] Relief of anxiety and physical pain are the mainstays of acute pain management. Management strategies can utilize nonpharmacological or pharmacological analgesic therapies.

A. Select analgesic regimens according to the anticipated severity and duration of the pain, the patient's physical status, available routes of administration, and the postoperative management plan (e.g., inpatient versus outpatient). Establish rapport and provide a supportive environment to alleviate anxiety. Consider use of preemptive analgesia to reduce operative anesthetic requirements and decrease postoperative pain in the early and late postoperative periods.

B. Provide appropriate nonpharmacological interventions. Cryotherapy can be applied intraoperatively to specific nerves. Hypnosis requires prior training of the patient and practitioner.

C. Consider nonsteroidal anti-inflammatory drugs (NSAIDs) for preemptive and postoperative analgesia. NSAIDs are equianalgesic at equivalent doses; select specific agent based on side effects, allergic potential, and preexisting organ function (e.g., renal function). Provide IV opioid via intermittent bolus or patient-controlled analgesia (PCA). PCA provides better analgesia, is more cost effective, and is associated with greater patient satisfaction. Select the opioid based on its duration of action, presence or absence of metabolites, and side effect profile. Opioids cause gut hypomotility and constipation in therapeutic doses; therefore, consider a bowel hygiene regimen. Other unwanted effects include nausea, dysphoria, respiratory depression, pruritus, and urinary retention. Avoid IM injections, because they are painful and drug absorption is unpredictable. Transdermal administration (e.g., fentanyl patches) is not suitable for acute postoperative pain management; it takes 12 to 18 hours to achieve therapeutic blood concentrations. Neuraxial opioid administration provides analgesia without autonomic, sensory, or motor blockade. Unwanted effects include pruritus, nausea, urinary retention, and respiratory depression. Partial agonists (e.g., buprenorphine) and mixed agonist-antagonists (e.g., nalbuphine) may be used as sole analgesics, but their utility is limited by an analgesic ceiling and antagonism to full agonist opioids if these should be required. Local anesthetics provide excellent intraoperative and postoperative analgesia with low morbidity. They can be applied topically (e.g., EMLA® cream), by infiltration into skin or joints, or via nerve block, plexus block, and neuraxis block. Their duration of action can be prolonged by the addition of adjunctive drugs (e.g., clonidine) and by placing a catheter and administering the local anesthetic by continuous infusion or repeated bolus dosing. Do not exceed maximum recommended local anesthetic doses. Inhalation of nitrous oxide in oxygen by fitted facemask provides excellent analgesia within 30 seconds. Consider this mode of analgesia for short procedures such as dressing changes, closed reduction of fractures, bone marrow aspiration, either alone or combined with other analgesic interventions (e.g., local anesthetics). Do not exceed a nitrous oxide in oxygen concentration of 70%. Nonanesthesiologists should not exceed a nitrous oxide concentration of 50%. Monitor adequacy of oxygenation and scavenge waste gases to avoid pollution. Adjuncts include ketamine, an anesthetic drug that also has analgesic effects. The analgesic dose (0.2 mg/kg IV) is approximately one fifth the anesthetic induction dose. Ketamine is associated with increased production of airway secretions and dysphoria. To avoid these effects, administer ketamine in combination with low doses of an antisialogogue and a benzodiazepine, barbiturate, or opioid.

D. Acute pain services can be extremely helpful in optimizing analgesic regimens. Consider consultation in any patient who has acute pain that persists at or above 5/10 VAS for greater than 24 hours and who expresses a desire for better pain relief. Special populations (e.g., opioid addicts, nonverbal patients) can be challenging, because therapy is guided by accurate self-report. When absent or unreliable, use patient function as a guide to appropriate analgesic therapy. If pain is limiting function, increased analgesia will improve function. If pain is not limiting function, increased analgesia will cause functional deterioration.

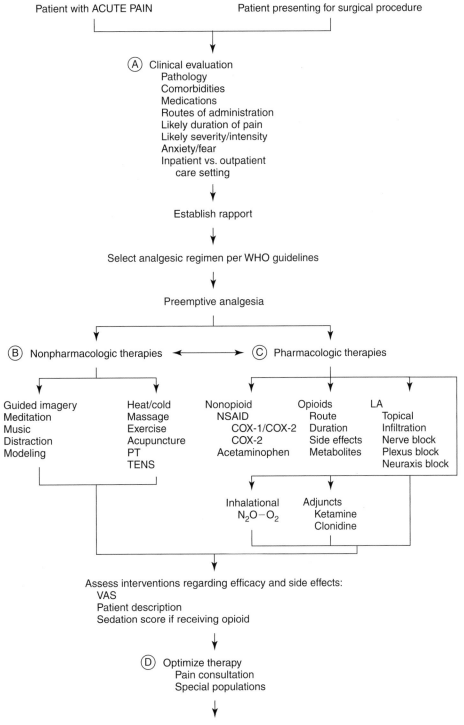

Patient with acute postoperative pain

Patient with ACUTE PAIN   Patient presenting for surgical procedure

(A) Clinical evaluation
        Pathology
        Comorbidities
        Medications
        Routes of administration
        Likely duration of pain
        Likely severity/intensity
        Anxiety/fear
        Inpatient vs. outpatient
            care setting

Establish rapport

Select analgesic regimen per WHO guidelines

Preemptive analgesia

(B) Nonpharmacologic therapies ←→ (C) Pharmacologic therapies

Guided imagery	Heat/cold	Nonopioid	Opioids	LA
Meditation	Massage	NSAID	Route	Topical
Music	Exercise	COX-1/COX-2	Duration	Infiltration
Distraction	Acupuncture	COX-2	Side effects	Nerve block
Modeling	PT	Acetaminophen	Metabolites	Plexus block
	TENS			Neuraxis block

Inhalational   Adjuncts
N_2O-O_2 Ketamine
                     Clonidine

Assess interventions regarding efficacy and side effects:
    VAS
    Patient description
    Sedation score if receiving opioid

(D) Optimize therapy
        Pain consultation
        Special populations

Goal = function not limited by pain or side effects
Usually correlates with VAS pain score ≤3/10
Multimodal approach usually superior to monotherapies

REFERENCES

1. American Pain Society: *Principles of analgesic use in the treatment of acute pain and cancer pain,* ed 5, Glenview, IL, 2004, American Pain Society.
2. Agency for Health Care Policy and Research: *Acute pain management in infants, children and adolescents,* Clinical Practice Guideline No. 1, AHCPR Publication No. 92-0020, Rockville, MD, 1992, Agency for Health Care Policy and Research.
3. Agency for Health Care Policy and Research: *Management of cancer pain: clinical practice guideline,* No. 9. AHCPR Publication No. 94-0592., Rockville, MD, 1994, Agency for Health Care Policy and Research.
4. Kissin I: Preemptive analgesia, *Anesthesiology* 93 (4):1138–1143, 2000.
5. Murat I, Gall O, Tourniaire B: Procedural pain in children: evidence-based best practice and guidelines, *Reg Anesth Pain Med* 28 (6):561–572, 2003.

Postoperative Nausea and Vomiting (PONV)

NIVINE H. DORAN, M.D.

Postoperative nausea and vomiting (PONV) is a common complication during recovery from surgery. The overall incidence of PONV is approximately 30% but can be as high as 70% in high-risk patients. Although severe complications are extremely rare, PONV is considered the most unpleasant side effect in patient satisfaction surveys. Severe vomiting can lead to electrolyte imbalance, dehydration, pulmonary aspiration, and wound dehiscence.

A. Thoroughly review the medical history, operative procedure, and anesthetic technique. Patient-related factors associated with a higher incidence of PONV include younger age, females (especially during menses), patients with a large body habitus, and non-smokers. A history of motion sickness or prior incidence of PONV may place the patient at higher risk. The operative site and type of surgery has been implicated in increasing the risk of PONV, including procedures involving the oropharynx, auditory and ophthalmic systems, and abdominal cavity (especially laparoscopic). Use of inhalational agents, including N_2O, and opioids leads to a higher incidence of PONV than a total intravenous anesthetic technique (TIVA) using propofol. Regional or major conduction anesthesia has a lower risk of PONV than general anesthesia, but the risk is not eliminated.

B. The benefit of prophylaxis for PONV in terms of absolute risk reduction will be dependent on the preoperative risk of the patient. Risk stratification with a multimodal approach to therapy is effective in limiting, if not eliminating, PONV. Choose antiemetics of differing mechanisms of action when combining agents for prophylaxis or treatment of PONV.

C. Evaluate other etiologies of PONV. Pain and hypotension have been associated with PONV. Adequate pain relief, despite use of opioids, has been known to decrease nausea and vomiting. Adequate hydration is mandatory, intraoperatively as well as postoperatively. The intraoperative use of oxygen at 80% with general anesthesia significantly reduced the incidence of PONV compared to 30%.

D. If a patient has persistent PONV, consider hospital admission and full evaluation of other medical conditions. Such conditions include acute myocardial infarction (MI), sepsis, and intracranial hypertension (HTN). Nausea and vomiting may be related to concurrent medications taken by the patient. Excessive doses of aminophylline and digoxin can lead to nausea. Patients on chemotherapeutic agents can experience nausea unrelated to the surgical procedure.

REFERENCES

1. Apfel CC, Laara E, Koivuranta M, et al.: A simplified risk score for predicting postoperative nausea and vomiting: conclusions from cross-validations between two centers, *Anesthesiology* 91 (3): 693–700, 1999.
2. Gan TJ: Postoperative nausea and vomiting—can it be eliminated? *JAMA* 287 (10):1233–1236, 2002.
3. Macario A, Weinger M, Carney S, et al.: Which clinical anesthesia outcomes are important to avoid? The perspective of patients, *Anesth Analg* 89 (3):652–658, 1999.
4. Apfel CC, Korttila K, Abdalla M, et al.: A factorial trial of six interventions for the prevention of postoperative nausea and vomiting, *N Engl J Med* 350 (24):2441–2451, 2004.
5. Stadler M, Bardiau F, Seidel L, et al.: Difference in risk factors for postoperative nausea and vomiting, *Anesthesiology* 98 (1):46–52, 2003.

POSTOPERATIVE NAUSEA AND VOMITING

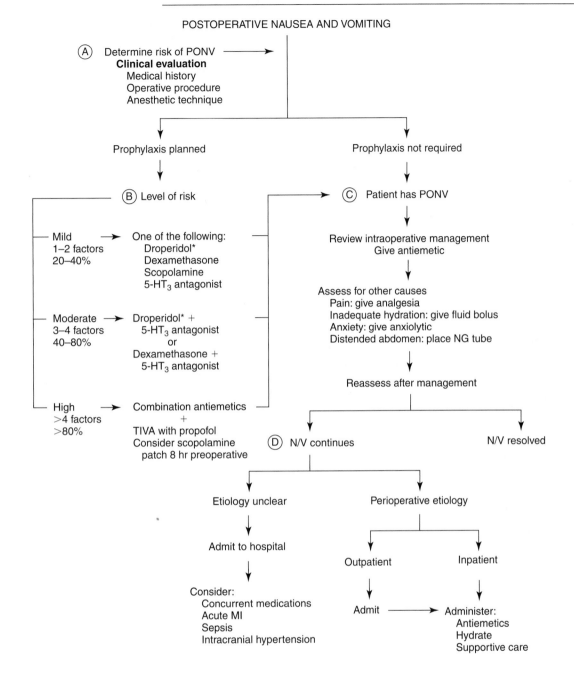

(A) Determine risk of PONV
Clinical evaluation
  Medical history
  Operative procedure
  Anesthetic technique

Prophylaxis planned

Prophylaxis not required

(B) Level of risk

(C) Patient has PONV

Mild → One of the following:
1–2 factors   Droperidol*
20–40%   Dexamethasone
             Scopolamine
             5-HT₃ antagonist

Review intraoperative management
Give antiemetic

Assess for other causes
  Pain: give analgesia
  Inadequate hydration: give fluid bolus
  Anxiety: give anxiolytic
  Distended abdomen: place NG tube

Moderate → Droperidol* +
3–4 factors   5-HT₃ antagonist
40–80%   or
           Dexamethasone +
             5-HT₃ antagonist

Reassess after management

High → Combination antiemetics
>4 factors   +
>80%   TIVA with propofol
        Consider scopolamine
          patch 8 hr preoperative

(D) N/V continues

N/V resolved

Etiology unclear

Perioperative etiology

Admit to hospital

Outpatient

Inpatient

Consider:
  Concurrent medications
  Acute MI
  Sepsis
  Intracranial hypertension

Admit ———→ Administer:
              Antiemetics
              Hydrate
              Supportive care

*Note: FDA warning due to risk of fatal cardiac arrhymia.

Delayed Awakening or Delirium

CAROL E. CAMPBELL, M.D.

A common situation in clinical anesthesia is management of the patient who fails to awaken from a general anesthetic or who emerges with a change in neurological status. Evaluation emphasizes rapid diagnosis and treatment of reversible conditions or prevention of further neurological injury.

A. Review relevant factors including preoperative status of the patient (preexisting conditions), intraoperative events (cardiac arrhythmias, hypertension [HTN], hypotension, treatment with vasopressors), and type of surgery (risk for neurological injury).

B. The DSM-IV-TR diagnosis of delirium is based on four key features: acute change in mental status from the preoperative state, inattention, disorganized thinking, and altered level of consciousness.[1] Predictors for postoperative delirium include age >70 years; alcohol abuse; decreased orientation preoperatively; poor physical status; preoperative electrolyte and glucose abnormalities; and vascular, aortic, or thoracic surgery.[2] The incidence of postoperative delirium is >10% in the elderly population and is associated with poorer surgical outcomes, major complications (e.g., myocardia infarction [MI], cardiac arrest, or respiratory failure), increased length of stay, and discharge to skilled nursing facilities.[3]

C. Determine which medications the patient has received. Prolonged drug effect is the most common, etiology of delayed awakening. Anesthetic requirements vary with age, ethnicity, size, and physical status of the patient; a relative anesthetic overdose can occur even with an experienced practitioner. Perioperative administration of benzodiazepines or opioids can prolong emergence. Nonanesthetic agents that affect cognitive function include tranquilizers, antihypertensives, anticholinergics, clonidine, and H_2 blockers.[3] Penicillin-derived antibiotics, amphotericin B, and immunosuppressive agents can induce changes in mental status.[4] Patients with renal or hepatic insufficiency are particularly at risk for adverse drug interactions. Consider sequelae from drug abuse in all patients regardless of age. Approximately 10 to 15% of elderly people take hypnotic drugs regularly, and 15 to 18% abuse alcohol.[5]

D. Assess oxygenation, ventilation, and metabolic state. Postoperative hypoxia is exacerbated by anemia, hypotension, or low cardiac output (CO). Significant hypercapnia can exist in the presence of normal oxygen (O_2) saturation. Carbon dioxide (CO_2) narcosis and delayed awakening can occur when CO_2 increases above 90 to 120 mm Hg. When $PaCO_2$ levels reach 150 to 250 mm Hg, cerebral function is significantly decreased, as with a general anesthetic.[6] Look for surgically induced electrolyte abnormalities (such as hyponatremia that may occur with transurethral surgery and hypocalcemia that may occur with thyroid and parathyroid surgery). Other predisposing conditions for delayed awakening or delirium include respiratory diseases, fever, hypotension, azotemia, hyperamylasemia, metabolic acidosis, hyperbilirubinemia, and elevated liver enzymes.[7] Mental changes occur in the preeclamptic or eclamptic patient from increased ICP, seizures, intracranial hematoma, or hypermagnesemia from magnesium therapy.

E. Postanoxic ischemic encephalopathy can be related to intraoperative hypotension treated with inotropic drugs, documented circulatory arrest, asphyxia, or hemorrhagic shock.[4] The risk for perioperative stroke increases with age (0.03 to 0.08% for the fourth decade to 3 to 4% for the eighth decade).[8] In general, deliberate hypotension is well tolerated, even in the at-risk patient.[8] Problems occur when BP falls outside the upper and lower limits for cerebral autoregulation. Conditions associated with hemorrhagic infarcts (i.e., BP above cerebral autoregulatory limits) include carotid endarterectomy, post–AVM removal, preeclampsia, and, perhaps, anticoagulation therapy. Conditions associated with acute perioperative ischemic stroke (i.e., BP below cerebral autoregulatory limits) include cardiac arrhythmias (especially atrial fibrillation), acute MI, cardioversion, embolic phenomena, diabetic dysautonomia, and previous cerebrovascular accidents.[9] Surgical procedures with increased risks for cerebral embolism include coronary artery bypass grafting (CABG), orthopedic (especially joint replacements), valvular, peripheral vascular, and aortic surgeries.

Patient with DELAYED AWAKENING OR DELIRIUM

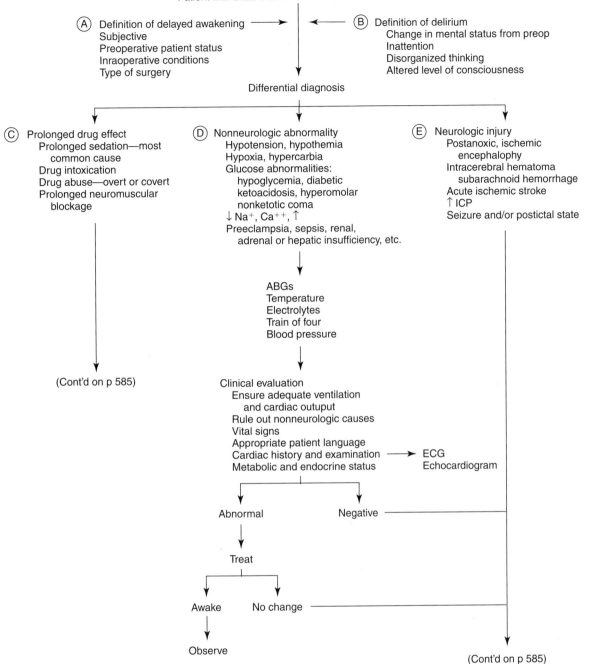

(A) Definition of delayed awakening　　　→　　　←　　(B) Definition of delirium
　　Subjective　　　　　　　　　　　　　　　　　　　　　　　Change in mental status from preop
　　Preoperative patient status　　　　　　　　　　　　　Inattention
　　Inraoperative conditions　　　　　　　　　　　　　　　Disorganized thinking
　　Type of surgery　　　　　　　　　　　　　　　　　　　Altered level of consciousness

Differential diagnosis

(C) Prolonged drug effect
　　Prolonged sedation—most
　　　common cause
　　Drug intoxication
　　Drug abuse—overt or covert
　　Prolonged neuromuscular
　　　blockage

(D) Nonneurologic abnormality
　　Hypotension, hypothemia
　　Hypoxia, hypercarbia
　　Glucose abnormalities:
　　　hypoglycemia, diabetic
　　　ketoacidosis, hyperomolar
　　　nonketotic coma
　　$\downarrow$ Na$^+$, Ca^{++}, $\uparrow$
　　Preeclampsia, sepsis, renal,
　　　adrenal or hepatic insufficiency, etc.

(E) Neurologic injury
　　Postanoxic, ischemic
　　　encephalophy
　　Intracerebral hematoma
　　　subarachnoid hemorrhage
　　Acute ischemic stroke
　　$\uparrow$ ICP
　　Seizure and/or postictal state

ABGs
Temperature
Electrolytes
Train of four
Blood pressure

(Cont'd on p 585)

Clinical evaluation
　　Ensure adequate ventilation
　　　and cardiac outuput
　　Rule out nonneurologic causes
　　Vital signs
　　Appropriate patient language
　　Cardiac history and examination　　→　ECG
　　Metabolic and endocrine status　　　　Echocardiogram

Abnormal　　　　　　　　　　　　Negative

Treat

Awake　　　No change

Observe

(Cont'd on p 585)

F. Review perioperative medications and preoperative neurological status. Give small doses of anesthetic reversal drugs for diagnostic purposes. In addition to monitoring vital signs and temperature, maintain ventilation and CO. Treat any metabolic and electrolyte abnormalities, as well as any cardiac cause for decreased mental status (arrhythmias, MI). Consider other causes for decrease in cognitive function, such as sepsis; hypothyroidism; hyperthyroidism; and adrenal, renal, or hepatic insufficiency.

G. Aggressively rule out neurological causes of delayed awakening when nonneurological causes are eliminated or focal neurological deficits occur. If increased ICP is suspected, intubate and hyperventilate the patient while maintaining tight BP control. Obtain neurosurgery or neurology consults. Patients may require expedited neurosurgical exploration or stroke therapy (i.e., tissue plasminogen activator within three hours of onset of ischemic stroke) to prevent permanent neurological deficits.[10]

REFERENCES

1. American Psychiatric Association Task Force DSM-IV: Delirium, dementia, and amnestic and other cognitive disorders. In: *Diagnostic and statistical manual of mental disorders, text revision, DSM-IV-TR*, Washington D.C., 2000, American Psychiatric Association.

2. Bohner H, Hummel TC, Habel U, et al.: Predicting delirium after vascular surgery: a model based on pre-and intra operative data, *Ann Surg* 238 (1):149–156, 2003.

3. Parikh SS, Chung F: Postoperative delirium in the elderly, *Anesth Analg* 80:1223–1232, 1995.

4. Wijdicks EF: Neurological complications in critically ill patients, *Anesth Analg* 83:411–419, 1996.

5. O'Keeffe ST, Chonchubhair A: Postoperative delirium in the elderly, *Br J Anaesth* 73:673–687, 1994.

6. Mecca RS: Postoperative hypercarbia, *Curr Rev Clin Anesth* 19 (9):93–104, 1998.

7. Aldemir M, Ozen S, Kara IH, et al.: Predisposing factors for delirium in the surgical intensive care unit, *Crit Care* 5 (5):265–270, 2001.

8. Kim J, Gelb AW: Predicting perioperative stroke, *J Neurosurg Anesth* 7:211–215, 1995.

9. Bladin CF, Chambers BR: Frequency and pathogenesis of hemodynamic stroke, *Stroke* 25:2179–2182, 1994.

10. Adams HP, Adams RJ, Brott T, et al.: Guidelines for early management of patients with ischemic stroke: A scientific statement from the Stroke Council of the American Stroke Association, *Stroke* 34 (4):1056–1083, 2003.

Patient with DELAYED AWAKENING OR DELIRIUM

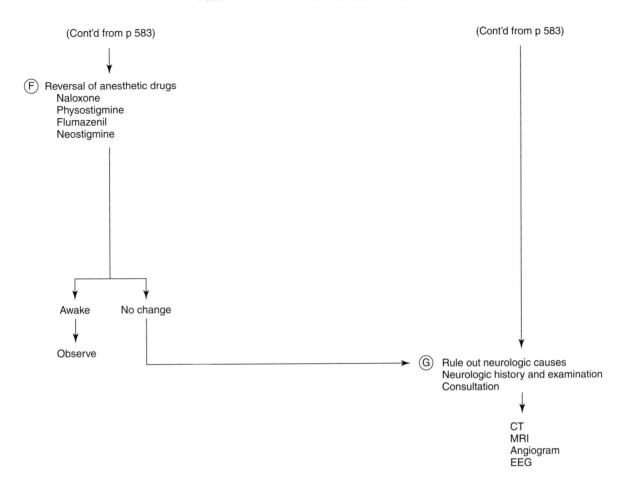

Postoperative Hypotension

CAROL E. CAMPBELL, M.D.

Hypotension is a common occurrence in the PACU. Postoperative hypotension is defined as BP that is 20 to 30% less than its chronic preoperative level.[1,2] The degree of hypotension that is associated with an increased risk of complications depends on the baseline BP and the presence of preexisting end-organ disease. Severe postoperative hypotension is most likely to occur within 1 day of surgery.[3] Complications include ischemia or infarction of the cerebrum, optic nerves, myocardium, kidneys, bowel, or spinal cord.[4–7] Orthostatic hypotension is common after general anesthesia, even with minor surgery, and increases the risk of morbidity postoperatively.[8]

The etiology of postoperative hypotension can be classified into one of three broad categories: decreased preload, decreased contractility, and decreased afterload. A decreased preload may be due to hypovolemia, vasodilation, surgical maneuvers that restrict venous return, elevated intrathoracic pressures, patient positioning, pericardial tamponade, and pulmonary embolus. Decreased contractility may be due to the effects of inotropic depressant drugs, arrhythmias, cardiomyopathies, congestive heart failure (CHF), myocardial ischemia, myocardial infarction, hypoxemia, valvular heart disease, or an abrupt increase in afterload. Decreased afterload may be due to vasodilation, sepsis, anaphylaxis, or endocrine abnormalities (Addisonian crisis, hypothyroidism, or hypoglycemia). Clinically, the search for the etiology of postoperative hypotension should be directed toward finding and treating life-threatening causes.

A. Evaluate the adequacy of ventilation (physical examination, ABG). Postoperative hypotension may be a reflection of hypoxemia or hypercarbia, either of which may be life-threatening.

B. Evaluate the urgency of the situation. Postoperative hypotension may be a reflection of ominous conditions. Emergently treat situations presenting with evidence of end-organ damage to prevent further sequelae. Perform a physical examination of the patient to determine the need for further laboratory studies. Search for evidence of myocardial ischemia or infarction by assessing patient history, ECG, and central monitoring (pulmonary artery [PA] catheter). Look for signs and symptoms of histamine release (bronchospasm, urticaria, or edema); these may indicate the presence of an anaphylactic/anaphylactoid reaction. Examine the chest for the presence of tracheal deviation or decreased breath sounds to rule out pneumothorax or tension pneumothorax. Distant heart sounds may indicate the presence of pericardial tamponade. Confirm the diagnosis of pericardial tamponade by noting equalization of right atrium, right ventricle (RV), and PA pressures and decreased ECG voltage. Echocardiography is diagnostic.

C. Perform a more thorough evaluation prior to treatment in situations that present no evidence of end-organ damage. Review the past medical history for the presence of autonomic dysfunction, medications that may contribute to hypotension, and baseline disease states. Review the intraoperative anesthetic record to reveal potential causes for hypotension. Be aware that antinociceptive doses of clonidine, an alpha$_2$ agonist, administered intrathecally or epidurally may produce significant hypotension and bradycardia.[9] Immediate postoperative hypotension is more common in patients receiving epidural or spinal anesthesia than in those receiving general anesthesia.[10] This hypotension is due to the significant and prolonged vasodilatory changes resulting from regional techniques. In healthy patients without significant associated disease, the most common cause of postoperative hypotension is hypovolemia, usually resulting from inadequate fluid or blood replacement.

D. If questions exist regarding volume status, consider placing invasive central monitors. If the CVP is decreased, the healthy, hypovolemic patient should respond to a fluid challenge. When there is a poor response to fluid challenge or an increased CVP in the setting of hypotension, or when the patient has known cardiac risk factors, consider placing a monitor of cardiac output, such as a PA catheter. The indices derived and measured with a PA catheter may be used to direct inotropic, vasodilator, or vasopressor therapy.

REFERENCES

1. Mecca R: Systemic hypotension after surgery, *Curr Rev Clin Anesth* 19 (24):265–280, 1999.
2. Harris SN: Hypotension, hypertension, perioperative myocardial ischemia, and infarction. In: Benumof J, Saidman L, editors: *Anesthesia and perioperative complications*, ed 2, St. Louis, 1999, Mosby.
3. Thompson JS, Baxter BT, Allison JG, et al.: Temporal patterns of postoperative complications, *Arch Surg* 138 (6):596–602, 2003.
4. Mecca RS: Post anesthesia recovery. In: Kirby RR, Gravenstein N, Labato EB, et al., editors: *Clinical anesthesia practice*, ed 2, Philadelphia, 2002 W.B. Saunders.
5. Bhardwaj A, Long DM, Ducker TB, et al.: Neurologic deficits after cervical laminectomy in the prone position, *J Neurosurg Anesthesiol* 13 (4):314–319, 2001.
6. Dunker S, Hsu Y, Sebag J, et al.: Perioperative risk factors for posterior ischemic optic neuropathy, *J Am Coll Surg* 194 (6):705–710, 2002.
7. Asensio JA, Forno W, Castillo GA, et al.: Posterior ischemic optic neuropathy related to profound shock after penetrating thoracoabdominal trauma, *South Med J* 95 (9):1053–1057, 2002.

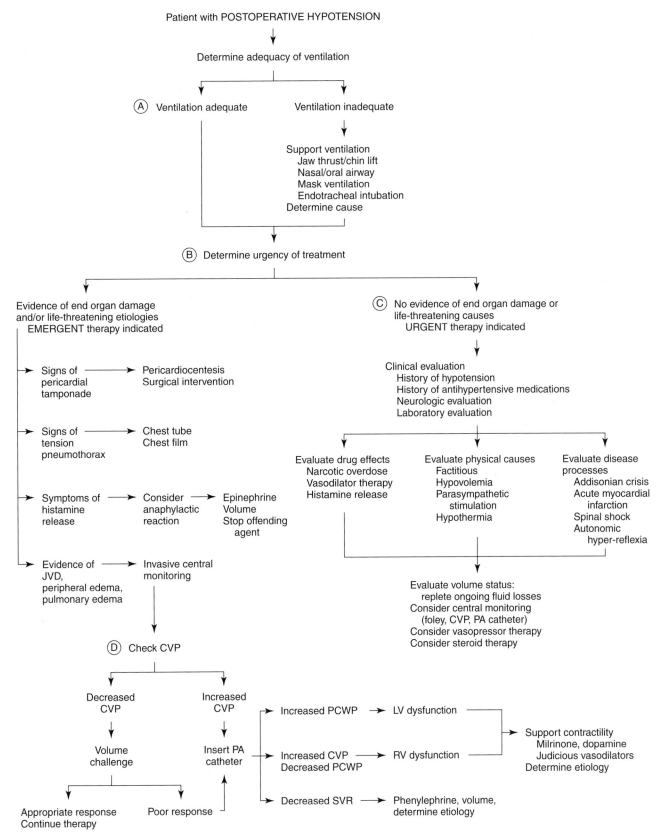

8. Cowie DA, Shoemaker JK, Gelb AW: Orthostatic hypotension occurs frequently in the first hour after anesthesia, *Anesth Analg* 98 (1):40–45, 2004.

9. Puskas F, Camporesi EM, O'Leary CE: Intrathecal clonidine and severe hypotension after cardiopulmonary bypass, *Anesth Analg* 97 (5):1251–1253, 2003.

10. Demirel CB, Kalayci M, Ozkocak I, et al.: A prospective randomized study comparing perioperative outcome variables after epidural or general anesthesia for lumbar disc surgery, *J Neurosurg Anesthesiol* 15 (3):185–292, 2003.

Postoperative Hypertension (HTN)

CAROL E. CAMPBELL, M.D.

Postoperative hypertension (HTN) is a common occurrence.[1,2] Postoperative HTN is defined as BP that is more than 20% above preoperative levels, or an absolute value of arterial BP above age-corrected limits.[3] The BP at which complications arise depends on a patient's chronic preoperative BP, the presence of preexisting end-organ damage, and the ability of the surgical closure(s) to withstand arterial pressure elevation. Evaluation of postoperative HTN should be directed toward establishing etiology. Prompt diagnosis and therapy can prevent further potential complications including myocardial ischemia, myocardial infarction, intracerebral hemorrhage, and wound hematoma.[4]

A. Evaluate the adequacy of ventilation. Postoperative HTN may be a reflection of hypoxemia or hypercarbia, both of which may be life-threatening. Auscultate to rule out pneumothorax, tension pneumothorax, and atelectasis. Search for evidence of myocardial ischemia or infarction. Evaluate the neurological status for signs of cerebrovascular compromise. Supplement the physical examination with focused laboratory studies (e.g., ABG to evaluate for hypercarbia).

B. Determine the urgency of the situation. Be aware that the rate of increase in BP is probably more significant than the actual BP level. Classic signs of hypertensive encephalopathy include decreased level of consciousness, headache, and mild to moderate CNS dysfunction.[2] Emergently treat situations for which there is evidence of end-organ damage (e.g., myocardial ischemia, myocardial infarction, intracerebral hemorrhage). When there is no evidence of end-organ damage, treat after more thorough evaluation.[2] Review the past medical history for HTN, antihypertensive medications, and baseline disease states. Review the anesthetic record for other possible causes of HTN. Patients with cerebral vasospasm may be deliberately rendered hypertensive.

C. Etiologies for postoperative HTN can be divided into four broad categories: pain, drug interactions, physical causes, and concomitant disease states. Develop a differential diagnosis within each category and direct the treatment toward an identifiable etiology.[5]

However, prior to treating HTN, confirm the accuracy of the BP by checking arm position, cuff size, and cuff placement.[6,7] If an arterial line transducer is not properly zeroed or calibrated or there is an excessive quantity of resonance, then systolic pressure may be overestimated.[8] If acute ischemic stroke is the probable etiology of the HTN, antihypertensive medications should be avoided unless the systolic BP is greater then 220 mm Hg or the diastolic BP is greater than 120 mm Hg because the area of cerebral ischemia may be increased.[4] Options for immediate control of BP include IV infusions of sodium nitroprusside, nitroglycerin, metoprolol, esmolol, nicardipine, fenoldopam, or trimethaphan. Treatment options for a more gradual control of BP include beta blockade (labetalol), alpha blockade (phentolamine), and calcium channel blockade (verapamil or nifedipine).

REFERENCES

1. Varon J, Marik PE: The diagnosis and management of hypertensive crises, Chest 118:214–227, 2000.
2. Murray MJ: Perioperative hypertension: evaluation and management. In: 53rd annual refresher course lectures, clinical updates and basic science review program, Park Ridge IL, 2002, American Society of Anesthesiologists.
3. Joint National Committee on Prevention, Detection, Evaluation and Treatment of High Blood Pressure: The sixth report of the joint national committee on prevention, detection, evaluation, and treatment of high blood pressure, Arch Intern Med 157:2413–2448, 1997.
4. Adams HP, Adams RJ, Brott T, et al.: Guidelines for early management of patients with ischemic stroke a scientific statement from the stroke council of the American Stroke Association, Stroke 34 (4): 1056–1083, 2003.
5. Stoelting RK, Miller RD: Post anesthesia care unit. In: Basics of anesthesia, New York, 2000, Churchill Livingstone.
6. McAlister FA, Straus S: Evidence based treatment of hypertension. Measurement of blood pressure: an evidence based review, Br Med J 322:908–911, 2001.
7. Harris SN: Hypotension, hypertension, perioperative myocardial ischemia and infarction. In: Benumof JL, Saidman LJ, editors: Anesthesia and perioperative complications, ed 2, St. Louis, 1999, Mosby.
8. Mecca RS: Postanesthesia recovery. In: Kirby RR, Gravenstein N, Labato EB, et al., editors: Clinical anesthesia practice, Philadelphia, 2002 W.B. Saunders.

Patient with POSTOPERATIVE HYPERTENSION

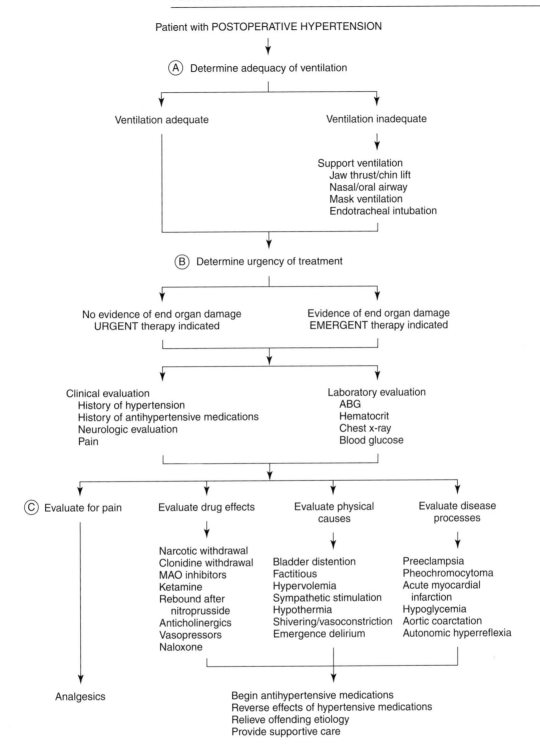

(A) Determine adequacy of ventilation

Ventilation adequate

Ventilation inadequate

Support ventilation
Jaw thrust/chin lift
Nasal/oral airway
Mask ventilation
Endotracheal intubation

(B) Determine urgency of treatment

No evidence of end organ damage
URGENT therapy indicated

Evidence of end organ damage
EMERGENT therapy indicated

Clinical evaluation
History of hypertension
History of antihypertensive medications
Neurologic evaluation
Pain

Laboratory evaluation
ABG
Hematocrit
Chest x-ray
Blood glucose

(C) Evaluate for pain

Evaluate drug effects

Evaluate physical causes

Evaluate disease processes

Narcotic withdrawal
Clonidine withdrawal
MAO inhibitors
Ketamine
Rebound after
  nitroprusside
Anticholinergics
Vasopressors
Naloxone

Bladder distention
Factitious
Hypervolemia
Sympathetic stimulation
Hypothermia
Shivering/vasoconstriction
Emergence delirium

Preeclampsia
Pheochromocytoma
Acute myocardial
  infarction
Hypoglycemia
Aortic coarctation
Autonomic hyperreflexia

Analgesics

Begin antihypertensive medications
Reverse effects of hypertensive medications
Relieve offending etiology
Provide supportive care

Prolonged Postoperative Apnea

CAROL E. CAMPBELL, M.D.

LOIS L. BREADY, M.D.

The initial management of the postoperative apneic or hypoventilating patient should include an assessment of the adequacy of both oxygenation and ventilation followed by appropriate supportive ventilatory management. Further evaluation proceeds in a systematic fashion beginning with a review of the past medical history and pertinent physical examination of the patient, including assessment of neuromuscular blockade and neurological function. The anesthetic record and other perioperative records may give a clue to medications or untoward intraoperative events that may influence the postoperative course. If apnea persists, examine pertinent laboratory values, including serum electrolytes, calcium, magnesium, sodium, blood glucose, acid-base status, ABG, and renal/hepatic function.

A. Review the records for narcotic analgesic dosages, including any premedication. Opioids can cause a direct dose-dependent inhibition of respiratory centers in the brainstem and increase $PaCO_2$. In the trauma patient, consider preinjury drug or alcohol ingestion. Naloxone, 0.1 to 0.2 mg IV, may reverse narcotic-induced respiratory depression but is not entirely innocuous. Nalbuphine may also reverse narcotic-induced respiratory depression. Flumazenil, 0.1 to 0.2 mg IV, may be titrated to reverse sedation caused by benzodiazepine administration. Physostigmine, 15 g/kg/IV, may reverse depression from sedatives or tranquilizers. Residual neuromuscular blockade may result from relative overdose or impaired excretion of nondepolarizing relaxant and may be avoided by monitoring neuromuscular blockade intraoperatively. Repeating anticholinesterase agents (neostigmine, 60 µg/kg up to 5 mg, or pyridostigmine 0.35 mg/kg up to 25 mg) may be effective. Residual succinyl-choline (SCC) effect can be seen in patients with abnormal pseudocholinesterase (PCE). Typically, deficiency of PCE activity (severe liver disease, malnutrition, pregnancy, postplasmapheresis, anticholinesterase therapy for myasthenia gravis [MG], echothiophate eye drops for glaucoma, or the use of metoclopramide) does not prolong SCC relaxation beyond 30 to 60 minutes. Neurally applied opiates, such as morphine, may cause a biphasic respiratory depression and delayed awakening after perioperative administration. The early phase reflects systemic absorption and produces respiratory depression and sedation of a similar magnitude to equipotent doses of parenterally administered narcotics. The later phase reflects the rostral spread in the CSF to depress the brainstem respiratory centers. Aminoglycoside antibiotics, as well as lithium, can prolong neuromuscular blockade and thus potentiate the risk for postoperative apnea. Reversal is inconsistent and unpredictable after receiving these drugs.

B. Certain patient profiles are associated with adverse respiratory events. Obese patients, obstructive sleep apnea patients, asthmatics, and smokers have a twofold to fivefold increased risk of manifesting postoperative respiratory events.[1,2] Patients who chronically retain carbon dioxide (CO_2) may hypoventilate when exposed to high FiO_2. Reduce FiO_2 when ABG results dictate. Damage to the CNS, such as increased ICP or CVA, and cervical cordotomy for chronic pain may cause apnea. Obtain neurological consultation and consider diagnostic neuroimaging. Renal or hepatic dysfunction may prolong the effects of many anesthetic agents and delay emergence. Patients with MG or other neuromuscular diseases may exhibit postoperative apnea; anticholinesterase therapy may be effective. Patients with hereditary hepatic porphyrias may develop porphyric attacks (manifested by neuromuscular weakness) after being given thiopental; support ventilation until the weakness resolves. Hysteria after general anesthesia can lead to dyspnea and hypoventilation or apnea.[3] Electrolyte derangements, including abnormalities in calcium, magnesium, sodium, and glucose, may contribute to delayed awakening. Correct abnormalities to facilitate return of motor and mental function.

C. Hypothermia exacerbates neuromuscular blockade. Chilled patients may become apneic even in the absence of muscle relaxants.[4] Rewarm to reverse these abnormalities. Intraoperative hyperventilation leads to loss of CO_2 from the body. Postoperatively, $PaCO_2$ may rise slowly, with a lack of respiratory stimulus for ventilation. Observe the capnogram intraoperatively to prevent this problem. However, it may be difficult to avoid this situation when hyperventilation is intentionally induced.

REFERENCES

1. Chung F, Mezei G: Adverse outcomes in ambulatory anesthesia, *Can J Anaesth* 46 (5):18–34, 1999.
2. Mecca RS: Postanesthesia recovery. In: Kirby RR, Gravenstein N, Labato EB, et al., editors: *Clinical anesthesia practice*, Philadelphia, 2002, W.B. Saunders.
3. Tanaka T, Sano H, Tanifuji Y: Dyspnea attack due to hysteria after general anesthesia, *Masui* 49 (5):555–558, 2000.
4. Delinger JK: Prolonged emergence and failure to regain consciousness. In: Gravenstein N, Kirby RR, editors: *Complications in anesthesiology*, ed 2, Philadelphia, 1996, Lippincott-Raven.

APNEIC OR HYPOVENTILATING PATIENT

↓

Support ventilation

Clinical evaluation ──────────→   ←────── Laboratory evaluation
    History of renal, hepatic, or   Serum electrolytes
        neuromuscular disease   Blood glucose
    Chart review for narcotics,   ABG
        sedatives, muscle relaxants,   Renal, hepatic function
        antibiotics   CXR
    Temperature in PACU   Consider CT scan
    Neurologic evaluation
    Neuromuscular stimulation
    Tidal volume

↓

Assess cause of
respiratory depression

Ⓐ Drug effects   Ⓑ Concomitant diseases   Ⓒ Physical factors

→ Benzodiazepines   → Chronic obstructive   → Hypothemia
    Narcotics   pulmonary disease
    Sedatives   ↓
                            ↓
    ↓   Warm patient
                            Adjust FiO$_2$
    Naloxone   Follow ABGs   → Prolonged
    Nalbuphine   hyperventilation
    Flumazenil   → Neurologic abnormality
    Physostigmine   ↓
                            ↓
                                                                ABGs
→ Neuromuscular   Neurologic consultation   Careful elevation
    blockade   Diagnostic imaging   of PaCO$_2$

    ┌────┴────┐   → Myasthenia gravis

Nondepolarizing Depolarizing   ↓
    relaxants   relaxants
                            Anticholinesterase
    ↓   ↓
                            → Porphyria
Repeat ACE   Support
              ventilation   ↓

→ Neuraxial   Support ventilation
    opiates   Consult hematologist

    ↓   → Renal dysfunction

    Naloxone   ↓
    (consider infusion)
                            Supportive care
→ Antibiotics
                            ↑
    ↓
                            → Hepatic dysfunction
    Support
    ventilation

Weaning from Mechanical Ventilation

ERIK A. BOATMAN, M.D.

Discontinuation of mechanical ventilation (MV) is an anesthetic art that balances patient performance, history, anatomy, and provider experience. Premature attempts can result in undue stress and risk difficulty with reintubation and prolongation of MV.[1] Duration of MV should be kept as short as necessary to minimize ventilator associated complications.[2,3] Fortunately, most patients can be rapidly weaned off MV.

A. When considering discontinuation of MV, first evaluate whether the reasons for institution of MV have been resolved. Next, assess for factors that may predispose to extubation failure[1,4] and address correctable issues. Carefully consider indicators of difficulty with reintubation, such as prior difficult airway, challenging anatomy, or local edema. Difficult intubation situations in the ICU are a major source of morbidity and mortality, especially when unanticipated. Have alternative airway tools, providers, and a surgical airway kit at the bedside prior to extubation of patients with a known difficult airway.

B. Several factors can demonstrate respiratory independence; however, individual extubation criteria (see Table 1) do not ensure successful extubation. In combination with a weaning protocol, the criteria provide supporting evidence. In recent studies, the most predictive criteria are the rapid shallow breathing index (RSBI) and the compliance, rate, oxygenation, pressure (CROP) integrated index.[2,5-8]

C. Implement weaning protocols when a patient meets several extubation criteria. These are designed to further demonstrate patient independence from the ventilator (as close as can be approximated while the patient remains intubated). Prepare the patient physically and mentally; eliminate or reverse all residual sedation, narcosis, and neuromuscular blockade. Choose a mode of weaning—most commonly SIMV, PSV, or T-piece/CPAP—although controversy exists as to which is best.[3,10,11]

D. Once a weaning protocol has been completed successfully, proceed with extubation. Optimize the patient for maximal pulmonary reserve immediately prior to extubation. After extubation, observe the patient closely for signs of impending respiratory embarrassment. Most problems with discontinuation of MV can usually be attributed to premature discontinuation, improper ventilator management, muscle atrophy, malnutrition, or strained cardiopulmonary reserve.[3]

E. All patients deserve a thorough consideration of freedom from MV. If several attempts at weaning make no progress, prepare the patient for chronic MV. Early discussion with the patient and family promotes eventual acceptance of this hard fact.

F. Occasionally, noninvasive methods can be successfully employed to provide positive airway pressure support for prevention of intubation or bridging from an artificial to a natural airway.[12]

REFERENCES

1. Rothaar, RC, Epstein SK: Extubation failure: magnitude of the problem, impact on outcomes, and prevention, Curr Opin Crit Care 9 (1):59–66, 2003.
2. Manthous CA, Schmidt GA, Hall JB: Liberation from mechanical ventilation: a decade of progress, Chest 114 (3):886–901, 1998.
3. Dries DJ, McGonigal MD, Malian MS, et al.: Protocol-driven ventilator weaning reduces use of mechanical ventilation, rate of early reintubation, and ventilator-associated pneumonia, J Trauma 56 (5):943–951, 2004.
4. Rady MY, Ryan T: Perioperative predictors of extubation failure and the effect on clinical outcome after cardiac surgery, Crit Care Med 27 (2):340–347, 1999.
5. Price JA, Rizk NW: Postoperative ventilatory management, Chest 115 (5 Suppl):130S–137S, 1999.
6. Chatila W, Jacob B, Guaglionone D, et al.: The unassisted respiratory rate-tidal volume ratio accurately predicts weaning outcome, Am J Med 101 (1):61–67, 1996.
7. Yang KL, Tobin MJ: A prospective study of indexes predicting the outcome of trials of weaning from mechanical ventilation, N Engl J Med 324 (21):1445–1450, 1991.
8. Tobin MJ, Perez W, Guenther SM, et al.: The pattern of breathing during successful and unsuccessful trials of weaning from mechanical ventilation, Am Rev Respir Dis 134:1111–1118, 1986.
9. Martinez A, Seymour C, Nam M: Minute ventilation recovery time: a predictor of extubation outcome, Chest 123 (4):1214–1221, 2003.
10. MacIntyre NR, Cook DJ, Ely EW Jr, et al.: Evidence-based guidelines for weaning and discontinuing ventilatory support: a collective task force facilitated by the American College of Chest Physicians; the American Association for Respiratory Care; and the American College of Critical Care Medicine, Chest 120 (6 Suppl):375S–395S, 2001.
11. Hubble CL, Gentile MA, Tripp DS, et al.: Deadspace to tidal volume ratio predicts successful extubation in infants and children, Crit Care Med 28 (6):2034–2040 2000.
12. Hore CT: Non-invasive positive pressure ventilation in patients with acute respiratory failure, Emer Med 14 (3):281–295, 2002.

TABLE 1
Individual Extubation Criteria

Mechanical function	Gas exchange function
FVC >10–15 mL/kg	PaO_2/F_IO_2 >200
FEV_1 >10 mL/kg	A-a gradient (with F_IO_2 = 1)
RR <25/min	<350 mm Hg
V_T >5 mL/kg	PaO_2/PAO_2 >0.34
RR/V_T <100/L (RSBI)	Q_S/Q_T <0.2
FRC >50% predicted	V_D/V_T <0.6
V_E <10 L/min	
NIF <−30 cm H_2O	**Other**
Thoracic compliance	UO >0.5 mL/kg/hr
Static >32 mL/cm	Arterial pH 7.35–7.45
Dynamic >21 mL/cm H_2O	Gastric intramural pH >7.30

FVC, forced vital capacity; FEV_1, forced expiratory volume in 1 second; RR, respiratory rate; V_T, tidal volume; RSBI, rapid shallow breathing index; FRC, functional residual capacity; V_E, minute volume; NIF, negative inspiratory force; PaO_2, arterial O_2 partial pressure; F_IO_2, fraction of inspired O_2; A-a, alveolar to arterial; PAO_2, alveolar O_2 partial pressure; Q_S/Q_T, shunt fraction; V_D, dead space ventilation

MECHANICALLY VENTILATED PATIENT

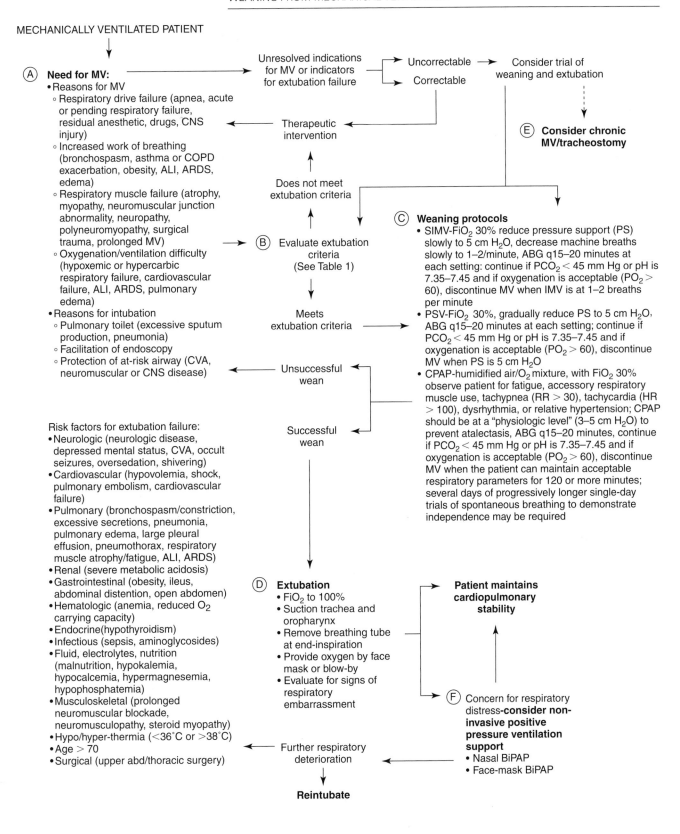

(A) **Need for MV:**
- Reasons for MV
  - Respiratory drive failure (apnea, acute or pending respiratory failure, residual anesthetic, drugs, CNS injury)
  - Increased work of breathing (bronchospasm, asthma or COPD exacerbation, obesity, ALI, ARDS, edema)
  - Respiratory muscle failure (atrophy, myopathy, neuromuscular junction abnormality, neuropathy, polyneuromyopathy, surgical trauma, prolonged MV)
  - Oxygenation/ventilation difficulty (hypoxemic or hypercarbic respiratory failure, cardiovascular failure, ALI, ARDS, pulmonary edema)
- Reasons for intubation
  - Pulmonary toilet (excessive sputum production, pneumonia)
  - Facilitation of endoscopy
  - Protection of at-risk airway (CVA, neuromuscular or CNS disease)

Risk factors for extubation failure:
- Neurologic (neurologic disease, depressed mental status, CVA, occult seizures, oversedation, shivering)
- Cardiovascular (hypovolemia, shock, pulmonary embolism, cardiovascular failure)
- Pulmonary (bronchospasm/constriction, excessive secretions, pneumonia, pulmonary edema, large pleural effusion, pneumothorax, respiratory muscle atrophy/fatigue, ALI, ARDS)
- Renal (severe metabolic acidosis)
- Gastrointestinal (obesity, ileus, abdominal distention, open abdomen)
- Hematologic (anemia, reduced O_2 carrying capacity)
- Endocrine(hypothyroidism)
- Infectious (sepsis, aminoglycosides)
- Fluid, electrolytes, nutrition (malnutrition, hypokalemia, hypocalcemia, hypermagnesemia, hypophosphatemia)
- Musculoskeletal (prolonged neuromuscular blockade, neuromusculopathy, steroid myopathy)
- Hypo/hyper-thermia ($<36°C$ or $>38°C$)
- Age > 70
- Surgical (upper abd/thoracic surgery)

Unresolved indications for MV or indicators for extubation failure → Uncorrectable → Consider trial of weaning and extubation

Correctable

Therapeutic intervention

(E) **Consider chronic MV/tracheostomy**

Does not meet extubation criteria

(B) Evaluate extubation criteria (See Table 1)

Meets extubation criteria

(C) **Weaning protocols**
- SIMV-FiO_2 30% reduce pressure support (PS) slowly to 5 cm H_2O, decrease machine breaths slowly to 1–2/minute, ABG q15–20 minutes at each setting: continue if $PCO_2 < 45$ mm Hg or pH is 7.35–7.45 and if oxygenation is acceptable ($PO_2 > 60$), discontinue MV when IMV is at 1–2 breaths per minute
- PSV-FiO_2 30%, gradually reduce PS to 5 cm H_2O, ABG q15–20 minutes at each setting; continue if $PCO_2 < 45$ mm Hg or pH is 7.35–7.45 and if oxygenation is acceptable ($PO_2 > 60$), discontinue MV when PS is 5 cm H_2O
- CPAP-humidified air/O_2 mixture, with FiO_2 30% observe patient for fatigue, accessory respiratory muscle use, tachypnea (RR > 30), tachycardia (HR > 100), dysrhythmia, or relative hypertension; CPAP should be at a "physiologic level" (3–5 cm H_2O) to prevent atelectasis, ABG q15–20 minutes, continue if $PCO_2 < 45$ mm Hg or pH is 7.35–7.45 and if oxygenation is acceptable ($PO_2 > 60$), discontinue MV when the patient can maintain acceptable respiratory parameters for 120 or more minutes; several days of progressively longer single-day trials of spontaneous breathing to demonstrate independence may be required

Unsuccessful wean

Successful wean

(D) **Extubation**
- FiO_2 to 100%
- Suction trachea and oropharynx
- Remove breathing tube at end-inspiration
- Provide oxygen by face mask or blow-by
- Evaluate for signs of respiratory embarrassment

Patient maintains cardiopulmonary stability

(F) Concern for respiratory distress-**consider non-invasive positive pressure ventilation support**
- Nasal BiPAP
- Face-mask BiPAP

Further respiratory deterioration

Reintubate

Neurologic Sequelae Following Regional Anesthesia

MICHAEL VERBER, M.D.

The precise risk of neurological damage from regional anesthesia (RA) is difficult to establish. Incidence is overestimated by patients and surgeons;[1,2] however, anesthesiologists may not see sequelae, which present days to weeks after the block. It is important to recognize the background risk of injury from certain procedures: 4.3% for total shoulder arthroplasty, up to 3% for total hip, and 0.8% after total knee arthroplasty.[3–5]

A. Perform and document a neurological examination preoperatively. Discuss the risks and benefits of RA with the patient and the surgeon, especially in patients with preexisting neurological disease. Absolute contraindications to RA include lack of informed consent or infection at the site of the block. Preexisting full systemic anticoagulation or significant coagulopathy is, for all but the most superficial peripheral nerves, another contraindication. Peripheral demyelinating disease is considered by some to be a contraindication. The performance of RA in adult patients under general anesthesia is an area of controversy, because the patient is unable to respond to pain; however, this is safe with children.[6,7]

B. Always administer RA using standard American Society of Anesthesiologists (ASA) monitoring and have resuscitative drugs and equipment immediately available. Confirm the identity of any injected substance with another individual. Never continue an injection if the patient complains of pain. In such cases, reposition the needle; if pain persists, abandon the procedure.

C. Document the postsurgical resolution of the block. If a long-acting agent has been used for a patient who will be discharged prior to resolution of the block, examine the surgical dressing to ensure that it is not causing compression. In addition, caution the patient to be aware of the position of the insensate extremity and to report immediately if the block fails to resolve within the expected time duration or if unexpected pain occurs. In patients discharged with continuous catheters, follow with telephone checks for the duration of catheter use; the risk of postdischarge injury is low.

D. RA complications have multiple etiologies including needle trauma to nerves or adjacent structures, direct or systemic local anesthetic toxicity, anaphylaxis, accidental injection of a toxic substance, contamination from disinfectants, unintended CNS blockade, infectious or compressive complications, and failure to achieve anesthesia. Postoperative neurological symptoms may be unrelated to RA and occur due to surgical, tourniquet or positioning injury, progression or unmasking of an underlying condition, nerve compression from postoperative swelling, casts or immobilizers, improper use of crutches, incidental injury to an extremity rendered insensate for postoperative analgesia, or the new onset of a neurological condition unrelated to either the anesthesia or surgery. The most common adverse reactions following peripheral nerve block is peripheral neuropathy;[8] after brachial plexus block, it is unintended intravascular injection;[9] after epidural it is unintentional subarachnoid injection.[10] Misplaced injections can be minimized by slow injection of sublethal aliquots and observation of and conversation with the patient between injections. The addition of epinephrine 2.5 μg/mL (1:400,000) may give early warning of intravascular injection but may increase the risk of neuritis and is not uniformly reliable.

E. Evaluate any suggestion of neurological compromise as soon as possible; it is imperative to diagnose remediable causes within the time limits of effective intervention. The majority of complaints will prove to have no specific findings or definitive treatment, and will rapidly resolve. With any serious condition, obtain bilateral electroneuromyographic studies. If there is profound sensory or any motor involvement, consult a neurologist or neurosurgeon immediately. Otherwise, consider referral if anticipated resolution does not occur. As noted, the great majority of neurological symptoms will resolve without any sequelae.

REFERENCES

1. Kuczkowski KM: Neurologic complication of labor analgesia: facts and fiction, *Obstet Gynecol Surv* 59 (1):47–51, 2004.
2. Weber SC, Jain R: Scalene regional anesthesia for shoulder surgery in a community setting: an assessment of risk, *J Bone Joint Surg Am* 84:775–779, 2002.
3. Lynch NM, Cofield RH, Silbert PL, et al.: Neurologic complications after total shoulder arthroplasty, *J Shoulder Elbow Surg* 5 (1): 53–61, 1996.
4. Wasielewski RC, Crossett LS, Rubash HE: Neural and vascular injury in total hip arthroplasty, *Orthop Clin North Am* 23 (2): 219–235, 1992.
5. Horlocker TT, Cabanela ME, Wedel DJ: Does postoperative epidural analgesia increase the risk of peroneal nerve palsy after total knee arthroplasty? *Anesth Analg* 79 (3):495–500, 1994.
6. Benumof JL: Permanent loss of cervical spinal cord function associated with interscalene block performed under general anesthesia, *Anesthesiology* 93 (6):1541–1544, 2000.
7. Giaufre E, Dalens B, Gombert A: Epidemiology and morbidity of regional anesthesia in children: a one-year prospective survey of the French-Language Society of Pediatric Anesthesiologists, *Anesth Analg* 83 (5):904–912, 1996.
8. Auroy Y, Benhamou D, Bargues L, et al.: Major complications of regional anesthesia in France: The SOS Regional Anesthesia Hotline Service, *Anesthesiology* 97 (5):1274–1280, 2002.

NEUROLOGIC SEQUELAE OF REGIONAL ANESTHESIA

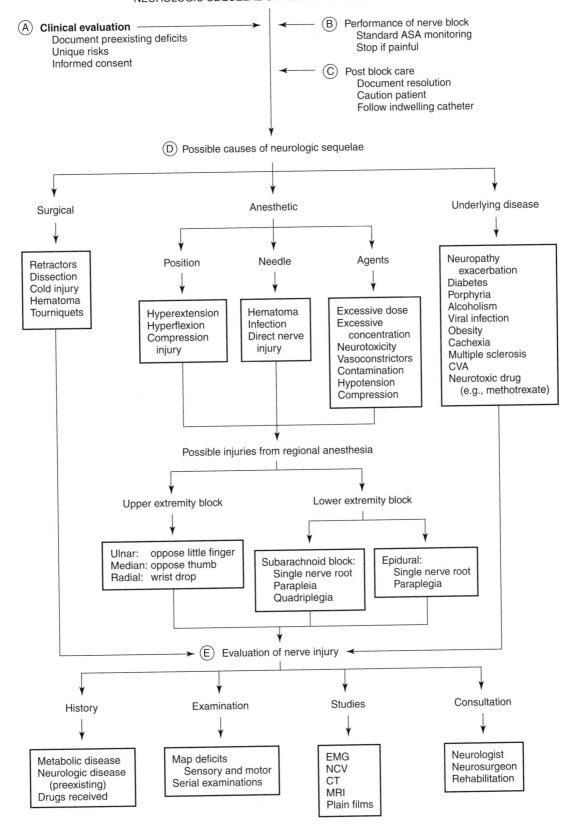

9. Brown DL, Ransom DM, Hall JA, et al.: Regional anesthesia and local anesthetic-induced systemic toxicity: seizure frequency and accompanying cardiovascular changes, *Anesth Analg* 81 (2):321–328, 1995.

10. Jenkins JG: Some immediate serious complications of obstetric epidural analgesia and anaesthesia: a prospective study of 145,550 epidurals, *Intl J Obstetric Anesth* 14 (1):37–42, 2005.

Perioperative Seizures

TOD B. SLOAN, M.D., PH.D.

Seizures are time-limited paroxysmal events that result from abnormal, involuntary, rhythmical neuronal discharges in the brain. The seizure usually lasts less than 5 minutes and may be preceded by a prodromal phase and can be followed by a prolonged postictal phase. Seizures involve loss of consciousness and may involve motor activity. They can be caused by transient alteration in brain metabolism or by inherited epilepsy. Seizures occurring during the perioperative period may have a variety of causes, including epilepsy, deranged physiology associated with a number of disease states, drugs, and CNS injury or structural lesions.[1,2] Prolonged seizures constitute status epilepticus and is a life-threatening situation.[3,4] Management involves acute care, diagnosis, and chronic management.

A. During the acute management of a patient during a seizure, conduct the following simultaneously: ensure an adequate airway; protect from aspiration and injury; and observe the type, location, and progression of the seizure (particularly noting whether the seizure has focal signs). Differentiate from other causes of altered consciousness (syncope, migraine, TIA, hypertensive encephalopathy) or motor activity (movement disorders) and hysterical or pseudoseizure. Attempts to physically restrain the patient or place objects in the mouth may be difficult during a violent seizure, and if forced cause more harm than good. Insert an oral airway (if this can be done easily) and use an Ambubag with oxygen (O_2) to assist ventilation. If the seizure is from a local anesthetic overdose, hyperventilation will increase the seizure threshold, otherwise this may lower the threshold. Establish an IV line to assist in drug delivery to treat or terminate a prolonged seizure.

B. Seizures from non-CNS lesions usually terminate with small doses of drugs. Consider sodium thiopental (0.5 to 1 mg/kg titrated to stop the seizure) or benzodiazepines (e.g., midazolam 0.5 mg increments or diazepam, usually up to 10 mg/70 kg, titrated to stop the seizure) to terminate a seizure. If deemed appropriate (after consultation with a neurologist or neurosurgeon), IV load with anticonvulsant (phenytoin, 15 to 18 mg/kg in saline at <50 mg/min; or phenobarbital, 120 to 240 mg given IV slowly and repeated every 20 to 30 minutes if needed to a total dose of 400 to 600 mg). If the cause of the seizure is not readily apparent, give 50 ml of dextrose 50% in water after blood has been drawn for diagnostic studies. If alcohol withdrawal is suspected, give thiamine, 100 mg slowly IV and 100 mg IM (followed by 100 mg IM every day for 3 days). If the seizure does not terminate or there is difficulty with ventilation, intubate the patient and use short acting neuromuscular block if needed (allow muscle function as marker of continued motor seizure).

C. Determine diagnosis by searching for causative and treatable etiologies. History and family review may indicate epilepsy (0.5 to 1% of the population). Seizures in an epileptic may be precipitated by hypoxemia or hypercarbia, especially in children. In these patients, assess compliance with chronic anticonvulsants and their blood levels. Fentanyl can evoke seizures in patients with complex partial epilepsy, and remifentanil has been reported to precipitate seizures.[5] Focal signs may indicate CNS injury or structural lesions (head injury, brain tumors). Evaluate the patient, the history, and the chart for disease states known to cause seizures: sepsis (blood, urine, CSF cultures), CNS infection (CSF culture), hyperthermia (temperature), diabetes (serum glucose), chronic renal failure (serum blood urea nitrogen [BUN], creatinine), hepatic failure (serum ammonia), malignant hyperthermia (temperature, blood gas, ECG), porphyria (urine porphyrins), collagen vascular disease, hypoparathyroidism (serum calcium), thyroid disease, and eclampsia[6] (pregnancy, hypertension [HTN], hyperreflexia, proteinuria). Head trauma, previous stroke, and CNS structural lesions (tumor, SAH, AVM) can cause seizures. Fever is the most common cause of seizures in children. Draw blood for analysis of sodium, magnesium, phosphate, calcium, and glucose, and ABGs for O_2, carbon dioxide (CO_2), and pH.

Patient with PERIOPERATIVE SEIZURE

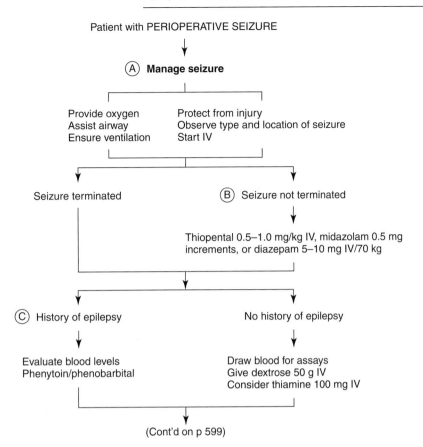

Ⓐ **Manage seizure**

Provide oxygen   Protect from injury
Assist airway   Observe type and location of seizure
Ensure ventilation   Start IV

Seizure terminated   Ⓑ Seizure not terminated

Thiopental 0.5–1.0 mg/kg IV, midazolam 0.5 mg
increments, or diazepam 5–10 mg IV/70 kg

Ⓒ History of epilepsy   No history of epilepsy

Evaluate blood levels   Draw blood for assays
Phenytoin/phenobarbital   Give dextrose 50 g IV
                                      Consider thiamine 100 mg IV

(Cont'd on p 599)

D. If the seizure occurs after surgery or anesthetic drug delivery, review the chart for surgical problems and procedures or for anesthetic agents known to cause or promote seizures in susceptible patients. These medications[7] include althesin, amitriptyline, anticholinesterases, antidepressants, antihistamines, enflurane, etomidate, iodinated contrast agents, ketamine, local anesthetics, oxytocin, meperidine, methohexital, propanidid, and propofol (frequently occurs in recovery period).[8] Lithium, bupropion and IV penicillin lower seizure threshold. Consider the possible presence of toxins (e.g., lead, mercury) and take specimens (urine and blood) if intoxication or withdrawal from addictive drugs is possible (alcohol, barbiturates, narcotics). Give specific treatment in addition to supportive care if the diagnosis is clearly identified.

E. Consult with a neurologist or neurosurgeon for further care (e.g., with head injury), diagnostic workup, or long-term management, particularly for management of recurrent seizures or the development of status epilepticus.

REFERENCES

1. Messing RO, Simon RP: Seizures as a manifestation of systemic disease, *Neurol Clin* 4:563–584, 1986.
2. Shneker BF, Fountain NB: Epilepsy, *Dis Mon* 49:426–478, 2003.
3. Chapman MG, Smith M, Hirsch NP: Status epilepticus, *Anesthesia* 56:648–659, 2001.
4. Kofke WA, Tempelhoff R, Dasheiff RM: Anesthetic implications of epilepsy, status epilepticus, and epilepsy surgery, *J Neurosurg Anesthesiol* 9 (4):349–372, 1997.
5. Haber GW, Litman RS: Generalized tonic-clonic activity after remifentanil administration, *Anesth Analg* 93 (6):1532–1533, 2001.
6. Stumpf DA, Frost M: Seizures, anticonvulsants, and pregnancy, *Am J Dis Child* 132:746–748, 1978.
7. Modica PA, Tempelhoff R, White PF: Pro- and anticonvulsant effects of anesthetics. Parts I and II, *Anesth Analg* 70:303–315, 433–444, 1990.
8. Mäkelä JP, Iivanainen M, Pieninkeroinen P, et al.: Seizures associated with propofol anesthesia, *Epilepsia* 34:832–835, 1993.

Patient with PERIOPERATIVE SEIZURE
(Cont'd from p 597)

Evaluate for cause of seizures

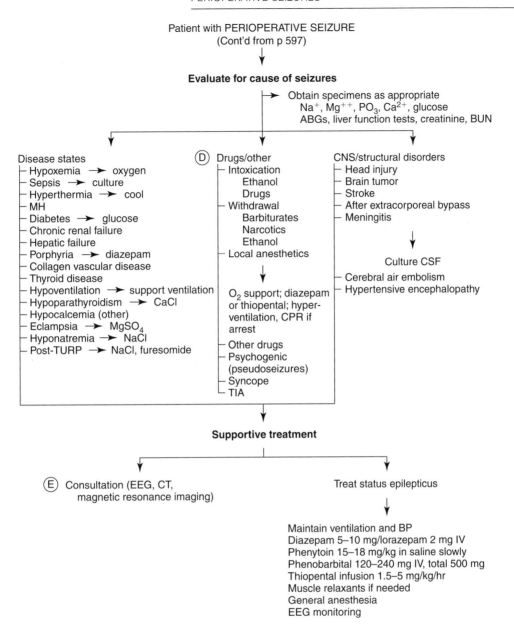

Obtain specimens as appropriate
Na^+, Mg^{++}, PO_3, Ca^{2+}, glucose
ABGs, liver function tests, creatinine, BUN

Disease states
— Hypoxemia → oxygen
— Sepsis → culture
— Hyperthermia → cool
— MH
— Diabetes → glucose
— Chronic renal failure
— Hepatic failure
— Porphyria → diazepam
— Collagen vascular disease
— Thyroid disease
— Hypoventilation → support ventilation
— Hypoparathyroidism → CaCl
— Hypocalcemia (other)
— Eclampsia → $MgSO_4$
— Hyponatremia → NaCl
— Post-TURP → NaCl, furesomide

Ⓓ Drugs/other
— Intoxication
  Ethanol
  Drugs
— Withdrawal
  Barbiturates
  Narcotics
  Ethanol
— Local anesthetics

O_2 support; diazepam
or thiopental; hyper-
ventilation, CPR if
arrest

— Other drugs
— Psychogenic
  (pseudoseizures)
— Syncope
— TIA

CNS/structural disorders
— Head injury
— Brain tumor
— Stroke
— After extracorporeal bypass
— Meningitis

Culture CSF
— Cerebral air embolism
— Hypertensive encephalopathy

Supportive treatment

Ⓔ Consultation (EEG, CT,
magnetic resonance imaging)

Treat status epilepticus

Maintain ventilation and BP
Diazepam 5–10 mg/lorazepam 2 mg IV
Phenytoin 15–18 mg/kg in saline slowly
Phenobarbital 120–240 mg IV, total 500 mg
Thiopental infusion 1.5–5 mg/kg/hr
Muscle relaxants if needed
General anesthesia
EEG monitoring

Postoperative Oliguria

ERIK A. BOATMAN, M.D.

SUSAN GARWOOD, M.B., CH.B., BSC, F.R.C.A.

Blood flow to the renal parenchyma can be estimated by urinary output (UO). Normally this output is 0.5 to 1 mL/kg/hr. Oliguria is defined as UO < 0.5 mL/kg/hr or < 400 ml/day, or < 10 ml/hr/m². Perioperative oliguria, while common, rarely implies acute renal failure (ARF).[1] However, the consequences of perioperative oliguria, if ignored, can be catastrophic. In the perioperative setting, ARF can have up to a 90% mortality rate,[2] thus demanding immediate attention and a focus on prevention. When encountering postoperative oliguria, traditionally the causes have been divided into three categories: prerenal, renal, and postrenal. While the etiology of low UO may seem complex, the application of the following systematic approach can lend itself to rapid identification of etiology and therapy.

A. Identification of patients at risk and maneuvers to prevent renal failure is extremely important. Those with preexisting renal disease are at greatest risk of postoperative oliguria and ARF. In multiple studies, preoperative renal dysfunction was the single consistent predictor of postoperative renal failure (RF).[3] Intraoperative events can exacerbate or create renal stressors and certain surgeries can also strain renal function. Preventative measures should be undertaken to prevent renal damage prior to or during imposed periods of renal stress. Many preexisting conditions predispose to or cause oliguria and several drugs can cause RF through a variety of mechanisms.[4]

B. Prerenal causes of oliguria reduce blood flow to the kidney. If uncorrected, prerenal insults cause permanent damage due to hypoperfusion or hypoxia. Hypovolemia appears to be an especially common etiology in acute postoperative RF. Correction with fluid is, perhaps, the most efficient and evidence-based intervention,[5,6] often in the form of a crystalloid challenge. If excessive volume is a concern, it may be helpful to provide oncotic pressure with an infusion of colloid, albumin, or blood product. If there is no response to a volume challenge, other prerenal causes must be considered and eliminated.

C. If no prerenal cause for oliguria can be found, postrenal causes must be eliminated. The most common postrenal causes of oliguria tend to be easily correctable. Obstructions to urinary flow should be interrogated as well as iatrogenic causes. Finally, patient history may provide some insight as to an etiology.

D. Once prerenal and postrenal causes have been eliminated, oliguria may be a sign of renal parenchymal damage. Intrinsic renal causes of postoperative oliguria can be difficult to diagnose and treat. To aid in diagnosis, a set of baseline renal function labs, which

TABLE 1
Indices Differentiating Prerenal from Intrinsic RF[7]

	Prerenal failure	Intrinsic RF
Osmolality (mOsm/kg H₂O)	—	<400
U/P osmolality	—	<1.5
U/P creatinine	>40	<10
U/P urea	>14	<10
U Na	<20	>40
RF index	<1	>1
FE$_{Na}$	<1%	>1%
FW clearance	≤20 ml/hr	≥20 ml/hr
Creatinine clearance	>25 ml/min	<25 ml/min

U, urine; P, plasma; Na, sodium; RF, renal failure; FE$_{Na}$, fractional excretion of sodium; FW, free water

include renal and serum chemistries and osmolality must be evaluated. Intrinsic RF as demonstrated by laboratory study (see Table 1) or clinical suspicion should prompt an aggressive management course, including early nephrology consultation. Careful review of preoperative comorbidities and medications, intraoperative course, and fluid management should take place to search for a potential renal insult or preexisting condition. Opinions on pharmacological and therapeutic interventions for the management of ARF are widely varied. None, however (other than preoperative aggressive fluid management), have proved their value beyond theoretical interest. Fenoldopam,[7,8] loop diuretics, mannitol, and dopamine have been used for prevention or treatment of ATN and atrial natriuretic peptide analogues, adenosine blockers, calcium antagonists all have theoretical value but have been insufficiently studied.[9] Management beyond this point should be directed by a nephrologist.

REFERENCES

1. Sladen RN: Oliguria in the ICU; a systematic approach to diagnosis and treatment, *Anesthesiol Clin North America* 18 (4):739–752, viii, 2000.
2. Novis BK, Roizen MF, Aronsen S, et al.: Association of preoperative risk factors with postoperative acute renal failure, *Anesth Analg* 78:143–149, 1994.
3. Sadovnikoff N: Perioperative acute renal failure, *Int Anesthesiol Clin* 39 (1):95–109, 2001.
4. Perazella MA: Drug induced renal failure: update on new medications and unique mechanisms of nehrotoxicity, *Am J Med Sciences* 325 (6):349–362, 2003.
5. Lameire NH, DeVriese AS, Vanholder RA: Prevention and nondialytic treatment of acute renal failure, *Curr Op in Crit Care* 9 (6):481–490, 2003.
6. Garwood S, Hines RL: Renal function monitoring, *Int Anesth Clin* 34:175–194, 1996.

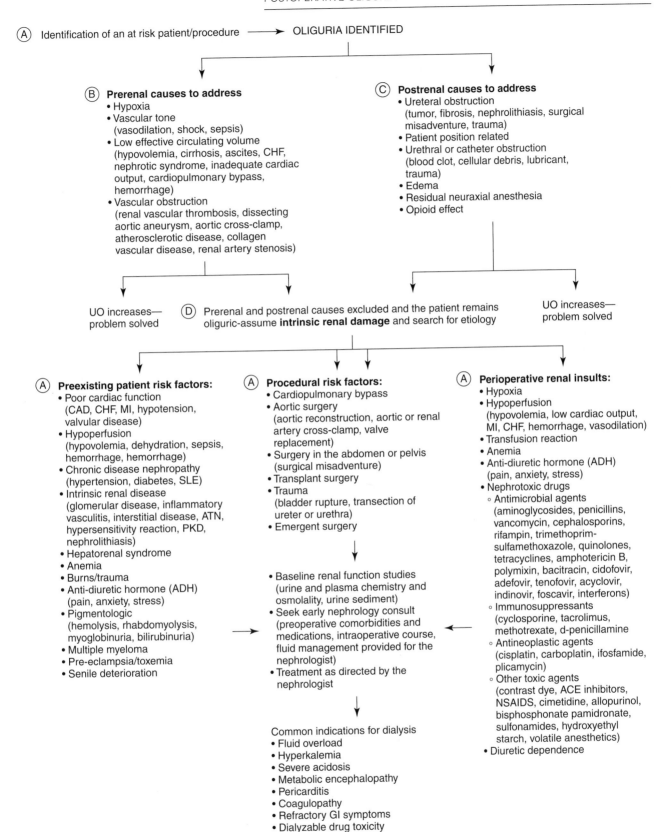

Ⓐ Identification of an at risk patient/procedure ⟶ OLIGURIA IDENTIFIED

Ⓑ **Prerenal causes to address**
- Hypoxia
- Vascular tone (vasodilation, shock, sepsis)
- Low effective circulating volume (hypovolemia, cirrhosis, ascites, CHF, nephrotic syndrome, inadequate cardiac output, cardiopulmonary bypass, hemorrhage)
- Vascular obstruction (renal vascular thrombosis, dissecting aortic aneurysm, aortic cross-clamp, atherosclerotic disease, collagen vascular disease, renal artery stenosis)

Ⓒ **Postrenal causes to address**
- Ureteral obstruction (tumor, fibrosis, nephrolithiasis, surgical misadventure, trauma)
- Patient position related
- Urethral or catheter obstruction (blood clot, cellular debris, lubricant, trauma)
- Edema
- Residual neuraxial anesthesia
- Opioid effect

UO increases—problem solved

Ⓓ Prerenal and postrenal causes excluded and the patient remains oliguric-assume **intrinsic renal damage** and search for etiology

UO increases—problem solved

Ⓐ **Preexisting patient risk factors:**
- Poor cardiac function (CAD, CHF, MI, hypotension, valvular disease)
- Hypoperfusion (hypovolemia, dehydration, sepsis, hemorrhage, hemorrhage)
- Chronic disease nephropathy (hypertension, diabetes, SLE)
- Intrinsic renal disease (glomerular disease, inflammatory vasculitis, interstitial disease, ATN, hypersensitivity reaction, PKD, nephrolithiasis)
- Hepatorenal syndrome
- Anemia
- Burns/trauma
- Anti-diuretic hormone (ADH) (pain, anxiety, stress)
- Pigmentologic (hemolysis, rhabdomyolysis, myoglobinuria, bilirubinuria)
- Multiple myeloma
- Pre-eclampsia/toxemia
- Senile deterioration

Ⓐ **Procedural risk factors:**
- Cardiopulmonary bypass
- Aortic surgery (aortic reconstruction, aortic or renal artery cross-clamp, valve replacement)
- Surgery in the abdomen or pelvis (surgical misadventure)
- Transplant surgery
- Trauma (bladder rupture, transection of ureter or urethra)
- Emergent surgery

- Baseline renal function studies (urine and plasma chemistry and osmolality, urine sediment)
- Seek early nephrology consult (preoperative comorbidities and medications, intraoperative course, fluid management provided for the nephrologist)
- Treatment as directed by the nephrologist

Common indications for dialysis
- Fluid overload
- Hyperkalemia
- Severe acidosis
- Metabolic encephalopathy
- Pericarditis
- Coagulopathy
- Refractory GI symptoms
- Dialyzable drug toxicity

Ⓐ **Perioperative renal insults:**
- Hypoxia
- Hypoperfusion (hypovolemia, low cardiac output, MI, CHF, hemorrhage, vasodilation)
- Transfusion reaction
- Anemia
- Anti-diuretic hormone (ADH) (pain, anxiety, stress)
- Nephrotoxic drugs
  - Antimicrobial agents (aminoglycosides, penicillins, vancomycin, cephalosporins, rifampin, trimethoprim-sulfamethoxazole, quinolones, tetracyclines, amphotericin B, polymixin, bacitracin, cidofovir, adefovir, tenofovir, acyclovir, indinovir, foscavir, interferons)
  - Immunosuppressants (cyclosporine, tacrolimus, methotrexate, d-penicillamine)
  - Antineoplastic agents (cisplatin, carboplatin, ifosfamide, plicamycin)
  - Other toxic agents (contrast dye, ACE inhibitors, NSAIDS, cimetidine, allopurinol, bisphosphonate pamidronate, sulfonamides, hydroxyethyl starch, volatile anesthetics)
- Diuretic dependence

7. Mathur VS, Swan SK, Lambrecht LJ, et al.: The effects of fenoldepam, a selective dopamine receptor agonist, on systemic and renal hemodynamics in normotensive subjects, *Crit Care Med* 27 (9): 1832–1837, 1999.
8. Tumlin JA: Fenoldopam mesylate blocks reductions in renal plasma flow after radiocontrast dye infusion: a pilot trial in the prevention of contrast nephropathy, *Am Heart J* 143 (5):894–903, 2002.
9. Dishart MK, Kellum JA: An evaluation of pharmacologic strategies for the prevention and treatment of acute renal failure, *Drugs* 59 (1):79–91, 2000.

Postdural Puncture Headache (PDPH)

DAVID C. MAYER, M.D.

FRED J. SPIELMAN, M.D.

Postdural puncture headache (PDPH) is one of the most common complications associated with epidural and spinal anesthesia. In a closed-claim study of obstetric anesthesia by the American Society of Anesthesiologists (ASA), PDPH was the second most common reason for litigation.[1] An acute reduction in CSF volume may initiate downward settling of intracranial contents when the patient assumes the upright position. Headache probably results from traction of blood vessels and pressure on pain-sensitive vessels in the meninges from descent of the brain. The trigeminal nerve is the pathway of pain above the tentorium cerebelli, while the vagus and upper cervical nerves provide the pathways for pain in the neck and occipital region. Other cranial nerve involvement is common. The loss of CSF leads to compensatory mechanisms to maintain normal intracranial volume, including vasodilation of cerebral vessels, enlargement of the pituitary, and engorgement of cerebral venous sinuses. This vasodilatory component is also felt to be one of the pain mechanisms.

A. Assess the patient. Symptoms of PDPH usually present within 24 to 48 hours after the dural puncture. The magnitude and rapidity of CSF loss and the rate by which it reforms govern the incidence, rapidity of onset, and severity of PDPH. The most common manifestations of PDPH are shown in Table 1. The headache is frequently in the occipital region, radiating to both temples and the forehead, and is described as a sharp, shooting pain, aggravated by coughing or sudden movement. Reversible cranial nerve involvement of the cochlear, vestibular, and abducens nerves is also associated with CSF volume loss.[2] The differential diagnosis includes cortical vein thrombosis, migraine, hypertension (HTN), meningitis, and metabolic abnormalities. Obtain magnetic resonance imaging (MRI) studies to make the diagnosis in difficult cases. Typical MRI findings are sagging of the brain and diffuse meningeal enhancement.[3] The size and configuration of the needle puncturing the dura is a major factor in determining the incidence of PDPH. Atraumatic spinal needles (Whitacre, Sprotte) result in fewer PDPHs, as low as 1%, compared with cutting needles (Quincke). Spinal needle selection should be based on the risk factors and the expected difficulty of block placement. Females are twice as likely to develop PDPH as are men. PDPH is rare in children and the elderly; it is most common in women of childbearing age. Obese patients have a decreased incidence of PDPH.[4] The immediate onset of postural headache during epidural placement using loss of resistance to air may be related to migration of air into the cerebral ventricles and cisterns.[5]

TABLE 1
Manifestations of PDPH[2]

Symptom	Percentage
Headache	97
Neck pain	87
Nausea, vomiting (vestibular)	69
Auditory (cochlear)	36
Ocular	36

Patient with POSTDURAL PUNCTURE HEADACHE

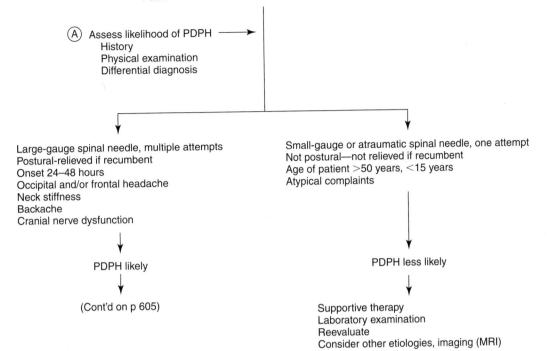

A Assess likelihood of PDPH ⟶
     History
     Physical examination
     Differential diagnosis

Large-gauge spinal needle, multiple attempts
Postural-relieved if recumbent
Onset 24–48 hours
Occipital and/or frontal headache
Neck stiffness
Backache
Cranial nerve dysfunction

PDPH likely

(Cont'd on p 605)

Small-gauge or atraumatic spinal needle, one attempt
Not postural—not relieved if recumbent
Age of patient >50 years, <15 years
Atypical complaints

PDPH less likely

Supportive therapy
Laboratory examination
Reevaluate
Consider other etiologies, imaging (MRI)

B. The symptoms of PDPH can be mild and remit within 2 to 3 days, but some patients will suffer from debilitating pain for weeks. Treat early for the best outcome.[6] Several regimens and special procedures have been employed in the management of PDPH. Maintain adequate hydration for maximal CSF production (hydration does not lead to CSF production above normal). Patients may be predisposed to volume depletion from blood loss, decreased oral intake, and vomiting. Bedrest minimizes the symptoms of PDPH, but several studies have shown no relationship between the length of time spent supine and the incidence, severity, or duration of the PDPH. Provide symptomatic relief, consisting of various analgesics, sedatives, and, if necessary, antiemetics.

C. The therapeutic goals ideally include replacing intracranial volume, sealing the leak, and controlling or reversing cerebral vasodilation. Vasoconstrictors, such as sumatriptan, caffeine, and theophylline, have been suggested as therapeutic agents, but none have proven effective in large studies. Epidural blood patch (EBP) is the most successful treatment modality for PDPH, likely due to two mechanisms. Blood injected into the epidural space increases ICP via a mass effect, while adherent clot at the dural rent is likely to slow down or prevent further leakage. The pressure-patch theory is confirmed by MRI studies after EBP.[7] MRI studies suggest that 20 ml of blood will cover as much as six vertebral segments, with most of the spread in the cranial direction. After EBP, patients should remain supine for at least 1 hour prior to assessing the success of the procedure. Success rates of higher volume EBPs (>15 ml) should be greater than 80%.[2] Common side effects of EBP include paresthesias, radiculitis, neck ache, back pain, and transient bradycardia. Significant complications are remarkably uncommon. Some success has been achieved with prophylactic blood patch via an existing epidural catheter, but this should not be performed until the local anesthetic blockade has completely regressed. Contraindications to EBP include septicemia, local infection, thrombocytopenia, and defects in coagulation. Injection of dextran or other substances into the epidural space requires further evaluation.

REFERENCES

1. Chadwick HS: An analysis of obstetric anesthesia cases from the American Society of Anesthesiologists closed claims project database, *Int J Obstet Anesth* 5:258–263, 1996.
2. Safa-Tisseront V, Thormann F, Malassine P, et al.: Effectiveness of epidural blood patch in the management of post-dural puncture headache, *Anesthesiology* 95:334–339, 2001.
3. Mokri B: Low cerebrospinal fluid pressure syndromes, *Neurol Clin* 22 (1):55–74, vi, 2004.
4. Spielman FJ, Mayer DC, Criswell HE: The relationship between body mass index and postdural puncture headache in parturients, *Anesthesiology* 98:A99, 2003.
5. Somri M, Teszler C, Vaida S, et al.: Postdural puncture headache: an imaging-guided management protocol, *Anesth Analg* 96: 1809–1812, 2003.
6. Weeks SK: Postpartum headache. In: Chestnut DH, editor: *Obstetric anesthesia: principles and practice*, ed 3, St. Louis, 2004, Mosby.
7. Beards SC, Jackson A, Griffiths G, et al.: Magnetic resonance imaging of extradural blood patches: appearances from 30 min to 18 h, *Br J Anaesth* 71:182–188, 1993.

Patient with POSTDURAL PUNCTURE HEADACHE

(Cont'd from p 603)

↓

Ⓑ Treatment

Supportive/reassurance ←   Ⓒ Definitive

↓

Hydration
Analgesics
Antiemetics
Caffeine
Bed rest

Contraindications
present ←

Review for contraindications to
epidural blood patch:
  Sepsis
  Local infection
  Coagulation defects

↓

No contraindications

↓

EBP >15 cc
Supine
Reevaluate at 1 hr

Postoperative Hepatic Dysfunction (PHD)

JOANNE BAUST, M.D.

Postoperative hepatic dysfunction (PHD) is a fairly common postoperative complication, particularly following major intraabdominal surgery. Most cases are asymptomatic, with mild elevation of serum transaminases or bilirubin and resolution in a few days. Determination of cause is often difficult and requires a careful, detailed review of the patient's past medical history, perioperative laboratory studies, and perioperative events. Review the operative procedure, anesthetic technique, medications, and any blood products given. Examine the anesthetic record for episodes of perioperative hypoxemia, hypotension, or reduced cardiac output (CO).

A. Preexisting hepatic dysfunction (e.g., viral or alcoholic hepatitis, cirrhosis) may be unmasked by perioperative insults. Marked elevation of serum transaminases and positive serologic tests for hepatitis (A, B, or C), CMV, EBV, and herpes simplex virus (HSV) may confirm acute viral hepatitis. The incubation period for these viruses is 2 to 3 weeks; perioperative blood transfusion is unlikely to be a cause of acute postoperative hepatitis unless the virus has been present and incubating preoperatively. Liver biopsy may confirm the presence of a fatty liver or alcoholic hepatitis. Elective surgery in patients with know viral or alcoholic hepatitis or cirrhosis should be postponed until their condition is medically optimized because of the greatly increased morbidity or mortality associated with these disease states.

Patient with POSTOPERATIVE HEPATIC DYSFUNCTION

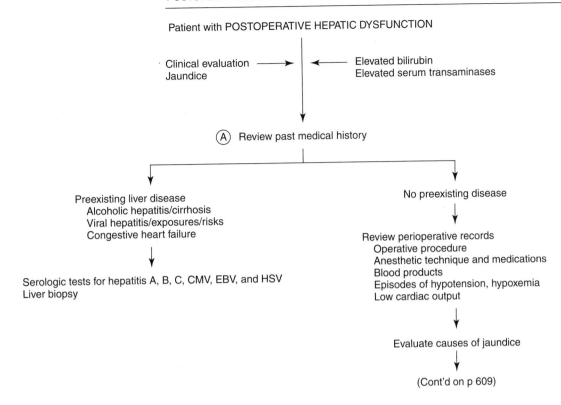

Clinical evaluation   Elevated bilirubin
Jaundice   Elevated serum transaminases

(A)   Review past medical history

Preexisting liver disease
     Alcoholic hepatitis/cirrhosis
     Viral hepatitis/exposures/risks
     Congestive heart failure

No preexisting disease

Serologic tests for hepatitis A, B, C, CMV, EBV, and HSV
Liver biopsy

Review perioperative records
     Operative procedure
     Anesthetic technique and medications
     Blood products
     Episodes of hypotension, hypoxemia
     Low cardiac output

Evaluate causes of jaundice

(Cont'd on p 609)

B. Postoperative jaundice can be due to increased bilirubin production, hepatocellular injury, or biliary obstruction. Causes of increased bilirubin production include multiple blood transfusions, hematoma resorption, and hemolysis. There are many causes of hemolytic anemia, including postcoronary bypass or valve replacement, transfusion reactions, pulmonary or fat emboli, and drug administration (quinidine, procainamide, or cephalosporins). Patients with sickle cell disease or other hemoglobinopathies and glucose-6-phosphate dehydrogenase deficiency may be prone to hemolytic anemia during perioperative stresses. Patients with Gilbert's or Dubin-Johnson syndromes may have increased bilirubin production. Renal failure may reduce the excretion of conjugated bilirubins independently of a hepatorenal syndrome.

C. Hepatocellular injury may be caused by exacerbation of preexisting liver disease, including advanced age and chronic total parenteral nutrition followed by perioperative episodes of hepatocyte hypoxia, systemic hypotension, and reduced hepatic blood flow. Shock, sepsis, and low CO states significantly contribute to PHD; the severity is related to the degree and duration of the insult. Vasopressors and PEEP also reduce hepatic blood flow. Hepatic resection, transplantation, and other major abdominal procedures are associated with a high incidence of PHD. Many nonanesthetic drugs produce liver dysfunction, including antibiotics (erythromycin, tetracycline, sulfonamides, and isoniazid), alpha methyldopa, chlorpromazine, and androgen and estrogen steroids.

Anesthetic drugs have long been implicated as a cause of PHD. All volatile anesthetics produce a dose-related reduction in hepatic blood flow (halothane > sevoflurane > isoflurane > desflurane) and transient hepatocyte hypoxia that may be recognized by a modest elevation in hepatic enzymes that rise then fall within 24 hours postoperatively. Propofol has little effect on changes in hepatic venous pressure and TIVA may be preferred when maintenance of these pressures are critical.

"Halothane hepatitis" involves 1 in 10,000 administrations but has been widely blamed for "unexplained" postoperative hepatic dysfunction. Two forms of toxicity have been identified. The first involves reductive metabolism of halothane during periods of hypoxia, creating toxic metabolites that cause direct hepatocyte destruction. The second form follows oxidative metabolism via cytochrome P450, creating the intermediate trifluoroacetic acid (TFA), which may be directly hepatotoxic but may also act as a hapten to stimulate an autoimmune reaction against hepatocytes (fevers, rash, eosinophilia) and relates to prior exposures to haloalkanes. Circulating antibodies to TFA may be detected for up to 3 months after exposure and may serve as a marker for this form of halothane hepatitis. Desflurane and isoflurane but not sevoflurane also are metabolized to TFA but in much smaller amounts than with halothane. Fulminant hepatic necrosis has been described following anesthesia with halothane and isoflurane but not sevoflurane. Cross-sensitivity between halothane, isoflurane, sevoflurane, and desflurane has been reported with elevations of hepatic enzymes 2 weeks postoperatively after remote prior exposures to inhalational agents. It has been suggested that all halogenated agents be avoided in patients with a history of this immune-mediated reaction.

D. Postoperative biliary obstruction is common, particularly after biliary, gastric, hepatic, or pancreatic surgery. "Benign postoperative cholestasis" is also associated with these procedures. Acute cholecystitis, a retained common bile stone and ascending cholangitis are also common. Ligation of the common bile duct requires immediate surgical repair. Some medications (e.g., narcotics) may cause bile duct obstruction and should be used cautiously.

E. Treatment of PHD is primarily supportive, including careful fluid management, alkalinization of the urine in hemolytic states for renal protection, and inotropic support for low CO states.

F. Patients recovering from PHD often have full return of normal hepatic function. If future anesthetics are required, carefully evaluate existing hepatic function and previous perioperative events. Avoid all halogenated agents in susceptible patients.

REFERENCES

1. Eger EI, Koblin DD, Bowland T, et al.: Nephrotoxicity of sevoflurane versus desflurane anesthesia in volunteers, *Anesth Analg* 84 (1):160, 1997.
2. Iwanaga Y, Komatsu H, Yokono S, et al.: Serum glutathione S-transferase alpha as a measure of hepatocellular function following prolonged anaesthesia with sevoflurane and halothane in paediatric patients, *Paediatr Anaesth* 10 (4):395, 2000.
3. Mandell MS, Durham J, Kumpe D, et al.: The effects of desflurane and propofol on portosystemic pressure in patients with portal hypertension, *Anesth Analg* 97 (6):1573, 2003.
4. Nishiyama T, Yokoyama T, Hanaoka K: Effects of sevoflurane and isoflurane anesthesia on arterial ketone body ratio and liver function, *Acta Anesthesiol Scand* 43:347, 1999.
5. Suttner SW, Schmidt CC, Boldt J, et al.: Low flow desflurane and sevoflurane anesthesia minimally affect hepatic integrity and function in elderly patients, *Anesth Analg* 91 (1):206, 2000.

Patient with POSTOPERATIVE HEPATIC DYSFUNCTION
(Cont'd from p 607)

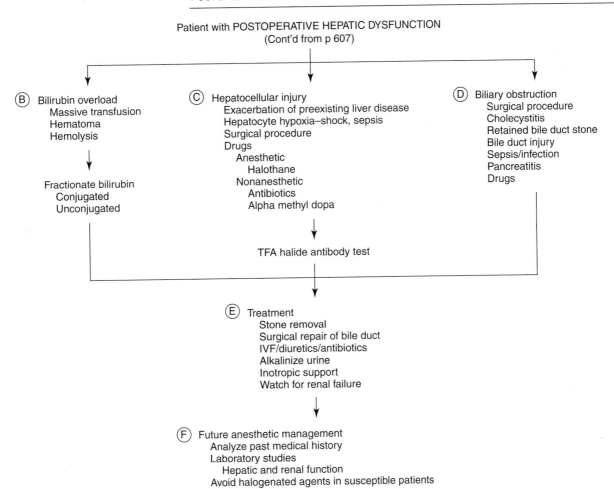

B Bilirubin overload
　　Massive transfusion
　　Hematoma
　　Hemolysis

Fractionate bilirubin
　Conjugated
　Unconjugated

C Hepatocellular injury
　　Exacerbation of preexisting liver disease
　　Hepatocyte hypoxia–shock, sepsis
　　Surgical procedure
　　Drugs
　　　Anesthetic
　　　　Halothane
　　　Nonanesthetic
　　　　Antibiotics
　　　　Alpha methyl dopa

TFA halide antibody test

D Biliary obstruction
　　Surgical procedure
　　Cholecystitis
　　Retained bile duct stone
　　Bile duct injury
　　Sepsis/infection
　　Pancreatitis
　　Drugs

E Treatment
　　Stone removal
　　Surgical repair of bile duct
　　IVF/diuretics/antibiotics
　　Alkalinize urine
　　Inotropic support
　　Watch for renal failure

F Future anesthetic management
　　Analyze past medical history
　　Laboratory studies
　　　Hepatic and renal function
　　Avoid halogenated agents in susceptible patients

Salivary Gland Swelling

DAVID PERCHES, M.D.

LOIS L. BREADY, M.D.

Salivary gland enlargement associated with general anesthesia is a little recognized perioperative complication first reported by Attas in 1968.[1] Swelling of the parotid or submandibular glands during or, more commonly, following general anesthesia has an estimated incidence of 0.2%.[2] When encountered, it can be frightening to both the anesthesiologist and the patient, yet the condition requires only supportive therapy unless airway compromise occurs. The typical clinical course is characterized by onset within 24 hours of general anesthesia, and spontaneous resolution usually occurs within 36 to 72 hours.

A. Review the medical history for evidence of preexisting salivary gland dysfunction or enlargement, such as recent viral or bacterial infection or malignancy. Note preoperative positive physical examination findings. If swelling is first observed postoperatively, review the anesthetic record for evidence of trauma during intubation or manipulation of the airway, and also note the type of procedure (i.e., a slightly higher incidence of salivary gland swelling has been noted after endoscopic procedures).

B. Once postoperative salivary gland swelling has been confirmed, assess adequacy of oxygenation and ventilation. If there is no airway compromise, conservative management (heat, analgesics if needed) is in order. However, if oxygenation or ventilation are impaired, secure the airway as a first priority. Supplemental oxygen (O_2) or intubation (if warranted) are the first steps, followed by ABG, chest x-ray (CXR), and electrolytes. Residual anesthetics, upper airway obstruction, chronic obstructive pulmonary disease (COPD), neurological disease, hypothermia, and myasthenia gravis (MG) are all factors that can further impair oxygenation or ventilation and must be addressed if present.

C. Swelling of submandibular glands has been reported to occur before induction of anesthesia, during maintenance, and for up to 24 hours following anesthesia. The glands are usually nontender and rubbery in consistency, and may be either unilaterally or bilaterally enlarged. Although no clear etiology has been defined, there are three major proposed mechanisms[3]: (1) The neurogenic or reflex arc theory is the most widely accepted mechanism. An afferent limb originating from sensory innervation of the tongue, mouth, or pharynx causes stimulation of an efferent impulse through the glossopharyngeal nerve. This is thought to cause vasodilation and hyperemia of the glands as a result of parasympathetic stimulation. (2) The physical obstruction theory proposes that there is blockage of the salivary ducts with acute retention of saliva caused by swelling of the epithelial lining or muscle spasm physically obstructing the duct. (3) The capillary hydrostatic pressure theory suggests that straining or bucking on the endotracheal tube (ETT) leads to venous engorgement, resulting in increased hydrostatic pressure and acute exudation of fluid from the vascular compartment. (However, swelling of salivary glands has been seen in cases in which there was no coughing or straining on the ETT.)

Rarely, a single theory fully explains an episode of submandibular gland swelling. Each of the three postulated mechanisms may play some role. In addition, no association has been found with age, gender, race, type of surgery, past medical history, premedications, or anesthetics used.[4-6] Fortunately, salivary gland swelling after general anesthesia is usually a self-limited process, and conservative management and reassurance are sufficient. If the patient appears toxic or if airway compromise is present, consult with an otolaryngologist.

REFERENCES

1. Attas M, Sabawala PB, Keats AS: Acute transient sialadenopathy during induction of anesthesia, *Anesthesiology* 29:1050–1052, 1968.
2. Matsuki A, Wakayama S, Oyama T: Acute transient swelling of the salivary glands during and following endotracheal anaesthesia, *Anaesthesist* 24:125–128, 1975.
3. Guyton DC: Oral, nasopharyngeal, and gastrointestinal systems. In: Gravenstein N, editor: *Manual of complications during anesthesia*, Philadelphia, 1991, J.B. Lippincott.
4. Dembo JB: Bilateral parotid sialadenopathy associated with general anesthesia: a case report discussion, *J Oral Maxillofacial Surg* 51:330, 1993.
5. Gombar KK, Singh B: Bilateral parotid sialadenopathy associated with general anesthesia: a case report, *J Oral Maxillofac Surg* 51:328–330, 1993.
6. Jacobson B: Transient swelling of the parotid glands following general anesthesia: "anesthesia mumps," *AANA J* 46:41–43, 1978.

Patient with POSTOPERATIVE SALIVARY GLAND SWELLING

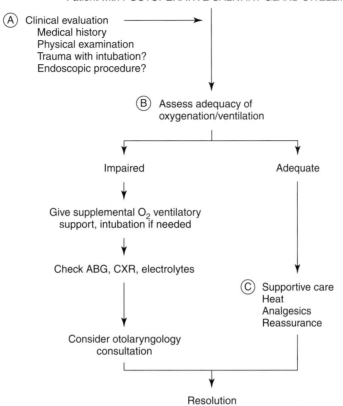

Dental Injuries Associated with General Anesthesia

ANTHONY S. POON, M.D., D.D.S., PH.D.

W. CORBETT HOLMGREEN, M.D., D.D.S.

Dental injuries represent the most common source of complaint and claims made against the anesthesiologist.[1] The incidence of anesthesia-related dental injury reported in the literature ranges from 0.02 to 0.7%,[1,2] although in one study where diagnoses of dental injuries were made by a dentist who examined the patients preoperatively and postoperatively, the incidence was found to be as high as 12%.[3] Damage to the teeth occurs most commonly during oral endotracheal intubation with direct laryngoscopy, when inadvertent impact or pressure is exerted via the blade of the laryngoscope. However, extubation, biting on an oral airway or grinding of teeth during emergence and recovery can cause dental trauma. The teeth most likely to be injured during anesthesia are the maxillary central incisors, with the left central incisor being at highest risk. The risk is increased fivefold when a preexisting dental disease exists.[4] Dental caries, periodontal disease, dental attrition or erosion, developmental tooth anomalies such as amelogenesis or dentinogenesis imperfecta, systemic disorders, such as certain types of leukemia, can all increase the risk of anesthesia-related dental injury. Teeth that have been extensively restored, nonvital or endodontically treated teeth are invariably weakened and thus prone to fracture. The risk of sublaxation or avulsion is increased in the lone-standing tooth, orthodontically treated teeth, crowded anterior teeth, in patients with mandibular retrognathism ("overbite"), as well as in children during their mixed-dentition phase. Dental veneers, crowns, bridges, and implants are also prone to fracture or dislodgement during anesthesia.

A. The risk for dental injuries can be minimized by careful preoperative dental assessment and management, proper intubation techniques, protective mouthguards, and the use of modified laryngoscope blades or alternative methods of intubation. Patients are carefully questioned and examined to identify any loose, carious, cracked, chipped, restores, or malpositioned teeth. Existing restorations and dental prostheses including crowns, bridges or implants should be documented and their condition noted. Present the risk of dental surgery to the patient and included in the consent for surgery and anesthesia.

B. Dental injuries range from minor cracking of the enamel to complete avulsion of the tooth. Regardless of how trivial the damage may appear, any dental injury, when noticed should be relayed to the patient and a referral to the dentist made. In the event of coronal fracture or complete avulsion, all efforts should be made to locate and retrieve the dislodged fragment or tooth to prevent subsequent aspiration. Chest and abdominal radiographs are needed when loose pieces are not accounted for despite an extensive search. While all dental injuries are treated definitively by the dental surgeon as soon as circumstances allow, immediate action can and should be taken by the anesthesiologist when sublaxation or avulsion of a tooth occurs, to improve the prognosis by the affected tooth. A subluxed (loosened) tooth can usually be reduced to its original position without much difficulty. Apply brief (30 to 60 second) but firm finger pressure to the alveolus around the tooth. Place a splint to stabilize it; supplies available in the OR include Thermasplint ™ and Stomadhesive. The splint, with the adhesive side applied to the enamel surface, is adapted around the teeth such that they are "sandwiched" between the folded splint (Figure 4). Hold firm digital pressure. The splint will remain in place until the patient is examined by the dentist as soon as circumstances allow. Inform the patient of the presence of the splint and take precautions to avoid its dislodgement and aspiration.

C. An avulsed permanent tooth (Figure 1) should be replanted as soon as it can safely be performed. The shorter the interval between avulsion and replantation, the better the prognosis.[5] Only the crown of the avulsed tooth should be handled; damage to the periodontal ligament cells on the root surface via handling has a negative impact on the prognosis. The tooth can be gently rinsed with clean water before replantation. The alveolar socket should be debrided by gentle saline irrigation without removal of the blood clot (Figure 2).[5] The avulsed tooth is then replanted, and firm digital pressure applied briefly to compress the socket (Figure 3). A splint will be prepared and placed as described earlier. If immediate replantation is not feasible, the tooth should be placed in a balanced salt solution within 15 minutes for storage and replanted as soon as possible. Primary ("baby") teeth should not be replanted. In case of alveolar bone or jaw fracture, immediate consultation with the appropriate surgical specialty (oral and maxillofacial surgery, otolaryngology) is advised.

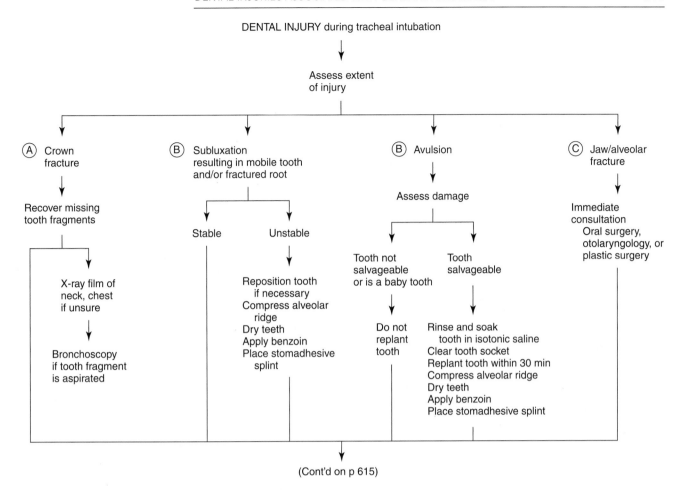

(Cont'd on p 615)

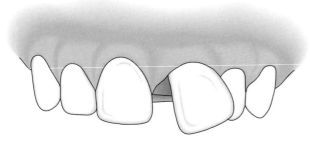

FIGURE 1 Tooth avulsion.

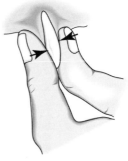

FIGURE 3 Digital replantation of tooth.

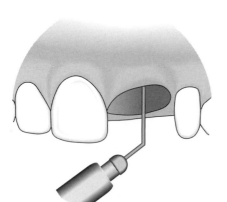

FIGURE 2 Irrigation and removal of debris from the tooth socket.

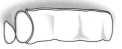

FIGURE 4 Application of a Stomadhesive strip to serve as a temporary splint.

D. After a dental injury has occurred, the patient must be informed and a dental consultation obtained as soon as possible.

REFERENCES

1. Owen H, Waddell-Smith I: Dental trauma associated with anaesthesia, *Anesth Intensive Care* 28:133, 2000.
2. Chadwick RG, Lindsay SM: Dental injuries during general anaesthesia, *Anesthesia* 180:255, 1996.
3. Chen JJ, Susetio L, Chao CC: Oral complications associated with endotracheal general anaesthesia, *Anaesth Sinica* 28:163, 1990.
4. Lockhart PB, Feldbau EV, Gabel RA, et al.: Dental complications during and after tracheal intubation, *JADA* 112:480, 1986.
5. Abubaker AO, Giglio JA, Mourino AP: Diagnosis and management of dentoalveolar injuries. In: Fronseca RJ, editor: *Oral and maxillofacial surgery*, Philadelphia, 2000, W.B. Saunders.

DENTAL INJURY during tracheal intubation

(Cont'd from p 613)

↓

(D) Inform patient

↓

Dental consultation

Management of a Needlestick

ARNOLD J. BERRY, M.D., M.P.H.

Despite exposure prevention, accidental needlesticks and other sharp injuries may occur.[1-3] Contaminated percutaneous injuries represent a greater risk of occupational transmission of blood-borne pathogens than mucocutaneous exposures.[4] The Centers for Disease Control and Prevention (CDC) guidelines for prevention of transmission of the blood-borne pathogens, hepatitis B virus (HBV), hepatitis C virus (HCV), and human immunodeficiency virus (HIV), to health care workers (HCWs) include strategies for handling contaminated needles: needles should not be recapped, bent, broken, or removed from disposable syringes and should be placed in puncture-resistant containers conveniently located in the work area.[5,6]

The rate of transmission of infection after a contaminated needlestick injury differs among the three blood-borne pathogens. Because a high concentration of HBV may be present in the blood of carriers, the risk of clinical hepatitis B may be as high as 31% after a percutaneous exposure when the source patient is both hepatitis B surface antigen (HbsAg) and e-antigen positive.[7] For HCV, the rate of percutaneous transmission is widely quoted as 1.8%[8] (range 0 to 10%), but more recent data from larger surveys suggest that it is 0.5%.[9] The overall rate of infection after an HIV-positive needlestick injury is 0.3%,[2] but the risk may be increased when a larger volume of blood (deep injury, large-diameter hollow needle, previously in the source patient's vein or artery) or blood with a high viral titer is transferred (source patient with end-stage AIDS).[10]

A. When an accidental needlestick occurs, have the wound washed with soap and water.[4] There is no evidence that an antiseptic solution is required or reduces the risk of infection. Bleach or disinfectants are not recommended for application to the skin. Report the injury (clinical supervisor, employee health department) as soon as possible so that medical follow-up (evaluation, counseling, and treatment) can begin. The Occupational Safety and Health Administration (OSHA) Blood-borne Pathogen Standard requires that employers provide access to medical follow-up for occupational exposures.[11] Employers must also comply with federal and state requirements for record keeping and for reporting the injury.

B. Appropriate follow-up depends on the likelihood that the source patient is carrying a blood-borne pathogen. Groups with a high prevalence of infection include homosexual men, sexual partners of infected persons, IV drug users, patients on hemodialysis, and individuals with hemophilia.

C. Test the source patient in compliance with federal and state privacy laws and regulations. Informed consent is usually required. Infection may sometimes be confirmed from the source individual's medical or laboratory records; observe federal and state privacy laws when accessing this data. If the information is not available, perform serologic testing. Under some circumstances, the source patient may be unknown (e.g., injury produced by a needle protruding from a sharps container), may not be available for testing, or may refuse testing.

D. HBV carriers are hepatitis B surface antigen (HBsAg) positive on serologic testing. During the follow-up period, the HCW can continue patient care duties but should be counseled not to donate blood, plasma, body fluids, or tissues until it is confirmed that he or she has not become infected with HBV.

E. Hepatitis B immune globulin (HBIG) is prepared from human plasma with a high titer of anti-HBs, the antibody that confers immunity against HBV infection. HBIG provides passive immunity in about 75% of cases and may be more effective when combined with hepatitis B vaccine.

F. Hepatitis B vaccine is recommended for all HCWs who have contact with blood or body fluids and should be administered as early as possible in their career. OSHA regulations require that employers offer hepatitis B vaccine to HCW.[11] Three doses of recombinant hepatitis B vaccine administered into the deltoid muscle at time 0, 1, and 6 months induce adequate levels of protective antibodies in up to 95% of healthy individuals.

G. Anesthesia personnel should be tested for anti-HBs 1 to 2 months after completion of the initial hepatitis B vaccine series. Individuals who develop immunity after vaccination (anti-HBs >10 mIU/mL) have adequate protection against clinical HBV infection.

H. A small number of vaccinees do not develop sufficient titer of anti-HBs after the three-dose series and remain at risk for HBV infection. Inadequate immunogenicity (anti-HBs <10 mIU/mL) is more likely with the following conditions: obesity, advanced age, male gender, subcut vaccine administration, smoking, and immune deficiency. Some nonresponders may produce antibodies with additional doses of hepatitis B vaccine.

I. For nonresponders who have not completed a second three-dose vaccine series, it is recommended that one dose of HBIG be used followed by the hepatitis B vaccine series. If a second vaccine series had been administered but the individual failed to respond, two doses of HBIG should be used.

J. Adequate immunity after hepatitis B vaccination is indicated with anti-HBs >10 mIU/ml; lower titers are inadequate.

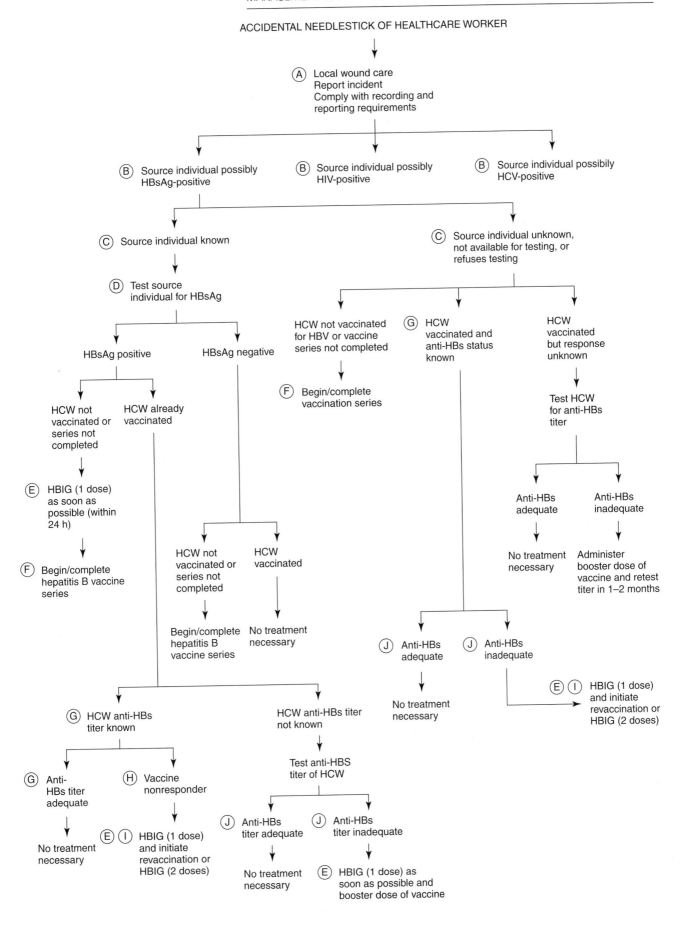

K. Evaluate the HCW as soon as possible (within hours) after potential exposure to HIV. Anti-HIV (the serum antibody to HIV) should be evaluated at baseline to determine the infection status at the time of exposure.

L. The source patient has asymptomatic HIV infection or is known to have a low viral load (<1500 RNA copies/ml).

M. The source patient has a known high viral load or has symptomatic HIV infection, acquired immune deficiency syndrome (AIDS), or acute seroconversion.

N. The source patient is of unknown HIV status (e.g., a deceased person without blood samples available for testing) or cannot be tested.

O. A source may be unknown if a contaminated needle or sharp device has produced the injury but the origin of the device cannot be determined.

P. If the source patient can be identified but the HIV status is unknown at the time of the exposure, the HCW should consider starting postexposure prophylaxis (PEP) until the HIV status can be determined. If the source patient is confirmed to be HIV-negative, PEP can be discontinued.

Q. The percutaneous exposure is judged to be less severe (e.g., produced by a solid needle and a superficial injury).

R. The percutaneous exposure is judged to be more severe (e.g., produced by a large-bore hollow needle, producing a deep puncture wound, visible blood on the device, or the needle was used in the patient's artery or vein).[10]

S. Based on the effectiveness of antiretroviral drugs in preventing HIV transmission from mother to infant, on animal models, and on epidemiologic data,[10] the CDC has recommended that PEP for exposed HCW after some types of occupational exposures to HIV.[4] Because there is limited knowledge on the efficacy and safety of PEP, especially in otherwise healthy individuals without preexisting HIV, the exposed HCW should be informed of the potential risks and benefits of the drugs. If PEP is used, treatment should be initiated promptly, preferably within 2 hours of the exposure, but can be started even after 36 hours. If tolerated, PEP should be administered for 4 weeks. Since some PEP failures have been associated with use of only one antiretroviral drug, minimum PEP should be a two-drug regimen usually consisting of two nucleoside analogues. For exposures that suggest an increased risk for HIV infection, an expanded three-drug regimen (such as two nucleoside analogues with a protease inhibitor) is recommended. An individual with expertise in antiretroviral drugs or other source (National Clinicians' Postexposure Prophylaxis Hotline, 888-448-4911) should be consulted for more complex situations such as when the source patient is taking antiretroviral agents or has HIV with known antiretroviral resistance. The exposed HCW should be reevaluated within 72 hours of the initial event, especially if additional information regarding the source patient becomes available.

T. Consider PEP indicates that the use of PEP is optional and a decision should be made after discussion between the exposed HCW and the treating clinician. When the source patient cannot be tested,

the risk of HIV may be based on the prevalence of the disease in the patient population of the health care institution or the community it serves.

U. The exposed HCW should be counseled to refrain from activities that may transmit HIV during the follow-up period (sexual abstinence or use of condoms, and refrain from donating blood, plasma, body fluids, or tissues). It is not necessary to modify the work duties of a HCW exposed to HIV. The HCW should be counseled that if they develop symptoms of an illness that is compatible with an acute retroviral syndrome, serologic testing for HIV should be performed.

V. Follow-up testing of exposed HCW should be performed to evaluate any toxicity from PEP and to determine whether HIV infection has occurred (use of enzyme immunoassay to test for anti-HIV). Most infected individuals seroconvert within 12 weeks after exposure and routine testing beyond 6 months is usually not recommended. When the source patient is coinfected with HIV and HCV, the exposed HCW should be followed with antibody testing for 12 months. The confidentiality of the HCW must be protected during the follow-up process.

W. The exposed HCW should have baseline testing for anti-HCV and alanine aminotransferase (ALT) activity. Positive anti-HCV results by enzyme immunoassay should be confirmed using recombinant immunoblot assay. Immune globulin is not recommended for PEP after HCV exposure. (Anti-HCV does not produce immunity against HCV.) Although interferon has been used successfully for treatment of chronic hepatitis C, there is insufficient data to recommend its use as PEP. Because there are no proven therapies to prevent hepatitis C after occupational exposures, recommended management is directed toward identification of infection and referral of the individual for early treatment of acute hepatitis.[4] It is not necessary to alter the exposed HCW's patient care duties during the follow-up period. The exposed HCW should be counseled not to donate blood, plasma, body fluids, or tissue, but they do not need to modify sexual practices during follow-up.

X. Follow-up testing for anti-HCV and ALT should be performed at 4 to 6 months. The average time between exposure to HCV and seroconversion is 8 to 10 weeks but may be longer in some cases. Testing for HCV RNA may be performed at 4 to 6 weeks if an earlier diagnosis is required.

REFERENCES

The most current recommendations from the CDC and other sources of information for treatment of exposed HCW can be accessed at *http://www.cdc.gov/niosh/topics/bbp*. Recommendations for pregnant personnel are not included in this review.

1. Berry AJ, Greene ES: The risk of needlestick injuries and needlestick-transmitted diseases in the practice of anesthesiology, *Anesthesiology* 77:1007, 1992.
2. Greene ES, Berry AJ, Arnold WP, et al. Percutaneous injuries in anesthesia personnel. *Anesth Analg* 83:273, 1996.
3. Greene ES, Berry AJ, Jagger J, et al.: Multicenter study of contaminated percutaneous injuries in anesthesia personnel, *Anesthesiology* 89:1362, 1998.

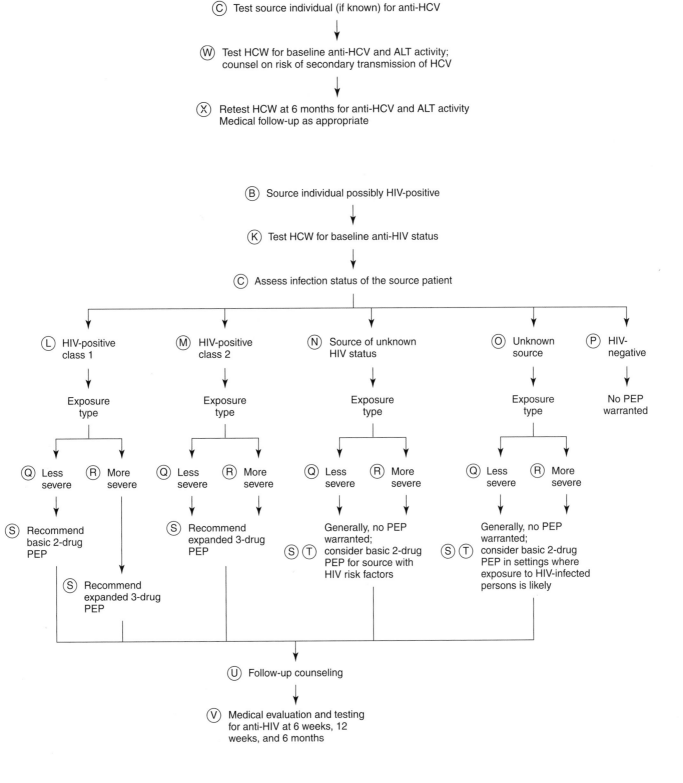

4. Marcus R, CDC Cooperative Needlestick Surveillance Group: Surveillance of health care workers exposed to blood from patients infected with the human immunodeficiency virus, *N Engl J Med* 319:1118, 1988.

5. Centers for Disease Control: Guidelines for prevention of transmission of human immunodeficiency virus and hepatitis B virus to health-care and public-safety workers, *MMWR* 38 (S-6):1, 1989.

6. Centers for Disease Control and Prevention: Updated U.S. Public Health Service guidelines for the management of occupational exposures to HBV, HCV, and HIV and recommendations for postexposure prophylaxis, *MMWR* 50 (No. RR-11):1, 2001.

7. Werner BG, Grady GF: Accidental hepatitis-B-surface-antigen-positive inoculations: use of e antigen to estimate infectivity, *Ann Intern Med* 97:367, 1982.

8. Lanphear BP, Linnemann CC, Cannon CG, et al.: Hepatitis C virus infection in healthcare workers: risk of exposure and infection, *Infect Control Hosp Epidemiol* 15:745, 1994.

9. Jagger J, Puro V, DeCarli G: Occupational transmission of hepatitis C virus (letter), *JAMA* 288:1469, 2002.

10. Cardo DM, Culver KH, Ciesielski C, et al.: A case-control study of HIV seroconversion in health-care workers after percutaneous exposure, *N Engl J Med* 337:1485, 1997.

11. Occupational Safety and Health Administration: Occupational exposure to bloodborne pathogens; Needle-sticks and other sharp injuries; Final Rule (29 CFR Part 1910.1030), *Federal Register* 66:5318, 2001.

The information contained in this manuscript are based on guidelines from the Centers for Disease Control and Prevention and published in *MMWR* 50 (No. RR-11), 2001.

CHRONIC PAIN MANAGEMENT

COMPLEX REGIONAL PAIN SYNDROME
(CRPS)

MYOFASCIAL PAIN (MFP)

LUMBOSACRAL RADICULOPATHY

CANCER PAIN

Complex Regional Pain Syndrome (CRPS)

JAMES N. ROGERS, M.D.

SOMAYAJI RAMAMURTHY, M.D.

Complex regional pain syndrome (CRPS) is defined as a chronic pain condition thought to be the result of central or peripheral nervous system dysfunction.[1-3] Pain is typically located in an extremity after an injury. There are two types of CRPS. Type I CRPS is pain associated with tissue injury but with no evidence of nerve injury. Type II CRPS is associated with clear nerve injury. Older terms for CRPS include "reflex sympathetic dystrophy" and "causalgia." The pain is often out of proportion to the degree of initial injury and can occur weeks after the injury. It is most common in adults but has been reported in children. CRPS is divided into three stages. In Stage I, disproportionate burning pain persists after healing. It is associated with hyperpathia, hypoesthesia, hyperesthesia, or dysesthesias. The skin may be warm, red, and dry. Later, it may become cold, cyanotic, and sweaty, with edema, dependent rubor, and reduced joint mobility. Stage II lasts 3 to 6 months, with proximal and distal spread of pain beyond the area of the initial injury. Hair growth slows, nails become deformed, joints thicken, and range of motion decreases. Osteoporosis begins to develop. In Stage III, the skin and boney changes become irreversible. Pain is severe and may involve the entire limb. Atrophy can be marked. There is often severe mobility limits to the affected joints. Limbs may become distorted.

A. Perform a clinical evaluation. Diagnostic signs include vasomotor instability, often with marked difference in skin temperature between the affected and opposite extremity, and exaggerated sympathogalvanic reflex. Sudeck's atrophy, the bone demineralization associated with CRPS, appears patchy radiographically, resembling disuse osteoporosis. Triple-phase bone scan comparing both sides shows increased radionuclide uptake on the affected side, reflecting high turnover osteoporosis. Relief of pain after sympathetic blockade can be diagnostic in patients with a large component of sympathetic nerve involvement.

B. Aim treatment at relieving painful symptoms and improving function. Physical therapy is important to maintain joint range of motion and limb function. A gradually increasing exercise program along with desensitization techniques can be helpful, particularly in Stages I and II. When pain limits physical therapy, consider continuous regional blockade of the extremity to provide analgesia during physical therapy.

C. CRPS can have profound psychological effects on patients and their families. Depression is common. Recommend psychotherapy to help the patient deal with the stress of chronic, persistent pain and disability.

D. Consider medications, such as antidepressants, antiepileptics, corticosteroids, and opioids, to provide symptomatic relief. Topical anesthetics may be beneficial, working directly on affected skin, nerves, and muscles.

E. Sympathetic nerve blocks may provide significant pain relief. In severe cases of CRPS, surgical or chemical sympathectomy may be necessary. Other invasive procedures for intractable cases of CRPS may include epidurally implanted spinal cord stimulators or intrathecal drug infusion pumps.

REFERENCES

1. Birklein F: Complex regional pain syndrome, *J Neurol* 252 (2): 131–138, 2005.
2. Wasner G, Schattschneider J, Heckmann K, et al.: Vascular abnormalities in reflex sympathetic dystrophy (CRPS I): mechanisms and diagnostic value, *Brain* 124 (Pt 3):587–599, 2001.
3. Raj PP: *Practical management of pain*, ed 3, St. Louis, 2000, Mosby.

Patient with COMPLEX REGIONAL PAIN SYNDROME

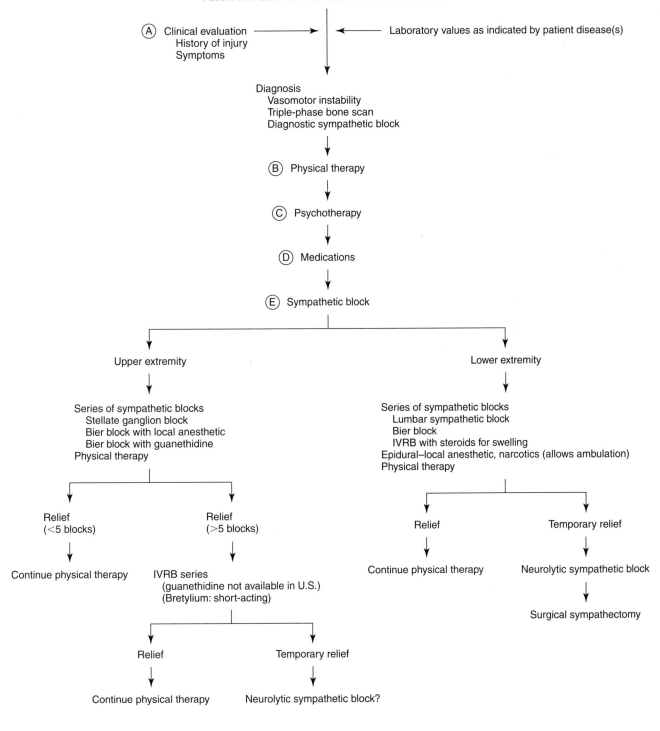

Myofascial Pain (MFP)

JAMES N. ROGERS, M.D.

SOMAYAJI RAMAMURTHY M.D.

Trigger point (TP) or myofascial pain (MFP) is extremely common in adults and children.[1,2] MFP can begin acutely with muscle strain or insidiously secondary to chronic muscle fatigue. The pain can last for years and can result in limited range of motion and permanent disability. It produces diffuse, aching musculoskeletal pain associated with multiple discrete and predictable tender points. It usually occurs in the third to fourth decade, more commonly in females. Management goals are to decrease pain, improve function, and prevent permanent disability. MFP is thought to be the result of reflex muscle spasms, muscle fatigue, and ischemia resulting from muscle injury. Afferent pain signals secondary to the muscle spasm enter the spinal cord along the dorsal columns, and communication with internuncial neurons leads to hyperactivity of anterior and anterolateral horn cells, resulting in more spasm and vasoconstriction.

A. Perform a history and physical examination. Clinical characteristics include a history of muscle injury or overactivity, a hyperirritable locus within a taut band of skeletal muscle called a TP with a referred pattern of pain and weakness. Compression of the TP reproduces the pain. Myopathies, arthritis, and inflammatory musculoskeletal disorders (e.g., tendonitis, bursitis) are included in the differential diagnosis.

B. Management involves alleviating pain and maintaining function and range of motion of the involved muscle(s). TP location is fairly constant and can be linked to a variety of pain syndromes. Consider TP injections (TPI) with local anesthetic, which can relieve pain and be diagnostic. After pain is relieved, institute a muscle-stretching exercise program to break the spasm cycle. Alternative techniques include ischemic compression of the TP, massage, deep heat, biofeedback, and acupuncture. A useful technique for neck MFP is the spray-and-stretch technique using vapo-coolant spray. Precise localization of the TP is not necessary when using this technique. A combination of some or all of these techniques may be necessary in patients with chronic, intractable pain. Early treatment is usually more effective and long lasting. A series of injections may be required when pain is chronic.

REFERENCES

1. Raj PP: *Practical management of pain*, ed 3, St. Louis, 2000, Mosby.
2. Bonica JJ: *The management of pain*, vol 1, ed 2, Philadelphia, 1990, Lea and Febiger.
3. Morris CR, Bowen L, Morris AJ: Integrative therapy for fibromyalgia: possible strategies for an individualized treatment program, *South Med J* 98 (2):177–184, 2005.

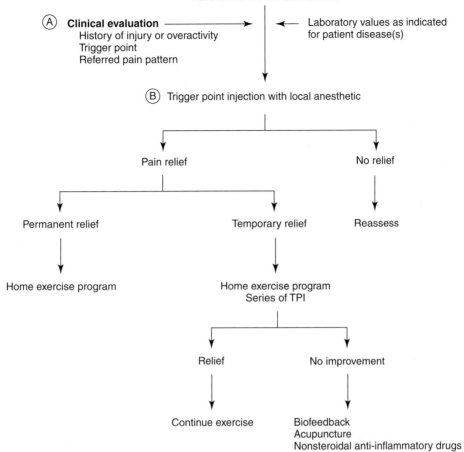

Patient with MYOFASCIAL PAIN

Ⓐ **Clinical evaluation** ⟶   ← Laboratory values as indicated
    History of injury or overactivity   for patient disease(s)
    Trigger point
    Referred pain pattern

Ⓑ Trigger point injection with local anesthetic

Pain relief   No relief

Permanent relief   Temporary relief   Reassess

Home exercise program   Home exercise program
                                      Series of TPI

                          Relief   No improvement

                   Continue exercise   Biofeedback
                                             Acupuncture
                                             Nonsteroidal anti-inflammatory drugs

Lumbosacral Radiculopathy

JAMES N. ROGERS, M.D.

SOMAYAJI RAMAMURTHY, M.D.

Low back pain is the most common complaint of patients presenting to a pain clinic.[1,2] Approximately 20% of the U.S. population experiences back pain each year. The typical patient will present with a history of previous episodes of back pain, lasting days to weeks. Following a twisting movement and a popping sensation, new and severe symptoms occur, subsequently replaced by sharp, shooting, radicular pain to the legs. The majority of these patients present to a pain clinic after already having sought medical care elsewhere, often from numerous health care providers and often following a wide variety of unsuccessful therapies. Therapy therefore can be complicated and often frustrating in this difficult class of patients.

A. Perform a clinical evaluation. Radicular pain from nerve root irritation is often described as toothache-like, sharp, and shooting to the ankle, foot, or toes. The most common cause is a herniated lumbar disc. The most common roots involved are L-5 and S-1. Straight-leg raising reproduces the shooting pain. Sensory loss, muscle weakness, and hyporeflexia of involved deep-tendon reflexes may be present. The pattern of pain, weakness, numbness, and loss of reflexes is fairly consistent. Pain on reversed-leg raising indicates a higher level of lumbar involvement. Paresthesias often are more widespread than the pain. The radicular pain may also be the result of spinal stenosis, tumor infiltration or metastasis, herpes zoster, or arachnoiditis. Obtain CT, magnetic resonance imaging (MRI), or myelograms to identify the site of nerve root compromise.

B. Attempt conservative therapy first, consisting of bed rest, mild analgesic medications, and avoidance of painful activities; it is often the most successful treatment. Consider adding local heat, a lumbar brace, and muscle relaxants. Oral corticosteroids have proved of some benefit in some patients, but such therapy should be brief. In obese patients, encourage a weight loss program. When pain is relieved, consider an exercise program to strengthen the abdominal muscles and stretch the spine extensors; this may decrease the risk of recurrence.

C. When conservative therapy has been unsuccessful, perform epidural steroid injection (ESI). ESI reduces inflammation and inhibits the action of nociceptive agents. If there is significant improvement after 2 weeks, no further injections are necessary. If initial improvement is not maintained, repeat ESI to a maximum of three injections, 2 weeks apart. Systemic absorption occurs, resulting in adrenal suppression for up to 3 weeks. Complications include unintentional spinal tap, meningitis, arachnoiditis, transient bladder paralysis, and sclerosing pachymeningitis. Use steroid suspensions, such as methylprednisolone or triamcinolone diacetate, to minimize the risk of arachnoiditis. Approximately two thirds of patients with acute discogenic disease will benefit from ESI.

D. Surgical intervention may be necessary in selected patients, although many patients who present to a pain clinic will already have undergone surgery. Consider physical therapy and psychological intervention to strengthen coping mechanisms in patients in whom other therapies have been unsuccessful.

REFERENCES

1. Bonica JJ: *The management of pain,* vol 2, ed 2, Philadelphia, 1990, Lea & Febiger.
2. Benzon HT, Molloy RE: Outcomes, efficacy, and complications from management of low back pain. In Raj PP, editor: *Practical management of pain,* ed 3, St. Louis, 2000, Mosby.

Patient with LUMBOSACRAL RADICULOPATHY

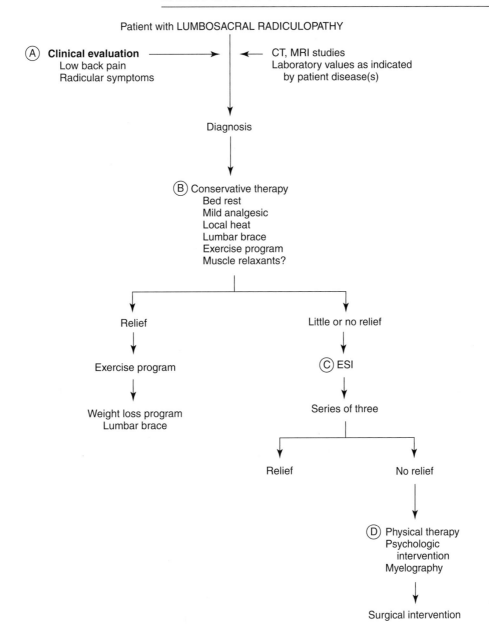

Cancer Pain

MYRDALIS DIAZ-RAMIREZ, M.D.

DAVID V. NELSON, PH.D.

Pain is a multidimensional (biological-sensory, affective-emotional, behavioral, cognitive, spiritual, cultural-environmental) experience. This is particularly evident in the diverse manifestations of cancer pain. The assessment and treatment of cancer pain flows from this conceptualization.[1] Cancer pain may be due to the disease process itself as well as specific cancer treatments. It may be influenced by stress, adjustment difficulties, and environmental, spiritual, or existential issues. The pain can be somatic, visceral, or neuropathic. It is classified as acute, chronic, or intermittent. Cancer treatments may contribute, for example, to peripheral neuropathy, abdominal cramps, joint pain, bone pain, and incisional pain.[1] Approximately 30 to 50% of people with cancer experience pain while undergoing treatment; 70 to 90% with advanced cancer experience pain.[2] Pain may be associated with a variety of other symptoms and conditions, including physiological and cognitive dysfunction, as well as affective disturbances. Adequate treatment of cancer pain requires adequate assessment. The primary mode of assessment is verbal self-report or close observation of patients who are unable to communicate.

A. Perform a history and physical examination, including neurological evaluation. Ask the patient to characterize the pain. Review current medications and treatments.
B. Determine the cause of the pain. If the pain is a symptom of the cancer, treatment specific for the cancer can relieve pain. For example, chemotherapy, radiation therapy, and surgery are performed to cure or palliate the cancer. They can also sometimes be performed to decrease multiple symptoms, including pain. Pharmacological therapy, however, is the mainstay of cancer treatment.[3] The American Pain Society and World Health Organization (WHO) have published principles and guidelines for the management of cancer pain.[3,4] The WHO guidelines include a stepladder for determining increasing aggressiveness of pharmacotherapy. The ladder identifies a patient with mild to moderate pain and begins treatment with nonopioid analgesics, with or without adjuvants. Adjuvant therapy may include antidepressants, antiepileptics, caffeine, stimulants, local anesthetics, glucocorticoids, radionuclides, skeletal muscle relaxants, antispasmodics, antihistamines, benzodiazepines, phenothiazines, and biphosphonates.[5] Opioids are added as the patient responds to other therapies or the pain worsens. They are generally prescribed on a fixed schedule with supplemental breakthrough medication available on an as-needed basis. The oral route is preferred with sublingual, transdermal,

suppository, subcut, and IV preparations available. IV patient-controlled analgesia (PCA) may help optimize pain control. Physiological dependence is almost certain to occur with the use of opioids. However, addiction (i.e., uncontrolled escalation of drug use) is rarely a problem in appropriately medicated patients without previous history of personal or family drug abuse. Pseudo-addiction may occur if the dosage is inadequate; this should not be mistaken for true addiction. Address tolerance by increasing dosages within safe limits or employing drug rotation.

While 70 to 90% of cancer pain can be effectively treated using the WHO ladder system, it does not take into account other useful treatment modalities. For example, physical therapy is useful to promote function and avoid deactivation, deconditioning, and atrophy. Transcutaneous electrical nerve stimulation (TENS), massage, manipulation, mobilization, ice, or heat may help in selected cases. Psychological-behavioral therapies include relaxation strategies (e.g., controlled breathing regulation, progressive relaxation, or visualization), distraction techniques, guided imagery, hypnosis, self-hypnosis training, cognitive-behavioral therapies, and supportive-educational therapies. They can help reduce emotional and physiological distress and may be effective in reducing levels of pain.[6]

C. Consider interventional therapies when noninvasive treatments fail to provide adequate pain relief. These may include diagnostic and therapeutic blocks, neurolytic blocks, intrathecal drug delivery, or neurosurgery. Sympathetic blockade (e.g., splanchnic or celiac plexus blocks) can be useful for treatment of visceral pain. If diagnostic blocks are effective, consider neurolytic blocks with alcohol or phenol. Intrathecal opioids are beneficial in patients who respond to opioids, but are unable to tolerate the doses required or side effects when conventional routes of delivery are used.

Complementary and alternative medicine therapies have some validated and experimental uses. Examples include acupuncture, Chinese medicine, nutritional and herbal remedies, and electromagnetic brainwave stimulation.[7]

REFERENCES

1. Hewitt DJ: The management of pain in the oncology patient, *Obstet Gynecol Clin North Am* 28 (4):819–846, 2001.
2. Seal C, Cartwright A: *The year before death*, Brookfield, VT, 1994, Ashgate Publishing Company.
3. American Pain Society: *Principles of analgesic use in the treatment of acute pain and cancer pain*, ed 5, Glenview, IL, 2003, American Pain Society.

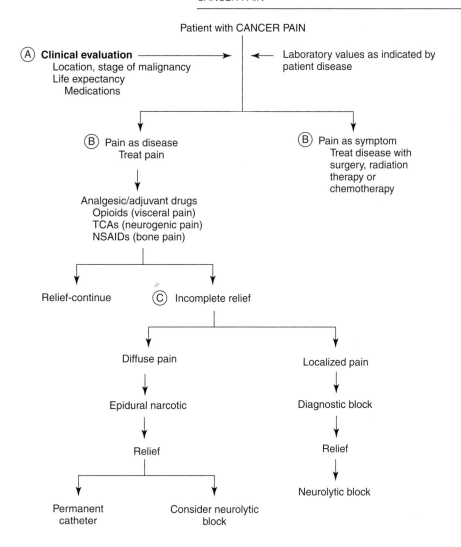

Patient with CANCER PAIN

(A) **Clinical evaluation** ⟶ ⟵ Laboratory values as indicated by
Location, stage of malignancy   patient disease
Life expectancy
Medications

(B) Pain as disease   (B) Pain as symptom
Treat pain   Treat disease with
                                        surgery, radiation
                                        therapy or
                                        chemotherapy

Analgesic/adjuvant drugs
Opioids (visceral pain)
TCAs (neurogenic pain)
NSAIDs (bone pain)

Relief-continue   (C) Incomplete relief

Diffuse pain   Localized pain

Epidural narcotic   Diagnostic block

Relief   Relief

Permanent   Consider neurolytic   Neurolytic block
catheter   block

4. World Health Organization: *Cancer pain relief*, ed 2, with a guide to opioid availability, cancer pain relief, and palliative care. Report of the WHO Expert Committee (WHO Technical Report Series, No. 804), Geneva, Switzerland, 1996, WHO.
5. Vielhaber A, Portenoy RK. Advances in cancer pain management. *Hematol Oncol Clin North Am* 16 (3):527–541, 2002.
6. Crichton P, Moorey S: Treating pain in cancer patients. In: Turk DC, Gatchel RJ, editors: *Psychological approaches to pain management: a practitioner's handbook*, ed 2, New York, 2002, Guilford Press.
7. Vickers AJ, Cassileth BR: Unconventional therapies for cancer and cancer-related symptoms, *Lancet Oncol* 2 (4): 226–232, 2001.

INDEX